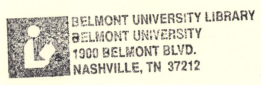

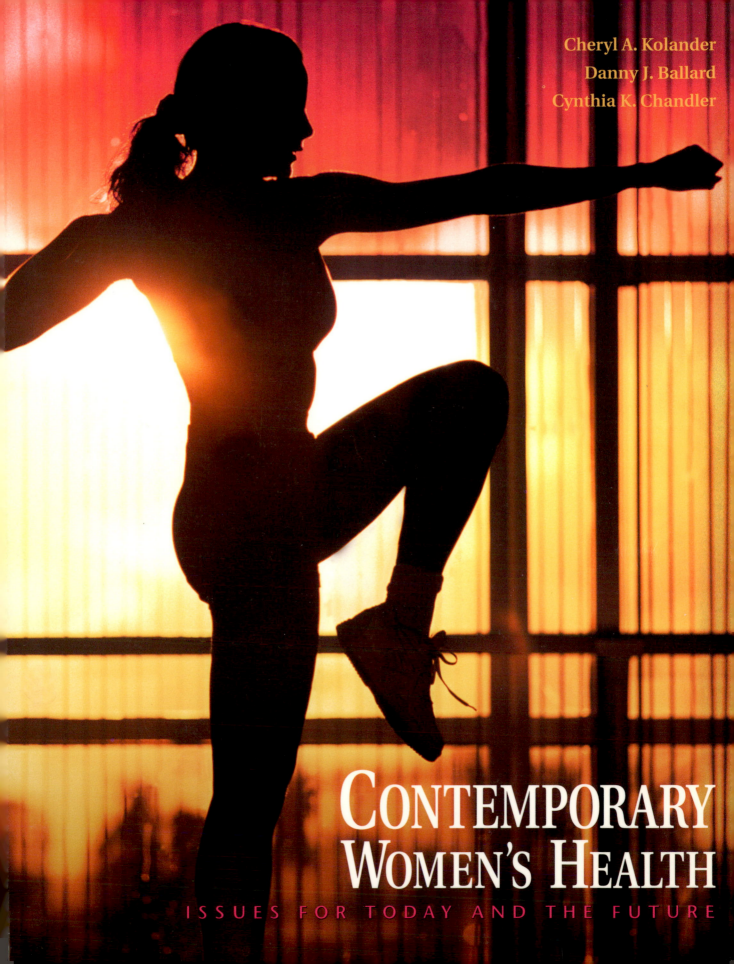

Cheryl A. Kolander
Danny J. Ballard
Cynthia K. Chandler

CONTEMPORARY
WOMEN'S HEALTH

ISSUES FOR TODAY AND THE FUTURE

C O N T E M P O R A R Y

Women's Health

C O N T E M P O R A R Y

Women's Health

Issues for Today and the Future

Cheryl A. Kolander, HSD, CHES
Department of Health Promotion, Physical Education, and Sport Studies
University of Louisville
Louisville, Kentucky

Danny J. Ballard, EdD, CHES
Department of Health and Kinesiology
Texas A&M University
College Station, Texas

Cynthia K. Chandler, EdD, LPC
Department of Counselor Education
University of North Texas
Denton, Texas

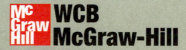

Boston   Burr Ridge, IL   Dubuque, IA   Madison, WI   New York   San Francisco   St. Louis
Bangkok   Bogotá   Caracas   Lisbon   London   Madrid
Mexico City   Milan   New Delhi   Seoul   Singapore   Sydney   Taipei   Toronto

WCB/McGraw-Hill

A Division of The McGraw·Hill Companies

CONTEMPORARY WOMEN'S HEALTH: ISSUES FOR TODAY AND THE FUTURE

This book is printed on acid-free paper.

1 2 3 4 5 6 7 8 9 0 DOW/DOW 9 3 2 1 0 9 8

ISBN 0-8151-0626-2

Vice president and editorial director: *Kevin T. Kane*
Publisher: *Edward E. Bartell*
Executive editor: *Vicki Malinee*
Senior developmental editor: *Michelle Turenne*
Senior marketing manager: *Pamela S. Cooper*
Senior project manager: *Gloria G. Schiesl*
Senior production supervisor: *Mary E. Haas*
Designer: *K. Wayne Harms*
Supplement coordinator: *David A. Welsh*
Compositor: *Shepherd, Inc.*
Typeface: *10/12 Garamond Book*
Printer: *R. R. Donnelley & Sons Company/Willard, OH*

Interior design: *Kaye Farmer*
Cover photo: *David Hall/Sharpshooters*

The credits section for this book begins on page 450 and is considered an extension of the copyright page.

Library of Congress Cataloging-in-Publication Data

Kolander, Cheryl A.
    Contemporary women's health : issues for today and the future /
Cheryl A. Kolander, Danny J. Ballard, Cynthia K. Chandler. — 1st ed.
        p.   cm.
    Includes index.
    ISBN 0-8151-0626-2
    1. Women—Health and hygiene.   I. Ballard, Danny J.
II. Chandler, Cynthia K. III. Title.
RA778.K72445   1999
613'.04244—dc21   98-24961
                                                      CIP

www.mhhe.com

Dedications

*To my nieces and nephews as they seek to make their own
contributions to improving the status of women.*

CAK

*To my loving husband and son, Jim and Brad, who make
all of life worthwhile; and to my beloved parents, Hershell
and Fay Ramsey—my first and best teachers.*

DJB

*To my family and friends whose support and guidance
have helped me to become the person I am.*

CKC

Brief Contents

Preface xiii
About the Authors xvii

Part One
IN THE BEGINNING 1

CHAPTER ONE
Why Study Women's Health? 2

CHAPTER TWO
Developing a Healthy Lifestyle 14

CHAPTER THREE
Life Transitions: Infancy to Early Adulthood 32

CHAPTER FOUR
Life Transitions: Middle to Late Adulthood 55

Part Two
MENTAL AND EMOTIONAL WELLNESS 69

CHAPTER FIVE
Enhancing Emotional Well-Being 70

CHAPTER SIX
Managing the Stress of Life 92

Part Three
CONTEMPORARY LIFESTYLE AND SOCIAL ISSUES 118

CHAPTER SEVEN
Eating Well 119

CHAPTER EIGHT
Keeping Fit 152

CHAPTER NINE
Avoiding Tobacco Use 174

CHAPTER TEN
Using Alcohol Responsibly 194

CHAPTER ELEVEN
Using Other Psychoactive Drugs 219

CHAPTER TWELVE
Becoming a Wise Consumer 240

CHAPTER THIRTEEN
Preventing Abuse Against Women 268

Part Four
SEXUAL AND RELATIONAL WELLNESS 294

CHAPTER FOURTEEN
Building Healthy Relationships 295

CHAPTER FIFTEEN
Examining Gynecological Issues 313

CHAPTER SIXTEEN
Selecting Birth Control Methods 332

CHAPTER SEVENTEEN
Planning for Pregnancy and Parenting 354

Part Five
COMMUNICABLE AND CHRONIC CONDITIONS 377

CHAPTER EIGHTEEN
Preventing AIDS and Other Sexually Transmitted Diseases 378

CHAPTER NINETEEN
Managing Cardiovascular Health and Other Chronic Conditions 400

CHAPTER TWENTY
Reducing Your Risk of Cancer 426

Credits 450
Index 452

Contents

Preface *xiii*
About the Authors *xvii*

Part One

IN THE BEGINNING 1

CHAPTER ONE

Why Study Women's Health? 2

Authors' Perspective 2
  Focus on Women's Health 2
  Emphasis on Health Promotion 3
  Cultural Awareness 3
International Concerns 4
Women's Social Movement 4
History of Women's Health Research 7
  Nurses Health Study 7
  Women's Health Initiative 7
To Help You Use This Text 8
  Health Tips 8
  Viewpoint 8
  FYI 8
  Journal Activity 9
  Her Story 9
  Assess Yourself 9
  Healthy People 2000 Objectives 9
  Assess Yourself: Personal Health Inventory 11

CHAPTER TWO

Developing a Healthy Lifestyle 14

What Is Healthy? 14
  Life Expectancy 15
  Leading Causes of Death 15
Whole Person Concept 15
  Mind, Body, and Spirit 16
  Dimensions of Wellness 16
  Holistic Wellness Model 16
Achieving Optimum Wellness 16
  Assess Yourself: Rate Your Wellness 18
World Wellness 19
Wellness Versus Illness 19
  Education 19
  Prevention 21
  Treatment 21
Learning and Behavior 22
  Hierarchy of Needs 22

Theories and Models of Behavior Change 23
  Field Theory 23
  Health Belief Model 24
  The Transtheoretical Model 25
  Theory of Reasoned Action 25
  Theory of Planned Action 25
  Theory of Personal Investment 26
  Self-Efficacy 26
  Social Cognitive Theory 26
Planning Your Lifestyle Change 26
  Personal Inventory 26
  Helpful Attitude 27
  Plan of Action 27

CHAPTER THREE

Life Transitions: Infancy to Early Adulthood 32

Theories of Development 32
The Phases of Life 35
  Childhood 35
  Adolescence 39
  Assess Yourself: Gay and Lesbian Rights 43
  Young Adulthood 46

CHAPTER FOUR

Life Transitions: Middle to Late Adulthood 55

Phases of Life 55
  Middle Adulthood 55
  Late Adulthood 59
  Assess Yourself: Palmore's Facts on Aging Quiz 61

Part Two

MENTAL AND EMOTIONAL WELLNESS 69

CHAPTER FIVE

Enhancing Emotional Well-Being 70

The Emerging Self 70
  Sociocultural Influences 70
  Mindful Self-Exploration and Integration 71
Life Skill Development 73
  Assertiveness Training 73
  Effective Communication 75
  Effective Problem Solving 76
  Image Building 77
  Image and the Media 78

Assess Yourself: The Appearance Shemas Inventory (ASI) 79
Eating Disorders 79
Self-Esteem Enhancement 80
Resolving Grief over Loss 80
Depression 82
Types of Depression 83
Psychosocial Stressors and Depression 83
Hormonal Effects on Depression 84
Positive Experiences Versus Depression 84
Developmental Issues and Depression 84
Multicultural Issues of Depression and Suicide 85
Predictors of Suicide 86
The Counseling Option 86
Emotions and Health 86

CHAPTER SIX

Managing the Stress of Life 92

Concepts of Stress 93
Stress and Perception 93
Positive Versus Negative Stress 95
The Stress Response 95
Fight-or-Flight Response 95
General Adaptation Syndrome 96
Anatomy and Physiology of Stress 96
Endocrine System 96
Autonomic Nervous System 96
Distress and the Body 97
Stress and "Dis-ease" 97
Stress-Related Disorders 97
Stress and Lifestyle 99
Major Life Events 99
College Stress 99
Daily Life Hassles 100
Impact of Multiple Roles 100
Assess Yourself: Stress Checklist 101
Destructive Qualities of Stress 102
Multicultural Issues 102
Spiritual Beliefs 102
Ability to Acculturate 102
Racial Issues 102
Age Factors 102
Financial Stress 103
The Impact of Technology 103
The Workforce 103
Employment and Health 104
Working Against Stereotypes 104
Environmental Stress 105
Stress and Trauma 105
Coping Skills for Stress: Prevention, Management, and Treatment 105
You Are What You Think 105
Stress and Nutrition 107
Use of Herbs 108

Massage and Reflexology 108
Acupressure and Acupuncture 109
Exercise 109
Time Management 109
Body Awareness 109
Relaxation Exercises 110
Biofeedback 111
Meditation 112
Yoga 112
Proper Breathing 112

Part Three

CONTEMPORARY LIFESTYLE AND SOCIAL ISSUES 118

CHAPTER SEVEN

Eating Well 119

Eating Well and Eating Wisely 119
Assess Yourself: Determining Your Food Choices 120
Guidelines to Good Eating 121
Dietary Guidelines for Americans 121
Food Guide Pyramid 123
Recommended Dietary Allowance 124
Necessary Nutrients 125
Carbohydrates 125
Protein 126
Fats 127
Vitamins 128
Minerals 128
Pregnancy and Breast-Feeding 133
Energy Needs During Pregnancy 134
Nutrient Requirements During Pregnancy 134
Assess Yourself: Foods for Folacin 136
Breast-Feeding 136
Physical Activity 136
Caloric Intake 136
Nutrients 137
Vegetarianism 137
Benefits of Vegetarianism 137
Concerns of Vegetarianism 137
Nutrition and the Consumer 138
Additives 138
Organic Foods 140
Natural Foods 140
Assess Yourself: What Do You Know About the Foods You Eat? 141
Food Labeling 141
Managing Weight Through Nutrition 143
Underweight, Overweight, and Obesity 143
Weight Loss 145

Eating Disorders 146
   Anorexia Nervosa 147
   Bulimia Nervosa 147

CHAPTER EIGHT
Keeping Fit 152

Benefits of Fitness 152
Health-Related Components of Fitness 154
   Cardiorespiratory Endurance 154
   Assess Yourself: Calculate Your Target Heart
     Rate 155
   Flexibility 155
   Muscular Strength and Endurance 157
   Body Composition 158
Other Exercise Considerations 159
Personal Fitness Programming 159
   Fitness Assessments 160
Design Your Personal Fitness Program 163
   Getting Started 163
   Staying Involved 165
   Avoiding Injuries 165
Joining a Fitness Club 166
Special Considerations 166
   Exercise and the Menstrual Cycle 166
   Exercise and Pregnancy 167
Compulsive Exercise 168
Managing Weight Through Exercise 170

CHAPTER NINE
Avoiding Tobacco Use 174

Tobacco: Looking Back 174
Women and Tobacco 175
   Prevalence of Tobacco Use 175
   Why Women Smoke 175
   Assess Yourself: Could You Become a Smoker? 177
Substances in Tobacco 177
Adverse Health Effects 178
   Other Physical Consequences 179
Addiction 181
Environmental Tobacco Smoke 181
   Effects on Adults 182
   Effects on Children 182
Smoking and Pregnancy 183
Smoking Cessation 184
   Behavioral Changes 184
   Nicotine Replacement Devices 184
Benefits of Smoking Cessation 186
   How to Stop Smoking! 186
Caffeine 187
   What Is Caffeine? 187
   Effects of Caffeine 188
   Caffeine Products 188
   Effects of Caffeine on Health 189

Caffeinism 190
Caffeine Research 190

CHAPTER TEN
Using Alcohol Responsibly 194

Women and Alcohol 194
   Alcohol: The Beverage 195
   Why Liquor Is Quicker for Women 197
Women and Alcohol: A Unique Relationship 197
   Alcohol Consumption 198
   College-Aged Women and Alcohol 199
   Associated Effects 200
   Alcohol and Pregnancy 205
Addiction and Dependency 206
   Dependency: What Is It? 207
Alcoholism 208
   Demographics 208
   Is Alcoholism a Disease? 208
   Indicators of Alcoholism 209
   How to Help 209
   Assess Yourself: Do You Have a Drinking
     Problem? 210
   A Family Disease 210
What Can Be Done? 211
   Resources 212
   Intervention 212
   Types of Treatment 212
Prevention 214
As We Go to Press . . . 215

CHAPTER ELEVEN
Using Other Psychoactive Drugs 219

Where Did All These Drugs Come From? 219
Addiction and Dependency 220
   Dependency: What Is It? 220
Prescription Drugs 220
   Understanding Drug Labels 221
   Commonly Prescribed Drugs 221
   Using Prescription Drugs Safely 225
Over-the-Counter (OTC) Drugs 225
   Assess Yourself: Safety Tips When Taking
     Medications 226
   OTC Drugs Used by Women 226
   Prescription and OTC Drug Use During
     Pregnancy 229
Illicit Drugs 230
   Drug Use and Pregnancy 230
   Cocaine and Crack 231
   Marijuana 232
   Heroin and Methadone 233
Illicit Drugs and Societal Problems for Women 235
   Women, Drugs, and HIV Infection 235
   Women, Drugs, and Homelessness 236

CHAPTER TWELVE

Becoming a Wise Consumer 240

Consumerism: What Is It? 240
How We Consume 240
Choosing a Health-Care Provider 241
   Health-Care Providers 242
   Reporting Unprofessional Treatment 245
Health-Care Delivery 245
Home Health Tests 246
   What Are They? 246
   Assess Yourself: Improving Your Chances for Accurate Test Results 247
Alternative Health Care 247
   Herbalism 248
   Acupuncture 248
   Chiropractic Care 249
   Massage 250
   Holistic Medicine 251
   Other Types of Alternative Health Care 252
   Health Quackery 252
   Protecting Yourself 252
Beauty-Enhancing Products and Procedures 252
   Products 252
   Assess Yourself: Assessing Alternative Health-Care Claims and Products 253
   Procedures 254
   Breast Augmentation 255
Effects of Advertising 256
   Types of Advertising Techniques 257
   Unrealistic Portrayals of Women 258
   Realistic Portrayals 259
Financial Considerations 259
   Health Insurance 259
   Medicare and Medicaid Services 261
   Social Security 261
Taking Action 262
   Agencies 262
   Credit Reports 262
   Righting a Wrong 263

CHAPTER THIRTEEN

Preventing Abuse Against Women 268

The Reality of Violence Against Women 268
The Extent of the Problem 270
Why Do Women Stay? 270
Types of Abuse 271
   Childhood Abuse 271
   Abuse and Adult Women 273
Incidences of Violence and Abuse 278
Common Elements in All Types of Abuse 280
   Minimization 280
   Directionality 280

Trivialization 280
   Blaming the Victim 280
Characteristics of Battered Women 280
   Personal Beliefs 280
   Personal Feelings 280
   Codependency 281
   Perception of Partner 281
Consequences of Abuse 281
   Physical Consequences 281
   Emotional and Psychological Consequences 282
   Spiritual Consequences 282
   Social Consequences 283
Moving Toward Change 283
   Why Women Stay in Abusive Relationships 283
Leaving the Abusive Relationship 283
   Deciding to Leave 283
   Developing a Safety Plan 284
   Locating Safe Shelter 284
   Locating Other Resources 284
Healing from Abuse 285
How to Help 286
Moving Forward 287
   Building Resiliency 287
   Self-Caring 287
   Assess Yourself: Recognizing and Meeting Personal Needs 288
   Meeting Needs 288
Preventing Abuse 288
   Personal Level 288
   Community Level 289
   State and Federal Levels 289

Part Four

SEXUAL AND RELATIONAL WELLNESS 294

CHAPTER FOURTEEN

Building Healthy Relationships 295

Gender-Role Attributes and Sociological Factors 295
   Gender-Role Attributes 295
   Sociological Factors 296
Forming Relationships 297
   Stages of Dating 297
   Assess Yourself: Are You Compatible as a Couple? 298
Theories of Love 299
   Sternberg's Triangular Theory 299
   Lovestyles 300
Traits of a Successful Relationship 300
Types of Relationships 301
   Marriage and Committed Relationships 301
   Cohabitation 302

Interracial Couples 303
Lesbian Couples 304
Single Lifestyle and Parenthood 305
Troubled Relationships 305
Love Addiction 306
Terminating a Relationship 306
Potential Sources of Conflict 306
Resolving Conflicts—Fighting Fair 309

CHAPTER FIFTEEN

Examining Gynecological Issues 313

Female Reproductive Anatomy 313
External Genitalia 313
Internal Genitalia 316
Breasts 316
Menstruation 318
Menarche 318
Dysmenorrhea 320
Amenorrhea 321
Toxic Shock Syndrome 322
Pelvic Examination and Pap Test 322
Pelvic Examination 322
Pap Test 322
Premenstrual Syndrome 323
*Assess Yourself: Physical and Emotional Symptoms
and PMS 324*
Human Sexual Response Cycle 324
Orgasms 325
Aging and Sexual Response 325
Menopause 326
Perimenopause 327
Hormone Replacement Therapy 327

CHAPTER SIXTEEN

Selecting Birth Control Methods 332

Access to Family Planning 332
Selecting Birth Control Methods 333
Contraceptive Choices 334
Abstinence 334
Fertility Awareness Methods 334
Barrier Methods 336
Hormonal Methods 339
Other Birth Control Methods 342
Selecting a Birth Control Method 345
Abortion 346
Defining Abortion 347
The Grief and Acceptance Process 349
Political Debate 349
Right to Life and Pro-Choice 350
*Assess Yourself: Attitudes Toward Induced
Abortion 351*
Human Dimension 351

CHAPTER SEVENTEEN

Planning for Pregnancy and Parenting 354

Pregnancy Today 354
Pre-Pregnancy Planning 354
Conception 355
Early Signs of Pregnancy 356
Home Pregnancy Tests 356
Fetal Development 357
Ectopic Pregnancy 357
Prenatal Care and Delivery 357
Primary Care Services 358
Labor and Delivery 360
Birthing Options 360
Birthing Positions 363
Breast-Feeding 363
Maternal and Infant Mortality 364
Infertility 365
Fertility Drugs 366
Artificial Insemination 366
Surrogacy 368
In Vitro Fertilization 368
Donor Eggs and Egg Retrieval 369
Multiple Births 369
Adoption 370
Foster Care 370
Parenting 370
*Assess Yourself: How Do You Rate Your
Competence to Be a Parent? 371*

Part Five

COMMUNICABLE AND CHRONIC
CONDITIONS 377

CHAPTER EIGHTEEN

**Preventing AIDS and Other Sexually Transmitted
Diseases 378**

The Primary Burden of STDs 378
Assess Yourself: Assess Your STD Risk 380
Discussing Common Sexually Transmitted Diseases 380
Chlamydia 380
Gonorrhea 382
Syphilis 383
Herpes Simplex Virus (HSV) 384
Human Papilloma Virus 385
Hepatitis B Virus 386
Reproductive Tract Infections 387
Pelvic Inflammatory Disease 387
Vaginitis 388
AIDS 390
Susceptibility to HIV 390

Defining HIV/AIDS 391
Contracting AIDS 392
Symptoms of HIV 392
Diagnosis of HIV 392
Treatment of HIV 393
HIV and Children 393
Prevention Strategies 394
Abstinence 394
Monogamy 394
Engaging in Less Risky Behaviors with Partners 395
Oral Contraceptives 395
Male Condoms 395
Female Condoms 395

CHAPTER NINETEEN

Managing Cardiovascular Health and Other Chronic Conditions 400

Leading Cause of Death in Women 400
Cardiovascular Diseases 402
Normal Cardiovascular Functioning 402
Types of Heart Disease 403
Risk Factors 406
Protective Factors Against Heart Disease 409
Assess Yourself: Risks for Women 410
Screening and Diagnosis 412
Stroke 412
Risk Factors for Stroke 412
Treatment 413
Disability from Stroke 414
Osteoporosis 414
Assess Yourself: Determine Your Risk for Osteoporosis 414
Protective Factors Against Osteoporosis 414
Risk Factors for Osteoporosis 415
Measuring Bone Density 416
Diabetes Mellitus 416
Insulin-Dependent Diabetes Mellitus (IDDM) 416
Non-Insulin-Dependent Diabetes Mellitus (NIDDM) 416
Gestational Diabetes 417
Epilepsy 417
Psychosocial and Economic Considerations 418
Pregnancy and Antiseizure Drugs 418
Arthritis 418
Osteoarthritis 419
Rheumatoid Arthritis 419
Systemic Lupus Erythematosus (SLE) 419

Multiple Sclerosis 420
Signs and Symptoms 420
Diagnosis and Treatment 420
Alzheimer's Disease 421
Signs and Symptoms 421
Risk and Protective Factors 421
Treatment 421
Role of Caregiver 422

CHAPTER TWENTY

Reducing Your Risk of Cancer 426

The Big "C" 426
Defining Cancer 426
Classifications of Common Malignancies 427
Causes of Cancer 430
Lifestyle Factors Implicated in Cancer 430
Environmental Factors Implicated in Cancer 431
Contributing Factors 431
Current Research Regarding Causes and Treatment 431
Molecular and Cellular Causes of Cancer 431
Assess Yourself: What Is Your Cancer Risk? 432
Cell Cycle Research 432
Gene Mutation Research 433
Adjuvant Treatment 433
Immunotherapy Research 433
Bone Marrow Transplant Research 433
Cancer at Selected Sites: What You Need to Know 433
Lung Cancer 433
Breast Cancer 435
Uterine Cancer 439
Ovarian Cancer 440
Skin Cancer 441
Colorectal Cancer 442
Actions to Take When Cancer Is Diagnosed 443
Social Support 444
Complementary Treatment in Cancer Management 445
Magnetic and Electronic Devices 445
Food Remedies 445
Spiritual and Meditation Practices 446
Choosing a Treatment Plan 446

Credits 450
Index 452

Preface

Women serve as the major decision makers and users of health-care services, but making wise health decisions today can be difficult. Only recently have we begun to understand that many of the decisions made by health-care providers have been based on research related to men. Research extrapolated data from studies using men as subjects and assumed that women would respond to similar treatment protocols. Thus, making the right choices for women's health can be challenging both for a woman and her health-care provider. The lack of research using women as subjects directly impacts the ability to make informed decisions. Fortunately, women are demanding more attention to their unique health needs. An increase in the amount of media attention and funding for research specific to women's health issues during the last decade is a testimonial to the increasing concern about women's health.

APPROACH

Contemporary Women's Health: Issues for Today and the Future has been written specifically to incorporate an interactive format with the most current, up-to-date material available about women's health. Although some topics in this text are similar to those found in personal health textbooks, most emphasis is placed on "women-only" issues. A variety of activities and reflective exercises have been designed to help women assess their current health status and plan for changes in their health behaviors.

We believe that learning should be dynamic and occurs when students integrate the issues as well as the facts for a vast array of health topics. Our emphasis is health promotion so we have addressed the social, economic, and political issues as well as the educational dimension. The format of this text encourages students to examine their current health knowledge, attitudes, and behaviors and explore possibilities to impact change and improvement in the health status of all women.

AUTHORSHIP

Contemporary Women's Health was written by three women university professors with considerable college teaching experience in health education and counselor education. As a result of long-term, continuous interaction with college women, we have developed a text that meets the complex needs of women as they explore their current health status and find ways to improve their quality of life. When we first discussed the possibility of writing this text, the only book available was *Our Bodies, Ourselves*. Since that time, the number of articles, research, and textbooks about women's health have proliferated. However, the format we have chosen lends itself well to classroom interaction, discussion, and problem solving related to the whole person, not just the physical aspect of women's health. We have written this text for women, thus the personal pronouns are from a female perspective. We hope that men, as well as women, will benefit from reading this text and gain a deeper understanding of the uniqueness of women's health issues.

AUDIENCE

This text is designed to be used by instructors and students in health education, nursing, and women's studies. The range of topics covered and the inclusion of viewpoints and activities makes this textbook appropriate for traditional and nontraditional students. We attempted to maintain sensitivity to diversity issues such as race, ethnicity, sexual orientation, and global health issues whenever possible.

FEATURES

Emphasis on Health Promotion

We believe that primary prevention remains the best method to curb rising health-care costs and reduce premature death. We encourage you to participate in the *Journal Activities* provided throughout the chapters.

Create your own personal journal to use with the text to record your reflections on the varied and complex health issues that are discussed, and how you may be impacted. Based on what you have read in the text, your journal entries should incorporate strategies for improving your quality of life and relationships.

Chapter 2, Developing a Healthy Lifestyle, includes health behavior change models to help you assess the conscious and unconscious factors contributing to women's health status. Many times we have a desire to change a particular behavior, and we are more likely to be successful in our efforts if we follow a plan. The health behavior change models will help you design a plan for change yielding more potential for success.

The *Assess Yourself* activities in each chapter present exercises and inventories also useful in developing your own personal plan for change.

Emphasizes Becoming a Wise Health-Care Consumer

Chapter 12, Becoming a Wise Consumer, examines practical issues and information that women need to know for making informed decisions with topics such as cosmetics and beauty products, the effects of advertising in the health-care industry, and home health tests.

Examines Emotional Health

Unique coverage of emotional health including skill development, assertiveness training, and resolving grief is presented to give students practical information to be used in developing positive self-esteem, decision making, and image building. Coverage of life transitions from childhood through late adulthood is also examined, and presents discussions of important topics such as body image, self-identity, social identity, family values, and life goals.

Integration of Multicultural and Global Issues

The culture of women is both unique and diverse. Women as a population have special needs and concerns that are universal to all women but different from men. At the same time, women around the world have a diversity of needs and concerns that arise because they come from many differing countries, ethnicities, value systems, and socioeconomic conditions. We have attempted to consider this complex mixture of women's health issues and have integrated this content in the text as well as in many of the various boxed materials.

The bumper sticker that adorns many cars, "Think globally, act locally," provides a thought-provoking message. We need to expand our consciousness regarding adequate health care and services for all women, and we strive to be more sensitive to the diversity of cultural perspectives.

Prevention of Violence Against Women

Chapter 13, Preventing Abuse Against Women, discusses topics such as date rape, acquaintance rape, sexual harassment, and child abuse while encouraging women to empower themselves against abuse by providing tips, helpful suggestions, and potential resources.

An Applied Approach

The events of today make up the history for tomorrow. Women's history is built from the stories of real-life women. *Her Story* are brief boxed vignettes about women, all based on real-life events, and intended to demonstrate how women's health is evolving. Each concludes with several follow-up questions to allow the student to apply the chapter content to discussions and possible solutions. The triumphs and tragedies, the successes and failures, and the gains and losses that women experience create the culture of women. As time passes, these same experiences will reflect the history of women, where they have been, and for what they are striving.

Healthy People 2000 Objectives

Each chapter includes an update of how far we have come in achieving the *Healthy People 2000 Objectives,* particularly those objectives most relevant to women. Progress toward achieving the goal based on the *Midcourse Review and 1995 Revisions* is quantified at the end of each objective. When the data show a negative value, it indicates movement away from the targeted goals; a positive value indicates movement toward the targeted goals.

Full-Color Design

To enhance the teaching-learning process, the full-color design accentuates the visual appeal of the text and makes more difficult illustrative concepts easier to understand.

Pedagogical Features

Although this text is designed to provide the most important and most current health information and research about women, the student will easily be able to apply the knowledge directly to herself. This process is made easy with the following helpful features in every chapter.

- *Chapter objectives* identify the goals at the beginning of each chapter.
- *Health tips* are boxed and provide steps to change and enhance health behaviors.
- *FYI* boxes highlight additional facts and events that impact the status of women.
- *Her Story* boxes provide brief vignettes of actual cases with follow-up questions to help students apply what they have just learned.
- *Viewpoint* boxes highlight controversial issues and ask students to reflect upon their own opinions.
- *Journal Activities* encourage students to record their reflections on the health issues discussed, how they are personally impacted, and identify strategies for improving health.
- *Assess Yourself!* activities provide interactive exercises and inventories to help students determine their own need for behavior change.
- *Definition* boxes are provided to reinforce new terms and provide pronunciation guides when appropriate.
- *Chapter summaries* are bulleted to reinforce content for test preparation.
- *Review questions* help students apply the concepts learned in the chapter.
- *Resources* provide a variety of additional materials including national organizations and hotlines (when available), videotapes and audiotapes, websites (when available), and suggested readings.
- *References* cite the most current resources available.

ANCILLARY

An *Instructor's Manual and Test Bank* contains chapter overviews, objectives, additional activities and resources, and more than nine-hundred test items. Twenty-five transparency masters are located at the back of the manual. Additional information about ancillaries is available from your WCB/McGraw-Hill sales representative.

ACKNOWLEDGMENTS

We wish to thank our professional colleagues who provided input, insight, and thoughtful consideration during the initial focus group. They include:

Lynne Fitzgerald
Morehead State University

Georgia L. Keeney
University of Minnesota at Duluth

Susan Cross Lipnickey
Miami University (Oxford, OH)

N. Gayle Schmidt
Texas A&M University

We want to also thank the reviewers for their excellent comments and suggestions that are evident throughout the pages of this text:

Linda C. Campanelli
American University

Sandra K. Cross
University of North Carolina at Pembroke

Eileen R. Fowles
Illinois Wesleyan University

June M. Goemer
St. Cloud State University

Becky K. Koch
Ohio State University

Susan Cross Lipnickey
Miami University (Oxford, OH)

Margaret V. Pepe
Kent State University

Laurie Pilotto
formerly of Hawkins County Health Dept.

Ellen D. Schulken
University of Maryland

We appreciate the care and attention to detail that were provided by the knowledgeable and experienced editors of this edition. Vicki Malinee and Michelle Turenne encouraged us and gently prodded us along throughout the entire process. Their insight regarding the qualities needed to make this a successful product were invaluable. Our gratitude must also be expressed for the excellent production of our text spearheaded by Gloria Schiesl, our Project Manager.

Recognition must also be given to the many women who touched our lives with their personal stories: Thank you for sharing your stories. We have a number of friends who have offered encouragement throughout this process: Joni, Bobbie, Roxanne, Carol, Nancy, Michael Ann, Michel, Patsy, Andree, Kathleen, Merita, Kathy, Betty, Suzanne, Sherry, Mary, Donna, Doffie, Bev, and Ben. Special thanks to Patricia Benson and Jim Robinson for their assistance through the various stages of this process. And we especially thank the numerous women, young and old, who have taken our classes, shared their stories, and provided further insight into the lives of women. ∞

CAK
DJB
CKC

About the Authors

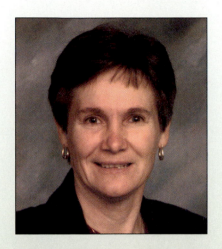

CHERYL A. KOLANDER

Cheryl A. Kolander is a professor of health education at the University of Louisville. She received her doctoral degree from Indiana University at Bloomington. She has taught health education at the university level for fifteen years, and makes regional and national presentations concerning women's health. Her research interests are women's health, alcohol and drug education, and spiritual wellness. ∽

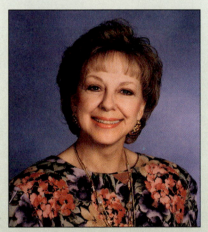

DANNY J. BALLARD

Danny J. Ballard is an associate professor of health education at Texas A&M University. She received her doctoral degree from Oklahoma State University. She has been an educator for more than thirty years, currently teaches courses in women's health issues, and makes regional and national presentations about women's health. Her research interests are women's health, worksite wellness, professional preparation, and school health. ∽

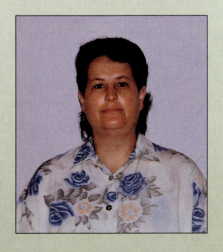

CYNTHIA K. CHANDLER

Cynthia K. Chandler is an associate professor of counselor education at the University of North Texas. She received her doctoral degree from Texas Tech University. She is the founder and director of the UNT Biofeedback Research and Training Laboratory, and teaches numerous courses in counseling. She is also a Licensed Professional Counselor and a Licensed Marriage and Family Therapist. Her research interests are in stress management, women's emotional health concerns, and holistic health and wellness. ∽

IN THE BEGINNING

Part One

CHAPTER ONE
Why Study Women's Health?

CHAPTER TWO
Developing a Healthy Lifestyle

CHAPTER THREE
Life Transitions: Infancy to Early Adulthood

CHAPTER FOUR
Life Transitions: Middle to Late Adulthood

One

Why Study Women's Health?

■ chapter objectives

When you complete this chapter you will be able to:
- Discuss the relevance of having a text dedicated to women's health concerns.
- Describe three common types of health action.
- Explain the significance of cultural and international diversity and women's health.
- Cite important events in the history of the women's social movement and in the history of women's health.

AUTHORS' PERSPECTIVE

Focus on Women's Health

Why do we need a text on women's health? An obvious reason is that women and men are different. In addition, many general health texts tend to relay information from studies based primarily on the male standard. A text geared specifically to women's health concerns will help to ensure that women's health issues are fairly represented.

By dedicating an entire text to women's health, there is opportunity to provide a comprehensive presentation of the vast number of issues and concerns that exist. Many health texts focus only on physiological conditions, whereas this text also incorporates the mental, emotional, and spiritual health dimensions as well.

A text dedicated to women's health sends a message to the public that women are important. Too often, issues regarding the welfare of women are completely ignored and when they are given consideration it is often as an afterthought. Only through long and difficult struggles have women made some progress toward being given equal consideration by the larger society, and yet significant discrimination toward women still exists.

A text dedicated to women's health is not meant to subjugate the importance of men's health concerns. It is meant to serve as a forum through which a presentation of issues regarding women's health can be understood and viewed as important and significant in and of themselves. Many aspects of women's health are uniquely different from those of men and need to be given ample consideration. Through a text specific to women's issues, information regarding women's status can be shared, examined, and addressed.

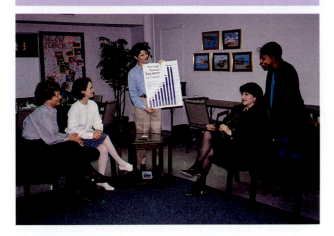

Women have some health issues that are very different from men.

But the Difference

was, she thought, a good woman
looks after others' interests such as grinding
corn, sewing skirts from old curtains,
hunter gathering, whereas a good
poet doesn't give a bugger, stuffs
herself on chocolate and champagne, sucks
dry the gourd of desire, thus releasing
the good poetry locked within. But being

quite well read as well as good she knew
only too clearly the statistics on obesity,
cirrhosis and hepatitis B and so forwent
these pleasures though not without certain

feelings of regret and moral complacency. But
she had a problem and it was this: the good
man whom she loved, who did not know
she was sacrificing good poetry for good

womanhood, who sat up late each evening
in their clean kitchen wrapped in a warm
scarf, writing his memoirs, unaware
of what he had nearly missed.

By Janet Fisher

Education is the keystone to progress. Education about women is the door through which women can be empowered. The performance of research studies regarding women must be emphasized. Information about the status of women must be made public and the public must pressure politicians to make women's issues a priority. The health of the world, a country, a city, or a community rests on the health and well-being of its women and children, not just on its men.

Emphasis on Health Promotion

Why is the concept of health promotion so important to the health field? The concept of health promotion is not limited to the idea that health is a condition we lose from time to time and try to gain back, but rather, health promotion includes the idea that health is something to be nurtured and by doing so we can prevent the onset of much illness and disease. Three common types of health action are: proactive care, health care maintenance, and reactive care. *Proactive care* involves designing and living a lifestyle that reduces the risks of illness, and also improves one's current health status. *Health care maintenance* is the continuation of what one is doing to maintain one's current health status. *Reactive care* is the treatment of any illness, disorder, or disease that may develop. The greatest emphasis in health promotion is placed upon proactive care.

Proactive health care serves to reduce health care costs with the prevention of the onset of many illnesses, disorders, and diseases, thereby avoiding the great expense involved in their treatment. Proactive health care is a holistic lifestyle model as opposed to a medical model. The traditional medical model is primarily reactive, and attends to the individual's needs after an unhealthy condition has developed. Holistic health care considers the interaction of the mind, body, and spirit: One area cannot be affected without the other areas also being affected. Understanding this interactive process is vital in providing proactive care to yourself and to others. Holistic health care incorporates all that we know about health, and utilizes this information to keep the body, mind, and spirit healthy.

Cultural Awareness

Why is it important to be sensitive about cultural issues in the health field? One reason is that, historically, a majority of human subject studies have been performed only with Caucasian, middle-class, and young to middle-aged male subjects. Research is expensive and because of limited funds for continuing research, applications of research outcomes to individuals not represented in the study remain purely hypothetical. A case in point: The National Institute of Health (NIH) was placed under congressional investigation in 1990 for failing to include female subjects in health studies that dictated diagnostic and

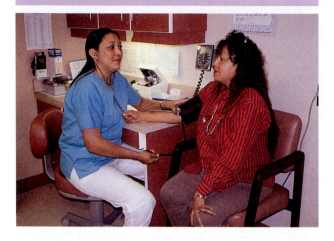

Flora Archuletta, a nurse at the Indian Health Center, has a special interest in Native American women's health issues.

prescriptive guidelines for both men *and* women. "The NIH excuse for not using females in such studies—that additional costs and complications are incurred with women subjects because of their numerous physiological differences in comparison with men—is the very reason women should have been included."[1]

Gender bias is common in health research. Some medications prescribed for women have not been actually tested on women, and some diagnostic and treatment guidelines for women are based on studies performed strictly with male samples.

Ethnic bias is also very present in health research. Studies that do incorporate women as subjects typically limit the subject pool to Caucasian, middle-class, and young to middle-aged females. Ethnic minorities remain significantly underrepresented in health research.

Socioeconomic bias is prevalent in the health field. The provision of continuous, high-quality health care is often limited to the middle and upper class, that is, those who have plenty of money or can afford health insurance. Social programs for the underprivileged, such as Social Security, Welfare, Medicaid, and Medicare are limited and frequently targeted by politicians for budget cuts. The poor are often deprived of adequate health care, the middle class can usually manage to at least maintain good health care and the wealthy can take the greatest advantage of the most up-to-date health information and medical treatment. In addition, even when health care is available, educational efforts about certain health risks or the availability of medical treatment is usually targeted toward the upper and middle class via restricted avenues such as a doctor's office or specialized magazines. Lower income families may never even know that a health service or a health risk exists unless special efforts are made to reach out to this population. (See *FYI:* "United States.")

Another cultural issue of concern is geographic differences. The majority of inner-city families are poor and they are often not aware of health services or cannot afford them. Rural families frequently do not have quick access to hospitals or specialists and thus adequate health care may not be available when needed. Or the family may have to drive a long distance to receive emergency health care or special services. Urban and suburban families are the most fortunate regarding the availability and affordability of quality health care.

INTERNATIONAL CONCERNS

Our text is based primarily on studies of women in the United States of America; however, women around the globe share many of the same concerns. All over the world there are women living in poverty, experiencing discrimination and violence, having limited access to birth control information and materials, lacking accessible child care services, developing diseases and disorders specific to women, suffering with low self-esteem and distorted body image, and facing serious gynecological health concerns.

There are many issues that are more specific to the time, place, and culture in which women live. Countries may have differing policies and attitudes toward women. In addition, religious or family traditions of certain countries place a special emphasis on certain images and roles women are expected to fulfill. The level of technological development, or the state of war versus peace in a country may also influence the status of women and their health. It is our special obligation to pay attention to world events regarding the health and well-being of women, and of all persons, who share our planet.

WOMEN'S SOCIAL MOVEMENT

The social stigmas attached with being a woman have significant influence on a woman's life development, including areas such as self-image, career choices and advancement, family relations, and personal

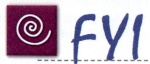

FYI   *United States: A Nation of Diverse Needs²*

- African Americans make up 12 percent of the U.S. population, constituting the largest minority group. Life expectancy for this group has lagged behind that for the total population throughout this century.
- Hispanic Americans compose the second largest minority group in the United States constituting about 8 percent. Due to the variety of Hispanic subgroups, such as Mexican Americans, Puerto Ricans, Cuban Americans, Central and South American immigrants, Hispanics experience the most varied set of health issues facing a single minority population.
- The third largest minority group is Asian and Pacific Islander Americans, more than 11 million in number. The diversity among this group is profound with over 30 different languages spoken, an equal number of distinct cultures, and incomes ranging from poverty level to above the national average.

- Descendants of the original residents of North America, American Indians and Alaska natives, number about 1.6 million, composing the smallest minority group. This group encompasses numerous tribes and over 400 nations, one-third living on reservations and about 50 percent in urban areas.
- Estimates of the number of persons with chronic, significant disabilities range from 34 million to 43 million. Persons with disabilities are at a higher risk for future problems because of their existing serious or chronic physical or mental disability.
- Nearly 1 of every 8 Americans lives in a family with an income below the poverty level. For all of the chronic diseases that lead the nation's list of killers, low income is a special risk factor.

Women represent many different cultures.

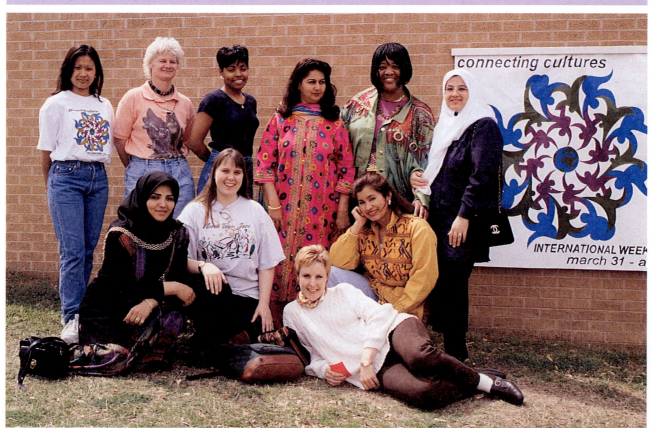

significance. One cannot isolate the personal well-being of the individual woman from the context of being a member of the larger culture of women. Therefore, it is important to address the transitions that women have passed through in recent history.

The U.S. women's movement began during the late 1700s and early 1800s as a general concern for education, out of which grew a specific concern for the education of women.[3] Women activists played a major role in improving the plight of others, including support for the abolitionists in eliminating slavery and extending constitutional rights to African Americans. Suffrage efforts were successful in obtaining the right to vote for women in 1920 with the passage of the Nineteenth Amendment.

Before women succeeded in obtaining the right to vote, women were mostly considered in the context of their husbands or fathers. In almost all instances, only the male head of the household was allowed to own property, borrow money, or sign legal documents. In fact, the social stigma towards women and children was that they were considered the property of men.

Prior to the 1900s, men could determine the fate of their wives, daughters, and children without women having much say in the matter. One case in point, Robert Todd Lincoln, the son of former U.S. President Abraham Lincoln, was pursuing a successful political career in city and state politics in Chicago, Illinois as well as in national politics. His mother, Mary Lincoln, had turned to what was then considered to be "outside of the mainstream" spiritualism, which included seances and attempts to communicate with the dead, as a way of resolving her grief after the assassination of her husband. Robert became embarrassed by his mother's actions and had her placed in an insane asylum and took over her financial estate. Mary Lincoln remained there for several months until a woman lawyer took on her case at no cost and was successful in getting Mrs. Lincoln released by convincing the court with her opinion that "Mary Lincoln is no more insane than you or I." Mary Lincoln lived the remainder of her days with a sister and, supposedly, never forgave her son for what he did to her.

The women's movement of the 1960s projected attention to issues such as job and wage discrimination. Due to these consciousness-raising efforts, the government added the category of sex discrimination to Title VII of the 1964 Civil Rights Act. Out of Title VII came the Equal Employment Opportunity Commission (EEOC), a body delegated to protect women and other minorities from discrimination in the workforce.

In 1966, the National Organization for Women was started along with women's liberation groups. In 1972, as a response to the concentrated efforts of these groups, the Ninety-second Congress voted overwhelming approval of a constitutional amendment known as the Equal Rights Amendment (ERA). The proposed amendment read as follows:

> Sec. 1. Equality of rights under the law shall not be denied or abridged by the United States or by any state on account of sex.
> Sec. 2. The Congress shall have the power to enforce by appropriate legislation the provisions of this article.
> Sec. 3. The Amendment shall take effect two years after the date of ratification.[4]

Support for the ERA in the 1972 Congress was evidenced by the following quotes:

> In the movement toward social liberation we have taken on the task of improving the status of blacks, Indians, Spanish-speaking Americans, other minority groups; but in the process we have overlooked another important group that has suffered from many forms of discrimination—women—which is all the more amazing because they are a (statistical) majority rather than a minority group. [Senator Gurney, Congressional Record, March 21, 1972. S-4393]
>
> All the ERA seeks to do is to say to the Supreme Court of the United States—"WAKE UP!—This is the 20th Century. Before it is over, judge women as individual human beings." [Congresswomen Martha Griffiths, principal sponsor of the Amendment; Congressional Record, October 6, 1971, H-9264]

The ERA failed to achieve the necessary 38 state ratification and was not incorporated into law. The failure of the ERA took the wind out of the sails of the once forceful women's movement. Though little has been heard regarding any united movement for women since the failure of the ERA, efforts are still being applied in specific areas to increase and maintain awareness about the extent of women's social, emotional, and physical concerns. For example, in the 1970s Affirmative Action assisted women in battling discrimination and obtaining higher paying jobs. In addition, in the 1980s, sexual harassment had been determined to be illegal in the work place and this gave women the ability to fend off sexual innuendos and threats without repercussions that could lead to job demotion, loss of promotion, or loss of a job.

In spite of some progress being made in past years, the following issues for women still require major attention as we approach the twenty-first century: enhancing self-esteem, promoting a healthy and realistic body image, countering the implied obligation to fulfill a sacrificial caretaker role, halting the expectation that women follow stereotypic traditional career choices requiring greater supervision and offering lower salaries, curbing violence against women, continuing the battle against gender-role socialization along with job and wage discrimination, and establishing standards of emotional, physical, and spiritual well-being that are specific to women and not derived from comparisons with men.

HISTORY OF WOMEN'S HEALTH RESEARCH

Women have long been underrepresented in medical research.[5] Historically, women's health research focused on diseases affecting fertility and reproduction; a focus reflective of the value society placed on women, that of primarily a reproductive organism. Other disease research has focused disproportionately on men. Despite this imbalance, new drug therapies tested on men, once approved, were prescribed to women without comparable trials of clinical safety or efficacy. For example, a few years ago a study revealed that aspirin helps prevent heart attacks in men. Women were not included in this study even though heart disease is the number one killer of U.S. women. Yet aspirin is now recommended to both men and women as a preventive measure for heart attacks. Women have been excluded from medical research for at least two reasons: (1) concerns about pregnancy during a trial and (2) concerns that women's changing hormone levels during menstrual cycles might skew test results. We now know that there are no significant reasons to exclude women in medical research. In most cases both sexes respond similarly to many therapies; however, there may be exceptions. For example, women may need lower dosages, or therapies may need to be specific to women.

Nurses Health Study

The first comprehensive effort to clinically study health issues for women was the Nurses Health Study.[5] The Nurses Health Study began in 1976, enrolling about 121,000 nurses. In 1989, a second group of 116,000 was enrolled in the Nurses Health Study II. The groups, designated NHS I and NHS II, were followed by means of a biennial mail questionnaire that inquired about lifestyle and health problems. The study continues to gather data from women nurses that contributes greatly to our understanding of women's health issues. Findings from the study are cited where appropriate in later chapters of the text.

Women's Health Initiative

To respond to the crucial need for the involvement of women in medical research, the NIH in 1990 established the Office of Research on Women's Health (ORWH). The earliest undertakings of the ORWH included the development of a research agenda to identify and address gaps in the biomedical community's knowledge of women's health, and the strengthening and revitalization of already-existing NIH guidelines and policies for the inclusion of women and minorities in clinical studies.[5]

The Women's Health Initiative (WHI) is a long-term, national study that focuses on strategies for preventing heart disease, breast and colorectal cancer, and osteoporosis in postmenopausal women.[5] These chronic diseases are the major causes of death, disability, and frailty in older women of all races and socioeconomic backgrounds. This $628 million, 15-year project, sponsored by the NIH, will involve 164,500 women aged 50–79, and is one of the most definitive, far-reaching clinical trials of women's health ever undertaken in the United States. Recruitment of subjects for the study began in 1991; 64,500 women will be studied to address health issues that include menopause, hormone replacement therapy, dietary modification and calcium and vitamin supplements, and, in the observational portion of the study, 100,000 women will be studied to examine the relationship between lifestyle, health and risk factors, and specific disease outcomes. The Women's Health Initiative should provide some valuable data regarding women's health concerns over the next several years.

h e a l t h   t i p s

Personal Health and Safety Tips

To achieve proactive health care in your daily life, the following is a sample of recommendations that you should regularly practice. Can you think of any others?

- Avoid all tobacco use.
- Drink alcoholic beverages in moderation.
- Use over-the-counter and prescription drugs properly; be sure to read labels and use only as directed.
- Avoid use of illegal drugs.
- Consume a nutritionally balanced diet.
- Exercise regularly.
- Minimize the effects of stress through exercise, proper rest, and stress reduction techniques.
- Practice safer sex techniques if you are in an intimate relationship.
- Never drink alcohol and drive.
- Never accept a ride from a stranger.
- Wear a seat belt whenever you are in a car; make sure all your passengers do the same.
- Be sure that children are properly restrained in the back seat of the car, and in age-appropriate child safety seats or belts.
- Know how to change a flat tire on your car and make sure the spare tire is inflated at all times.
- Always count to three and look both ways before proceeding into an intersection with your vehicle after a stoplight has turned green.

- Always keep doors and windows locked in your home or dorm room.
- Be sure that smoke and carbon monoxide detectors work properly.
- Keep toxic substances, for example medications and cleaning fluids, out of the reach of children.
- Bend your knees whenever you lift a heavy object; lift with your legs and not your back. Ask for assistance or use a lifting device if the object is too heavy.
- Be very careful when climbing onto a ladder; make sure it is level and secured well. Be sure to have someone help you when you climb on a high ladder to keep it steady below.
- Wear protective eye wear when engaging in activities that might endanger your eyes; for example, when working with machinery or during sporting activities such as racquetball.
- Wear protective ear wear, muffling headphones, or ear plugs when around loud noises such as loud machinery.
- Do not turn the volume up high when using stereo headphones to listen to music.
- Make sure that someone you trust knows where you are going and when you are expected to arrive; stay in touch with them so they can monitor your whereabouts.

TO HELP YOU USE THIS TEXT

Health Tips

Throughout the text, practical *Health Tips* are provided. These helpful tips are recommendations that will enhance your personal health journey. Although some of these tips may seem obvious, others may be new ideas to you. See *Health Tips:* "Personal Health and Safety Tips" for examples.

Viewpoint

We have attempted to provide a text on women's health that is comprehensive and unbiased. In cases when a controversy is presented in the textbook, the major issue is highlighted in a box labeled *Viewpoint*. This is an opportunity for you, the reader, to become informed of differing opinions or controversies and formulate an opinion of your own. The term "viewpoint" is symbolic in that just as you might travel across the countryside, you might stop from time to time to ponder a scenic view and take in the breadth and scope of the landscape before you. This is also true of life. It is important to pause from time to time, examine the views before you, and formulate your own ideas. Take a look at the information in *Viewpoint:* "1995 Women of the Year." Do you agree or disagree with what it may be suggesting?

FYI

On occasion, throughout the text, a particular item of information will be highlighted in a box labeled *FYI,* meaning "for your information." This is much like a news flash that serves to capture your attention. *FYI*

Viewpoint

1995 Women of the Year[6]

Do you agree that these women are heroes?
- Myrlie Evers-Williams. For her commitment to revitalizing the oldest civil rights associaton in the United States, the NAACP.
- Candace Gingrich (sister of the U.S. Congressional Speaker of the House, Newt Gingrich). For speaking up and out for lesbian and gay rights.
- Oseola McCarthy. For her act of extraordinary generosity; even though she never made more than poverty wages, she bequeathed most of her life savings, $150,000, to a local university.
- Mimi Ramsey. For selflessly striving, despite her own pain from childhood trauma, to end the mutilation of female genitalia of young girls practiced regularly in her native country, Ethiopia, and in many other countries.
- Aung San Suu Kyi. Through a private act of sacrifice, for helping to keep the dream of democracy alive in her native Burma.
- Willow Farey. For believing in the right of girls to be treated with honesty and respect by standing up to a high school teacher who sexually harassed her and a number of other female students.
- Prema Mathai-Davis. For organizing the YWCA Week Without Violence program; thereby reminding America that violence need not be a way of life.

JOURNAL ACTIVITY

Women's Health Issues and the News

What current local, state, national, or international women's health issues can you find in the newspaper, news magazines, on television or radio, or by surfing the Internet? How do these issues impact you directly and indirectly? Write down your thoughts about these questions in your personal health journal.

---

boxes emphasize a certain piece of information that is interesting or may be especially helpful to you. Examples appear in *FYI:* "Women's World Report."

Journal Activity

A *Journal Activity* may be suggested at various times throughout the text. It is our hope that you will keep a written journal and incorporate many of the text's activities within the journal. A written journal can provide insight into your life that might not otherwise be gained. Writing down thoughts, feelings, and behaviors serves not only as a personal diary but presents an opportunity for repeated examination of yourself. This exercise can place pieces of information together like a jigsaw puzzle and help you get a clearer picture of who you currently are, and where you are going. A journal can be a companion and a friend on your life journey. Try com-

pleting *Journal Activity:* "Women's Health Issues and the News" as a way of getting started on your own personal journey through your exploration of women's health. Other types of journal activities could be to write poetry or songs, or create other art forms that depict life issues reflecting or impacting your personal health journey.

Her Story

As the authors of this text, we want to present a realistic picture of issues regarding women's health. We have chosen to incorporate case examples based on real-life events. In many instances, the names of the individuals involved in the events may have been changed to protect their identity; however, in more publicized cases, the true identities will be used. These real-life events, or case examples, have been called *Her Stories.* This a takeoff from "history" or "his story." Consider each *Her Story* as a page out of women's health history.

Assess Yourself!

From time to time you will come across an *Assess Yourself!* This type of exercise is provided to assist you in organizing information about yourself that might be helpful in making informed decisions about your personal lifestyle. Take *Assess Yourself!:* "Personal Health Inventory" now, and then take it again when you have finished reading this textbook to compare your results.

Healthy People 2000 Objectives

In 1990 a document titled *Healthy People 2000: National Health Promotion and Disease Prevention Objectives* was published.[20] This document has formed the strategic plan for improving the health of

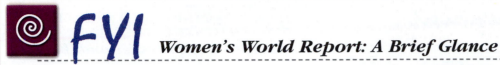

FYI   *Women's World Report: A Brief Glance*

1996

- The most experienced U.S. astronaut is Dr. Shannon Lucid, a 53-year-old mother of three grown children, who lived aboard the Russian space station, Mir, for several months. She set two space duration records: one for the most logged hours for any woman, and the other for the most logged hours for any U.S. astronaut.[7] This comes 13 years after the first U.S. woman astronaut, Sally Ride, flew into space aboard the space shuttle Challenger on June 18, 1983.[8]
- Violent protests marred the Miss World pageant in Bangalore, India. Before the pageant finals began, about 1,000 demonstrators denouncing beauty contests as demeaning to women tried to block roads leading to the site of the pageant.[9]

1995

- Women workers in Asia, Russia, and Eastern Europe hired by international shoe manufacturers are exploited.[10]
- Ireland's senate debated information on abortion; the controversy focused on the right of Irish women to obtain information about foreign abortion clinics.[11]

1994

- March 8, 1994, was International Women's Day. The day received little media attention, and the state of women internationally remains grim. For example, genital mutilation continues in the Middle East and Africa, as does sexual slavery in Thailand, and the burning of brides for their dowry in India.[12]

- Approximately 60 women die every hour in developing countries as a result of what may be unwanted pregnancies, according to the International Women's Health Coalition.[13]

1993

- The International Astronomical Union has asked the help of its members in choosing names for topographic structures on the surface of the planet Venus, which were discovered by the space probe Magellan. The planet's regions will be named after famous women and mythological heroines and goddesses.[14]
- Women's tennis has become almost as popular as men's tennis. Some tournaments, such as the Matinee Limited International, attract higher rating than men's competitions. However, women still do not win as much prize money as men tennis players.[15]

1992

- Prime Minister Kiichi Miyazawa apologized in January 1992 to Korean women used as sex slaves by Japanese soldiers during World War II. However, Japan continues to refuse to compensate the women, numbering between 80,000 and 200,000 women, who were sent to Japanese military camps around Asia, where they were raped by soldiers.[16]
- Men significantly outnumber women in India and China. Females are aborted, killed at birth, or left to die of diseases without medicine and food because parents prefer male offspring. In these cultures, women are unwanted because they can neither benefit their parents financially nor carry family names because of inflexible social traditions.[17]

---

the public in the United States. The three primary goals for the nation that were presented in this document were: Goal I—increase the span of healthy life for Americans; Goal II—reduce health disparities among Americans; and Goal III—achieve access to preventive services for all Americans. An important follow-up document was published in 1996 titled *Healthy People 2000: Midcourse Review and 1995 Revisions.*[21] Objectives presented in these documents are identified in the remaining chapters as *Healthy People 2000 Objectives.* Each objective relates to the specific subject areas.

Her Story

Deborah

Deborah's four daughters each clutched a single red rose and wiped away tears as they joined nearly 100 people last night for a candlelight vigil to remember their mother. It was the one-month anniversary of Deborah's shooting death and they were gathered to speak out against domestic violence. The four daughters were left without parents after Deborah's estranged husband shot her before turning the gun on himself.[18]

- Do you know someone who is or has been a victim of domestic violence?
- What would you say to them?
- Would you encourage them to seek help from the community?

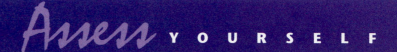

Personal Health Inventory[19]

Circle the number for each item that best describes you.

Cigarette Smoking

Note! If you never smoke, enter a score of 10 for this section and go to the next section on Alcohol and Drugs.

	Almost Always	Sometimes	Almost Never
1. I avoid smoking cigarettes.	2	1	0
2. I smoke only low tar and nicotine cigarettes or I smoke a pipe or cigars.	2	1	0

Smoking Score: _____

Alcohol and Drugs

1. I avoid drinking alcoholic beverages or I drink no more than 1 or 2 drinks a day.	4	1	0
2. I avoid using alcohol or other drugs (especially illegal drugs) as a way of handling stressful situations or the problems in my life.	2	1	0
3. I am careful not to drink alcohol when taking certain medicines (for example, medicine for sleeping, pain, colds, and allergies), or when pregnant.	2	1	0
4. I read and follow the label directions when using prescribed and over-the-counter drugs.	2	1	0

Alcohol and Drug Score: _____

Eating Habits

1. I eat a variety of food each day, such as fruits and vegetables, whole grain breads and cereals, lean meats, dairy products, dry peas and beans, and nuts and seeds.	4	1	0
2. I limit the amount of fat, saturated fat, and cholesterol I eat (including fat on meats, eggs, butter, cream, shortenings, and organ meats such as liver).	2	1	0
3. I limit the amount of salt I eat by cooking with only small amounts, not adding salt at the table, and avoiding salty snacks.	2	1	0
4. I avoid eating too much sugar (especially frequent snacks of sticky candy or soft drinks).	2	1	0

Eating Habits Score: _____

Exercise/Fitness

1. I maintain a desired weight, avoid being overweight and underweight.	3	1	0
2. I do vigorous exercise for 15–30 minutes at least 3 times a week (examples include running, swimming, brisk walking).	3	1	0
3. I do exercises that enhance my muscle tone for 15–30 minutes at least 3 times a week (examples include yoga and calisthenics).	2	1	0
4. I use part of my leisure time participating in individual, family, or team activities that increase my level of fitness (such as gardening, bowling, golf, and baseball).	2	1	0

Exercise/Fitness Score: _____

Stress Control

1. I have a job or do other work that I enjoy.	2	1	0
2. I find it easy to relax and express my feelings freely.	2	1	0
3. I recognize early, and prepare for, events or situations likely to be stressful for me.	2	1	0
4. I have close friends, relatives, or others to whom I can talk about personal matters and call on for help when needed.	2	1	0
5. I participate in group activities (such as church and community organizations) or hobbies that I enjoy.	2	1	0

Stress Control Score: _____

Safety

1. I wear a seat belt while riding in a car.	2	1	0
2. I avoid driving while under the influence of alcohol and other drugs.	2	1	0
3. I obey traffic rules and the speed limit when driving.	2	1	0
4. I am careful when using potentially harmful products or substances (such as household cleaners, poisons, and electrical devices).	2	1	0
5. I avoid smoking in bed.	2	1	0

Safety Score: _____

Interpretation: There is no total score for this inventory. Compare your individual scores for each topic with the scales below.

9–10 Excellent! Your answers show that you are aware of the importance of this area to your health.

6–8 Your health practices in this area are good, but there is room for improvement.

3–5 Your health risks are showing! You should seek out information on changing your behaviors in this area.

0–2 Your answers show that you may be taking serious and unnecessary risks with your health in this area. It is definitely time to take the steps to change your behaviors. Seek out information and assistance about behavior change.

CONCLUSION

Women have health needs and concerns that are unique to their gender. Thus, it is important to have a health text dedicated specifically to women. The culture of women has evolved, like all cultures do. Who women are today and the issues they face have developed over time as a result of both positive and negative events throughout history. That is why this text addresses the importance of women's health issues within the context of social, political, and medical arenas.

We hope you enjoy using this text as much as we enjoyed writing it. The topic of women's health is vast and we do not suppose that we have covered everything that can be covered regarding the subject. We do hope that we addressed most of the major issues. We now leave it to you to continue the journey and advocate for greater awareness and attention to the field of women's health. ∞

Chapter Summary

- There are three common types of health action: proactive care, health care maintenance, and reactive care.
- Holistic health care incorporates all that we know about health and utilizes this information to keep the body, mind, and spirit healthy.
- A major cultural bias is the absence of adequate representation of women and ethnic minorities in medical research.

- Women around the globe share many of the same health concerns. However, cultural differences significantly impact the type and severity of these concerns.
- The status of women's health must be examined from cultural, political, and social perspectives.

Review Questions

1. Why do we need a text specific to women's health issues?
2. Can you name and describe three common types of health action?
3. How would you describe holistic health care?
4. Why is cultural sensitivity necessary in health care?
5. Can you name the various types of culture bias in health care?
6. What are some health issues that are shared by women around the globe?
7. What are some major social and political events in the history of the U.S. women's movement?
8. What is the Nurses Health Study?
9. What is the Women's Health Initiative?

Resources

Organizations and Hotlines

Office of Research on Women's Health
National Institutes of Health
Building 1, Room 201
9000 Rockville Pike
Bethesda, MD 20892

Women's Health Initiatives
U.S. Dept. of Health and Human Services
NIH Federal Building, Room 6A09
Bethesda, MD 20892
Telephone: (800) 54-WOMEN or 800-549-6636

National Health Information Center
U.S. Dept. of Health and Human Services
Referral Specialist
P.O. Box 1133
Washington, DC 20013-1133
Telephone: (800) 336-4797 or (301) 565-4167

U.S. Federal Information Phone Directory
Telephone: (800) 688-9889

U.S. Dept. of Health and Human Services
Public Health Service, Information Office
Washington, DC
Telephone: (301) 433-2403

U.S. Public Health Service Publication Clearinghouse
Telephone: (800) 358-9295

U.S. Government Printing Office and Bookstore
Telephone: (202) 512-1800

Parklawn Library for Government Documents
Washington, DC
Telephone: (301) 443-2673

Health Research and Services Administration
Washington, DC
Telephone: (301) 443-2086

Agency for Healthcare Policy and Research
Washington, DC
Telephone: (301) 594-1364

U.S. Government Book Store
Dallas, Texas
Telephone: (214) 767-0076

Websites

Office of Research on Women's Health, NIH
http://www.aamc.org/research/adhocgp/women.htm

Office on Women's Health, Public Health Service
http://phs.os.dhhs.gov/progorg/ophs/owh.htm

Women's Health Initiative
http://www.wellweb.com/survey/whi.htm

National Health Information Center
http://nhic-nt.health.org/

National Institutes of Health
http://info.rutgers.edu/orsp/nihsite.1.html
http://www.nih.gov/
http://web.fie.com/fedix/nih.html

National Center for Health Statistics
http://www.cdc.gov/nchswww/nchshome.htm

U.S. Dept. of Health and Human Services
http://www.os.dhhs.gov/

U.S. Public Health Service
http://phs.os.dhhs.gov/phs/phs.html

References

1. Chandler, C. 1991. The psychology of women: Approaching the twenty-first century. *Individual Psychology* 47 (4): 487.

2. Public Health Service. 1990. *Healthy People 2000: National Health Promotion and Disease Prevention Objectives.* Washington, DC: U.S. Dept. of Health and Human Services.

3. Snyder, E.C. 1979. The anatomy of the women's social movement. In *The Study of Women: Enlarging Perspectives of Social Reality,* edited by E. C. Snyder, New York: Harper & Row.

4. Rawalt, M. 1979. Constitutional rights for women—the equal rights amendment (p. 125). In *The Study of Women: Enlarging Perspectives of Social Reality,* edited by E. C. Snyder, New York. Harper & Row: 124-42.

5. Women's Health Initiative. Website: 2 March 1997, http://www.nih.gov/od/odp/whi/factsht.htm

6. Women of the year. 1995. *Ms. Magazine* (January-February): 41-64.

7. Walters, B. The 10 most fascinating people of 1996. ABC Television Broadcast, 6 December 1996.

8. Congratulations Dr. Lucid. Maximov Online, Website: December 1996, http://www.maximov.com/Mir/lucid.html

9. Associated Press. Violent protests mar Miss World pageant. *Denton Record Chronicle,* Denton, Tex., 24 November 1996, p. 7A.

10. Enloe, C. 1995. The globetrotting sneaker. *Ms. Magazine* 5 (March-April): 10-15.

11. Clarity, J. Ireland's Senate debates information on abortion. *New York Times,* 13 March 1995, International Pages, p. A2.

12. Pollitt, K. Subject to debate. *The Nation* 258 (4 April 1994): p. 441.

13. Steele, I. Moving beyond birth control. *World Press Review* 41 (August 1994): 44.

14. Sky & Telescope. Venus: The name game. *Sky & Telescope* 86 (September 1993): 14-15.

15. Deacon, J. Queens of the court: Women's tennis enjoys a surge in popularity. *Maclean's* 106 (16 August 1993): 46-47.

16. International News. Japan: Small comfort for "comfort women." *Ms. Magazine* 2 (March-April): 11.

17. Mahony, R. 1992. On the trail of the world's "missing women." *Ms. Magazine* 2 (March-April): 12.

18. Tharp, R. Vigil held for victim of domestic violence. *Star-Telegram,* Ft. Worth, Tex., 10 December 1996, p. B6.

19. Assessment adapted from *Health Style: A self test.* U.S. Department of Health and Human Services (PHS) 81-50155.

20. Public Health Service, 1990. *Healthy People 2000.*

21. U.S. Department of Health and Human Services. 1996. *Healthy People 2000: Midcourse Review and 1995 Revisions.* Boston, Mass.: Jones & Bartlett.

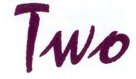

Developing a Healthy Lifestyle

■ chapter objectives

When you complete this chapter, you will be able to:
- Define the dimensions of wellness in regard to the whole person concept.
- Describe the health continuum, from wellness to illness, and appropriate intervention strategies.
- Describe theories of learning and models of behavior change.
- Apply the phases of lifestyle change to your own life: behavioral assessment, goal setting, behavioral contracting, initiation of behavior change, and periodic evaluation of progress.

WHAT IS HEALTHY?

Do you consider yourself to be healthy? What do you compare yourself with to decide that you are healthy? How old do you feel? How long do you expect to live? These are not easy questions to answer primarily because living is a very complex process. Your health is dependent upon your personal lifestyle choices as well as upon uncontrollable elements, such as genetics, environmental conditions, the technological development of your country, your gender, your ethnicity, cultural issues, age-specific risks, and the potential for accidents.

This whole book serves as a guide for lifestyle assessment and enhancement for women. The ideas presented in this chapter are meant to prepare you for the material presented in later chapters. And although much of the information in this chapter may be applied to anyone, you can use this information to help you understand how you, personally, make lifestyle choices. Think of this chapter as a presentation of the basic philosophies of health and behavior change. You may note that this chapter includes some of the classical theories and models on which current ideas about healthy lifestyle choices are formed.

Some people live to be over 100 years old and some die in infancy. There are just too many factors to consider in determining just how long you will actually live. Life expectancy figures are important in that they provide researchers with overall, statistical averages for tracking health concerns, but statistical averages do not consider the individual. The most important consideration for you is what you are doing to achieve a lifestyle that is enjoyable for you, and a lifestyle that will prolong your enjoyment as much as possible.

This chapter presents average life expectancy figures, and it also describes established models for

HEALTHY PEOPLE 2000 OBJECTIVES

- Reduce human exposure to toxic agents by decreasing the release of hazardous substances from industrial facilities: 65 percent decrease in carcinogens, 50 percent decrease in the most toxic chemicals. 1995 progress toward goal: minus 80 percent
- Increase to at least 85 percent the proportion of people who receive a supply of drinking water that meets the safe drinking water standards established by the Environmental Protection Agency. 1995 progress toward goal: minus 40 percent
- Establish curbside recycling programs that serve at least 50 percent of the U.S. population and continue to increase household hazardous waste collection programs. 1995 progress toward goal: 60 percent
- Increase years of healthy life to at least 65 years. 1995 progress toward goal: minus 30 percent
- Increase the proportion of all degrees in the health professions and allied and associated health profession fields awarded to members of underrepresented racial and ethnic minority groups. 1995 progress toward goal: blacks 20 percent of target achieved; Hispanics 55 percent of target achieved; American Indians/Alaska natives 35 percent of target achieved.

Table 2.1

Life Expectancy for Women of the World[2]

NATION	YEARS OF LIFE
Japan	82
France	81
Spain	80
Australia	80
United States of America	79
Poland	75
Argentina	75
Hungary	74
Mexico	73
Romania	73
Malaysia	73
Republic of Korea	73
China	71
Turkey	70
Brazil	69
Tunisia	68
Philippines	67
South Africa	66
Egypt	62
India	60
Nigeria	53
Bangladesh	52
Mozambique	48

healthy living. The health models presented in this chapter serve as a basis for you to understand your own personal life concerns and can aid in the design of a lifestyle that suits you the best as you proceed through the remainder of this book.

Life Expectancy

The expectation of life at birth in 1994 in the United States was an average of 75.7 years, but slightly lower than the record high of 75.8 years in 1992.[1] As compared to 1993, in 1994 life expectancy for the white population increased by 0.1 years for females (79.6) and 0.2 years for males (73.2). For the black population, life expectancy at birth increased 0.4 years for females (74.1) and 0.2 years for males (64.9). During 1994, an estimated 2,268,000 deaths occurred in the United States, and in 1995 an estimated 2,312,203 deaths occurred. Table 2.1 provides a comparison of life expectancies among women living in westernized and Third World countries.

Leading Causes of Death

Heart disease, cancer, and stroke continued to be the top three causes of death in 1995 for all Americans.[3] Accidents were the leading cause-of-death for persons until age 24. HIV infection was the leading cause-of-death for those persons aged 25–44 years. Cancer was the leading cause-of-death for those aged 45–64 years, whereas heart disease was the leading cause-of-death for those aged 65 years and over. HIV/AIDS has risen rapidly over the past few years and in 1995 was the eighth leading cause of death for all Americans. Table 2.2 summarizes the leading causes of death in the United States. The number one leading cause of death for U.S. women overall in 1995 was heart disease.

WHOLE PERSON CONCEPT

Your health status is not limited to the physical realm because you also have emotions, thoughts, and spirit. These all work together to bring about

Table 2.2

U.S. Deaths by Causes in 1995[3]

CAUSE	NUMBER
Diseases of the heart	738,781
Malignant neoplasms	537,969
Cerebrovascular diseases	158,061
Chronic obstructive pulmonary diseases	104,756
Accidents and adverse effects	89,703
(Motor vehicle accidents	41,786)
(Other accidents	47,917)
Pneumonia and influenza	83,528
Diabetes mellitus	59,085
HIV infection	42,506
Suicide	30,893
Chronic liver disease and cirrhosis	24,848
All other causes	442,073
All causes	2,312,203

your state of well-being. Each of these interacts with the other, so, if you are affected in one area, the other areas will also be impacted. When examining your lifestyle it is important to look at the whole picture of your health.

Mind, Body, and Spirit

One comprehensive conceptual model of individual health involves all three of the following elements: psyche, soma, and spirit (mind, body, and spirit).[4] The psyche involves your emotional, attitudinal, and mental state. Soma, or body, refers to your physical status. Spiritual health is your philosophy about living for yourself and living with others. Have you thought about yourself in these three different ways?

There are two major categories of factors that influence your status as a whole person: endogenous factors and exogenous factors. **Endogenous factors** are those events that occur within you. Examples of endogenous factors would be the presence or absence of illness, a positive or negative attitude, ability to have intimacy, and so on. **Exogenous factors** are external events that influence you, such as the type of personal relationships you have, the weather, stressful events, and so on. Endogenous and exogenous events interact to create an impact on your whole person. Can you think of some things occurring within and around you that impact your health?

Dimensions of Wellness

Wellness has been described as consisting of six major dimensions: physical, emotional, social, occupational, intellectual, and spiritual.[5,6] Do you think it is possible to pay attention to all six dimensions in your life? Some feel that this may be one ultimate goal of wellness. You may not be able to pay attention to all six at once, but you can take turns on each one at different times in your life, depending upon which is most important to you at the time. (See *FYI:* "Descriptions of Wellness.")

Holistic Wellness Model

Another way to conceptualize health is as five primary dimensions of wellness—physical, emotional, social, occupational, and intellectual—and two basic components within each dimension, a personal component and a spiritual component (see Fig. 2.1).[8] The personal component is striving for the satisfaction of your own personal needs, such as nutrition, exercise, shelter, income, relaxation, recreation, education, and personal achievement. The spiritual component is striving for a relationship or connection with other persons and things, such as family, friends, community, country, world, and higher power. This includes enhanced awareness, knowledge, and love of others. Sometimes an issue or event is not clearly in one area but rather may coexist in more than one wellness dimension and in more than one component, spiritual or personal, at a time.

Developing a healthy lifestyle is a process. It is a goal worth working toward, but it can often be a life goal. Total attention to all wellness dimensions at the same time is very difficult to achieve. Thus, the holistic wellness model is not a mandate, but it is a guide for living.

ACHIEVING OPTIMUM WELLNESS

You must decide for yourself how you want to design your lifestyle. Life events and demands may pull you in one direction or another, and balance may not be possible until the events and demands are worked through. As a woman, your style of living is going to look different from that of a man. In fact, everyone's

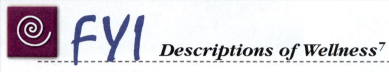

Descriptions of Wellness[7]

- *Physical wellness* is the willingness to take time each week to pursue activities that increase physical flexibility and endurance. A physically well person understands and employs the relationship between nutrition and body functioning.

- *Emotional wellness* is an awareness and acceptance of a wide range of feelings for oneself and others. It includes an ability to freely express and manage feelings effectively. An emotionally well person functions autonomously, yet is aware of personal limitations and the value of seeking interpersonal support and assistance.

- *Social wellness* is the willingness to actively participate in and contribute to efforts that promote the common welfare of one's community. A socially well person lives in harmony with fellow human beings, seeks positive interdependent relationships with others, develops healthy sexual behaviors, and works for mutual respect and cooperation among community members.

- *Occupational wellness* is the personal satisfaction and enrichment one experiences through work. The occupationally well person has integrated a commitment to work into a total lifestyle, and seeks to express personal values through involvement in paid and unpaid activities that are rewarding to the individual and valuable to the community.

- *Intellectual wellness* is self-directed behavior that includes continuous acquisition, development, creative application and articulation of critical thinking, expressive and intuitive skills, and abilities toward the achievement of a more satisfying existence.

- *Spiritual wellness* is the willingness to seek meaning and purpose in human existence, to question everything, and to appreciate the intangibles that cannot be explained or understood readily. A spiritually well person seeks harmony between that which lies within the individual and the forces that come from outside the individual.   ∞

FIGURE 2.1 Holistic wellness model.

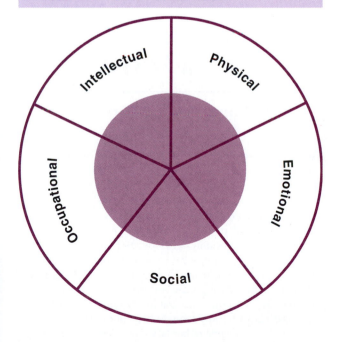

■ Personal component

■ Spiritual component

lifestyle is unique and different. Wellness models can be used to assess your lifestyle based on an ideal. However, it is ultimately up to you to decide how you want your life to be the same or to be different. (See *Journal Activity:* "Your Personal Wellness Guide" and then complete *Assess Yourself!:* "Rate Your Wellness.")

Even if you currently have an illness or disease you can still achieve the optimum level of wellness that is right for you. For example, individuals living with the HIV virus or AIDS can design a lifestyle to maximize their own health potential and contribute to their longevity. (See *Viewpoint:* "Is There Healing Potential in Healthy Living?")

endogenous factors (en **dodge** en us)—those events that occur within the individual.

exogenous factors (ex **odge** en us)—external events that influence the individual.

JOURNAL ACTIVITY

Your Personal Wellness Guide

Use the following guide to become more aware of your own personal wellness. Read the following questions and record your ideas. A few samples have been provided to get you started. Some of the dimensions and components may overlap. You may want to include a third category for behaviors that include both personal and spiritual components equally.

- How do you participate in physical wellness?
  Examples:

Personal Component	*Spiritual Component*
nutrition, vitamins	donate to a food bank
regular exercise	charity walk-a-thon
get a massage	support a sick friend

- How do you participate in emotional wellness?
  Examples:

Personal Component	*Spiritual Component*
have a positive attitude	avoid blaming others
seek personal therapy	listen and be supportive
express your needs	respect needs of others

- How do you participate in social wellness?
  Examples:

Personal Component	*Spiritual Component*
ask to be included	invite others along
ask for honesty and respect	be honest and respectful
receive community assistance	be a community volunteer

- How do you participate in occupational wellness?
  Examples:

Personal Component	*Spiritual Component*
be in a job you like	help others get a job
develop your skills further	teach job skills to others
invest your money	recycle products

- How do you participate in intellectual wellness?
  Examples:

Personal Component	*Spiritual Component*
read and learn	lead a reading group
be creative or artistic	encourage creativity
broaden your experience	share your experience

Assess YOURSELF

Rate Your Wellness

Refer to the holistic wellness model in Figure 2.1. Rate how well you believe you are attending to the personal and spiritual components for each of the five dimensions of wellness as explained in the Journal Activity. You will have ten separate ratings, one for the personal component and one for the spiritual component in each of the five wellness dimensions. Use the following scale: 1=not enough attention, 2=enough attention, 3=too much attention. Now ask yourself the following questions:

- Is one wellness dimension attended to more than another? If so, why?
- Do you have balanced focus on both the personal and spiritual components of each wellness dimension? Or, is one component given more attention than the other? If so, why?
- What adjustments, if any, would you like to make in your spiritual or personal focus, or in each wellness dimension to be more balanced?
- Do you have any areas in conflict? If so, how can this conflict be resolved?
- Are you ready and/or able to make a commitment today to focus more on a particular area?

Viewpoint

Is There Healing Potential in Healthy Living?

In 1985, Niro was diagnosed with AIDS-related complex, now known to be an early or a middle stage of HIV disease. She suffered from diarrhea, thrush, weakness, sweats, aches, and pains. She says she cured herself through a combination of mind-body exercises, natural foods, and physical exercise. Today there is no trace of the infection in her body. Her case defies rational explanation. Niro, who is now a grandmother and recently remarried, plans to establish a center to heal AIDS patients through a combination of meditation, mind-body techniques, natural foods, and exercise.[9]

Did Niro's healthy lifestyle help her to achieve optimum wellness in spite of her HIV diagnosis? Can optimum healthy living cure as well as prevent deadly disorders?

By participating in a charity walk, these women help themselves and their community.

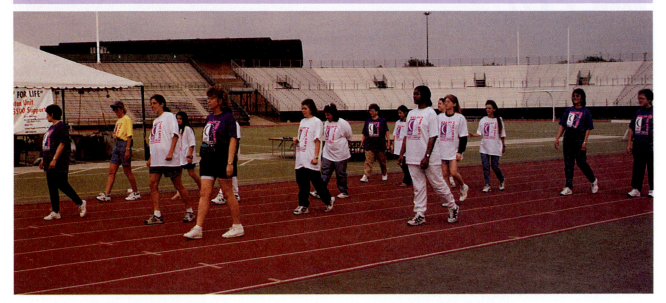

WORLD WELLNESS

There are six primary environmental issues for world wellness: air, water, energy, food, toxins, and nature.[10] These are described further as air quality, water quality, sustainable energy and recycling, sustainable agriculture, hazardous material and waste management, and protection of wilderness areas and rain forests. The basic essentials of life include air, water, food, activity, and sex. Because the earth sustains us, the world must be kept in good shape in order for humans to continue to survive.

It is vital that we attend to the issues of world health in addition to individual health in order for life to continue. So what does world wellness have to do with women's health? Well, the world is often referred to as *Mother Earth,* and she does nurture our survival. The *Mother Earth* concept is perhaps the earliest and strongest female archetype that exists for women. (See *FYI:* "One Woman's Contribution to World Wellness," *Health Tips:* "Enhancing World Wellness," and *Journal Activity:* "Your World Wellness Guide.")

> *Mother Earth,*
> I feel your support beneath my feet,
> sometimes firm, fluid or soft, but
> too often forgetting to acknowledge that
> without you I would be no-where.

> You feed, wash, clothe and caress
> and breathe life into my soul, yet
> this is what you do, so why should
> I make such a big deal of it?

> Gifts given lend license to do
> as I please with them; my air to
> cloud, my water to taint, my land
> to destroy, my animals to kill.

> You must love me very much to be
> so giving to an ungrateful child.
> And tomorrow, if I remain the same,
> would you still be there for me?
>
> *By Cynthia Chandler*

WELLNESS VERSUS ILLNESS

Health is viewed along a continuum of wellness to illness with a whole myriad of possibilities in between. Health intervention is defined as the act or fact of interfering so as to modify.[11] Health interventions fall into at least three categories: education, prevention, and treatment. (See Fig. 2.2.)

Education

Health education involves research and study in the causes, prevention, and treatment of disorders and diseases. It also involves the publication and distribution

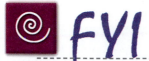 **FYI**   *One Woman's Contribution to World Wellness*

Melissa Crabtree does her part to heal and preserve the environment. At 28 years of age, she is an active environmentalist. She teaches others to appreciate and love the environment by interacting with it on a very personal level. During the spring, she is a white-water river raft guide. In the winter, she is a cross-country ski guide and works on a ski patrol. In the summer she teaches canoeing and sea kayaking. Melissa is also a songwriter and performs her music about the environment across the country at women's music festivals and nightclubs.   ∽

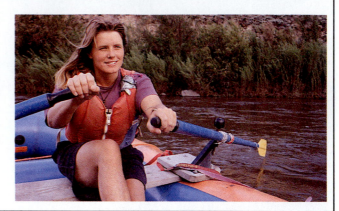

health tips

Enhancing World Wellness

It is very easy to participate in world wellness. There are small things you can do every day that can have a big impact.

- ■ Turn out the lights in every room you are not using.
- ■ Do not throw litter on the ground.
- ■ Join a community litter-cleanup group.
- ■ Recycle newspaper, paper, plastic, bottles, and aluminum.
- ■ Use biodegradable soaps and detergents; many of these are available in your local grocery store or health food store.
- ■ Plant a garden and grow food.
- ■ Plant and care for a tree.
- ■ Drive environmentally safer vehicles, that is, low exhaust output and safer air-conditioning systems.
- ■ Share a ride or carpool.
- ■ Take short showers, or take baths instead of showers.
- ■ Fix water drips and leaks as soon as possible. Water is more precious than gold.
- ■ Use less water in your toilet tank with each flush by setting the water level lower.
- ■ Do not purchase products from companies that regularly violate environmental protection laws.

JOURNAL ACTIVITY

Your World Wellness Guide

How are you contributing to world wellness in each of the six areas listed?
- Maintaining and/or improving air quality
- Maintaining and/or improving water quality
- Saving energy and/or recycling
- Growing and/or saving food
- Preventing and/or reducing toxins and pollutants
- Preserving and/or enhancing nature

of this information to the public. Paramount to education is the concept of health promotion. Health promotion efforts include:

- Dissemination through literature and workshops of information regarding healthy lifestyles, enhancement of life quality, and illness prevention
- Provision of information about early warning signs of disorders and diseases
- Provision of information regarding community services for assessment, such as health checkups

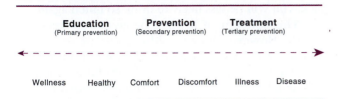

FIGURE 2.2 Health interventions continuum.

| Education
(Primary prevention) | Prevention
(Secondary prevention) | Treatment
(Tertiary prevention) |

Wellness   Healthy   Comfort   Discomfort   Illness   Disease

- Assistance in the development of personal health programs in each of the wellness dimensions

The American Cancer Society has an extensive education program. They publish pamphlets about the warning signs of breast cancer, posters of women using breast self-examination, and even poems written by and about survivors of breast cancer.

Prevention

Preventive health action is defined as measures serving to avert the occurrence of illness or disease.[11] According to the public health service model for prevention, services may be directed toward the individual (host), toward the source (agent), and toward the environment that encourages and supports, or sustains the source. This is referred to as the epidemiological model. **Epidemiology** is the study of the relationships of the various factors determining the frequency and distribution of diseases in a human community.[11] For example, let us consider three preventive measures regarding the health risks of using tobacco for women. One, an educational campaign is directed toward women explaining the increased risk of cancer and heart disease for women smokers. This preventive action is directed at the individual or host. Two, a legislative bill requires that tobacco products manufacturers place a statement on their products warning that use of that product may cause a health hazard. This preventive action is directed at the source or agent. Three, further legislation prohibits the advertisement of tobacco products via television. This preventive measure is directed at the environment that may otherwise support the use of the tobacco product, in this case, the advertising industry.

Prevention efforts can be divided into three types: primary, secondary, and tertiary. Primary prevention is an extension of health education. Based upon what we know, we can take steps to enhance the quality of life and prevent the development of illness. Primary interventions include efforts that assist with the prevention of most discomfort, disorders, diseases, and premature death. This prevention can be accomplished by sufficient attention to those things that keep us healthy—such as proper diet, regular exercise, a positive attitude, stress management and relaxation, fostering relationships, avoidance of toxins and pollutants, avoidance of the abuse of drugs and alcohol; avoidance of tobacco, and looking both ways before crossing the street, among other things. The bottom line is to live smart and be well.

In spite of your best efforts, you could possibly still experience some degree of discomfort, disorder, or disease in your life. Secondary prevention identifies persons who are in the early stages of "unhealth," which may lead to the development of disorders or illnesses. Secondary prevention attempts are interventions used to stop unhealthy behaviors and seek any necessary treatment.

Tertiary prevention is the application of an intervention to treat an existing disorder or illness. This is for the purpose of preventing the disorder or illness from getting worse. Tertiary prevention can also involve rehabilitative efforts. Rehabilitation efforts attempt to facilitate recovery to the highest degree of health possible for an individual.

Treatment

Treatment interventions are applied to halt the progress of a discomfort, disorder, or disease and, if possible, move the individual away from discomfort and toward increased health. A woman who has entered menopause may experience extreme discomfort that accompanies this phase, such as hot flashes

epidemiology (ep ah **dee** me **ol** ah gee)—the study of relationships of the various factors determining the frequency and distribution of diseases in a human community.

and mood swings. She may want to seek the assistance of a health provider for the purpose of considering hormone replacement therapy, or instead she may want to seek the advice of an herbologist for herbs that can reduce the discomforts of menopause.

Health treatment can involve intervention by a mental health provider, a physical health provider, or both. Examples of mental health providers include trained professionals, such as mental health counselors, social workers, psychologists, drug and alcohol counselors, marriage and family therapists, and psychiatrists. Examples of physical health providers include trained professionals, such as physicians, nurse practitioners, nurses, dentists, rehabilitation therapists, osteopaths, chiropractors, herbologists, massage therapists, and physical therapists.

It is up to you to decide from whom you would like to seek treatment and what type of treatment you wish to receive. It is best to act as an educated consumer and be as familiar as possible with the current and most effective treatment or treatments for your condition. It is also advisable to seek an opinion from more than one health professional, whenever appropriate, to explore additional possibilities regarding diagnosis and treatment.

LEARNING AND BEHAVIOR

In considering learning behavior you must understand the role of primary reinforcers: positive, negative, and punishment.[12] A **positive reinforcer** is rewarding. If your behavior is followed by something perceived by you as rewarding, then you will more likely repeat that behavior. If you exercise and feel better, then you may be more likely to exercise more. A **negative reinforcer** is the removal of something uncomfortable and this too can be rewarding; thus, if your behavior is followed by the removal of something uncomfortable to you, then the likelihood that you will repeat that behavior increases. For example, if telling an individual to stop criticizing you unnecessarily should result in a positive outcome, you are more likely to assert yourself again. **Punishment** involves the presentation of something uncomfortable. Thus, when your behavior is followed by punishment, the likelihood of that be-

havior being repeated by you decreases. For example, if you drink too much alcohol and become very sick, you will be less likely to drink so much again.

The concept of learned behaviors is basically simple. However, how would you explain resistance to change even with the presentation of reinforcers? Resistance to change is often a result of the existence of secondary reinforcers. A **secondary reinforcer** is much less obvious but still has some influence over behavior. If you are experiencing difficulty in changing your behavior, then consider less obvious reasons that may be holding you back, such as an interfering belief or value. (See *Her Story:* "Danette.")

Hierarchy of Needs

The importance placed on a reinforcer is dependent upon the value that you give it. This can vary greatly from person to person. However, the "hierarchy of needs" is a way of exploring the motivating potential of a reinforcer.[13] People have at least five sets of goals, usually referred to as basic needs, that are common to all persons: physiological, safety, love, esteem, and self-actualization. These needs contribute to motivating actions or behavior. Maslow summarizes the hierarchy of needs as shown in Figure 2.3.

Physiological needs, the lowest level on the hierarchy, refer to such things as freedom from hunger, sufficient oxygen, adequate water, sufficient sleep, freedom of movement, and sexual activity. Safety needs refer to such things as protection from danger, non-isolation, sufficient trust to build relationships, freedom from fear, and freedom from deprivation. Love needs are comprised of such things as love, affection, and belongingness. Esteem needs refer to such things as the desire for respect from others, self-respect, self-esteem, achievement, adequacy, confidence, and independence. Self-actualization needs, the highest level on the hierarchy, is the need or desire to become everything one is capable of becoming, to strive for ideals, and to strive for success or life satisfaction.

Typically, you do not move up the hierarchy of needs until your lower needs are met sufficiently. However, there may be instances when upper-level needs take precedence over lower-level needs. (See *Her Story:* "Charlene.")

Her Story

Danette

Danette came into therapy complaining of extreme stress in her life. She played a major role as a caretaker to her children, spouse, and peers. She left no time for herself. She had anxiety and extreme headaches. The counselor suggested that she reprioritize her life, learn and use assertiveness skills, and incorporate time and stress management techniques. These skills and techniques were recommended to her by the therapist because they are known to be documented, effective strategies for assisting with Danette's kind of problem. However, Danette persisted in her complaints without trying the techniques even though she seemed to understand that they would in fact help her situation. The counselor suspected that Danette might have less obvious motives contributing to her resistance to change (secondary reinforcers), motives that Danette herself might not be completely aware of. Through continued exploration of Danette's values and belief systems, the counselor discovered that Danette be- lieved she was not a worthwhile person unless she sacrificed herself for others. It was further discovered that this was a very old belief that Danette learned as a child from her mother: "To be a good person you must always sacrifice yourself for others, otherwise you are a selfish person." This belief became integrated into Danette's lifestyle when she was rewarded with praise in childhood whenever she acted accordingly. When Danette realized that this old belief was creating difficulty for her, she decided to put it aside in certain situations so she could make healthier choices in her life.

- Is it sometimes necessary to put another's needs before your own needs?
- How can Danette determine when the act of putting another's needs before her own is too much sacrifice?
- What other ways can Danette be assured that the needs of others are being met without always having to be the one who meets the needs of these others?

FIGURE 2.3 Hierarchy of needs.

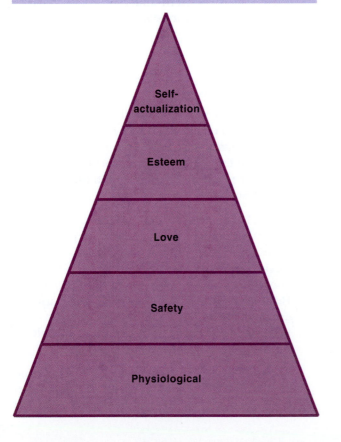

Self-actualization

Esteem

Love

Safety

Physiological

THEORIES AND MODELS OF BEHAVIOR CHANGE

There are many models and theories that suggest ways to change health behaviors. Some of these were developed many years ago but still present ideas that are very relevant today.

Field Theory

Field theory is a useful tool for determining the forces at work in situations involving change.[14] According to field theory, behavior results from two

positive reinforcer—presentation of a reward to increase the likelihood that a behavior will be repeated.

negative reinforcer—the removal of something uncomfortable to increase the likelihood that a behavior will be repeated.

punishment—the presentation of something uncomfortable to reduce behavior.

secondary reinforcer—a less obvious reinforcer that may be contributing to resistance to change.

Her Story

Charlene

Charlene, an 18-year-old college student, was diagnosed with an eating disorder called anorexia nervosa. Charlene was a member of the gymnastics team and she felt she needed to make her weight as low as possible to stay on the team. She was literally starving herself to death because of her belief that she was overweight and her fear that she would get kicked off of the team. Her body weight became dangerously low and, starved for nutrition, it began to rob her muscles and organs of vital nutrients. Her situation had become life threatening. In this case, Charlene placed a higher priority on esteem needs than on physiological needs. Thus, she was motivated to behavior based on the area of her life in which she believed there was the greatest need. Charlene's belief was not well grounded in reality, because she was an anorexic who was willing to starve her body in an effort to feel better about herself.

- How can education and counseling about the concept of the hierarchy of needs be used to help Charlene?
- How can you relate each level in the hierarchy of needs to your own life and the decisions you have made about your health and well-being?

---

sets of forces: change or driving forces and resisting or restraining forces. "Change forces" pressure the individual or group to move toward a goal. "Resisting forces" push against change and hinder progress. When change forces and resisting forces are equal, one is stuck in immobility. **Force-field analysis** involves the process of identifying and understanding change forces and resisting forces for the purpose of removing obstacles and facilitating movement toward a desired goal. If it can be determined where behavior change is blocked, then resolution of the problem creating the block will allow behavior change to proceed. It is also necessary to continue to increase change forces while reducing resisting forces because changes brought about without increasing driving forces are likely to be temporary.

The action-planning procedure for field-theory involves five phases of learning and change called the unfreezing-to-refreezing theory: unfreezing, problem diagnosis, goal setting, new behavior, and refreezing. "Unfreezing" is becoming ready to consider change through a shift in attitude. "Problem diagnosis" provides a better understanding of why current behaviors exist, what purposes they currently serve, the negative consequences of a currently existing behavior, and the expected positive outcome resulting from behavior change. "Goal setting" is crucial in planning the behavior change. Some ultimate goals may take a great deal of time to reach, and frustration and impatience could begin to reduce motivation. Therefore, goal setting must involve short-term and long-term goals with healthy, intrinsic rewards for each degree of accomplishment. "New behaviors" are tried and tested as possible avenues toward goal achievement. "Refreezing" occurs when a new behavior becomes an integrated, routine, ongoing, and stabilized part of the person's lifestyle. Refer to *Her Story:* "Charlene."

How can force-field analysis help Charlene change her behavior from starvation to healthy nutrition, and still allow her to be a competitor on the gymnastics team?

Health Belief Model

The health belief model is a widely used psychosocial approach to explaining health-related behavior.[15] The health belief model provides a means to analyze forces that influence health behavior. It also has implications for program planning and implementation. The model postulates that:

1. Health behavior of all kinds is related to a general health belief that one is susceptible to health problems.
2. Health problems have undesirable consequences.
3. Health problems and their consequences usually are preventable.
4. Barriers or costs have to be overcome if health problems are to be overcome.

The health belief model consists of three distinct phases that lead to proactive health: individual perception, modifying factors, and likelihood of action.

Individual perceptions are of two basic types: perceived susceptibility and perceived severity. "Perceived susceptibility" is the subjective perception of risk of contracting an unhealthy condition. "Perceived severity" is the perception of the nature of the condition such as degree of accompanying discomfort, disability or injury, potential death, or other negative consequences. "Perceived threat" is considered the combination of susceptibility and severity. In the case of Charlene, the perceived threat of not being able to stay on the gymnastics team was greater to her than the perceived harm she may do to her body by starving herself. Her perceptions were distorted and she was not in touch with reality. It is necessary to have accurate and realistic perceptions about yourself and what you wish to accomplish in order to achieve healthy behavior change.

The decision to engage in a behavior is influenced by modifying factors. These can be demographic variables, such as age, gender, and educational level; sociopsychological variables, such as personality and peer pressure; and structural variables, such as knowledge about the condition or disease. With some guidance from her coach, a friend, or a counselor, Charlene would be able to alter her perceptions and recognize the severity of the threat to her body and make some healthy adjustments in her eating behavior.

Likelihood of action takes place when the individual acknowledges personal susceptibility to undesirable consequences. The desire to lower susceptibility or reduce the threat must also be present. Ultimately, the resulting action is related to an individual's estimation of the benefits from the action minus the barriers to the action. If Charlene could recognize that her susceptibility to becoming ill, because she was not eating, was much more important than that of not making the gymnastics team because of her weight, then she would be more likely to change her actions and to eat a balanced and nutritious diet instead of starving herself.

The effectiveness of the health belief model may be based on three essential factors: (1) the readiness of the individual to consider behavioral changes; (2) the existence and potency of forces in the environment that influence change and make it possible; (3) the behaviors themselves.[16] Each of these three factors is impacted by the personality and immediate environment of the individual, as well as past experiences with health service providers, health promoters, and health educators.

The Transtheoretical Model

The transtheoretical model of change, or sometimes referred to as the multi-component stage model, suggests that you will experience several stages as you attempt to change your health behavior over time.[17] The first stage is precontemplation, the time when you are not seriously thinking about changing during the next six months. The second stage is contemplation, when you are seriously thinking about behavior change during the next six months. The third stage is action, the six-month period following an overt modification of a behavior. The fourth stage is maintenance, the period after action until the unwanted behavior is permanently modified or terminated. The final stage is termination, when you are no longer tempted by the unwanted behavior, and you feel confident in your ability to resist relapse.

Theory of Reasoned Action

The theory of reasoned action promotes three primary concepts that affect behavior change: your attitude toward performing the behavior, standard beliefs about what relevant others think you should do, and your motivation to comply with those others.[18] In other words, sometimes you may do certain things because other people who are important to you or have power over you think that you should do it. This concept is often referred to as the subjective norm. Doing things because others think you should can work in both positive and negative ways. For example, if Charlene's coach keeps encouraging her to lose more and more weight, then the coach may actually reinforce Charlene to be anorexic. However, if Charlene's coach encourages the athletes to maintain a proper, nutritious diet, then Charlene will be less likely to engage in unhealthy eating behavior.

Theory of Planned Action

The theory of planned action is similar to the theory of reasoned action with one addition. The theory of planned action adds the concept of perceived behavioral control, that is, the perceived ease or difficulty

---

force-field analysis—the process of identifying and understanding change forces and resisting forces for the purpose of removing obstacles and facilitating movement toward a desired goal.

of performing the behavior; it is assumed to reflect past experience as well as anticipated obstacles and impediments. The more favorable the attitude and subjective norm with respect to behavior, and the greater the perceived behavioral control, the stronger should be the individual's intentions to perform the behavior under consideration.[19]

Theory of Personal Investment

In this theory, the subjective meaning of a behavior is the critical determinant of your investment or engagement in the behavior. This theory contends that meaning has three interrelated facets: personal incentives associated with performing in a situation, thoughts about self, and perceived options available in a situation.[20] Charlene's incentive to lose weight was very high since she wanted to stay on the gymnastics team. However, she had limited perceptions about her options for accomplishing this task. It would have been better if Charlene had consulted with a health provider, especially a nutritionist, to determine, first, if losing weight was a healthy idea given her current body build, and second, if it was okay for her to lose weight, what methods would be most effective and most healthy for her to use.

Self-Efficacy

The perception of potential benefits of action is related to the concept of self-efficacy. **Self-efficacy** is the conviction that one can successfully execute the behavior or behaviors required to produce desired outcomes.[21] Let's say that you were, in fact, significantly overweight. Your ability to design and stick to a plan of behavior change would depend on your belief that you could do it. Self-efficacy suggests that people's beliefs in their ability to perform specific behaviors influences the following:[22,23]

- Choice of behavior and the situations that will be avoided or attempted
- Effort expended in a specific task
- How long one will persist with a task even when facing difficulties
- Emotional reactions such as positive emotions with perceived success or negative emotions with perceived lack of success

A strong sense of self-efficacy is essential for the promotion of healthy behavior change.

Social Cognitive Theory

According to the social cognitive theory, behavior is determined by expectations and incentives. Expectations include: (1) beliefs about how environmental events are connected; (2) opinions about the consequences of your own actions; and (3) expectations about your own ability to perform the behavior needed to influence outcomes (self-efficacy). Incentive is the perceived value of an outcome, such as improved health status or approval of others.[24] If you want and need to lose weight, ask yourself why. What would you be able to do or feel after losing the weight that you cannot do or feel now? The incentive to lose weight would be a motivating factor to persevere through the planned action to change. In addition, your expectations about your ability to lose weight and about what would be accomplished from the change in your body would influence actually being able to lose the weight you want.

Now that you have reviewed the various models and theories that suggest how behavior is changed, it is time to consider how you can develop your own individualized plan of action.

PLANNING YOUR LIFESTYLE CHANGE

You can manage many lifestyle changes through a self-help plan of action. This involves three primary steps: take a personal inventory, maintain a helpful attitude, and develop a plan of action. The plan should be realistic and developed with an attitude of appreciation for even the smallest of movements toward the goal. Patience is also a major key when persevering a lifestyle change.

Personal inventory. The first step in a self-plan is to take a personal inventory. This involves an evaluation of personal health habits and practices. (See *Journal Activity:* "Your Personal Inventory.")

JOURNAL ACTIVITY

Your Personal Inventory

Make a list of your existing health-promoting behaviors. Now make a list of your existing health-inhibiting behaviors. Consider two questions at this point: (1) Which behaviors present the greatest threat to your health, and (2) which behaviors do you need to target first?

Helpful Attitude

A realistic and positive attitude is paramount to successful behavior change. It is important not to set goals too high nor expect outcomes too quickly. Both of these attitudes can lead to discouragement and even termination of effort. It is also important to view behavior change as a lifestyle change rather than just a temporary goal. Otherwise, success that is achieved may be short-lived. Avoid an attitude of denial or deprivation; these can result in preoccupations of thought or impulsive actions that worsen the targeted behavior. Instead, find healthy substitutes for the things that you are reducing or eliminating from your life.

Plan of Action

Essential principles of lifestyle management when structuring a plan of action include: (1) assessing behavior, (2) setting specific and realistic goals, (3) formulating intervention strategies, and (4) evaluating progress.[25] (See Fig. 2.4.)

Assessment of current behaviors involves the process of counting, recording, measuring, observing, and describing. Assessment tools are usually daily logs, journals, and diaries. The assessment phase is completed when there is sufficient information to form a behavior profile, state specific goals, and customize a program that matches your unique circumstances and personality.

Goal setting involves establishing specific and realistic goals for behavior change. Specific goals are concrete, observable, and measurable. Realistic goals are reasonable and relate to personal circumstances. Goal setting should start off small to facilitate initial successes that will provide further motivation for continued participation in the personal lifestyle change program.

Intervention strategies should be personalized to fit your needs. Common intervention strategies include the use of stimulus control, healthy positive reinforcers, and positive behavior substitution and behavioral contracts. "Stimulus control" includes the reduction or elimination of the stimulus that encourages the original unhealthy behavior. For example, to help you stop smoking cigarettes, use nicotine patches that have gradually lower dosages of nicotine. The presentation of healthy positive reinforcers or rewards will increase the potential for healthy behaviors to be reported. For example, if you are attempting to overcome procrastination, you can re-

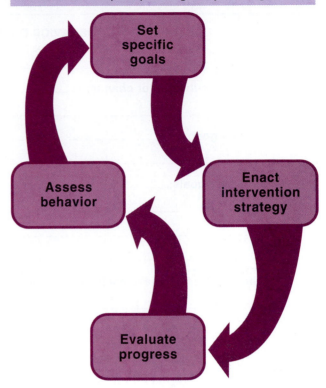

FIGURE 2.4 Steps in planning lifestyle change.

Set specific goals

Enact intervention strategy

Evaluate progress

Assess behavior

ward yourself with an activity you enjoy, such as a bike ride, after you complete a chore. Positive behavior substitution is the incorporation of a healthy behavior that is incompatible with the unhealthy behavior, such as walking instead of watching television or chewing gum instead of smoking.

A **behavioral contract** is a written agreement in a behavior change program. Most contracts state long-range and intermediate goals, target dates for completion, rewards, intervention strategies, names of friends and resources to serve as a support network, and witnesses to the agreement who serve as sources

self-efficacy (eff uk ah see)—the conviction that one can successfully execute the behavior or behaviors required to produce desired outcomes.

behavioral contract—a written agreement in a behavior change program that includes long-range and intermediate goals, target dates for completion, rewards, intervention strategies, and witnesses to the agreement.

FIGURE 2.5 Behavior change contract.

BEHAVIOR CHANGE CONTRACT

Name:_____ Date of Contract:_____

Identified health area for change:_____

_____

Long-term goal:_____

_____

Intermediate goals:_____

_____

_____

_____

Estimated time to achieve each intermediate goal:_____

_____

_____

_____

Rewards for achieving intermediate goals:_____

_____

_____

_____

Support network (persons and facilities):_____

_____

_____

_____

_____   _____
Signature of Participant   **Signature of Witness**

---

for encouragement. (See Fig. 2.5 for a sample contract, and then complete *Journal Activity:* "Behavior Change Contract.")

To evaluate your progress you must regularly monitor goal-related activities. Consistent monitoring provides information necessary for determining progress toward your goal. Periodic monitoring (weekly or monthly) is better than daily monitoring. Monitoring can be done in the form of charts, graphs, or lists or descriptions of behaviors and attitudes.

JOURNAL ACTIVITY

Behavior Change Contract

Write a behavior change contract in your journal. Keep a record in your journal of your activities related to the contract. Assess your progress periodically. Remember to reward yourself in healthy ways for demonstrating progress toward your goals. Don't forget to frequently seek out encouragement and guidance from your support system.

CONCLUSION

The information and activities in this chapter encourage you to understand and, if needed, change your lifestyle. The remaining chapters have additional information and activities to help you with your own personal health journey.   ∞

Chapter Summary

- Wellness encompasses the whole person concept including the following dimensions of health: physical, emotional, social, occupational, intellectual, and spiritual.
- The primary dimensions of world wellness are: air, water, energy, food, toxins, and nature.
- The three primary health-related intervention strategies are: education (primary prevention), prevention (secondary prevention), and treatment (tertiary prevention).
- The basic hierarchy of needs for humans are: physiological, safety, love, esteem, and self-actualization.

- The health belief model for behavior change consists of three distinct phases that lead up to proactive health: individual perception, modifying factors, and likelihood of action.
- A self-help plan involves three primary steps: taking a personal inventory, having the right attitude, and a plan of action.
- A plan of action involves the following steps: assessment, goal setting, intervention strategies, and evaluating progress.

Review Questions

1. Can you name and describe the five dimensions of wellness and give examples of components of each dimension as presented in the holistic wellness model?
2. What are the environmental issues for world wellness?
3. What are the three types of interventions utilized in the health services?
4. What are reinforcers?
5. Can you describe the hierarchy of needs?
6. Can you describe the components of field theory?
7. What are the major components of the health belief model?
8. Can you describe the transtheoretical model for change?
9. Can you describe the theory of reasoned action and the theory of planned action?
10. Can you describe the theory of personal investment?
11. What is self-efficacy and can you describe the social-cognitive theory?
12. Can you devise a self-help plan for behavior change?

Resources

Organizations and Hotlines

Women's Health America Group
P.O. Box 259690
Madison, WI 53725
Telephone: (800) 558-7046

Association for the Advancement of Health Education
1900 Association Drive
Reston, VA 22091
Telephone: (703) 476-3437

United States Environmental Protection Agency
401 M Street SW
Washington, DC 20460
Telephone: Information line: (202) 260-2080
Environmental justice hotline: (800) 962-6215

Centers for Disease Control and Prevention
Dept. of Health and Human Services, Information
Mail Stop D25
1600 Clifton Road, NE
Atlanta, GA 30333
Telephone: (404) 639-3286/3534
Immunization hotline: (800) 232-SHOT

American Nurses Association
600 Maryland Avenue, SW
Suite 100 West
Washington, DC 20024-2571
Telephone: (800) 274-4ANA

Association of American Physicians and Surgeons
1601 North Tucson Boulevard, Suite 9
Tucson, AZ 85716
Telephone: (800) 635-1196

American Hospital Association
Information
1 North Franklin Street
Chicago, IL 60606
Telephone: (800) 242-2626

American Public Health Association Clearinghouse
1015 15th Street, NW
Washington, DC 20005
Telephone: (202) 789-5600

Audiotapes

1. *Inner Healing.* Duluth, MN, 1995, Whole Person Associates (Phone: 800-247-6789).
2. *Personal Empowering.* Duluth, MN, 1995, Whole Person Associates (Phone: 800-247-6789).
3. *Healthy Balancing.* Duluth, MN, 1995, Whole Person Associates (Phone: 800-247-6789).
4. *Spiritual Centering.* Duluth, MN, 1995, Whole Person Associates (Phone: 800-247-6789).
5. *General Wellness.* Duluth, MN, 1995, Whole Person Associates (Phone: 800-247-6789).

Websites

World Health Organization
http://www.who.ch/

Agency for Health Care Policy and Research Clearinghouse
http://www.ahcpr.gov/

Bureau of Health Professions
http://www.hrsa.dhhs.gov/bhpr/bhpr.html

Women's Health America Group
http://www.womenshealth.com/

Centers for Disease Control
http://www.cdc.gov/

Environment Hotlist
Environmental Ecological Resources
http://www.mev.etat.lu/envhot.html

U.S. National Park Service
http://www.nps.gov

National Institute of Environmental Health Sciences
http://www.niehs.nih.gov/

Rural Information Center Health Service
http://www.nal.usda.gov/ric/richs/orhp.htm

American Health Assistance Foundation
http://www.ahar.org/

American Nurses Association
http://www.ana.org/

American Institute for Preventive Medicine
http://aipm.healthy.net/

Suggested Readings

Borysenko, J. 1988. *Minding the body, mending the mind.* Toronto: Bantam Books.

Chopra, D. 1991. *Perfect health: The complete mind/body guide,* New York: Harmony Books.

Dossey, B. M., L. Keegan, L. G. Kolkmeier, and C. Guzzetta. 1989. *Holistic health promotion: A guide for practice.* Rockville, MD.: Aspen

Greene, B., and Winfrey, O. 1996. *Make the Connection: Ten steps to a better body and a better life,* New York: Hyperion.

Kabat-Zinn, J. 1990. *Full catastrophe living: Using the wisdom of your body and mind to face stress, pain, and illness.* New York: Delacorte Press.

Moyers, B. 1993. *Healing and the mind.* New York: Doubleday. (Also available as a series of videotapes.)

Myss, C. 1996. *Anatomy of spirit.* Westminster, Md.: Random House.

Siegel, B. 1992. *Love, medicine and miracles.* New York: Harper and Row.

References

1. National Center for Health Statistics. 1994. *Annual summary of births, marriages, divorces and deaths: United States, 1994.* Washington, D.C.: Center for Disease Control.

2. Bonita, R., and A. Howe. 1996. *World Health Statistics Quarterly* 49 (2): 134–41.

3. National Center for Health Statistics. 1995. Births and deaths, United States, 1995. *Monthly Vital Statistics Report* 45 (3S2): Center for Disease Control.

4. Allen, R., and R. Yarian. 1981. The domain of health. *Health Education* 12 (4): 3–5.

5. Hettler, W. 1979. *Six dimensions of wellness.* Stevens Point, Wisc.: National Wellness Institute, University of Wisconsin.

6. Hettler, W. 1990. Six dimensions of wellness. *Guidepost: American Counseling Association,* 33 (September): 1.

7. Opatz, J. 1986. Stevens Point: A long-standing program for students at a midwestern university. *American Journal of Health Promotion* 1 (1): 60–67.

8. Chandler, C., J. Holden, and C. Kolander. 1992. Counseling for spiritual wellness: Theory and practice. *Journal of Counseling and Development* 71 (2): 168–75.

9. Gavzer, B. 1997. I saw I had a future. *Parade Magazine* (April 6): 4–7.

10. Hettler, W. 1991. Environmental issues for world wellness. *Guidepost: American Counseling Association* 33 (17): 17.

11. *Mosby's Medical, Nursing and Allied Health Directory,* 1994 4th ed. St. Louis, Mo.: Mosby.

12. Skinner, B. F. 1953. *Science and Human Behavior.* New York: Macmillan.

13. Maslow, A. H. 1943. A theory of human motivation. *Psychological Review* 50 (July): 370–96.

14. Lewin, K. 1961. Quasi-stationary social equilibria and the problem of permanent change. In *The Planning of Change.* Edited by W. G. Bennis, K. D. Benne, and R. Chin. New York: Holt, Rinehart & Winston.

15. Rosenstock, I. M. 1991. The health belief model: Explaining health behavior through expectancies. In *Health behavior and health education: Theory, research and practice.* Edited by K. Glanz, F. M. Lewis, and B. K. Rimer. San Francisco: Jossey-Bass.

16. Dignan, M., and P. A. Carr. 1987. *Program planning for health education and health promotion.* Philadelphia: Lea and Febiger.

17. Prochaska, J., and C. DiClemente. 1992. Stages of change in the modification of problem behaviors. *Progress in Behavior Modification,* 28, 1992, 183–218.

18. Fishbein, M., and I. Ajzen. 1975. *Belief, attitude, intention and behavior: An introduction to theory and research.* Reading, Mass.: Addison-Wesley.

19. Ajzen, I. 1988. *Attitudes, personality and behavior.* Chicago: Dorsey Press.

20. Maehr, M., and L. Braskamp. 1986. *The motivation factor: a theory of personal investment.* Lexington, Mass.: Lexington Press.

21. Bandura, A. 1986. *Social foundations of thought and action.* Englewood Cliffs, N.J.: Prentice-Hall.

22. Lyn, L., and K. R. McLeroy. 1986. Self-efficacy and health education. *Journal of School Health* 56 (2): 317–21.

23. Schunck, D. H., and J. P. Carbonari. 1984. *Self-efficacy models.* In *Behavioral Health: A Handbook of Health Enhancement and Disease Prevention.* Edited by J. D. Malarazzo and others. New York: John Wiley & Sons, pp. 230–47.

24. Rosenstock, I., V. Strecher, and M. Becker. 1988. Social learning theory and the health belief model. *Health Education Quarterly* 15: 175–83.

25. Anspaugh, D. J., M. H. Hamrick, and F. D. Rosato. 1997. *Wellness: Concepts and applications,* 3rd ed. St. Louis: Mosby.

Three

Life Transitions: *Infancy to Early Adulthood*

■ chapter objectives

When you complete this chapter you will be able to:
- Explain the transitional theories of psychosexual, psychosocial, cognitive and moral development, and the biases they present about women.
- Describe the major issues for women moving through early life transitions; including biological, educational, social, and political issues.

THEORIES OF DEVELOPMENT

From about 1905 to 1978, the psychology profession made significant contributions to the long-held societal belief that women were inferior to men. However, in 1979 a female psychologist, Carol Gilligan,[1] began to challenge the views of earlier psychologists who had neglected the specific concerns of women or had negatively stereotyped women by judging their differences from men as being a state of inferiority. For example, in 1905, Sigmund Freud, who is considered to be the father of psychology, designed the theory of psychosexual development around the experiences of the male child, depicting women as envying that which they missed, such as a penis. From Freud's view, differences between men and women resulted from women's developmental failure to meet the male standard.[2] (See *FYI:* "Freud's Stages of Psychosexual Development.")

In 1968, another prominent psychologist, Erik Erikson, did recognize gender differences by noting that in males the ability to develop an identity precedes intimacy development, but the development of intimacy occurs along with identity development in females. This tendency for women to identify themselves through their relationships with others remains strong for most women throughout their life. Despite Erikson's observation of gender differences, his life-cycle stages consistently depicted the male pattern as the standard for healthy psychosocial development.[2] (See *FYI:* "Erikson's Stages of Psychosocial Development.")

Jean Piaget did not acknowledge the value of the female pattern in his theory of cognitive development in 1932. Piaget equated normal child development with male development and considered females to be far less developed in capacities that would allow them to deal adequately with the reali-

HEALTHY PEOPLE 2000 OBJECTIVES

- Reduce pregnancies among females aged 15–17 to no more than 50 per 1,000 adolescents. 1995 progress toward goal: -20 percent
- Reduce to no more than 30 percent the proportion of all pregnancies that are unintended. 1995 progress toward goal: data unavailable
- Reduce the infant mortality rate to no more than 7 per 1,000 live births. 1995 progress toward goal: 60 percent
- Increase to at least 75 percent the proportion of mothers who breast-feed their babies in the early postpartum period and at least 50 percent the proportion who continue breast-feeding until their babies are 5 to 6 months old. 1995 progress toward goal: 10 percent
- Reduce the death rate for children by 15 percent to no more than 28.6 per 100,000 children aged 1–14, and for infants by approximately 30 percent to no more than 7 per 1,000 live births. 1995 progress toward goal: data unavailable
- Reduce the death rate for adolescents and young adults by 15 percent to no more than 83.1 per 100,000 people aged 15–24. 1995 progress toward goal: data unavailable
- Reduce the death rate for adults by 20 percent to no more than 341.5 per 100,000 people aged 25–64. 1995 progress toward goal: data unavailable

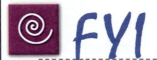

FYI

Freud's Stages of Psychosexual Development

A person who receives too much or too little gratification at any stage might become fixated at that stage and this incomplete development, or fixation, would then be the source for dysfunctional or unhealthy patterns of behavior later on in life.

- Oral stage—(birth to 1 year) the child seeks gratification via the mouth, such as chewing, sucking, tasting.
- Anal stage—(ages 2–3 years) the child's focus is primarily on anal activity, such as eliminative functions.
- Phallic stage—(ages 4–5 years) the focus shifts to the genital area and exploration of the body through manipulation.
- Latency stage—(ages 6 to puberty) the child's focus shifts from self to other persons, cultivating relationships.
- Genital stage—(ages puberty to adulthood) the primary focus is on seeking sexual stimulation and satisfaction through relation to another.

ties of adult life. Piaget based his assumption on his observations of adolescent children playing games. Boys focused more on a resolution of conflicts by following established rules to the letter; while girls were more tolerant in their attitudes, were more easily reconciled to innovative solutions, and were more willing to make exceptions if the rules did not seem to result in fair outcomes relative to the situation. Piaget determined that the female pattern of conflict resolution lacked the necessary legal sense that was essential to moral development, thus he determined that girls were inferior to boys.[2] Piaget failed to recognize that the approach that girls took to conflict resolution, although different from boys, was an equal or sometimes more favorable approach to resolving the conflict depending upon the circumstances of the particular situation. (See *FYI:* "Piaget's Stages of Cognitive Development.")

Lawrence Kohlberg, in 1969, derived his theory of moral development without considering the potential benefits of gender differences.[2] Kohlberg explains that gender differences develop because girls play games that are less likely to involve strict rules, such as hopscotch and jump rope. And, he observed, when conflicts over rules do develop in girls' games, the games often end. Rather than elaborating a set of rules to settle the dispute, girls subordinate the continuation of the game in favor of the continuation of relationships. This type of solution to conflict resolution was considered inferior by Kohlberg. Thus, when Kohlberg developed a scale to measure moral development, he utilized an exclusively male subject group; so, when measured by Kohlberg's scale, women are consistently found to be deficient in moral development.

As a response to gender bias within the psychology profession, Gilligan proposed to the profession that a new psychology for women be developed that was independent of comparisons to male standards and that encouraged women to trust their own judgments about themselves. The psychology profession gradually began to respond to Gilligan's

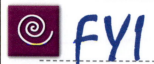

Erikson's Stages of Psychosocial Development

If the life task is mastered, a positive quality is incorporated into the personality. If the task during each stage is not mastered, the ego is damaged because a negative quality is incorporated into it.

- Trust vs. distrust—(0-1 year) learning to trust caregivers to meet one's needs or develop distrust if needs are not met.
- Autonomy vs. shame and doubt—(1-2 years) gain control over eliminative functions and learn to feed oneself; learn to play alone and explore the world and develop some degree of independence; or, if too restricted by caregivers, develop a sense of shame and doubt about one's abilities.
- Initiative vs. guilt—(3-5 years) as intellectual and motor skills develop, one explores the environment and experiences many new things and assumes more responsibility for initiating and carrying out plans; or caregivers who do not accept the child's own initiative instill a feeling of guilt over labeled misbehavior.
- Industry vs. inferiority—(6-11 years) learning to meet the demands of life, such as home and school, and develop a strong sense of self-worth through accomplishment and interaction with others; or, without the proper support and encouragement one begins to feel inferior in relation to others.
- Identity vs. role confusion—(12-19 years) develop a strong sense of self; or become confused about one's identity and roles in life.
- Intimacy vs. isolation—(twenties and thirties *for males only; and 12-19 years for females*) develop close relationships with others; or become isolated from meaningful relationships with others. (*Note: Intimacy develops in conjunction with identity in females and intimacy development follows identity development in males.*)
- Generativity vs. stagnation—(forties and fifties) assume responsible, adult roles in the community and teach and care for the next generation; or become impoverished, self-centered, or stagnant.
- Integrity vs. despair—(60 years and over) evaluate one's life and accept oneself for who they are; or despair because one cannot determine the meaning in one's life. ∞

*The italicized comments above, which recognize the female differences in development, do not appear in Erikson's traditional presentation of the psychosocial life-cycle stages. Although he acknowledged female differences in some of his writings, Erikson typically only presented the male model as the standard for development.

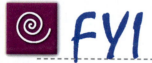

Piaget's Stages of Cognitive Development

Piaget believed that cognitive development was the combined result of the maturation of the brain and nervous system along with the person's adaptation to the environment.

- Sensorimotor stage—(birth-2 years) learn to coordinate sensory experiences with motor actions.
- Preoperational stage—(2-7 years) acquire language and manipulate symbols that represent the environment.
- Concrete operational stage—(7-11 years) greater capacity for logical reasoning limited to personal experience; also, can perform many mental operations, such as hierarchical classifications, class inclusion relationships and serialization (grouping objects), symmetry and reciprocity, and conservation (for example, the volume of a cup of water is consistent whether it is in a tall thin glass or a short fat one).
- Formal operational stage—(11 years and up) moving beyond personal experience and thinking in more abstract, logical terms. ∞

suggestion and a sensitivity to women's issues continues to evolve within the field. In fact, the American Psychological Association now has a subdivision dedicated entirely to the psychology of women.

THE PHASES OF LIFE

An examination of the biological, social, educational, and political issues associated with various life stages is important in understanding how your needs are different as you grow and age. You are who you are today because of your earlier life experiences. Your genetic and physical makeup were exposed to particular types of environments that influenced you to develop in certain ways. This is known as the nature-nurture interaction that determines development. There are many different theories about how this nature-nurture interaction works, but a summary of ideas from these various theories would suggest that development occurs because of an interaction of four primary elements: (1) your genetic potential; (2) your physical condition and abilities, some of which can be related to genetics; (3) the stimuli from your environment, such as people, places, and things; and (4) your freewill choice about how to respond to the environment.

Childhood

The brain of the child is not fully developed at birth. Neural connections will continue to form as the child experiences stimuli from the environment. The first three years of the child's life is vital for developing a neural network that may impact the child's later development. There are "windows of opportunity" for learning that will close for the child by age 3 to 5 years. If the child has not yet built the necessary neural pathways that will assist in continued growth in these areas, then later development in certain areas of the child's life will be stagnated. These neural pathways form after birth as a result of exposure to stimuli from the child's surroundings. From the time of birth and forward, it is very important that the child receive love, physical nurturance, and proper nutrition, and experience language and a variety of sounds, colors, smells, and age-appropriate eye-hand motor-coordination activities. (See *Health Tips:* "Tips for Talking to Your Infant.")

The concept of "missed windows of opportunity" was demonstrated in the 1980s by the tragedy of the

health tips

Tips for Talking to Your Infant[3]

To stimulate neural development, parents need to talk to their children in age-appropriate ways during their first year of life. For example:

- First month—low level of stimulation; talk in a conversational way, but filter out distracting noises such as radio.
- Months 1 to 3—introduce high-contrast pictures or objects (such as black, white, and red toys); describe what you are showing her; the brain is starting to discriminate speech patterns so talk in an animated voice.
- Months 3 to 5—show more complex pictures that match real objects in the baby's environment (such as board books); use motion when showing objects to attract attention to the object.
- Months 6 to 7—the baby is becoming more alert to cause and effect and what objects do, so demonstrate and talk about how to do things, such as turning a doorknob and opening a door.
- Months 7 to 8—she is associating sounds with objects and activities; point out sounds like running water at the sink or a doorbell ringing.
- Months 9 to 12—sensory and motor skills are beginning to coordinate in a more mature way; let the child turn on a faucet or a light switch under supervision to learn association and coordination.

children of Romania. The Romanian dictator declared that the government could do a better job of raising children. Children were removed from their families at a very early age and placed in large group homes. For the first few years of their lives, most of the children received no more daily contact or activity than being quickly fed, having their diaper changed, and then placed back in their cribs. By the time the dictatorship fell in Romania several years later, the damage had already been done. The children in the group homes were emotionally, mentally, and physically disabled. Many had learning disabilities and many had even lost the ability to make personal attachments. Several families in the United States adopted some of these Romanian children and have had to spend endless hours and monies in rehabilitation efforts, many of which are helpful, but the children will probably never reach the potential they might have if they had had the proper care in infancy.

Infant Mortality Infant death at the time of birth is still a major concern. However, there seems to be some progress being made in this area. According to the Centers for Disease Control, the infant mortality rate of 8.0 per 1,000 live births reached a record low in 1994, the lowest final rate ever recorded for the United States. The infant mortality rate for black infants (15.8) was 2.4 times the rate for white infants (6.6).

Children and Mortality The leading cause of death for Americans aged 1 through 14 years in 1995 was accidents, primarily motor vehicle accidents. As of 1995, gunfire was the second leading cause of death among Americans aged 10 to 19, according to the Child Defense Fund.[4] Firearm deaths are increasing faster among youths than any other age group. In 1993, a child died every 92 minutes from gunfire, and was most often murdered. An analysis of the 5,751 childhood gunfire deaths in 1993 showed that 3,661 were homicides, 1,460 were suicides, 526 were accidents, and 104 were of unknown origin. Over half of the victims were Caucasian. Gunfire was determined to be the fourth leading cause of death for the age group of 5 through 9 years and the second leading cause of death for the age group of 10 to 19 years. But gunfire was the leading cause of death in 1993 for black males aged 15 to 19.

Nutrition Nutrition is a vital component to healthy development. For infants, breast-feeding is advantageous in that it is typically nutritionally superior to formulas and to cow's milk.[5] Breast milk contains the right proportion of vitamins, proteins, minerals, calories, fats, and several additional amino acids. It is also easier to digest for most infants and contains antibodies that help to protect the child from disease and infection. It is estimated that over 50 percent of mothers breast-feed their babies in the hospital but only 20 percent are still breast-feeding when their babies are 6 months old. This number goes down to only 6 percent by the time the infant is 1 year old.[6] In comparison to all mothers in the United States, breast-feeding is less common among African American women, women with less than a high school education, women in poverty, and women who have never worked outside of the home.[7]

As of 1997, the major goal of UNICEF and the World Health Organization is to promote breast-feeding; and the U.S. Surgeon General strongly recommends breast-feeding. (See *FYI:* "Benefits to Breast-Feeding.") The American Academy of Pediatrics recommends that babies be breast-fed for 6 to 12 months; solid foods can be introduced when the baby is 4 to 6 months old, but a baby should drink breast milk, or at least infant formula, for a full year; and as long as the baby is eating age-appropriate solid foods, a mother can nurse for a couple of years if she wants.[8]

If you choose to breast-feed your baby, follow these very important precautions: Don't drink alcohol, don't smoke, don't drink caffeine, and avoid birth control pills and certain other types of medications that can be dangerous to your infant. These are the same types of precautions that you would take if you were pregnant with the child. Not all women can breast-feed. In such cases, it is vital that the baby drink a formula rich in the necessary nutrients the infant needs to flourish.

As children get older their bodies need a balanced diet of protein, minerals, vitamins, carbohydrates, fats, roughage, and water.[9] These nutrients can be derived from the basic food groups: fruits; vegetables; breads, cereals, rice, and pasta; milk products; and meat, poultry, fish, beans, eggs, and nuts. Nutritional information is covered in greater depth in chapter 7.

Physical Activity Physical play activity is necessary in the development of the child. Play activity is a way of releasing excess energy and enjoying social contact and having fun; thus, all children need frequent periods of physical activity.[10]

The 1984 *National Children and Youth Fitness Study* concluded that, "Today's children are less physically fit than were children in the 1960s." The study determined that, in the mid 1980s, children tended to have more body fat; were less fit in terms of heart rate, muscle strength, lung capacity, and physical endurance; and had higher levels of cholesterol or high blood pressure. Possible reasons for these less physically fit children included a less active schedule, more television watching or video game playing, fewer physical education classes in school, the availability of "fast foods" high in fat and cholesterol, and decreased participation in out-of-school physical activities, such as walking, bicycling, skating, swimming, and so forth. Exercise is vital for children to be healthy. More information about healthy fitness activities is presented in chapter 8.

Children must be encouraged to participate in physical activity, but must also be encouraged to ap-

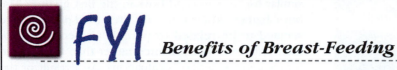

FYI *Benefits of Breast-Feeding*

FOR INFANTS

- Contains the right amount of nutrients.
- Provides lactoferrin to allow optimal absorption of iron, and thus, less incidence of iron deficiency.
- Provides lipases that assist in digestion of fats; this helps to lower the incidence of gastrointestinal upsets.
- Fewer allergic problems due to protective enzymes in the breast milk.
- Fewer bacterial and fungal infections due to protective antibodies in the breast milk.
- Healthier teeth and jaws, fewer cavities, and less orthodontic work required than bottle-fed babies.
- Less frequency of illness than bottle-fed babies.
- Breast milk contains the precursors for the baby to manufacture its own choline. This B vitamin is important for normal development and function of the brain.

FOR MOTHERS

- Stimulation of sucking the breast nipple causes the uterus to contract, making postnatal hemorrhage less likely, and the uterus shrinks back to its normal size more quickly.
- More rapid and sustained weight loss so the body returns to prepregnancy weight more quickly.
- May reduce the likelihood of developing breast cancer for mothers who breast-feed for at least 6 months.
- The pleasure experienced from the baby suckling enhances the emotional bond between mother and baby.
- Can delay the return to ovulation and menstruation, thus preventing pregnancy in the first six months as long as exclusive nursing is practiced.

proach the task with the attitude of having fun. An overemphasis on performance, rather than participation, can cause physical and psychological harm to the child. Overtraining a child can lead to physical injuries, and pressure to win can create excessive amounts of emotional stress.[11,12]

Education Introducing children to language and comprehension activity very early in life is necessary for the development of cognitive abilities and communication skills. A variety of age-appropriate toys and activities is preferable because they will provide opportunity for diverse stimulation and enhance cognitive development in many ways. Activities and toys classified as educational are designed to stimulate the development of specific cognitive and motor abilities.

The provision of gender-specific toys only must be avoided. A child exposed to toys and activities that stimulate the development of both masculine and feminine traits within the child will assist in the development of a child with a broader range of knowledge and skills—both nurturing skills and mechanical skills. Research shows that adult ratings of toys can be very gender specific. Toys rated as "boy toys" also received high ratings in the promotion of symbolic or fantasy play, competition, constructive-

ness, handling, sociability, and aggressiveness; "girl toys" were rated higher on manipulability (ease of removing and replacing parts), creativity, nurturance, and attractiveness.[13] It is important to remember that limiting the child to toys that follow only traditional gender roles will also limit the scope of the child's development.

Socialization Fostering the potential development of both masculine and feminine traits in a child is important because it avoids the limitations associated with sex-role stereotyping or gender-role socialization and promotes the potential benefits of androgyny. **Gender-role socialization** is the tendency for parents to interact with the child or to limit the experiences of the child in ways that seem more "suitable" to traditional roles, such as encouraging girls to associate more with staying home and

> **gender-role socialization**—the tendency to interact with a child or to limit the experiences of a child in ways that seem more suitable to traditional roles relative to the child's gender.

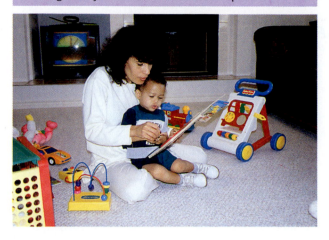

Reading with your child nurtures development.

caretaking and encouraging boys to venture out in the world and problem solve.[14] **Androgyny,** a concept whose importance was first emphasized by Sandra Bem in 1974, is the balance of masculine and feminine traits within the individual.[15] Adults who were more androgynous were shown to have more characteristics associated with better mental health than adults who were less androgynous.

Partly as a result of Bem's androgyny research in the mid 1970s, there was an emphasis on research in the 1980s in the study of the propensity of gender-role socialization by parents toward their children. The research determined that most boys were socialized to develop a system that presumes or anticipates mastery, efficacy, and instrumental competence, whereas most girls were socialized toward fostering proximity, discouraging independent problem solving by premature or excessive intervention by parents, restricting exploration, and discouraging active play.[16] In one study, mothers' speech with their male toddlers included more questions, numbers, verbal teaching, and action verbs than the speech with their female toddlers.[17] Another study showed that, when working on a jigsaw puzzle and memory tasks with 6-year-old sons and daughters, parents were more likely to attempt to teach general problem-solving strategies to the sons but to make specific solution suggestions to the daughters.[18] Other research discovered that, after tracking 1,100 children semester by semester over the first three grades of school, the boys developed higher expectations for their performance in mathematics than the girls did, despite the fact that arithmetic marks and general aptitude were

similar for the girls and boys in the first grade.[19] The boys' higher expectations for their own performance seemed to be related to parents' expectations for their children's performance rather than to past performance or teachers' evaluations. As a result of the findings of the gender-role socialization research of the 1980s, teachers and parents were cautioned to not limit the opportunity for a child's development because of sex-role stereotyping.

Toy manufacturers in the 1990s responded to a desire expressed by parents to have their children, regardless of gender, develop more balanced traits, both nurturing and mechanical. A stroll down the aisle of a major toy store today will show a greater diversity of types of toys, especially those designed to develop a variety of social, cognitive, and motor skills for both girls and boys. However, it is still up to parents to encourage their children to play with a diversity of toys so that both girls and boys may develop as many skills as possible to prepare them for the challenges of life as both potential caregivers and career professionals.

Nurturance   Nurturing the child from the moment of birth is extremely important. An infant child will fail to thrive if it does not receive soothing touch. Cradling an infant or holding and hugging a child in a gentle and appropriate fashion are healthy ways to nurture. Speaking to infants or young children in a low tone and easy manner is nurturing. Responding to the infant's or child's attempts to communicate back also assists in the development of their sense of well-being.

It is often difficult for working parents to provide sufficient nurturance to their child during work hours. Thus, it is vital that any substitute caregiver supplement these interactions during the parent's absence. However, the parents must also establish the provision of nurturing time to their child as a priority in their lives.

Children are highly susceptible to victimization. The incidence of child abuse is very high; 3.1 million children are reported annually to Child Protective Services as being abused or neglected, with thousands dying as a result.[20] Child abuse comes in many forms: emotional, physical, sexual, and neglect. Much of the child sexual abuse that occurs is among female children by their own fathers. If you suspect abuse of a child, you should consult with your community Child Protective Services. In addition, you can teach your children to be wary of strangers who might otherwise abduct and abuse your child.

Family The family serves as the first social structure of which the child is a member and from which a sense of significance or meaningfulness is derived. The perceptions and resulting assumptions that children have about individuals and society, based on the early family experience, will continue to have a major influence on how they interact with persons and systems throughout their life. Thus, the family environment plays a critical role in the development of the child.

An encouraged child seems to thrive better than a discouraged one. Children can become discouraged by a parent who is either authoritarian or permissive. An *authoritarian parent* uses force to curb the child's freewill and restrict the child's autonomy. A *permissive parent* is overaccommodating to the child, providing no rules or boundaries and accepting the child's impulses and behaviors without shaping the child's behavior. A healthy parenting style is considered to be authoritative. An *authoritative parent* seeks to direct the child's activities in a rational manner, encouraging discussion and exerting control when the child does disobey, but without being overly restrictive. An authoritarian or permissive parenting style tends to discourage children and this may lead to mistaken beliefs and misbehavior by the child. Authoritative parenting methods incorporate an encouraging attitude into the parenting style. Within this framework, the parents are still the recognized authority. However, children feel more secure in that they are listened to and respected by their parents. An authoritative parent takes the time to explain things to help the child learn reasoning skills, appropriate respect for boundaries, and understand logical consequences for behavior.

Adolescence

Adolescence begins around the time of the initiation of puberty, usually about ages 12 or 13 years, and extends to about ages 18 or 19 years. In 1994, the total U.S. population was 260.3 million and those who were under 18 years of age totaled 26.1 million; thus, children and adolescents together represent almost 10 percent of the total U.S. population.[21]

The adolescent period is also referred to as the "teenage" years. These years are fraught with inconsistencies in behavior as adolescents struggle to free themselves from dependency on the family and establish an identity of their own. The adolescent vacillates between: being rebellious versus conforming,

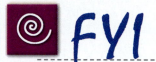

FYI

Adolescent Developmental Tasks

According to Erik Erikson's adolescent development theory, eight major tasks are to be accomplished during adolescence:

1. Accepting and using your body effectively.
2. Achieving emotional independence from parents and other adults.
3. Achieving a social sex role.
4. Achieving new and more mature relations with age-mates of both sexes.
5. Desiring and achieving socially responsible behavior.
6. Acquiring a set of values and an ethical system as a guide to behavior.
7. Preparing for an economic career.
8. Preparing for a committed relationship and family life. ⌥

seeking social contact versus isolation, experiencing intense infatuation versus falling out of love, being self-centered versus loving, being materialistic versus idealistic, having confidence versus self-doubt, having enthusiasm versus indifference. (See *FYI:* "Adolescent Developmental Tasks.")

Puberty The conclusion of childhood is facilitated by changes in the physiology of the body brought about as the result of hormonal influences. Women experience their bodies becoming much fuller in the breasts, hips, and thighs and their life is changed forever with the initiation of the monthly menstrual cycle. Biologically speaking, all of these changes occur to prepare the female body for potential reproduction.

With the onset of the menstrual cycle, many women will experience premenstrual syndrome (PMS), which is a set of symptoms that arrive three to five days before the onset of menstruation. PMS can involve both physical and emotional problems, for example, bloating, cravings, headaches, cramping,

androgyny (an **drodge** en ee)—the balance of masculine and feminine traits.

health tips

Eating Healthy to Avoid PMS[22]

Poor nutrition and low-quality foods contribute directly to the incidence of PMS. Some foods are known to worsen your problems.

FOODS TO AVOID

- Refined carbohydrates such as white bread, cakes, cookies, refined breakfast cereals, crackers, candy, and chocolate
- Foods that are high in fats, including dairy products and red meat
- Synthetic foods that are highly processed and full of chemical additives
- Caffeinated drinks such as coffee, tea, and soda
- Alcohol
- Salt and heavily salted foods

FOODS TO ADD TO YOUR DIET

- Complex carbohydrates, such as whole grain bread, brown rice, whole grain pasta, and whole grain cereals
- Plenty of fresh fruits and vegetables
- Low-fat protein sources, such as fish, chicken, and vegetarian proteins
- Vegetable oils (rich in essential fatty acids)

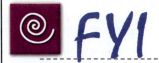

Types of PMS[22]

Women who suffer from PMS tend to experience groupings of symptoms. For this reason, PMS symptoms are categorized under four main headings:

- *Type A.* A stands for anxiety. This type of PMS is most notable for its emotional symptoms of anxiety, irritability, and mood swings.
- *Type C.* C stands for carbohydrate cravings (you fall into this category if you would kill for chocolate in the week before your period!) Along with the sugar cravings are exhaustion and headaches (all symptoms of low blood sugar).
- *Type D.* D stands for depression. This is accompanied by mental confusion, an inability to think clearly, and poor memory.
- *Type H.* H stands for hyperhydration, which is like waterlogging. You suffer from Type H PMS if you swell up like a balloon, none of your clothes fit you, and your rings cut into your fingers when your periods are due. The fluid retention will also cause your breasts to swell and become very tender.

You may find that your PMS symptoms fall into one or a combination of these categories, although Type A is the most common accounting for 80 percent of PMS sufferers.

anxiety, irritability, or depression. (See *Health Tips:* "Eating Healthy to Avoid PMS" and *FYI:* "Types of PMS.") The PMS syndrome has been a source for discriminating against women; many women were prohibited from positions of professional responsibility before the 1970s, and the biased reasoning was, "that women were not emotionally stable enough to be responsible in the workplace." More information on the menstrual cycle and PMS is provided in chapter 15.

The combination of biological readiness, increased sex drive, and the adolescent tendency to take risks can lead to unexpected pregnancy. The United States has one of the highest rates of teenage pregnancy and childbearing among industrialized nations.[23] (See Tables 3.1 and 3.2.) The rate of unmarried women who have a child is highest among African American women.

The ability to create a human life from an egg waiting in the woman's ovaries is a tremendous feat. This is why many culture archetypes throughout his-

tory revere the female aspect as that which gives life. However, in many ways, women have also suffered because of their life-giving ability. Throughout history, and even today, control over this special ability of women is still dictated: when and how she can, must, or should utilize this ability. Thus, the blessing of life-giving can also be a tremendous burden. There is often societal pressure on women to reproduce even if it means sacrificing their own goals of education or career achievement.

An unplanned pregnancy can be traumatic for a woman, especially if she is a young, unmarried woman. Options are available to women who have unplanned pregnancies, from having the child, to giving the child up for adoption, to terminating the pregnancy by abortion. However, some religious and social groups condemn the abortion option for women, believing instead that a woman should be forced to endure the physical and emotional stress of

Table 3.1

Unmarried Mothers in the United States
(from July 1993 to June 1994)[24]
(Numbers in thousands)

TOTAL BY AGE (YEARS)	NUMBER WHO HAD A CHILD	NUMBER AND PERCENT WHO WERE UNMARRIED	
White			
15–19	294	194	66.0
20–24	702	215	30.6
25–29	856	87	10.2
30–44	1,255	84	6.7
Total	*3,107*	*580*	*18.7*
Black			
15–19	87	78	89.7
20–24	189	152	80.4
25–29	144	69	47.9
30–44	147	76	51.7
Total	*567*	*375*	*66.1*
Hispanic			
15–19	108	71	65.7
20–24	161	50	31.1
25–29	181	28	15.5
30–44	195	28	14.4
Total	*645*	*177*	*27.4*
Asian/Pacific Islander			
Total (15–44 yrs)*	112	18	16.1

*Specific data unavailable.

Table 3.2

Unmarried Mothers in Selected Countries [25]

Country	% BORN TO UNWED MOTHERS 1980	% BORN TO UNWED MOTHERS 1992
Sweden	40	50
Denmark	33	46
France	11	33
United Kingdom	12	31
United States	18	30
Canada	13	29
Germany	8	15
Netherlands	4	12
Italy	4	7
Japan	1	1

carrying the child to term, even if she does not want to. Some antiabortion groups have resorted to terrorist-type tactics such as harassing or threatening doctors who perform abortions, or intimidating patients as they attempt to enter or leave abortion clinics. Some of these physicians have actually been killed or injured, and some U.S. abortion clinics have been bombed or set on fire. More about planned and unplanned pregnancy will be presented in chapters 16 and 17.

Body Image   The biological effects of puberty dictate that the woman's body become fuller and retain greater fat stores. However, today's society pressures a woman to go against the natural inclination of her own biology and strive for "thinness." This is impossible to achieve for most women, and those who do so often compromise some aspects of their health to maintain the image. This is a very sensitive area for the adolescent woman, who is dealing with the changes in her own body as well as societal expectations about her physical appearance. More about body image issues is presented in chapter 5.

An emphasis on fitness must be maintained during adolescence. This can be accomplished through encouragement to participate in health and nutrition courses, physical education classes, organized sports, and recreational outings. Fitness activities in adolescence often carry through in some way or another into adulthood. Thus, a development of interest in fitness participation during the adolescent years can influence fitness patterns throughout the rest of your life. More about fitness issues and techniques is provided in chapter 8.

There are many more opportunities for women's participation in organized team sports today than there were twenty-five years ago. In 1971, one of twenty-seven girls participated in high school sports; today, in 1997, one of three does.[26] This rise in women's participation in sports is, for the most part, a result of the passage of Title IX—legislation passed in 1972 that required equal opportunities for females in school sports programs.

Self-Identity Adolescence is a difficult time for identity issues. Adolescents are no longer willing to universally accept the beliefs and values that their parents hold, yet they have not yet formulated a clear set of values and beliefs of their own. Adolescence is a time for experimentation. During this time, parents hope that their adolescent child's trial-and-error learning does not endanger the child in any way. Any important messages a parent wants their children to hear to help prepare them for their adolescent trials should be communicated before the onset of the adolescent period because it is less likely that once a child reaches adolescence he or she will be as open to hearing these messages.

Adolescents identify most with their own peer group. The desire to gain acceptance and prestige within the group makes the adolescent susceptible to peer pressure. Unhealthy influences that are commonly exerted on adolescents by their own peers are to: disobey parents, skip school, drink alcohol, abuse drugs, engage in sexual activity (often unprotected sex), drive fast, drive under the influence of alcohol or drugs, and attempt other types of risky behaviors. (See *FYI:* "Positive Peer Pressure," as an example.) Adolescent acting-out behaviors seem to be attempts at proving oneself in the presence of others or proving that one has what it takes to make it through to adulthood; adolescence is the period for the "rite of passage" into adulthood.

To help adolescents make informed choices about their life, important information about their personal safety must be provided before and during adolescence. Education in the following areas is beneficial for this purpose: the hazards of alcohol and drug use and abuse, the effects of smoking and other

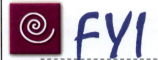

Positive Peer Pressure

The *Best Friends* program was started a few years ago by Elaine Bennett in the public elementary and junior high schools of the Washington, D.C. area. *Best Friends* is designed to use peer pressure in a positive way to help young girls say "no" to teenage sex and say "no" to drugs and alcohol abuse forever.[27] Although the Washington, D.C. area has a teenage pregnancy rate of 26 percent, the girls in the *Best Friends* program have a pregnancy rate of only 2 percent. The program uses curriculum to educate girls in areas such as decision making, AIDS, drug and alcohol abuse, and health and fitness programs. The program presents standards and sends consistent messages to help young women resist the negative peer pressure to use drugs and have sex that so many young teenagers endure. They participate in activities together and build positive friendships that give them the strength to resist participation in negative health behaviors. The program also involves the young women in community song and dance presentations in which they celebrate their fight against negative peer pressure. As of 1997, the *Best Friends* program has been embraced by seventeen school systems nationwide.   ∞

tobacco use, and sex education such as pregnancy risks, birth control methods, risks for getting sexually transmitted diseases, and safer sex practices.

For an adolescent woman, there is a strong focus on her potential abilities as a mate and mother. For girls, physical maturation, such as the development of breasts and a more sexually mature appearance, is associated with early pressures in the direction of the traditional female role. An adolescent woman is aware that she is being judged according to her sexual attractiveness and pleasing personality, and the pressure is on to have both. It is difficult to develop an individual identity free of these pressures. In addition, parents may place harsher restrictions on adolescent girls to protect them from premature pregnancy, thus growing up is associated with a loss of freedom rather than increased opportunities.[28]

Adolescence can be especially trying for homosexual women (also referred to as gay women or lesbians). Today's society still does not universally accept this particular lifestyle. In fact, there is a high

Assess **Y O U R S E L F**

Gay and Lesbian Rights

Circle A for agree and D for disagree for each of the following items.

A   D   1.   It should *not* be legal to fire a gay or lesbian person from a job based solely on his or her sexual orientation.

A   D   2.   A gay or lesbian individual should *not* be denied custody of his or her children solely on the basis of sexual orientation.

A   D   3.   A gay or lesbian person should be allowed to designate his or her relationship partner as a recipient of spousal benefits on insurance benefit plans.

A   D   4.   A gay or lesbian couple should *not* be allowed to file joint income tax returns.

A   D   5.   A gay or lesbian couple should *not* be allowed to legally marry.

A   D   6.   A lesbian or gay person should *not* be allowed to adopt a child.

A   D   7.   A lesbian should *not* be allowed to use a sperm bank to inseminate sperm in order to get pregnant.

A   D   8.   Major television networks should *not* be able to show programs that depict lesbian or gay persons during prime-time hours (such as 7 to 9 P.M.).

A   D   9.   Grade school libraries and/or curriculum should include some books that depict families with gay members, such as gay parents.

A   D   10.   High school libraries and/or curriculum should *not* include some books about lesbian and gay persons.

A   D   11.   An adolescent who claims to be gay should be encouraged to seek mental health therapy to change his orientation to become less gay and thus, more heterosexual.

A   D   12.   A parent should *not* have the right to refuse his or her child, who is 17 years old or younger, room and board because the child is gay or lesbian.

A   D   13.   A parent should have the right to require a gay child, who is 17 years old or younger, to seek mental health therapy to become less gay and thus, more heterosexual.

A   D   14.   Lesbian and gay persons should be allowed to serve in the military without having to hide their sexual orientation.

A   D   15.   Multicultural awareness programs and courses designed to fight discrimination and bigotry should include information on gays and lesbians in the same way that they present information on other minority groups.

Scoring

If you answered the items in the following designated direction, then give yourself one point for each: (1) A; (2) A; (3) A; (4) D; (5) D; (6) D; (7) D; (8) D; (9) A; (10) D; (11) D; (12) A; (13) D; (14) A; and (15) A.

Interpretation

If your score was 8 or higher, then you are considered to have an attitude more in favor of gay and lesbian rights. The higher your score, the more in favor of gay and lesbian rights you are. If your score was 7 or less, then you are considered to be less in favor of gay and lesbian rights. The lower your score, the less in favor of gay and lesbian rights you are. The maximum score is 15 and the minimum score is 0.

incidence of violence toward homosexuals in the United States.[29,30] It is difficult to develop an identity when your family, friends, or society do not condone it, and oftentimes condemn it. **Homophobia** is the fear or dislike of a person who is homosexual. Many people in this country are homophobic, and thus, many homosexual women hide their true sexual orientation to keep from being ostracized or rejected.

Evaluate your awareness and attitudes toward gay and lesbian rights by completing *Assess Yourself!*—"Gay and Lesbian Rights."

homophobia (hoe **moe** foe bee ya)—the fear or dislike of someone who is a homosexual.

Her Story

Ellen DeGeneres

Ellen DeGeneres, a well-known comedian with her own situation-comedy television show, hid her lesbian identity from the public for most of her life out of fear that it would hinder her chances of success.[31] DeGeneres decided to "come out" on her television program at the end of April 1997. Some companies threatened to pull their commercial spots off of the program if DeGeneres became openly gay on her TV show.

Much of the American society still struggles with the idea of accepting lesbians as normal and healthy women.

- Do you know any gay persons, and if so, how do you feel about them?
- Or if you are gay, how do you think people who are not gay may feel about you as a gay person?

A lesbian adolescent may find it difficult to explore her attraction for other women during a time when it is most natural for her to do so. Lesbians often do not feel safe enough to begin the dating process with other women until they leave home and high school, and migrate to a community that is more supportive of this type of relationship or where it is at least easier to be inconspicuous. It is difficult for a lesbian to find role models for dating because much of this culture remains hidden. Thus, the lesbian is frequently forced to not only hide her desires and delay acting upon her attractions, but she has little opportunity to learn from others about how to establish and maintain a healthy lesbian relationship. (See *Her Story:* "Ellen DeGeneres.")

Any adolescent woman struggles to develop a sense of individual identity or **autonomy** without significantly alienating her peers, including those seen as potential dating partners. This struggle batters the woman's self-esteem. If she does not perceive herself as having achieved a significant, individual identity and also respect by her peers or dating partners, then she is likely to feel inadequate in one or more of these areas.

The emphasis on femininity is very pronounced during a woman's adolescence, a time when she is perceived as "coming of age." This can be a disappointing time for women in that they are expected, by many facets of society, to limit themselves to feminine roles. Women are often judged by how well they can fulfill the feminine stereotype. This is a double-edged sword. Much empirical research has indicated that society holds masculine traits in higher regard than feminine traits and that there is a higher correlation between self-esteem and masculine traits.[32] Thus, the double message for women is "you are only as good as you are feminine; however, you will never be seen as favorable as that which is masculine." The degree to which a woman resolves this conflict within herself will impact her sense of adequacy within society.

Any sense of inadequacy incurred in adolescence can follow a woman into adulthood unless significant insight is gained. Exploring and discussing various beliefs and values in an open and nonjudgmental atmosphere can assist an adolescent woman in the continuing process of developing her own beliefs and values. A woman must have courage to follow her own value and belief system and trust that she will attract friends and relationship partners that will be consistent with these, instead of trying to be whatever her friends or relationship partners want her to be.

Social Identity Adolescence is a time when young women are struggling to discover their place within the larger society. They feel pressured to some day achieve in all areas: as a wife or relationship partner, as a mother, and in a career. During adolescence, women are attempting to prepare for these three roles.

The identity development in adolescent women is based on their relatedness to others. Women develop in a context of attachment and affiliation. Indeed, women's sense of self becomes very much organized around being able to make and then to maintain affiliations and relationships. Women define themselves in terms of relations with others and they judge themselves in their ability to care.

Women tend to base their identity development on their relationships and certain environmental factors can create special circumstances. For example, one study of thirty lower socioeconomic-status adolescent urban black mothers found these girls' most consistent role models had been teenage mothers.[33] Thus, the mother-daughter relationship is an important factor in childbearing. Another study determined that, due to many sociocultural factors that have been implicated in affecting the identity development of adolescent women, adolescent childbearing among lower socioeconomic-status African American girls is a career choice and an alternative, normative life path within African American culture.[34]

Adolescence is a period that can put a strain on the mother-daughter relationship. Adolescent girls have to adjust to pubertal development, begin to achieve an individual identity, and gain acceptance from their families regarding their emerging independence. These changes may exert a special pressure on the relationship between adolescent daughters and their mothers. If conflicts should arise and they are not resolved adequately, the adolescent girl may resort to acting out, that is, she may engage in negative behaviors as a result of frustration regarding a mother-daughter conflict. Using drugs, engaging in sexual promiscuity, or breaking rules are all examples of conflict. The following are a few suggestions that a mother and daughter can try together to help resolve issues that arise from mother-daughter conflicts and adolescent acting-out.[35]

- The mother should explore her response to the changes in her adolescent daughter.
- Have the adolescent daughter explain her reasons for her actions.
- Mother and daughter discuss the implications for the acting out on the family.
- Ask other family members to explain why they think the adolescent is acting out.
- Explore the possibility that the mother may be resisting the daughter's development; this may impact behavior.
- Ask the adolescent daughter to explore her reactions to her mother's attitude toward her.
- Explore the future effect on the family if the adolescent continues to act out. Discuss the possibility of seeking professional assistance, such as family therapy, if acting-out behavior continues. Life skills development is vital during adolescence.

Education that addresses issues around self-esteem building, assertiveness, communication, healthy relationships, motherhood, and parenting are helpful at this time. These areas of skill development are discussed in more detail in chapters 5, 14, and 17.

Participation in extracurricular activities is a great way to develop skills. Many school- and community-sponsored programs are available in music, art, theater, youth politics and governance, and recreation. These programs also provide addi-

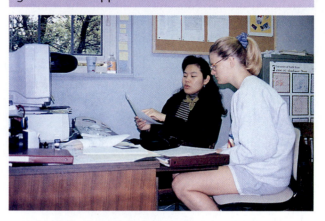

Angie and Suanthong work on a college research paper together. A college education can result in greater career opportunities for women.

tional opportunities for making friends and developing and exercising social skills.

A woman must be encouraged to pursue her career interests, not only so she will be prepared to provide for herself economically, but also so she can experience greater fulfillment. Many communities and high schools have interactive after-school and summer programs that offer teenagers apprenticeships to learn a career trade.

Education   Completing a high school education is vital for survival in today's society. Continuing on to vocational training or a college education is preferred today, due to the competition for jobs that exists in a technologically advanced society. An evolving society is slowly presenting more diverse achievement opportunities for women. Women are thriving in career areas that were either completely or mostly unavailable to them just a quarter of a century ago, such as business executives, astronauts, airline and fighter pilots, governors, mayors, senators, members of congress, firefighters and rescue workers, and so on. Even with more opportunities available for women, the financial rewards for women's educational and career achievements is still significantly below that of men.

> **autonomy** (awe **tohn** uh me)—maintaining an individual identity and self-direction.

Opportunities for a woman in high-paying careers are directly related to the level of education she receives; thus, a woman's standard of living can be dependent on her educational attainment. Unfortunately, these opportunities differ for women by ethnicity. In 1992, the U.S. Census Bureau reported that those women who received eight years of education or less were: 36.4 percent Mexican American, 13.2 percent African American, and only 8 percent white.

Young Adulthood

Young adulthood encompasses the ages of twenties and thirties. The emphases during this period of life are on career development and the establishment of a family.

Physical Status The average young adult woman is at her peak fitness level. She has reached full, physical maturity and little to no deterioration from the aging process is evident. Adults are typically not as physically active as adolescents, thus an effort must be made to maintain healthy nutrition and regular exercise.

Many women play professional sports. The attendance at women's sporting events is still significantly below that of men, as are the salaries for professional women athletes. However, women athletes are gradually beginning to see more commercial endorsements and public recognition for their work. For example, some of the best attended events at the 1996 Summer Olympic games in Atlanta, Georgia, were women's events in which many U.S. women won gold medals. There are many doors that still need to be opened for women athletes. Although men's ice hockey had been a part of the winter Olympic games for many years, women were allowed to compete in ice hockey for the first time in the 1998 Olympic games. The games were held in Nagano, Japan. The U.S. women's ice hockey team won the gold medal, Canada won the silver medal, and Finland took the bronze. In 1998, there was no professional women's ice hockey league in the United States.

The first nationally recognized women's sports magazine was published by the staff of *Sports Illustrated* in the spring of 1997; the name of the magazine is *Women Sport*. The staff of *Sports Illustrated* was counting on the support of their 450,000 female *SI* subscribers to help the success of the *Women Sport* magazine. The second issue of the *Women Sport* magazine was published in the fall of 1997. The planned publication schedule was significantly less frequent

Viewpoint

Women in Sports

The cover of the premier issue of *Women Sport* magazine created some controversy. It depicts a very pregnant Sheryl Swoopes holding a basketball. Swoopes won a national collegiate championship as well as an Olympic gold medal in her sport. Some comments by women about the cover of the magazine were positive—"It demonstrates the diverse capacities of women, to excel in sports and have children." Other comments by women about the cover were negative—"It erroneously suggests that women should only play sports if it does not interfere with the fulfillment of their role as mother and wife." What type of message do you think this cover sends to other women and to the public in general?

than the existing publication schedule of the weekly edition of *Sports Illustrated,* which focuses primarily on men's sports. Currently, a lack of subscriptions has postponed the publication of future issues of *Women Sport.* However, efforts that resulted in the publication of *Women Sport* should certainly be applauded. (See the accompanying *Viewpoint:* "Women in Sports.")

In young adulthood, many women are still preoccupied by their body shape and size. Any concern over body image that may have started as early as adolescence can persist into young adulthood, and when women reach physical maturity, some even consider cosmetic adjustments. The use of silicon breast implants was a popular approach to breast enlargement until implants were discovered to leak toxic substances into the body. Using cosmetic surgery as a way of feeling better about yourself is not usually the best approach. This type of medical procedure is extremely useful to those who have significant impairments from birth defects, accidents, or disease. However, for a woman to have cosmetic surgery because she wants to add an inch or more to her breast size or smooth out a couple of natural wrinkles that may come with aging can be a self-defacing decision. Learning to love one's body is an important step toward self-acceptance, self-confidence, and self-esteem. The decision to have cosmetic surgery should be considered carefully, and mental health counseling is recommended before engaging in cosmetic adjustments. (See *FYI:* "Hazards of Silicone Breast Implants.")

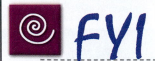

Hazards of Silicone Breast Implants[36]

Dow Corning Corporation, once the nation's leading maker of breast implants, today (May 15, 1995) filed for bankruptcy protection because of lawsuits over the devices. The filing freezes all suits against the company. Dow Corning and other makers of the implants face billions of dollars in damages from lawsuits. An estimated 500,000 to 2 million women have received the implants, and many blame them for health problems including lupus and hardening of the breasts. ∞

A young adult woman is at her healthiest stage for reproduction, and many women make decisions about having children during this phase of life. Also, there exists several options for having children, such as adoption or the use of sperm donors or sperm banks. Even many lesbians have children.

Some young adult women choose to delay childbirth or not to have children at all. This type of decision can be stressful for the woman for three primary reasons: (1) there is frequently social pressure to reproduce (mostly from parents who want grandchildren), (2) the woman may experience a sense of obligation to reproduce because she can (and may have resulting guilt for not utilizing her ability), and (3) there are limitations that the biological clock can impose if she delays reproduction for too long (such as the aging egg and increased risks of an unhealthy baby, and the gradual onset of menopause in middle adulthood). Though a woman may feel some pressure to have children, she must feel free to make the decision either way. Having children is an option for women and should *not* be viewed as an expectation. A woman can enjoy her unique gender capabilities without being obligated to participate in all of them.

A woman who chooses to plan for childbirth or chooses not to have children must consider the necessity for birth control when engaging in sexual intercourse with a male partner. This can be a difficult decision because some of the more effective birth control methods, such as birth control pills, can have negative side effects and involve health risks.

Women who are sexually active with a partner must consider safer-sex practices to prevent the transmission of sexually transmitted diseases; this goes for both heterosexual and homosexual women. More information about pregnancy, birth control methods, sexually transmitted diseases, and safer-sex practices is provided later in parts IV and V.

Family Values During young adulthood, women take on a different kind of relationship with their parents. The young adult sees older parents more as friends and consultants; however, the older parents may have some difficulty adjusting to this new view because they still see the young adult as their child and may tend to want to tell them what they "should" do.

In young adulthood, most women are seeking a relationship partner who can provide intimacy, and who may assist with the establishment and raising of a family if the woman chooses to have children. The idea of entering into a committed relationship is often a priority. If you rush into a relationship or if you settle for a partner who is not compatible with many of your values and ideas, then you are taking a great risk that the relationship will be fraught with extreme conflict or will not last.

According to the National Center for Health Statistics, in 1994, approximately 2,362,000 heterosexual couples married and 1,191,000 divorced. As of 1997, homosexual couples were not allowed to enter into a legal marriage contract, thus no official marriage and divorce records have been maintained on homosexual relationships. Most divorces occur within the first ten years of marriage. The median duration of marriage for divorcing couples in 1990 was 7.2 years. In 1990, the wife was awarded the custody of children involved in the divorce 72 percent of the time, joint custody was the second most common arrangement at 16 percent, and husbands were awarded custody 9 percent of the time.

Before you make a commitment with someone, it is a good idea to make a list of partner characteristics that you value, and judge potential partners on how many of these characteristics they meet. Being in a relationship is not just about being in love, it is also about compatibility, healthy communication, mutual respect and support, flexibility, and having fun. It is wise not to commit to someone on the expectation that they will change and be more of what you want them to be once you get them in the relationship. It is extremely unlikely that this will happen. More information about healthy relationships is discussed in chapter 14. Complete *Journal Activity:*

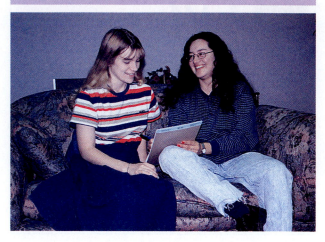

Developing friendships is a vital social skill.

"Valued Partner Characteristics" to help you determine the characteristics you value in a partner.

A young adult woman also needs friends outside of her relationship. Some levels of intimacy and trust can be exercised through friendships with others of both sexes. Also, spending time with friends can break the monotony of always being with your relationship partner. Friends can serve as good support mechanisms for the individual as well as for the relationship.

The young adult woman and, if she has one, her relationship partner face the decision of whether or not to have children. If they choose to have children, how many should they have, and how far apart? Once children arrive, decisions regarding the child must be made about day care, schools, house rules, and what type of family and spiritual values to influence upon the child.

In 1993, 29.9 percent of children under 5 years of age were cared for in day care or nursery schools; this figure is not much different for working married couples (30 percent) as compared to single working mothers (29.5 percent).[37] The average percent of family income spent on children for child care arrangements for families below the poverty income level was 21.1 percent; and for families whose income was above the poverty level, 7.0 percent of the family income was spent on child care arrangements.[38] The average weekly expenditures for persons making child care arrangement payments was $70 a week (or $280 a month).

When a child is taken care of by a parent who stays at home with the child, most of the time it is the woman who does so. However, this trend is shifting slightly, and in 1997, there were actually an estimated 2 million stay-at-home dads, but many of these had part-time or at home jobs.[39]

The responsibility of a child's upbringing is a very large and constant one. Knowledge about child care and effective parenting are vital for establishing a healthy, loving relationship with a child. Many schools and community agencies offer these type of educational opportunities for parents and prospective parents of all ages. Once a child arrives into the home, the welfare for that child must take priority over many other issues. However, with the right support, it is very possible for a woman to have children and pursue her own life goals. Table 3.3 shows the increasing number of working mothers in the U.S. workforce.

Life Goals   Human beings seek a sense of purposefulness in life. This is an extension of their spirituality. For young adult women, a sense of purpose is often achieved through establishing relationships and/or having children. In addition, it is a natural tendency for a woman to seek meaning and purpose through personal achievements that center on career and recreation. Young adulthood is the time when a woman begins to establish herself in her career. In addition, those areas of interest that are not part of her occupation can become hobbies. An occupation

Table 3.3

U.S. Women Who Had a Baby in the Past Year[40]

Year	Number (000s)	In the labor force (000s)	Percent in Labor Force
1994	3,890	2,066	53.1
1992	3,688	1,985	53.8
1990	3,913	2,068	52.8
1988	3,667	1,866	50.9
1986	3,625	1,805	49.8
1984	3,311	1,547	46.7
1982	3,433	1,508	43.9
1980	3,247	1,233	38.0
1978	3,168	1,120	35.3
1976	2,797	865	31.0

*Women aged 18–44 years.

Dentistry is an example of a profession in which a woman can own the business, set her own working hours, make good money, and provide jobs for others.

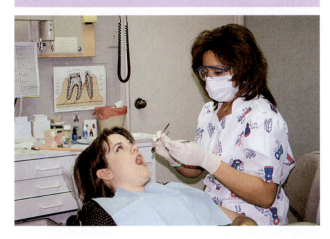

can be chosen on the basis of financial need, area of interest, or ideally, both. The more education a woman has, the greater the likelihood will be that she can become involved in a career that provides financial support and satisfies a great number of her interest areas.

Regardless of a woman's career choice, there will very likely be the presence of wage and promotion discrimination. (See Fig. 3.1.) As of 1997, in only 22 percent of dual income families did the woman get a higher salary than the man.[39] Overall, women

make the equivalent of about 70 cents for every dollar made by men. Women who make more than their male counterparts are often viewed as less feminine, which is meant as an insult in this context.[41]

Young adulthood is a time for financial planning. A woman needs to establish her own individual credit line, even if she shares some expenses and investments with her relationship partner. When a relationship is terminated due to a break up or death, the financial transition is less burdensome if a woman has established her own credit history. (See *Journal Activity:* "Setting Your Financial Goals.")

During young adulthood, many large purchases are made, such as a car and a house. It is also time to begin investing in a retirement plan and establishing other types of investments when possible, such as stocks and bonds, certificates of deposit, and so on.

CONCLUSION

Developmental theory has almost always emphasized the male standard and women have been ignored for the most part. That is why this chapter focused on some important life phases for women and the unique approach to life transitions that women have. In the past, women's differences from men have been viewed as inferior instead of as special in themselves. Women can do some very incredible things that men cannot do, and they can do some things better than men. But it is really not about who is better than whom, because both men and women make important

FIGURE 3.1 Average income by education attainment for women and men.

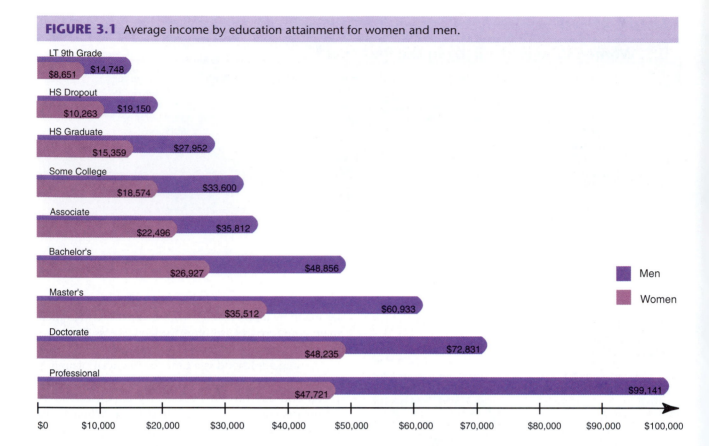

JOURNAL ACTIVITY

Setting Your Financial Goals

Examine some of the ideas presented below:[42]

Examples of short-term goals to be accomplished within 1–2 years:

- Pay off credit cards.
- Buy a new car.
- Change jobs.
- Start a college savings plan for yourself or your children.
- Make a down payment on a new home.

Examples of intermediate goals to be achieved within 2–15 years:

- Fund a college education for yourself or your children.
- Pay off your home mortgage.
- Buy a retirement home.
- Add rooms to your home.
- Become completely debt free.

Examples of long-term goals to be accomplished over a 15-year-plus period:

- Be able to retire.
- Start another business.
- Pay cash for a retirement home.

These are just some general examples. Your particular goals depend on your own hopes and dreams. You should start setting up a financial plan with short-term, intermediate, and long-term goals in young adulthood, but it is never too late to set up a financial plan with each of these types of goals. Take some time and write down a current financial plan for yourself with each of these types of goals in mind.

A woman's art can be a reflection of her unique culture. Angie Yazzie, a renowned master potter at the Taos Pueblo, displays her award-winning pottery.

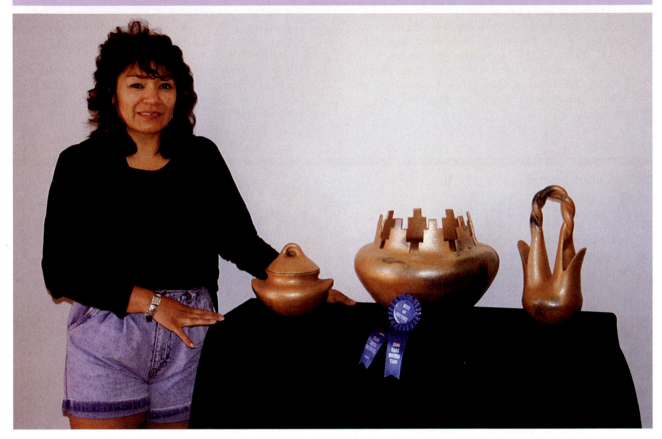

and necessary contributions. Neither sex is more significant than the other, and both are important for a healthy balance to exist in the world. Emphasizing women is important because there is historically and currently significantly less information published about women, and women's importance to world survival needs to be publicized. We will continue the adventure of exploring women's life transitions as we pick up the journey in the next chapter at middle adulthood and travel onward to late adulthood. ∞

Chapter Summary

- Sigmund Freud, a psychoanalyst, devised the stages of psychosexual development.
- Erik Erikson, a developmental psychologist, developed the stages of psychosocial development. He also developed the tasks to be completed during adolescence.
- Jean Piaget, a developmental psychologist, devised the stages for cognitive development.
- Lawrence Kohlberg devised the major premises for moral development.

- The developmental theories and ideas presented by Freud, Erikson, Piaget, and Kohlberg all tended to discriminate against the normal development of the female child, and gave preference to the development of the male child as the expected norm for both males and females.
- Carol Gilligan presented the first major ideas that served as the origins for a psychology of women.
- Infants and children have critical periods of development during which they must be exposed to a variety of

stimuli in order to learn significant developmental tasks or else their normal development will be hindered.

- Nutrition is a vital component to healthy development, as is exercise.
- An individual should be encouraged to develop both feminine and masculine traits to maximize their potential as a caregiver and career professional.
- Because the family is the first major social group from which a child learns, nurturing family interactions and positive parenting are vital for teaching the child social skills.

- A woman faces many negative messages in the media that can significantly impact the way she feels about her own body.
- Getting a good education is a key for career success. However, even with a college education, women will likely still experience some discrimination in job opportunities and salaries.
- A woman may acquire many complex social roles in her life that require a variety of social skills: daughter, sister, aunt, spouse, mother, grandmother, or great grandmother.

Review Questions

1. What are the stages of psychosexual development?
2. What are the stages of psychosocial development?
3. What are the stages of cognitive development?
4. Can you name the benefits of breast-feeding for the infant and for the mother?
5. What is gender-role socialization?
6. What are the psychosocial tasks to be accomplished during the period of adolescence?
7. What major roles are a young adult woman expected to play?

Resources

Organizations and Hotlines

League of Women Voters
1730 M Street, NW
Washington, DC 20036
Telephone: (202) 429–1965

National Organization of Parents, Families and Friends of Lesbians and Gays (PFLAG)
1012 Fourteenth, N.W., #700
Washington, DC 20005
Telephone: (202) 638–4200

Websites

National Organization for Women (NOW)
http://www.now.org/

National Lesbian and Gay Health Association
http://www.serve.com/nlgha/index.htm

LaLeche League International
http://www.zipmall.com/

Suggested Readings

Borysenko, J. 1996. *A woman's book of life.* New York: Riverhead Books.
Boston Women's Health Book Collective. 1992. *The new our bodies, ourselves.* New York: Touchstone.
Bricklin, M. 1993. *Prevention Magazine's nutrition advisor: The complete, up-to-date guide to healthy eating.* New York: MJF Books.
Gilligan, C. 1982. *In a different voice.* Cambridge, Mass.: Harvard University Press.
Lewis, J., and J. Bernstein. 1996. *Women's health: A relational perspective across the life cycle.* Boston: Jones & Bartlett.
Lewis, J., B. Hayes, and L. Bradley. 1992. *Counseling women over the life span.* Denver, Colo.: Love Publishing.
Peterson, A., and S. Rosenberg. 1997. *Every woman's guide to financial security.* Franklin Lakes, N.J.: Career Press.
Reuben, C., and J. Priestley. 1991. *What every woman should know about vitamins, minerals, enzymes, & amino acids.* San Francisco: Thorsons.
Sheehy, G. 1977. *Passages.* Bantam Books.
Sheehy, G. 1995. *New passages: Mapping your life across time.* New York: Random House.
Stein, D. 1992. *The natural remedy book for women.* Freedom, Calif.: Crossing Press.
Wharton, L. 1995. *The natural guide to women's health: How a woman can be healthy at any age.* New York: MJF Books.

References

1. Gilligan, C. 1979. Women's place in man's life cycle. *Harvard Educational Review* 49 (4): 431–46.

2. Gilligan, C. 1982. *In a different voice: Psychological theory and women's development.* Cambridge, Mass.: Harvard University Press.

3. Ellers, F. 1997. Parents need to learn how to talk too. *Louisville Courier-Journal* 24 April, E3.

4. Myers, L. 1996. Gunfire among leading causes of death for children, report says. *Louisville Courier-Journal* 9 April, B7.

5. Dermer, A., and A. Montgomery. 1997. Breastfeeding: Good for babies, mothers and the planet. *The Medical Reporter,* April, website: http://www.dash.com/netro/nwx/tmr0297/breastfeed0297.html

6 Martin, J. 1997. The politics of breastfeeding. *Parents Place,* April, website: http://parentsplace.com/readroom/articles/politics.html

7. U.S. Bureau of the Census. 1988. *Statistical abstract of the U.S., 1988,* 108th ed. Washington, D.C.: U.S. Government Printing Office, p. 64.

8. Williams, R. 1995. Breast-feeding best bet for babies. *FDA Consumer Magazine* (October).

9. Rice, F. P. 1992. *Human development: A lifespan approach.* New York: Macmillan.

10. DiPietro, J. B. 1981. Rough and tumble play. A function of gender. *Developmental Psychology* 17: 50–58.

11. Micheli, L. J. 1988. The incidence of injuries in children's sports: A medical perspective. In *Competitive sports for children and youth: An overview of research and issues.* Edited by E. W. Brown and C. F. Branta. Champaign, Ill: Human Kinetics, pp. 280–84.

12. Martens, R. 1988. Helping children become independent, responsible adults through sports. In *Competitive Sports for Children and Youth: An Overview of Research and Issues.* Edited by E. W. Brown and C. F. Branta. Champaign, Ill.: Human Kinetics, pp. 297–307.

13. Miller, C. L. 1987. Qualitative differences among gender-stereotyped toys: Implications for cognitive and social development in girls and boys. *Sex Roles* 16 (9/10): 473–78.

14. Lips, H. M. 1989. Gender-role socialization: Lessons in femininity. In *Women: A Feminist Perspective,* 4th ed. Edited by J. Freeman. Mountain View, Calif.: Mayfield, pp. 197–216.

15. Bem, S. L. 1974. The measurement of psychological androgyny. *Journal of Consulting and Clinical Psychology* 42 (2): 155–62.

16. Block, J. H. 1984. Psychological development of female children and adolescents. In *Sex Role Identity and Ego Development.* Edited by Jeanne H. Block. Jossey-Bass, pp. 126–42.

17. Weitzman, N., B. Birns, and R. Friend. 1985. Traditional and nontraditional mothers' communication with their daughters and sons. *Child Development* 56: 894–98.

18. Frankel, M. T., and H. A. Rollins, Jr. 1983. Does mother know best? Mothers and fathers interacting with preschool sons and daughters. *Developmental Psychology* 19 (5): 694–702.

19. Entwisle, D. R., and D. P. Baker. 1983. Gender and young children's expectations for performance in arithmetic. *Developmental Psychology* 19 (2): 200–209.

20. The National Exchange Club Foundation for the Prevention of Child Abuse, April 1997, website:http://rtpnet.org/~nec/trtwell.htm

21. U.S. Census Bureau, 1995. USA statistics in brief.

22. Wharton, L. 1995. *The natural guide to women's health: How a woman can be healthy at any age.* New York: MJF Books.

23. United Nations. 1992. *Demographic Yearbook 1990.* New York: United Nations, Department of International Economic and Social Affairs, Statistical Office, pp. 313–31.

24. U.S. Census Bureau. 1995. Percentage of women who have had a child in the last year who were unmarried: June 1990-1994. Washington, D.C.: U.S. Census Bureau.

25. U.S. Census Bureau. 1994. Births to unmarried women, selected countries: 1970 to 1992. *Statistical Abstract of the United States.* Washington, D. C.: U.S. Census Bureau.

26. Editorial. *Sports Illustrated,* 14 April 1997, p. 5.

27. CBS Television Network. Best Friends Program. CBS Sunday Morning, 27 April 1997.

28. Katz, P. A. 1986. Gender identity: Development and consequences. In *The social psychology of female-male relations.* Edited by R. D. Ashmore & F. K. Del Boca. Orlando, Fla.: Academic Press, pp. 21–67.

29. Herek, G. M. 1989. Hate crimes against lesbians and gay men. *American Psychologist* 44 (6): 949–55.

30. Comstock, G. D. 1991. *Violence against lesbians and gay men.* New York: Columbia University.

31. Roll over Ward Cleaver and tell Ozzie Nelson the news: Ellen DeGeneres is poised to become TV's first openly gay star. *Time Magazine,* 14 April 1997, pp. 78–86.

32. Burnett, J. W., W. P. Anderson, and P. P. Heppner. 1995. Gender roles and self-esteem: A consideration of environmental factors. *Journal of Counseling and Development* 73 (3): 323–26.

33. Williams, C. W. 1991. *Black teenage mothers: Pregnancy and childrearing from their perspective.* Lexington, Mass.: Lexington Books.

34. Merrick, E. 1995. Adolescent childbearing as career "choice": Perspective from an ecological context. *Journal of Counseling and Development* 73 (3): 288-95.

35. Trad, P. V. 1995. Adolescent girls and their mothers: Realigning the relationship. *The American Journal of Family Therapy* 23 (1): 11-24.

36. Associated Press. 1995. Dow Corning files for bankruptcy. *Denton Record Chronicle,* Denton, Tex. 15 May 1995, vol. 91, no. 286, p. 1.

37. U.S. Census Bureau. 1994. Percent of children under 5 in selected child care arrangements: 1977-1993.

38. U.S. Census Bureau. 1994. Weekly child care costs paid by families with employed mothers: 1985-1993.

39. CNN Headline News Network. At home dads. CNN Financial News, 12 April 1997.

40. U.S. Census Bureau. 1995. Percentage of women in the labor force who had a birth last year: 1976-1994.

41. Casamassima, C. 1995. Battle of the bucks. *Psychology Today* (March/April): 43-45, 67-68.

42. Peterson, A., and S. Rosenberg. 1997. *Every woman's guide to financial security,* 2nd ed. Franklin Lakes, N.J.: Career Press.

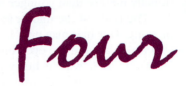

Life Transitions: *Middle to Late Adulthood*

■ chapter objectives

When you complete this chapter you will be able to:
- Explain the major life issues for women in middle to late adulthood, including: physical status, social influences, self-image, family issues, and life goals.
- Describe the physical, emotional, and social implications of menopause.

PHASES OF LIFE

Let's say that you have now turned 40 years old. Congratulations, you are at middle age. This is assuming that you only live to the estimated average life span for U.S. women, which is 79 years of age. However, you may live much longer than that. There are women in their nineties and older who live very active lives. But let's back up to age 40 first and see what life is like in middle adulthood.

Middle Adulthood

A woman is in middle adulthood when she is in her forties and fifties. This is often referred to as "middle age." Many women feel that middle age is a time when they can live a life freer of obligations and full of fun. This is a time when most women have raised their children (or their children are old enough not to need as much care), established themselves in their career, gained financial security including sav-

ing some money, and have more flexibility in their schedules for travel and recreation.

Physical Status The physical signs of middle age can be worn like a badge of courage; it says to others, "I have been there and done that already." Because of her years of accumulated experience, a middle-aged woman is often wiser and more emotionally mature than younger women.

The body of the middle-aged woman shows signs of aging. Her hair may gray in places, her face begins to wrinkle around the eyes and mouth, her skin is not as elastic as it was in her youth, and she does not have the same kind of physical stamina she once had. She will begin to feel some of the aches and pains associated with an aging body. When she exercises, she will feel sorer the next day because her body will not recover as quickly as it did in her youth.

The effects of the aging process on the woman's body are viewed by many as a loss of youthful beauty. Others have a healthy appreciation for the physical signs of aging. A woman can wear the physical signs of aging like a trophy that is earned from a life's work of achievements. Aging is a reflection of accumulated wisdom and experience. The middle-age woman has a special, mature beauty not available to younger women.

Because she may have less stamina than younger women, middle-aged women may find it more difficult to stay physically fit. However, fitness is no less important at this age than at any other. Participation in physical fitness activities is a must whether it be individual activities like walking, biking, and swimming, or group activities like dance aerobics, golf, or tennis.

A middle-aged woman finds it more difficult to keep the body fat down. Thus, significant adjustments in the diet may have to be made, such as a reduced calorie diet and the avoidance of foods containing animal fats and processed sugars. A health care provider may even recommend dietary supplements such as vitamins, iron, and calcium.

Menopause In middle adulthood, "m" stands for menopause, or the big "M" as it is fondly referred to. A middle-age woman is facing the onset of **menopause.** This is the time when her reproductive cycle is coming to an end and the balance of hormones in her body change. **Perimenopause,** which involves the early symptoms suggesting that the big "M" is near, can be present in a woman's life for a few years before the actual onset of menopause. Perimenopause typically occurs in women in their early to mid forties. It can involve any number of symptoms that may come and go for periods of time, such as an irregular menstrual cycle or flow, night sweats, hot flashes, or mood swings.

Menopause itself commonly occurs in women in their late forties to mid fifties. The menstrual cycle

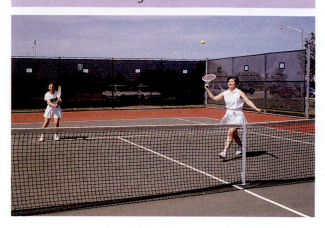

Staying fit through exercise is very important to the health of the middle-aged woman.

slows and eventually ceases, and the symptoms that were present during perimenopause become more prevalent. A menopausal woman can wake up in the middle of the night drenched in her own sweat, or have such intense hot flashes at any time so that she feels like ripping her clothes off and standing in a refrigerator. Between 63 and 75 percent of menopausal women experience hot flashes ranging in intensity from an occasional sensation of heat to frequent drenching sweats. Accompanying menopause are a number of other potential discomforts such as dryness and irritation in the vagina, urinary incontinence, chronic vaginal and bladder infections, insomnia, migraines, depression, anxiety, dry skin, bone-thinning problems (osteoporosis). Remember when you were moody and irritable while you were "PMS-ing" in your younger days? Well, you can break all of those old records for emotional intensity during your menopausal phase. Some women take hormone replacement therapy to counter the effects of menopause. Hormone replacement therapy entails some health risks, so some women may prefer to take natural herbs to decrease the negative symptoms of menopause. *Health Tips:* "Natural Remedies for the Ills of Menopause" lists suggestions for natural remedies to counter menopausal symptoms. Menopause and hormone replacement therapy are addressed in additional detail in chapter 15.

Family Values The middle-adult woman continues with the projects she began in young adulthood. If she has children, they are older now and she is assisting them with their movement toward and through adolescence and young adulthood. Or, her

health tips

Natural Remedies for the Ills of Menopause[1]

Consult with a health-care provider about using the following natural remedies to counter the symptoms of menopause:

- Take vitamin and mineral supplements such as vitamin E, a balanced high-potency B complex, and a multi-mineral formula of calcium and magnesium.
- Make dietary adjustments such as cutting out all refined carbohydrates, including white bread, white rice, white pasta, cookies, candies, sugar, and sugar-laden cereals; and replace them with unrefined carbohydrates, including whole grain bread, brown rice, whole wheat pasta, fresh fruits, and starchy vegetables such as potato, pumpkin, and yams. If you are on a three meal-a-day plan, change to six mini-meals a day.
- Participate in aerobic exercise such as walking, biking, jumping on a trampoline, or other aerobic activity.
- Try some herbal and homeopathic remedies such as belladonna for intense hot flashes; lachesis for hot flashes and headaches; pulsatilla for emotions and mild hot flashes; nat mur for vaginal dryness, depression, and tearfulness; bryonia for vaginal dryness and severe constipation; staphisagria for dry, thin vaginal membranes, as well as for anger and resentment; and chamomille for insomnia.

children may have gone out on their own by now and she struggles with the **empty-nest syndrome.** The empty-nest syndrome is a type of crisis for the middle-adult woman whose children have left home and the woman, whose life was once filled with activity for support and care of her children, now finds herself with a sense of less purpose.

Middle adulthood is a time for doing those things that a woman might have postponed because of other priorities. If a woman has delayed a career to have children, then she may be considering entering or reentering the workforce in middle age. Or on the other hand, if a woman has delayed having children because of her career, she may be having children in her forties in an effort to beat the onset of menopause, when her reproductive potential ends.

Other relationships for a middle-aged woman may also begin to take on a different shape. If her parents are still living, the middle-aged woman may

move into a supportive, caregiving role with them either emotionally, financially, physically, or all three depending on the state of her parents. Her relationship with her husband or partner has matured to a comfortable, familiar level, or perhaps she has a different relationship partner now than she did in young adulthood. It is not uncommon for women to seek a new relationship partner in middle adulthood, usually someone who is more compatible with who she is at this phase of her life.

A woman can play various roles in her life: daughter, sister, mother, grandmother, great-grandmother, and even great, great-grandmother. The role of grandmother commonly begins in middle adulthood. At middle age, a woman may be guiding her children to have and raise children of their own.

Financial Status A middle-aged woman often owns her own home, car, and maybe even her own business, and she is well on her way to paying into a retirement plan. A woman who is married or partnered may share some of the daily living expenses with her mate and also share in some of the major investments. Women in poverty or divorced or widowed women may find it difficult just to pay for daily living expenses and may not be able to set aside the monies necessary to invest in property, or to plan for retirement. These women will be especially vulnerable to financial stress when they reach late adulthood. If there are any major child care expenses for a woman in middle adulthood, it is more likely to be paying for a child's wedding or college education.

Life Goals Middle age is a time when a woman looks back upon what she has accomplished, evaluates her happiness, and makes significant adjustments based on what she wants from this next part of her life. She is an experienced and skilled worker

---

menopause—the hormonal shift that occurs in middle adulthood that signals the end of the reproduction cycle.

perimenopause—the early signs signaling the coming of menopause.

empty-nest syndrome—the sense of purposelessness for a middle-aged woman when all of her children have grown up and left home.

Four generations of women. A woman can play many roles in her life, such as daughter, mother, grandmother, and great-grandmother.

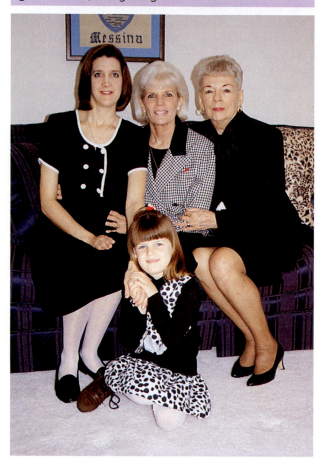

By middle age, a woman can own her own home.

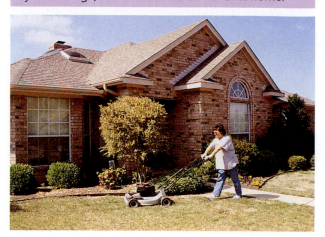

JOURNAL ACTIVITY

What Is It Like to Be in the Middle of Life?

If you are under the age of 40 years old, interview a woman who is in her forties or fifties; or if you are 40 or older, then write about what middle age is or was like for you. Ask about how middle adulthood was different from young adulthood in some of these areas: physically, emotionally, in a career, family issues, child care issues, financial issues and so on. Also, ask about the life goals and ambitions in middle adulthood of your interviewee.

and she has finely tuned her talents. She may be at the peak of her career with a flourishing business of her own. She may want to stay in the same job, or she may want something new and different. She may want to stay in her home, or she may decide to try a different home or move to a new part of the country or the world. A woman in middle adulthood is more aware that her life span is limited and she may want to get as much from what is left as she can before time runs out.

The evaluation process that occurs in middle adulthood is referred to as the **midlife crisis.** It is another extension of the spiritual dimension in human beings. A woman in this phase of her life is examining how she has come to fit into her family, her community, her country, the world, the cosmos. She is determining whether she has obtained the sense of meaningfulness and purposefulness that she

desires. She is looking at what else she wants to accomplish in her life and how she wants to relate to others and to the world. (See *Journal Activity:* "What Is It Like to Be in the Middle of Life?")

Sometimes a woman's relationship partner may go through a midlife crisis. If a divorce is the result, then the dreams and expectations of living one's life with that person are gone. A lifestyle that was used to a dual income now has to adjust to a single income. The emotional upheaval and sense of rejection from divorce can be devastating. Trying to get back into the dating game at the age of 40 or 50 may seem awkward, and the prospect of having to spend most of your time alone can be unpleasant. (See *Her Story:* "Renee.") In 1989, there were 4.5 million divorced women aged 45 or older in the United States and more than 1.6 million over the age of 65.[2] One-fourth of all divorced women subsist at the poverty level.

Sandy Seth raises miniature horses in New Mexico.

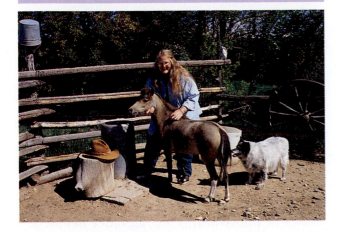

Valerie Graves is an accomplished professional artist.

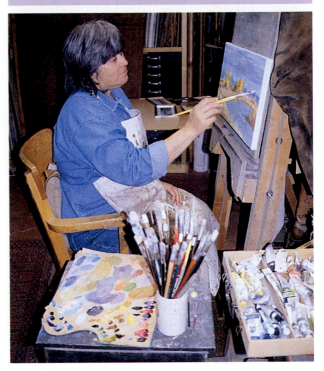

Her Story

Renee

When Renee was 44 years old, her husband wanted a divorce. He had fallen in love with a younger woman. Renee received very little money from the divorce settlement. After the divorce, Renee and her 12-year-old son moved across the country to the mountains of northern New Mexico to get a fresh start. Renee had often dreamed of living near the Rocky Mountains. They rented a small two-bedroom house in the country. She could only find part-time work as a drug-and-alcohol counselor, so they had to struggle to make it financially. Though things were rough, Renee enjoyed her new freedom and took up hiking and cross-country skiing. After a year of looking, Renee found a full-time job and things became a little easier financially. Renee's income is still low, especially compared to what she was used to before the divorce when the family had two incomes. Although Renee has been dating, three years later she is still not in a committed relationship. However, Renee loves northern New Mexico and is finding happiness there.

- Do you know someone with a similar story where their life changed drastically in middle adulthood?

women. By the year 2000, there will be 4 million more people in the United States over the age of 65 than in 1990, and the number of people living beyond age 85 is at record levels.[3] The population aged 85 and over is expected to grow from 3,000,000 in 1990 to 8,000,000 in 2030 and to 18,000,000 by the year 2050.[4] As life expectancy increases, the number of years of good health in comparison to chronic illness is important. How will American society support and care for its increasing numbers of elderly persons?

Aging women in developing countries remain a smaller proportion of the population than in developed countries.[5] Whereas women age 60 years and older account for around 20 percent of the female population in developed regions of the world, they account for only some 7 percent of women in developing countries. The equivalent proportions for men

Late Adulthood

When a woman reaches the age of 60, she moves into late adulthood; an individual in this phase of life is referred to by society as a **senior citizen.** In 1993, about 60 percent of America's nearly 33,000,000 elderly, that is, persons 65 years of age and over, were

midlife crisis—the life review and evaluation process that occurs in middle adulthood.

senior citizen—a person in late adulthood, usually 60 years of age or older.

60 years and over are nearly 15 percent in developed countries and 6 percent in developing countries.

It is important to encourage groups of older women to consider their own future health in order to alert health policy makers to potential problems. For example, in Latin America it is projected that 60 percent of women who were aged 45–49 years in 1990 will survive to age 75–79 in the year 2020. The health that these survivors can expect in their old age will depend on the social and physical environments in which they live over the next thirty years. Evaluate your knowledge about aging by completing *Assess Yourself!:* "Palmore's Facts on Aging Quiz."

Physical Status   The body of the senior woman demonstrates the continuation of the aging process. The hair can be mostly to all gray, more wrinkles appear in the skin, the skin has lost most of its elastic quality, age spots can appear on the hands and elsewhere, physical strength significantly declines, calcium loss may create a fragile bone structure, and as the woman gets older her spinal disks may compact, which causes her to loose some height.

"Seniorhood" is a time when women are at greater risk for disorders and diseases associated with aging. Some of the more common age-related diseases include: osteoporosis, arthritis, dementia and Alzheimer's, cancer, cardiovascular disorders, advanced gum disease, failing sight, and hearing loss. More about age-related disorders and diseases is discussed in chapter 15.

Exercise can postpone or diminish the symptoms of many disorders related to aging. Popular activities for fitness maintenance for senior women include: swimming, water aerobics, walking, biking, and light weight lifting. However, some women race cars and jet skis in their sixties and seventies. You should not stop having fun just because you get older. (See *Her Story:* "Aletha Keach.")

Over 4,000,000 elderly persons need assistance with one or more everyday activities. Chronic illnesses increase with age and are more common among women, who average more years of chronic illness than men. Among those age 85 and over, almost 25 percent live in a nursing home because of serious health problems.[8] Of the elderly living at a home, about 40 percent have a condition that limits their activities. Functional limitations are highest among elderly black women and those with relatively low incomes.

The appetite for a senior is often less than that of other age groups. A major problem that often exists for seniors is the maintenance of a healthy diet with the proper nutritional balance. Elderly persons have a different sleep cycle than they did when they were younger. Instead of requiring one period of 8 to 10 hours of continuous sleep in a 24-hour cycle as they did when they were younger, the elderly usually sleep for much shorter periods at a time, taking several naps in a 24-hour cycle.

Although heart disease is the leading cause of death for persons age 65 and over, unintentional injuries are the seventh leading cause of death among older adults.[9] In 1991, more than 10,000 people over age 65 died of unintentional injuries. The major causes of injury deaths among older people are motor vehicle crashes, falls, drownings, fires and burns, and poisonings. These high mortality rates are related to: decreasing ability to perceive and avoid hazards such as moving automobiles; musculoskeletal, perceptual, and balance difficulties that increase the likelihood of falls; greater likelihood that an incident will produce injury since older bodies are more frail; and poorer outcomes following an injury because older bodies do not heal as well.

Family Values   The senior woman has seen her children grow up. Her parents have probably passed away by now. Her role in her family is that of grandmother, great-grandmother, or elder aunt. She is mostly removed from having a direct impact on the caretaking of others. Many of the people she has known have passed on, and she is aware of her own advancing age. She has experienced a great deal of grief and loss in her life and faces the contemplation of living and dying on a frequent basis. The older adult woman may struggle to maintain a sense of meaning and purpose during this time of her life, especially because many of the persons who used to rely on her no longer need her or she is not as capable as she used to be.

An ancient female cultural archetype for a woman in late adulthood is the "wise crone." The crone recognizes the strength and wisdom of the elder woman along with her insatiable capacity for maternal love. The wise crone holds a position of great respect and admiration. Elder women in today's American society do not seem to get the respect they have earned as the elder, wise crone of the family. This is merely a matter of societal attitude. The elderly today are not valued as highly for their

Assess **Y O U R S E L F**

Palmore's Facts on Aging Quiz[6]

Circle the appropriate answer for each of the following questions. Compare your responses with the correct answers located after the quiz.

1. In old age, a person's height
   a. does not change.
   b. only appears to change.
   c. tends to decline.
   d. depends on how active one is.

2. As compared to younger persons, more older persons (65 or over) are limited in their activity by which type of illnesses?
   a. acute illnesses (short-term)
   b. colds and flu
   c. infections
   d. chronic illnesses

3. Which type of illnesses do older persons have less frequently than younger persons?
   a. chronic illnesses
   b. colds and flu
   c. infections
   d. acute illnesses

4. Compared with younger persons, older persons have
   a. more injuries in the home.
   b. have about the same number of injuries in the home.
   c. have less injuries in the home.
   d. are twice as likely to be injured in the home.

5. Older workers
   a. have higher rates of absenteeism than younger workers.
   b. cannot be depended upon.
   c. have about the same rates of absenteeism as younger workers.
   d. have lower rates of absenteeism than younger workers.

6. The life expectancy of African Americans at age 65
   a. is higher than that of whites.
   b. is lower than that of whites.
   c. is the same as that of whites.
   d. has never been determined.

7. Men's life expectancy at age 65 as compared to women's life expectancy
   a. is lower.
   b. tends to be returning to what it was in the 1940s.
   c. is about the same.
   d. is higher.

8. What percent of medical expenses for the aged does Medicare pay?
   a. nearly 50 percent
   b. nearly 70 percent
   c. nearly 100 percent
   d. about 15 to 20 percent

9. Social Security benefits
   a. automatically increase with inflation.
   b. are not subject to change.
   c. are not adjusted to meet inflation.
   d. are often cut back in times of inflation.

10. Supplementary Security Income (SSI)
    a. guarantees a minimum income for the needy elderly.
    b. provides extra income for all the elderly.
    c. supplements the income of the elderly in nursing homes.
    d. pays medical expenses for the elderly.

11. As far as the aged getting their proportionate share of the nation's income,
    a. most of the aged live below the poverty level.
    b. the aged are the poorest group in our society.
    c. the aged do get their proportionate share of income.
    d. the income gap between the aged and other adult groups continues to widen.

12. Compared to persons under 65, rates of criminal victimization among the elderly are
    a. higher.
    b. lower.
    c. much the same.
    d. steadily increasing.

13. Regarding crime and the elderly,
    a. they are more fearful of crime than are younger persons.
    b. they fear crime the same as other age groups.
    c. they are less fearful of crime than are younger persons.
    d. most elderly persons have no fear of crime.

14. The most law abiding of all adult age groups are
    a. the middle aged.
    b. persons in their thirties.
    c. young couples.
    d. the elderly.

Continued.

Assess **YOURSELF**

Palmore's Facts on Aging Quiz—Continued.

15. Regarding the number of widows and widowers among the aged,
    a. their numbers are about equal.
    b. there are nearly five times as many widows as widowers.
    c. there are about twice as many widowers as widows.
    d. the number of widows is rapidly increasing.
16. When it comes to voter participation rates,
    a. the aged seldom vote.
    b. those age 35–44 tend to have higher rates than the elderly.
    c. college students have higher rates than do the elderly.
    d. older people have higher rates than the rest of the population.
17. In reference to public office
    a. there is no relationship between age and public office.
    b. older people are seldom found in public offices.
    c. there are proportionately more older persons in public office.
    d. there are proportionately more younger persons in public office.
18. The proportion of African Americans among the aged is
    a. growing.
    b. declining.
    c. very small compared with other minority groups.
    d. staying about the same.
19. Participation in voluntary organizations
    a. usually does not decline among healthy older persons.
    b. drops among healthy older persons.
    c. rises among healthy older persons.
    d. is highest among the youth.

20. The majority of old people live
    a. alone.
    b. in institutions.
    c. with their spouses.
    d. with their children.
21. The rate of poverty among the elderly
    a. is lower than among those under 65.
    b. is higher than among those under 65.
    c. is the same as it is for other age groups.
    d. is high as a result of their having fixed incomes.
22. The rate of poverty among aged African Americans
    a. is less than that of whites.
    b. is about the same as that of whites.
    c. is about triple that of older whites.
    d. continues to increase.
23. Older persons who reduce their activity tend to be
    a. happier.
    b. not as happy as those who remain active.
    c. more well-adjusted than those who remain active.
    d. healthier.
24. When the last child leaves home, the majority of parents
    a. have serious problems of adjustment.
    b. have higher levels of life satisfaction.
    c. try to get their children to come back home.
    d. suffer from the "empty nest" syndrome.
25. The proportion of the widowed among the aged
    a. is gradually decreasing.
    b. is rapidly increasing.
    c. has remained the same in the last half century.
    d. is unrelated to increasing longevity.

Correct answers: (1) c, (2) d, (3) d, (4) c, (5) d, (6) c, (7) a, (8) a, (9) a, (10) a, (11) c, (12) b, (13) a, (14) d, (15) b, (16) d, (17) c, (18) a, (19) a, (20) c, (21) a, (22) c, (23) b, (24) b, (25) a.

life experiences, perhaps because the United States is so materialistic and technologically dependent. The elderly, who may not be up-to-date on the latest technological gadgetry, are viewed as out-of-touch. However, the elderly do have much to teach the younger generations, especially in the life areas of love, courage, perseverance, and emotional strength in the face of challenge and tragedy. The life stories of the

elderly provide excellent guidelines for living during any time period. (See *FYI:* "The Female Archetype of the Wise Crone.")

Marital status and living arrangements vary for the elderly. However, because of longevity factors, elderly men are much more likely to be married than elderly women. So elderly men are more likely to have a spouse who can take care of them if they be-

Her Story

Aletha Keach

Aletha Keach, 96 years old, is in pretty good shape as an instructor of yoga, nutrition, and reflexology at the Senior Center.[7] She attributes her vigorous, beautiful health to following a few simple principles of nutrition and fitness, and to an insatiable appetite for and interest in life. "I've always been interested in the world around me, in the people around me, in creating things, and in appreciating beautiful things like music. Life is having interesting things to learn and to do. I'm still getting interested in new things." She is a strong advocate of yoga and believes the slow and smooth stretching is good for everyone at any age. She teaches a Dynamic Health class in eight-week courses, three times a year at the Senior Center that incorporates yoga, reflexology, and nutrition. Her favorite exercise though is walking and she has organized walking clubs at several different sites. After participants have walked 100 miles at various sites, they are awarded a beret hand-knit by Ms. Keach. Knitting is one of many needle arts Ms. Keach practices and teaches. She is a trained seamstress and tailor, but has concentrated on the decorative arts with needlepoint, quilting, tatting and other outlets for her creative energies.

- Your community is most likely full of seniors with vast experiences and talents. How many do you know?
- Can you take some time from your schedule to interview or interact with some interesting seniors?
- How can you benefit from such interactions?

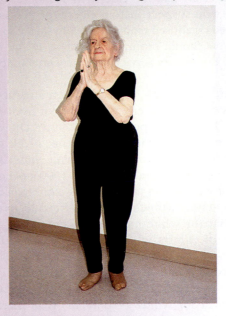

Aletha stays fit at age 96 by walking and practicing yoga.

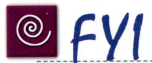

The Female Archetype of the Wise Crone[10]

The crone's title was related to the word "crown," and she represented the power of the ancient tribal matriarch, who made the moral and legal decisions for her subjects and descendants. As the embodiment of wisdom, she was supposed to have written the first tablets of the law and punished the first sinners. She also established the cyclic system of perpetual becoming by which every temporary living form in the universe blends eventually into every other form, nothing is unrelated, and there can be no hierarchy, better or worse, and no "we" and "they." ∞

come ill. Over 9,000,000 elderly live alone; 78 percent are women.[11]

There is a widespread perception in America that older persons are not sexually active. The reality is that many older people enjoy an active sex life that is often better than their sex life in early adulthood. A survey in 1992 showed that 37 percent of married people over age 60 have sex once a week or more and 16 percent have sex several times a week.[12]

It is a tragedy that many elderly persons are victims of neglect or abuse. In 1992, it was estimated that about 900,000 older Americans were abused by their own children, but some sources suggest that this figure is even higher.[13] The identified risk factors that contribute to elder abuse are: an unhealthy dependence by the perpetrator upon the victim, and vice versa; the disturbed psychological state of the perpetrator; the frailty, disability, or impairment of the victim; the social isolation of the family; or over-stressed caregivers with insufficient knowledge of or access to resources.[14,15]

Financial abuse of the elderly is another type of victimization. Children can steal from their parents relatively easily, and salespersons and repair companies can easily talk the elderly into unnecessary services. If you suspect that an elderly person is being neglected or abused emotionally, physically, or financially, you should report the incident to the Protective and Regulatory Services in your community.

Financial Status   There has been a reduction in the percentage of elderly who are poor from 35 percent in 1959 to 12 percent in 1990.[16] The elderly poor are disproportionately female, black or Hispanic, 75 years and older, and living alone. Among the elderly age 75 and older, the 1990 poverty rate for black women (44 percent) was more than double that for white women (17 percent) and over five times that for white men (8 percent). In 1990, 24 percent of elderly white females who lived alone were poor, compared with 58 percent of black elderly women and 50 percent of Hispanic elderly women. For elderly married couples, poverty rates were lower for whites (4 percent) than blacks (22 percent) or Hispanics (16 percent).

For many Americans, Social Security has turned into their sole retirement plan and primary retirement income. This was *not* its original purpose. The Social Security Tax that is applied to each of your paychecks throughout your life was originally levied to help ensure that when you reached an older age that you would not be completely destitute. With the increasing number of older persons that rely on Social Security, Social Security has become an ever-increasing burden on taxpayers of all ages. Social Security is constantly being examined by politicians with the intent of someday maybe even dissolving it completely. If you are currently under age 50, there is a good chance that, when you reach retirement age, Social Security will not be available to you, even though you will have spent years paying into it. If you are 50 or older, Social Security may be there for you in some degree, however we are not talking about very much money. The average monthly benefit for all retired workers in 1997 was $745. Social Security should not be your sole retirement plan. *You* must establish a retirement plan at an early age to prepare for a comfortable income after age 60 years (See *FYI:* "Social Security" and *Journal Activity:* "Retirement Planning.")

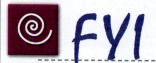

Social Security: Will You Benefit?[17]

You are entitled to retirement benefits if you have reached age 62 years. If you begin receiving Social Security at 62, you will not receive full benefits. For that to occur, you must refrain from taking benefits until the normal retirement age of 65. However, the "normal retirement age" will change in the years ahead.

- If you reach age 62 between the years 2000 and 2005, normal retirement age, starting at age 65, increases by 2 months per year for each of those years.
- Normal retirement age will be age 66, if you reach age 62 between 2005 and 2016.
- If you reach age 62 between 2016 and 2022, normal retirement age, starting at age 66, increases by 2 months a year for each of those years.
- Normal retirement age will be age 67, if you reach age 62 after 2022.

JOURNAL ACTIVITY

Retirement Planning

How much money should you set aside for retirement? The answer is, "as much as you need to generate enough income for the rest of your life." The earlier you start setting aside a percentage of your income for retirement the less you will have to set aside each year. However, if you wait until later in life, you will have to set aside a much larger proportion of your income per year in order to catch up. The following is a list of the estimated percentage of your income that you need to set aside per year until retirement age in order to have a retirement income that will last for the rest of your life:

Age You Begin	Percent of Income to set Aside Every Year[18]
20	10–15
30	15–20
40	20–30
50	30–40

Write down the amount of money you should begin setting aside every year for retirement based on your current age. If you already have begun a retirement investment, calculate the amount using the age that you did start setting aside for your retirement.

Life Goals The senior woman may be facing retirement issues. She usually quits working in her sixties and spends more time with recreation and travel. It is very important for the senior woman to stay active. The body and the mind will deteriorate more quickly if they are not exercised frequently. (See *Viewpoint:* "Over the Hill? Don't Bet on It!")

Viewpoint

Over the Hill? Don't Bet on It!

Drag racer Cleo Chandler came in eighth in the 1991 International Hot Rod Association Spring Nationals in spite of being 76 years old and a great-grandmother.[19] Do you think that a 76-year-old should be running around in a race car? Do you know a woman who is in her sixties, seventies, or even older who is an active and vibrant woman? What do you think keeps her active?

Participation in social groups is a popular way to stay active and involved in the community. Most communities have senior citizen centers to facilitate senior activities. Some seniors volunteer their time to others, for example, with reading groups for children at the library, visiting with and running errands for disabled persons, political activist groups, visiting lecturers at colleges, and so on. Maggie Kuhn was 65 years old when she cofounded the Gray Panthers to protest the Vietnam War. The Gray Panthers is still a powerful political lobbying force today. (See *Her Story:* "Maggie Kuhn.")

The elderly face certain stressors unique to their age group. The senior citizen is living on a fixed income based primarily on Social Security benefits and, if they have any, retirement savings. The senior has more medical problems because disorders and diseases are more prevalent in the aging body. Medical insurance is very expensive and social programs designed to assist with medical expenses for those with limited incomes,

Her Story

Maggie Kuhn

Maggie Kuhn was one of the founders of the Gray Panthers. She led a full and interesting life. The following are clips from just a few of her life experiences.[20] She was born in Buffalo, New York on August 31, 1905, in her grandmother's front bedroom; grew up in Cleveland; and graduated with honors from high school in 1922 and from college in 1926. She was sexually active with her boyfriend and utilized a diaphragm to prevent pregnancy. After college, she worked at the YWCA in Cleveland, Philadelphia, and later in New York, where she organized programs for working women, started classes on marriage and human sexuality, and provided programming for women workers assisting in the World War II effort. In 1950 she went to work for the Presbyterian Church for which she traveled extensively to teach social justice issues to clergy and laity; however, her salary was thousands less than that of men who had equal or lesser jobs. By age 41, she had two mastectomies. In 1958, she secured a mortgage and bought her own home in Philadelphia during a time when single women were not readily given loans because they were considered to be "undesirable risks." She commuted to work in New York City. In the 1960s, she developed a special interest in the problems of the elderly. During this period, the Presbyterian Church enforced its mandatory retirement policy upon her when she was 65 years old even though she did not yet desire retirement. In 1970 she, and five other active professional women who were facing retirement, founded the Gray Panthers to protest the Vietnam War and later to address numerous social issues specific to the elderly. These issues included minority discrimination by the Social Security system, discrimination of lending policies by banks, nursing home reform, health-care policies and concerns, home health-care advocacy, and combating the myths and stereotypes of old age. In 1976, she was diagnosed with uterine cancer and had a radical hysterectomy. In 1977, she was attacked by a man in a hotel corridor and forced into her hotel room where she was physically assaulted and robbed. She refused to let the mugging incident keep her from her work or her travels, but she never walked down a hotel corridor alone again. She had a number of romances, but chose to never marry or have children. She remained sexually active through her senior years and promoted the premise of sexual activity for the elderly. She remained active in social causes until she died in 1995.

- How well do you know the seniors in your life?
- Are you missing out on some really good life stories, and perhaps life lessons, by not taking more time to listen to the elder persons in your life?

such as Medicare and Medicaid, are susceptible to increased budget cuts from the federal government.

Final Wishes Many persons have a "living will." This is especially common among the elderly. A **living will** is a legal document that expresses a person's wishes concerning dying and life support, for instance, a desire not to be put on any artificial life support or to be resuscitated so as to not prolong pain and suffering if you are terminally ill. Without this document on file, the hospital can keep you or your loved one alive by artificial means no matter how severe the suffering may be. Most hospitals can provide you with a copy of a living will. However, the document must be completed before the onset of a major illness to be valid. Today, too many persons suffer in prolonged pain, and the cost of dying can destroy the financial status of other family members.[21]

Decisions about your funeral arrangements can be done in advance. (See *Journal Activity:* "How Do You Want to Be Remembered?") This is usually a good idea for many reasons. First, it assures that your own personal wishes will more likely be followed. Second, it saves the grieving family members the stress of taking care of these arrangements during a time of their own suffering. And third, decisions involving a large amount of money should be made well in advance to avoid any errors.

CONCLUSION

A middle-aged woman is considered to be at the halfway point of her life. It is a time to reflect upon her accomplishments and to look forward to enjoying the second half of her life, which is likely to be

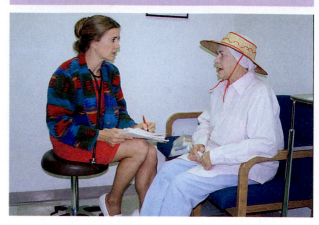

Dr. Ellen Warren, physician, examines her 72-year-old patient, Addie. Regular physical examinations are important for a woman's health care.

very different than the first half. The middle-aged woman faces the onset of menopause, which replaces that aspect of her identity related to reproductive potential. However, there is definitely life after menopause: The middle-aged woman is freer to explore her own goals and ambitions.

A senior woman can have a great deal of fun and accomplish as much as her willpower will let her. Many senior women are very active and outgoing, and selflessly contribute to their friends, family, and community. Some seniors would say that "a whole new life begins after 60!"

living will—documentation designating one's wishes to avoid resuscitation or artificial life support to prevent prolonged suffering and pain.

JOURNAL ACTIVITY

How Do You Want to be Remembered?

When you die, what kind of memorial ceremony, if any, would you like your surviving friends and family to experience? How do you want your body to be taken care of; by burial or cremation? What kind of epitaph would you like read at your memorial service or placed on your memorial? Take some time to think about and honor this part of your life. Enter your ideas about your current wishes for the end of your life. These ideas may change later on, but always make sure that someone close to you knows what your current desires are about your death. Also, do you want a "living will" so that no artificial means are used to keep you alive in the instances of brain death or advanced pain or suffering that accompanies a terminal illness? And what about the disposition of your personal belongings? Do you have a financial "legal will and testament" completed and on file? If not, perhaps you should begin preparing one. This document can be adjusted throughout your life as you acquire new assets and heirs.

Chapter Summary

- In middle adulthood, your children will need you less, and your parents may need you more.
- In middle adulthood, your relationship with your partner may be more familiar and comfortable, or your desired partner characteristics may have changed so that you may have or seek a new relationship partner.
- In middle adulthood, your physical body is changing rapidly and the onset of menopause replaces that aspect of your identity related to reproductive potential.
- The woman in middle adulthood can schedule more time for recreation and travel, and is often more secure and self-confident because of her accumulated life experience.

- Late adulthood is a time for retirement; if one does work, it is likely for the purpose of enjoyment.
- The senior adult is prone to have more health problems; and a senior woman is likely to find herself living alone.
- Many seniors choose to live in retirement communities so that they can rely on each other for support.
- The most vulnerable seniors are divorced or widowed women, and black or Hispanic women, because, statistically speaking, they tend to have more financial difficulties.

Review Questions

1. What are the physical and psychological symptoms experienced with menopause?
2. Can you describe the evaluation process that occurs in middle-age women (the midlife crisis)?

3. Why is it important to stay active as an older adult woman?
4. What types of myths and misconceptions exist about the older adult?

Resources

Organizations and Hotlines

American Association of Retired Persons
601 E Street, NW
Washington, DC 20049
Telephone: (202) 434-2277

Older Women's League
666 11th Street, NW
Suite 700
Washington, DC 20001
Telephone: (202) 783-6686

The Alliance for Aging Research
2021 K Street, NW
Suite 305
Washington, DC 20006
Telephone: (202) 293-2856

Alzheimer's Disease Education and Referral Center,
National Institute on Aging
P.O. Box 8250
Silver Spring, MD 20907-8250
Telephone: (800) 438-4380

National Institute on Aging Information Center,
National Institute on Aging
P.O. Box 8057

Gaithersburg, MD 20898-8057
Telephone: (800) 222-2225

Better Vision Institute
1800 North Kent Street
Suite 904
Rosslyn, VA 22209
Telephone: (703) 243-1508

Bureau of Aging and In-Home Services
P.O. Box 7083
Indianapolis, IN 46207-7083
Telephone: (800) 545-7763

Better Hearing Institute
P.O. Box 1840
Washington, DC 20013
Telephone: (703) 642-0580

Dial a Hearing Screening Test
Occupational Hearing Services
P.O. Box 1880
Media, PA 19063
Telephone: (800) 222-3277

Lighthouse National Center for Vision and Aging
111 East 59th Street
New York, NY 10022
Telephone: (212) 821-9200

Websites

American Association of Retired Persons
http://www.aarp.org

National Institute on Aging Information Center
http://www.nih.gov/nia/

Alzheimer's Association
http://www.alz.org/

Arthritis Foundation
http://www.arthritis.org/

Osteoporosis and Related Bone Diseases. National
Resource Center, National Institute of Arthritis and
Musculoskeletal and Skin Diseases
http://www.osteo.org/

Suggested Readings

Birkedahl, N. 1991. *Older and wiser: A workbook for coping with aging.* Oakland, Calif.: New Harbinger.

Dolan, K., and D. Dolan. 1995. *American guidance for seniors and their caregivers.* Obispo, Calif.: Impact Publishers.

Doress-Worters, P., and D. Siegal. 1994. *The new ourselves, growing older.* New York: Touchstone.

Estes, C. 1992. *Women who run with the wolves: Myths and stories of the wild woman archetype.* New York: Ballantine.

Ginsburg, G. 1995. *Widow: Rebuilding your life.* Tucson: Fisher Books.

Kuhn, M., C. Long, and L. Quinn. 1991. *No stone unturned: The life and times of Maggie Kuhn.* New York: Ballantine Books.

Powell, L., and K. Courtice. 1992. *Alzheimer's disease: A guide for families.* Reading, Mass.: Addison-Wesley.

Sheehy, G. 1992. *The silent passage: Menopause.* New York: Random House.

Sheehy, G. 1995. *New passages.* New York: Ballantine.

Smith, K. 1995. *Caring for your aging parents: A sourcebook of timesaving techniques and tips.* Obispo, Calif.: Impact Publishers.

Spencer, S., and J. Adams. 1995. *Life changes: Growing through personal transitions.* Obispo, Calif.: Impact Publishers.

Sullivan, D. 1994. *A senior's guide to healthy travel.* Franklin Lakes, N.J.: Career Press.

Teague, M., V. McGhee, D. Rosenthal, and D. Kearns. 1997. *Health promotion: Achieving high-level wellness in the later years,* 3rd ed. Madison, Wisc.: Brown & Benchmark.

Walker, S. 1995. *A caregiver's guide to activities with the elderly.* Obispo, Calif.: Impact Publishers.

References

1. Wharton, L. 1995. *The natural guide to women's health.* New York: MJF Books.

2. Peterson, A., and S. Rosenberg. 1997. *Every woman's guide to financial security,* 2nd ed. Franklin Lakes, N.J.: Career Press.

3. *Healthy People 2000: Midcourse Review and 1995 Revisions.* 1996. Boston: Jones & Bartlett.

4. Taeuber, C. 1993. Women in our aging society. *USA Today Magazine* (September) 42–44.

5. Bonita, R., and A. Howe. 1996. Older women in an aging world: Achieving health across the life course. *World Health Statistics Quarterly* 49 (2): 134–41.

6. Harris, D., and P. Changas. 1994. Revision of Palmore's second facts on aging quiz from a true-false to a multiple-choice format. *Educational Gerontology* 20: 741–54.

7. Trimble, J. Yoga instructor lives full life. *Denton Record-Chronicle,* Denton, Tex., 16 March 1997, 19–20A.

8. Taeuber, C. 1993. Women in our aging society. 42–44.

9. Stevens, J., and T. Thomas. 1996. *Major causes of unintentional injuries among older persons: An annotated bibliography.* Atlanta, Ga.: National Center for Injury Prevention and Control.

10. Walker, B. 1985. *The Crone: Woman of age, wisdom, and power.* San Francisco: Harper & Row, p. 14.

11. Taeuber, C. 1993. Women in our aging society. 42–44.

12. Mayo Foundation. 1993. Sexuality and aging. *Mayo Clinic Health Letter,* February. Rochester, Minn.: Mayo Foundation.

13. Clevenger, D. 1992. Family violence. *Facets* (March): 9–30.

14. Wolf, R. 1996. Understanding elder abuse and neglect. *Aging* (367): 4–13.

15. Van Hightower, N. 1997. *Understanding and treating survivors of family violence.* College Station, Tex.: Texas A & M Health Science Center.

16. Taeuber, C. 1993. Women in our aging society. 42–44.

17. Peterson and Rosenberg. 1997. Every woman's guide to financial security.

18. Ibid.

19. Karvonen, K. 1991. Go, Granny go!. *Sports Illustrated* 71 (October 21): 30A.

20. Kuhn, M., C. Long, and L. Quinn. 1991. *No stone unturned: The life and times of Maggie Kuhn.* New York: Ballantine Books.

21. The American way of dying. *U.S. News and World Report,* 4 December 1995, pp. 70–72 and 74–75.

MENTAL AND
EMOTIONAL WELLNESS

Part Two

CHAPTER FIVE
Enhancing Emotional Well-Being

CHAPTER SIX
Managing the Stress of Life

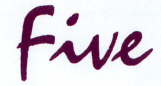

Enhancing Emotional Well-Being

▋ chapter objectives

When you complete this chapter you will be able to:
- Define and describe sociocultural influences on personal development.
- Demonstrate assertive communication.
- Demonstrate effective listening skills.
- Delineate the steps for effective problem solving.
- Perform activities for enhancing self-image and self-esteem.
- Describe the natural stages of the grief process.
- Identify the types of depression.

THE EMERGING SELF

How is it that you become the person that you are? How do you develop your values, beliefs, feelings, thoughts, and ideas about yourself, others, and the world around you? How does your personality emerge and what contributes to the happiness and unhappiness in your life? How do you decide when it is time to change, and to think, feel, believe, or behave differently about something or someone? Who do you decide to include in your social support system as persons who influence you and help you? These are important questions to consider as you explore your personal development and your emotional health.

Sociocultural Influences

Sociocultural influences (SCIs) may significantly impact your emotional health. Examples of SCIs include, but may not be limited to: family members, family history, family values, religious doctrine, media, school activities and personnel, community events, national events, world events, historical events, friends, famous persons, and significant others. These SCIs can impact you in many different ways. As you experience them in your life you will choose, either consciously or unconsciously, to integrate them into your self in some meaningful way. Once integrated, these SCIs can guide and direct your thinking, feeling, believing, and behaving. The

HEALTHY PEOPLE 2000 OBJECTIVES

- Reduce suicides to no more than 10.5 per 100,000 people. 1995 progress toward goal: 45 percent
- Reduce to 1.8 percent the incidence of injurious suicide attempts among adolescents aged 14 through 17. 1995 progress toward goal: -200 percent
- Reduce to less than 17 percent the prevalence of mental disorders among children and adolescents. (1995 revision) 1995 progress toward goal: data unavailable
- Reduce the prevalence of mental disorders (exclusive of substance abuse) among adults living in the community to less than 10.7 percent. 1995 progress toward goal: data unavailable
- Increase to at least 30 percent the proportion of people aged 18 and older with severe, persistent mental disorders who use community support programs. 1995 progress toward goal: data unavailable
- Increase to at least 45 percent the proportion of people with major depressive disorders who obtain treatment. 1995 progress toward goal: close to 40 percent
- Increase to at least 20 percent the proportion of people aged 18 and older who seek help in coping with personal and emotional problems. 1995 progress toward goal: close to 40 percent
- Increase to 50 the number of states with officially established protocols that engage mental health,
- alcohol and drug, and public health authorities with corrections authorities to facilitate identification and appropriate intervention to prevent suicide by jail inmates. 1995 progress toward goal: data unavailable
- Establish a network to facilitate access to mutual self-help activities, resources, and information by people and their family members who are experiencing emotional distress resulting from mental or physical illness. (1995 revision) 1995 progress toward goal: 256 percent
- Increase to at least 50 percent the proportion of primary care providers who routinely review with patients their patient's cognitive, emotional, and behavioral functioning and the resources available to deal with any problems that are identified. 1995 progress toward goal: data unavailable
- Increase to at least 75 percent the proportion of providers of primary care for children who include assessment of cognitive, emotional, and parent-child functioning, with appropriate counseling, referral, and follow-up, in their clinical practices. 1995 progress toward goal: data unavailable
- Reduce the prevalence of depressive (affective) disorders among adults living in the community to less than 4.3 percent. (1995 addition) 1995 progress toward goal: data unavailable

impact of these SCIs in your life can lead to life satisfaction and the pursuit or achievement of wellness, or they can lead you to some points of dissatisfaction or dysfunction. In fact, some SCIs can have a positive impact early on in your life but eventually lose their usefulness as you grow and change and thus may eventually begin to have a negative impact in your life. This is why it is important to be in touch with yourself, the impact that SCIs have on you, and when and how you need to alter your course to maintain or achieve greater degrees of life satisfaction and wellness. (See *Her Story:* "Ning.")

Mindful Self-Exploration and Integration

There are many things to be happy about in life, but there can also be varying degrees of unhappiness. It is important to understand how you developed happiness about yourself, other people, and things so you can maintain and continue to add to your happiness. It is equally important to understand how you might have developed unhappiness about yourself, other people, and things so you can change what led to that unhappiness.

Some SCIs are appropriate for some persons and inappropriate for others. You must decide for yourself which ones are best for you and in what ways you need to integrate their meaningfulness into your life in order to lead a more satisfactory and functional life. There are many possibilities for life dissatisfaction and dysfunction, but just a few warning signs might be low self-esteem, a poor self-concept, relationship conflict, prolonged unhappiness, depression, an eating disorder, dissatisfaction about your body, drug or alcohol abuse, and so on.

Her Story

Ning

Ning was unhappy in her college major. She came to the student counseling center for advisement. The career tests that she took all suggested that she would be much happier in a different area, in this case, theater arts. She confirmed to the counselor that she had wanted to be a theater major since high school, at which she starred in several school stage plays. When the counselor began to suggest that Ning change her major from premedicine to theater arts, Ning became very uncomfortable and said she just could not do that. With further probing, she explained that her parents fully expected her to be a physician and that she dare not change out of her premed major or they would be very upset with her. She described that her parents' definition of a successful career included medicine, but not the theater. The influence that Ning's parents had on her was so strong that Ning felt like she could not choose her own profession for fear of alienating the love of her parents and demonstrating disrespect toward them.

Ning decided to stay in counseling to explore how she developed her beliefs and values and to determine how these may be serving her well or not serving her so well in her life. This process of mindful self-exploration assisted Ning in making new choices in her life that would result in greater happiness for her. One choice was to develop a style of assertive communication with her parents that would help Ning to express her needs and desires in a better way but would also, in her opinion, not demonstrate disrespect for her parents, which was very impor-

tant to Ning. After talking to her parents and working through their differences of opinion, Ning chose to change her major to theater arts. She was much happier, and she felt that, although her parents were still somewhat disappointed in her choice, they now were more accepting of her desire to strive to do her best in a career for which she was more highly motivated to succeed.

- Have you ever had an internal conflict over something really important to you?
- How could mindful self-exploration help you to examine, understand, and potentially resolve this conflict?

Ning resolves those issues that led to her life dissatisfaction through the process of a mindful self-exploration of the sociocultural influences upon her life.

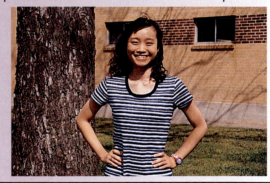

The integration of SCIs into yourself with a state of ongoing mindfulness can result in greater satisfaction and functioning and less dissatisfaction and dysfunction in your life. **Ongoing mindfulness** is the process of exploring your inner self and the impact that SCIs have on you. You are then more mindful, or consciously aware, of how you are integrating, and did integrate in your past, certain SCIs that led to particular beliefs, thoughts, feelings, and actions in your life. When dissatisfaction or dysfunction is discovered through this process of self-exploration, you can reorganize the meaningfulness of the SCIs and their impact on you. You can then reintegrate new beliefs, thoughts, feelings, or actions that can provide you with greater satisfaction and wellness. The reorganization of the impact of certain SCIs may involve tak-

ing the relevant SCI and discarding all or part of it from your life, or transforming its meaning into something different that may be more helpful to you. (See Fig. 5.1.)

Without mindful integration of SCIs, these can dictate your development and state of emotional well-being in ways not completely appropriate for who you are and thus, lead to your unhappiness. It is important to maintain, or regain when it is not present, a state of mindfulness about past and present SCIs and their impact on you. You can then discard inappropriate ones in order to lead a more satisfied and functional life.

Resistance to self-exploration and change can often be a result of your fear of trying something unfamiliar to you. You may also be afraid of appearing

FIGURE 5.1 The impact of sociocultural influences (SCI).

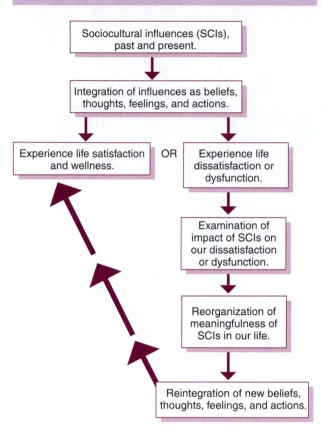

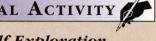

JOURNAL ACTIVITY

Mindful Self-Exploration

Identify three things you really like about yourself or your life and write each down on a separate piece of paper. Now do the same for three things you do not like about yourself or your life (assuming you can think of three things you are unhappy about). Below each item, write down the sociocultural influences you think you have integrated into your thinking, feelings, or belief processes that may have contributed to that particular happiness or unhappiness. (For example, family values, parental messages you received, messages about who you "should" be from television or other sources, religious beliefs, modeling persons you admired, and so on, might be included.) If you have trouble coming up with ideas, try asking a friend for some input.

to be disloyal to your family, friends, or familiar institutions (for example, your religious affiliation) because you want to be different from them. You may fear rejection by those important to you if you change the way you are. You may be uncomfortable with change and fear harm, failure, or destruction if you change. When your resistance to change gets in the way so that you find it too difficult to self-explore and reorganize yourself on your own, then you may want to seek assistance from someone else to help you, such as a mental health professional. Complete *Journal Activity:* "Mindful Self-Exploration" to determine your own mindfulness.

LIFE SKILL DEVELOPMENT

Life is a job and, ideally, life is a fun job. Life can be very challenging in that you can face some pretty tough demands at times. Certain life skills make it easier to cope with life demands. Examples of help-

ful life skills for emotional health include: assertiveness training, effective communication, problem solving, maintaining a healthy self-image, having good self-esteem, and resolving grief over loss. Life skills can be taught to any age group, including very young children. When children do not learn life skills early on, then these children may have a rougher time growing up emotionally healthy or staying emotionally healthy through their life span. It is never too late to learn helpful life skills. Many very good self-help books are on the market to assist with this process and a few are listed at the end of this chapter. In addition, schools, community organizations, and mental health agencies commonly offer one or more life-skill-building programs to the public.

Assertiveness Training

Assertiveness training is one of the most common personal improvement programs currently offered. Many health educators and mental health professionals have some experience and knowledge in training assertion skills to individuals and groups. Assertion

ongoing mindfulness—the process of exploring the impact that sociocultural influences have on you and your life development.

A personal growth group is a good outlet for sharing your concerns and getting support from your peers.

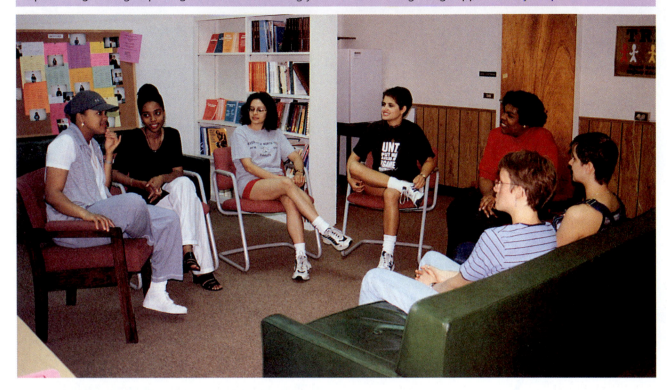

training teaches the differences between assertive, aggressive, and nonassertive behavior, and increases experience in applying responsible assertive behavior. *FYI:* "What Is Assertiveness?" explains what assertiveness is.

A need for assertion training is more prevalent for women than for men. This is because many messages from American society tend to encourage boys to be aggressive career professionals while encouraging girls to be passive caregivers and homemakers.

Assertive behavior is more common in working women than in homemakers. In a study regarding women's views about leisure time, homemakers were less likely than working women to feel assertive, competent, or independent during their leisure. They felt more constrained by lack of skills and opportunity, poor self-image, fear, personal values, and the belief that some leisure activities are only for men.[2]

Adventure-based activities can have a positive influence on assertiveness enhancement for women. Ropes course training is one such activity. Women must overcome obstacles, usually constructed in an

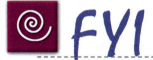

What Is Assertiveness?

Assertiveness, or assertion, is standing up for personal rights and expressing thoughts, feelings, and beliefs in direct, honest, and appropriate ways that do not violate another person's rights. Assertiveness involves the use of "I" messages; for example, "This is what *I* think." "This is what *I* feel." "This is how *I* see the situation." These types of messages express "who the person is" and is said without dominating, humiliating, or degrading the other person.

"Assertiveness involves respect—not deference. Deference is acting in a subservient manner as though the other person is right or better simply because the other person is older, more powerful, experienced, knowledgeable, or is of a different sex or race. Deference is present when people express themselves in ways that are self-effacing, appeasing, or overly apologetic."[1] With assertion, one must communicate respect for self and for others.   ⌘

outdoor wilderness area, that include crossing rivers on rope ladders, scaling high walls, swinging across chasms on ropes, rock climbing, or repelling down cliffs. Adventure-based courses have produced positive changes in women participants, such as increases in women's abilities to take risks, to practice assertive leadership, to solve problems effectively, and to feel more competent in general.[3,4] Participants in adventure-based courses for women report that feelings of power and achievement emerge in this setting.

In spite of the positive impact that assertiveness can have in your life, such as enhancing your success in a career and increasing your ability to meet your needs and the needs of significant others, there is some pressure exerted by society for women to not be assertive. For example, one study of 122 men, between the ages of 17 and 25 years, rated women described as independent and assertive as less physically attractive than women described as affectionate and compassionate.[5] What is especially significant about this study is that the two groups of women had been rated as equally physically attractive by a separate sample of men when no personality characteristics were described. It was only with the addition of the differentiating personality characteristics that men now found one group, the independent and assertive women, as less physically attractive than the other group.

Sending assertive messages is an important step for getting your needs met. *Health Tips:* "When Do You Need to Be Assertive?" and *FYI:* "Types of Assertive Messages" provide examples of when and how to be assertive.

Being an effective communicator is also important in creating positive and productive interactions.

Effective Communication

Components of effective listening involve: appropriate body language, minimal responses, paraphrasing, clarification, and summarization.[8] Effective listening begins with appropriate body language. When someone is talking, be attentive. Watch her or his face and, when appropriate, make eye contact. From time to time, make brief responses (one to two words only) to let the person know you are listening, for example, "I see" or "I hear you." Sometimes a brief head nod is appropriate. The purpose of minimal responses is to let the individual know you are listening without implying agreement at this point. When the individual

pauses, attempt to paraphrase what has been said; that is, in one or two sentences restate in your own words what has been told to you.

Occasionally, effective listening involves a need for clarification if you are having difficulty understanding the person talking. Clarification can be achieved through brief exploratory statements and open-ended questions. An exploratory statement is an attempt to request further information without disrupting the flow of communication by the other person. An example exploratory statement would be, "Tell me more about your need for space." Another example of an exploratory statement would be, "Please give me more details about how you see our relationship evolving." An example of an open-ended question would be, "When you said my being late for meetings causes a disruption, could you tell me in

health tips

When Do You Need to Be Assertive?

Applying assertive behavior may be required in many situations in order to get your needs met in a healthy manner. Here are just a few examples in which you may need to be assertive.[6]

- Maintaining assertion in the face of someone's aggression and personal attack.
- Being assertive with repair people who overcharge or do not properly do the work.
- Giving supervisory criticism.
- Presenting yourself at a task meeting where others ignore, discount, or put down your ideas.
- Negotiating salary increases, and dealing with changes in job title or job function.
- Being assertive with colleagues who make sexist, racist, or condescending remarks.
- Expressing feelings of hurt, anger, and disappointment with people who are close to you.

assertiveness—involves standing up for personal rights and expressing oneself in direct, honest, and appropriate ways that do not violate another person's rights.

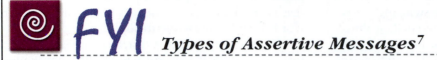

FYI — *Types of Assertive Messages*[7]

There are six basic types of assertive messages: *I want* statements help to clarify to both yourself and others what you really want. For example, "I want you to call when you are going to be late." *I feel* statements help express your feelings without attacking the other person. For example, "I feel embarrassed when you criticize my clothes in front of my friends." *Mixed feelings* statements name more than one feeling and explain where each is coming from. For example, "I enjoy going out and doing things with you, yet I feel it is unfair that you frequently do not bring enough money and ask me to pay for you." *Empathic assertion* presents some sensitive understanding about the other person and then expresses how you feel. For example, "I know you said that you are angry and do not want to talk about it. However, I feel we need to talk about it when you feel ready." *Confrontive assertion* is necessary when there are contradictions such as differences between what a person says and what she or he does. For example, "I know you said you would teach the newer students some of the beginning information as part of your internship, yet you consistently put them off, or do not show up for appointments. I want you to be more responsible and follow through on the tasks that you agreed to do." *I language assertion* is useful for expressing difficult negative feelings. For example, "When you cancel a weekend event with me because you say you are busy working and then I find out you went out with someone else, I feel rejected and humiliated. I need for you to be honest with me about why you do things or it could damage our friendship."

what ways so I might better understand your concern?" An open-ended question is usually formatted with what, when, where, or how.

When the individual stops talking, briefly summarize the main contents of what you think was communicated and then ask the person if he or she feels you understood. This effective listening process can then be followed by communication from you to the other person regarding your thoughts, ideas, or needs. Assertive communication can be useful at this point. The goal to effective listening is that each party be heard and understood. Then, via assertive communication, attempts can be made at caregiving, problem solving, conflict resolution, or negotiation and compromise. Complete *Journal Activity:* "Practice Effective Listening and Communication" to practice your listening skills.

Effective Problem Solving

Everyone appreciates the love, warmth, and potential companionship that can come from a relationship. Most people do not consider or adequately prepare for the disagreements or conflicts that will inevitably arise in any type of relationship, be it family, friends, relationship partner, or colleagues at work. Some individuals have misconceptions around conflict and disagreements that can impair adequate resolution.

JOURNAL ACTIVITY

Practice Effective Listening and Communication

Get a partner and practice effective listening and communication activities. Take turns being the listener and the communicator. Make a point to practice each part of the effective listening process: appropriate body language, minimal responses, paraphrasing, clarification, and summarization. Also, try some of the types of assertive communication. Each of these parts can be exercised in any order and more than once as needed. You and your partner can then give each other feedback about how well each of you did in listening and communicating to one another.

Many people incorrectly believe that a conflict must automatically be their fault, or that they must win a conflict, or that they should be able to handle a conflict so well that the problem never recurs.[9] Other similar kinds of misconceptions to avoid: a compromise means losing and being less powerful than the other person; conflict should be avoided at any cost; your solution is the only worthwhile one; all conflicts must be resolved; and one party must be right and one must be wrong in any conflict.

Effective problem solving is a step-by-step approach of planning and negotiating and involves all parties to be effected. A common model for problem solving and negotiation involves six basic steps: defining the problem; generating possible solutions; evaluating the solutions; making the decision; determining how to implement the decision; and assessing the success of the solution.[10] After assessing success, some adjustments might have to be made, but it is important that all involved parties have a say in any adjustments to the original agreement.

Image Building

A positive image of self is central to feeling good and being successful. A key element to building and maintaining a positive self-image is to focus on being what you want to be, that is, building an image from the inside out instead of trying to be what others want you to be.

Society presents many messages about the supposed "ideal image." This is a myth; there is no such thing as the "ideal woman." Every woman has something unique to offer on an emotional, physical, mental, social, occupational, and spiritual level. It is the differences you present that helps to make the world diverse and complete.

To enhance your self-image, start by loving yourself and accepting yourself as you are right now at this very moment. If you can do this, then any changes you want to make in yourself can be much more fun instead of seeming so hard and laborious. (See *Journal Activity:* "Loving Myself.")

A preoccupation with body image can reach elevations significant enough to be considered clinical in nature. Body dysmorphic disorder (BDD) is the classification of body image disturbance reserved for the non-eating disorder population. BDD is a preoccupation with an imagined defect in appearance that results in distress in social or other important areas of life functioning.[11] Preliminary evidence suggests that BDD is diagnosed with approximately equal frequency in women and in men. BDD behaviors include frequent mirror checking or avoidance of mirrors, frequent comparisons to others, and excessive grooming behavior. Dysmorphophobia is the label the Europeans have assigned to BDD and the term used by the World Health Organization and the *International Classification of Diseases* diagnostic reference.

JOURNAL ACTIVITY

Loving Myself

Write a love letter to yourself. Be sure to use your name and "I" messages. Write down things about yourself that you like. Tell yourself that you love yourself. Tell yourself that you really appreciate who you are and how hard you work. Describe examples of these things. Tell yourself that you do things for yourself because you want to and because you love yourself very much. Tell yourself that you trust yourself to do whatever is best for you and that you will remain open to any additional insights about what you need and when you need it. Write for about 20 minutes. Mail the letter to yourself and/or put it up where you will see it and read it several times a week. You may find this activity difficult at first. But, with practice, you can see very positive benefits in how you feel about yourself over time.

Do I Like Who I Am?

I spend too much time thinking,
do I really like who I am?
Am I pretty enough; am I smart enough?
Am I doing everything that I can?

Do I like myself in Winter
when ice-capped wonderlands abound?
I can wear my heavy sweaters
and camouflage each and every pound.

The Spring brings so much color;
flowers peeking their pretty petals out.
I dread shedding my winter layers
and revealing holiday eating bouts.

The warmth of Summer is delightful;
parks full of players, all over town.
How will I look in my swimming suit?
I'm frantic about those extra pounds.

The Autumn is so beautiful
It's so easy for the trees to change.
They are lovely in every season;
I wish that I felt the same.

Yes, I spend too much time thinking,
do I really like who I am?
Because I'm pretty, smart, and daring,
but, if I want to, I'll change, because I can.

By Cynthia K. Chandler

Image and the Media

Glamorous images projected in the media have contributed to harsh self-criticism by women regarding their own body image. Television, movies, and magazines can present images of women that seem real, but, in fact, are impossible to compete with. Many models and actresses have what is considered to be an ideal body image but, they also have all of the best clothes designers, hair dressers, and makeup staff. These professionals spend many hours sculpting a woman into a form that is, supposedly, "ideal," but pretty unrealistic most of the time. What they have created is an image of a woman that does not occur naturally in the world. One perfect example is the glamorization of Barbara Stanwyck, a well-known actress in the United States in the mid 1940s, 50s, and 60s. Ms. Stanwyck had a "figure fault" by Hollywood standards, her hips were considered to be too low in the back and thought to look odd when she was walking. A famous designer in Hollywood at the time, Edith Head created a new design for Ms. Stanwyck to hide this "flaw." The design created by Edith Head was a dress with a high midriff, as opposed to a well-defined waistline that would accentuate the hips. This new design resulted in a taller, sleeker-looking Barbara. The dress design was incorporated into Ms. Stanwyck's wardrobe and was presented in the 1941 movie *The Lady Eve.* After this, Barbara Stanwyck had a career boost by getting more glamorous roles. Edith Head's high midriff dress design was copied by many designers and purchased in abundance by women all over the country who wanted to camouflage their waistline or hips. The design was known as "The Lady Eve" dress.[12] This type of camouflaging of a woman's natural image has continued throughout history. More public efforts have been put into hiding a woman's natural image than in accepting the nature of a woman's uniqueness.

There have been instances where the media industry has been beneficial to the image of women. For example, the movie wardrobe of Marlene Dietrich, a famous actress of the 1930s, 40s and 50s, made wearing pants more socially acceptable for women at a time when dresses had been socially demanded.[13] It is important to remember that in the movie and fashion industry, what is "in" one day may be "out" the next. This should add emphasis to the point that diversity and uniqueness is what allows us to be individuals and still fit in.

For the most part, the media has contributed more to the fictional "ideal woman" image than the healthy "real woman" concept. In the 1990 movie *Pretty Woman,* the leading actress, Julia Roberts, was portrayed as having a beautiful and desirable perfect body type. What the general public did not know was that several models were used as stand-ins. When Ms. Robert's body was supposedly revealed, it was actually one of these body doubles that was being shown.[14] Thus, the "pretty woman" was not considered pretty enough for Hollywood standards. In fact, on the movie poster to advertise the film, Julia Robert's head was superimposed on another woman's body. The unsuspecting public was led to believe that the woman on this poster was actually Julia Roberts. Another example of how the media promotes a fictionalized presentation of how women "should be" is the cover girl on a 1990s modeling magazine who was actually computer generated. Different parts of different women, including different facial features, were put together to create a whole new woman. An unsuspecting public can be easily misled by media magic tricks.

The *glamorization* of women, or basing the desirability of a woman on her body shape, mainly thinness in the arms, legs, face, and waist, and largeness of breasts and hips (the hourglass figure), is thought to have begun in the 1830s, when the camera was invented.[15,16,17] This type of woman's figure was additionally popularized in the late 1800s by a male artist named Gibson who created the "Gibson girl" in a series of his paintings, which presented the supposed ideal woman.[18] Gibson's fictional depictions became very popular and women strived to model after them.

Modern media technology is now reaching newly developing countries, and these societies are being exposed to fictionalized presentations of the "ideal" woman's body image. As this media technology is made more available in these countries, we have seen the instigation and rise of eating disorders and other emotional distresses that accompany striving to become the fictional "ideal woman."[19,20]

There are ethnic differences in how women view body-image satisfaction. Caucasian-American women report greater levels of disordered eating and dieting behaviors and attitudes and greater body dissatisfaction than Asian Americans and African Americans.[21] Low self-esteem and high public self-consciousness were associated with greater levels of problematic eating behaviors and attitudes and body dissatisfaction.

There are some differences in how men and women view their own body. Women reportedly have lower body-image satisfaction than men, and

Assess **Y O U R S E L F**

The Appearance Schemas Inventory (ASI)[24]

Rank your beliefs about these items using the scale below from 1 to 5. Then determine your body-image satisfaction by completing the scoring section that follows.

1	2	3 Neither Disagree Nor	4	5
Strongly Disagree	Mostly Disagree	Agree	Mostly Agree	Strongly Agree

____ 1. What I look like is an important part of who I am.

____ 2. What's wrong with my appearance is one of the first things that people will notice about me.

____ 3. One's outward physical appearance is a sign of the character of the inner person.

____ 4. If I could look just as I wish, my life would be much happier.

____ 5. If people knew how I *really* look, they would like me less.

____ 6. By controlling my appearance, I can control many of the social and emotional events in my life.

____ 7. My appearance is responsible for much of what has happened to me in my life.

____ 8. I should do whatever I can to always look my best.

____ 9. Aging will make me less attractive.

____10. For women: To be feminine, a woman must be as pretty as possible.
For men: To be masculine, a man must be as handsome as possible.

____11. The media's messages in our society make it impossible for me to be satisfied with my appearance.

____12. The only way I could ever like my looks would be to change what I look like.

____13. Attractive people have it all.

____14. Homely people have a hard time finding happiness.

Scoring and Interpretation: Add your score for all items above. Now divide by 14 to get your average score. If your average score is 2.99 or higher, then your score is the same as persons who report having extreme body-image dissatisfaction and are seeking therapy. If your average score is 2.58 and below, then your score is the same as persons who do not seek therapy for extreme body-image dissatisfaction. Higher ASI scores, an average of 2.99 and above, are related to greater public self-consciousness, poorer social self-esteem, more social-evaluative anxiety, more depressive symptoms, and greater eating disturbance.

self-esteem is linked to body-image attitudes more for women than for men.[22] These differences can become evident as early as adolescence, in that adolescent males are found to feel more positive about their bodies than are adolescent females.[23]

Most women do not actually have unattractive and unacceptable bodies. It is more likely that society has been generating unfair messages to women about how they "should" and "should not" look so that most women feel that they may have unattractive bodies or features. The reality is that most women's sense of unattractiveness has been created by media bias. It is difficult to turn around a pattern of thinking that has endured for such a long time. Some progress has been made in countering the fictional images of a woman's body. However, society has a long way to go. In the meantime, the image of women will sustain harsh criticism as it continues to be based on biased and unrealistic thinking.

Rate your own feelings about your appearance in *Assess Yourself!:* "The Appearance Schemas Inventory."

Eating Disorders

Poor body image has been identified as the central factor in the development of eating disorders.[25] Eating disorders include anorexia nervosa and bulimia nervosa. Anorexia nervosa is starving oneself, sometimes even to death, because of a personal belief that one is unattractive or unlovable. Bulimia nervosa is eating and then vomiting soon afterward to get rid of the food in order to avoid weight gain. Ninety percent of all anorexics and bulimics are females.[26] Women who suffer from an eating disorder frequently have a poor self-concept. The treatment for eating disorders requires a combination of personal mental health counseling as well as nutritional guidance. Chapter 7 contains additional information on eating disorders.

Self-Esteem Enhancement

Self-esteem is based on the distance between the perceived self and the ideal self. The perceived self is how you currently see yourself. The ideal self is how you believe you "should" be. The greater the distance between the perceived self and the ideal self, the lower your self-esteem.

Self-esteem enhancement is the process of reducing the distance between the perceived self and the ideal self. In cases of low self-esteem, typically the ideal self is too unrealistic. Thus, the process here would be to bring the ideal self into reality, to make the view of the ideal self more realistic and less perfectionistic. Once the ideal self is more realistic, then you can have a healthier opinion about yourself and greater self-esteem. When you desire to make some changes, having good self-esteem is prerequisite to making healthier and more realistic decisions about change.

Individuals who have low self-esteem are often discouraged persons. Activities that help to instill a belief in oneself can raise self-esteem, bring the ideal self into a healthier perspective, and build success and confidence. Participation in adventure programs, sports, music and arts, and community service are just a few examples of activities that enhance self-esteem through the experience of success while having fun.

Low self-esteem can originate from discouraging messages we received from our parents. Parents serve as primary role models and message senders. For a woman, the most common primary role model is her mother. The presence of critical messages or the absence of encouraging messages from a woman's mother can create severe doubt in a woman's own judgment and ability throughout her life span.

> If we feel trapped by unfulfilled needs that arose out of childhood experiences, we first need to understand them as best we can. In terms of the self-concept, it is helpful to understand how much of any belief about ourselves is an accurate reflection of us and how much is the product of circumstance or other people's misperceptions.[27]

At some point in their life women have to ask, "Whom are we to believe?" An integral part of mov-

ing on is learning to trust our own judgments as much as or more than our parents.

Not only is it important to feel good about yourself, but it also may be important to let others know. Characters who were boastful or positive about themselves were rated by undergraduate college students as being more competent than characters who made negative statements about their self.[28] Thus, bragging about yourself may enhance the opinion that others have about you. (See *Journal Activity:* "I Am Awesome.")

The process of maintaining or enhancing self-esteem in women may vary across cultures. Conditions that impact self-esteem were compared for young Asian, black, and white women in America.[29] The best predictors of good self-esteem among Asian women included having children, having nonconflicting social networks, and positive life events. For black women, the best predictors of good self-esteem included educational opportunities and having nonconflicting social networks. For white women, the best predictors of good self-esteem included the absence of negative life events, the presence of nonconflicting social networks, and a good income.

Resolving Grief over Loss

During your life, you will lose someone or something very important to you. This will probably happen many times in your lifetime. Losing someone or something meaningful is very painful. Understanding the grief resolution process is an important life skill for coping with the pain accompanied by loss.

Grief is a normal response to loss. It does not matter what or who has been lost. The more meaningful the thing or person that is lost, then the more intense will be the sense of loss. People grieve in various ways. Some seek support and others grieve silently and alone. Some recover quickly whereas others are bereaved for a very long time. There is no one right way to grieve. However, the grief process must not consume your life to the degree that you become dysfunctional and risk losing additional things that are important and necessary, such as relationships and employment.

The support of close friends and family is helpful during bereavement. Sometimes it may become necessary to seek the assistance of a mental health professional experienced in facilitating the grief recovery process. Grief support groups are common. Individuals who participate in a community grief support group or professional grief counseling often recover more quickly from their bereavement. People tend to work through loss in healthier ways and integrate loss more effectively when assistance from others and a variety of resources are readily available. Resources form the basis of a support network consisting of three systems that focus on clarifying how you derive meaning from life through your beliefs and values, how you access support from those around you, and how you draw upon your own personal strengths and abilities.[30]

Recovering from loss does not necessarily mean that you will no longer experience any pain from the memory of the loss. It does mean that you will regain a sense of being okay and going on with your life. Recovery means that you are no longer consumed by the loss and can incorporate new beginnings and new ways of thinking into your life. The first six months after a loss are usually the most difficult. The formal bereavement or grieving process typically takes a good two years, although the sense of pain usually subsides gradually over this two-year period. Even after the two-year period, you may find certain dates related to the loss just as difficult, for example, the birthday of a deceased child, or the anniversary of the death of a spouse or relationship partner.

Some commonalities have been discovered in the grief process. One grief process model describes grief from the loss of a loved one as having three phases, each with its own set of characteristics, challenges, and choices: early mourning, mid-mourning, and late mourning.[31] The early mourning phase lasts from the time you first hear about the loss to the

final disposition of the body and personal belongings of the deceased. This phase can last as long as three to six weeks after the funeral. Challenges to face include getting through the funeral, dealing with funeral details, notifying family and friends, settling estate arrangements, and preparing for the transitions to come.

Mid-mourning is the phase of having to face the harsh reality of the loss. As others begin to get on with their lives, you will find it difficult to do so. You may suffer deep separation, feelings, pain, or anxiety. You may have difficulty in distinguishing fact from fantasy. You may have physical symptoms develop such as sleep disturbance, reduced appetite, anxiety attacks, headaches, stomachaches, and shortness of breath. Your health may be fragile during this phase and it is extremely important, difficult as it may be, to exercise and eat a nutritious diet. During this phase there can be a flood of emotions, intense sadness, and loneliness as well as feelings of guilt, depression, powerlessness, abandonment, anger and rage, fear, and panic. You may choose to be alone in order to grieve completely. However, it is also important to seek out and maintain a support system during this vulnerable time.

The late mourning phase focuses on getting on with your life. Your feelings will focus less on grief, although anger and sadness may still be prevalent, and more on attitudes and perceptions as they relate to moving on with your life. An attitude of acceptance has gradually evolved and an integration of the loss into your life-scheme has occurred.

Another grief process model involves five stages of grief: denial, anger, sorrow/despair/depression, bargaining, and acceptance.[32] These stages can be experienced in any order and more than once in the grieving process.

Denial is often the initial reaction, although it can be experienced again at any time. Denial is a buffer of protection against the shock and trauma of the loss. It allows us time to adjust to the event. This stage is accompanied by a feeling of numbness and disbelief. As is the case with each of these stages, it is important to work through the denial. From there, one must regain and maintain a presence of mind as

self-esteem—how good one feels about oneself; measured by the distance between the perceived self and the ideal (preferred) self.

soon as possible so one can function in the world realistically. Seeking and receiving support and understanding from others is very important during this time.

When you have lost someone or something important to you, you can become very angry. You may want to lash out and hurt others with your words and deeds. It is important to remember that what you are angry about is the loss, and you should not become destructive toward yourself or others as a result. Anger can be worked through by talking with others. Anger is a natural part of the grief process, and it needs to be expressed, but in a healthy manner.

Sorrow, despair, and/or depression is a natural and healthy way to express sadness from a loss. Crying is useful for releasing the sadness. Ritualistic ceremonies, such as funerals, wakes, and memorial services, are often held to facilitate opportunities for expressing sadness with others who are also feeling the loss or wish to support you in your loss. These ceremonies can assist with the transitions that are necessary from one stage to another in the grieving process.

Bargaining is a desperate attempt to stay in control. This stage is accompanied by our attempts to second guess the situation or try to reverse the loss. We might say things like "If only I had done this or that, then this would not have happened," or "If I promise this thing or that thing then everything will be okay again," etc. Although the bargaining stage does not necessarily have many healthy aspects, it is still a very common experience during bereavement. The persistent and gentle assurance and reassurance by those close to you that "there is nothing you could have done" or "there is nothing you can do now" will help you through this potentially destructive stage.

Acceptance is the final stage of grief, although it is possible to recycle through the previous stages again. Acceptance is the final goal of the grief process. In this stage, we come to accept the loss that has occurred. We come to terms with reality. We understand that our life will always be different having been impacted by the loss, but that we can and will go on. We can let go of our doubts and anger and lift our sadness. We can go on and live our lives fully again.

Grief has been described as the emotional experience of loss, whereas *mourning* has been described as the actual expression of loss, that is, those behaviors that take place as a result of the grief expe-

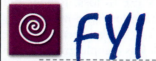

Prevalence of Depression

The U.S. Department of Health and Human Services reports in *Healthy People 2000: Midcourse Review and 1995 Revisions* that depression is a highly prevalent disorder, particularly among women. Primary care physicians often fail to recognize the symptoms of depression in their patients because the symptoms of depression often mimic those of physical illnesses. Depression is an emotional condition in the category of affective disorders (mood disorders). Depression is a significant public health problem that can be effectively treated. Approximately 80 percent of patients can be successfully treated, yet less than 40 percent of individuals with depression are treated by a health-care provider. Particularly disturbing is the high rate of affective disorders among females. The rate for females is 6.6 percent, which is nearly twice that of males at 3.5 percent. The overall rate is 5.1 percent. Depression is closely associated with suicide. More than 30,000 suicides occur each year. The ninth leading cause of death in 1992, suicide is the third leading cause of death among adolescents and young adults aged 15–24 years.

rience.[33] An actual loss or some memory of a previous loss can each serve as a trigger to experience the emotions of grief. These emotions then result in behaviors to mourn the loss. It is important to mourn the loss to reconcile the emotions of grief. Unreconciled or poorly reconciled grief experiences can lead to unhealthy behaviors.

DEPRESSION

A common emotional health concern for women is the presence of symptoms associated with depression. **Depression** is an emotional state of persistent dejection that may range from mild discouragement to feelings of extreme despair. These feelings are usually accompanied by loss of motivation, loss of energy, insomnia, loss of appetite, and difficulty in concentrating and making decisions.[34] Persons who have had a stressful or traumatic event often experience depression afterwards. (See *FYI:* "Prevalence of Depression" for a discussion of the prevalence of depression.)

Types of Depression

Individuals may have just a few characteristics associated with depression or they may have more severe symptoms indicative of a clinical depression. Clinical depression usually requires intervention by a trained mental health professional. The most common types of clinical depression are *major depressive episode, dysthymic disorder, major depressive disorder,* and *bipolar disorder* (commonly referred to as manic depression; see *FYI:* "Common Types of Clinical Depression"). In any given community, it is estimated that between 10 and 25 percent of women and 5 to 12 percent of men will develop a major depressive disorder sometime in their lifetime.[35] These prevalence rates for major depressive disorder seem to be unrelated to ethnicity, education, income, or marital status.

Psychosocial Stressors and Depression

Any individual can develop depression; however, women are twice as likely as men to be diagnosed with depression.[37,38] Some researchers believe that the higher incidence of depression in women is because they respond to depressing life events differently than men. Men tend to cut off the depression before it has serious consequences, whereas women tend to remain focused on their depressed mood in ways that prolong its duration and intensify its effects.[39]

Other researchers believe that women have higher incidences of depression than men because they experience more stress and discrimination than men. Women are subject to unique psychosocial stressors that can initiate depression and impede recovery. Examples include conflict between domestic and job demands, gender discrimination in financial and political venues, and pressure by society to maintain a prescribed body image. Body-image dissatisfaction has been linked to low self-esteem and higher rates of depression.[40] (See *Viewpoint:* "Are Women More Susceptible to Depression?".)

Stressful or threatening life events are commonly associated with the onset or presence of depression. Women who developed depression were more likely to reflect feelings of humiliation and being trapped following a severely threatening event.[41]

The interpersonal and psychological functioning of women can be significantly impaired from the ex-perience of childhood trauma. Childhood physical abuse, incest, and parental alcoholism have each been associated with higher rates of depression, higher sexual assault rates, lower self-esteem, and greater involvement with a chemically dependent partner.[42]

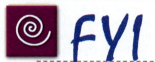

Common Types of Clinical Depression[36]

Major depressive episode involves the presence of at least five of the following symptoms for most of the day for at least a two-week period:
- Feel sad or empty
- Diminished interest or pleasure
- Weight loss
- Insomnia
- Feelings of worthlessness or inappropriate guilt
- Diminished ability to think or concentrate
- Recurrent thoughts of death or suicide

   Dysthymic disorder involves the presence of at least two of the following symptoms for most of the day for at least two years (one year for adolescents and children):
- Poor appetite or overeating
- Insomnia
- Low energy or fatigue
- Low self-esteem
- Poor concentration or difficulty making decisions
- Feelings of hopelessness

   Major depressive disorder is typically the reoccurrence of a major depressive episode (two or more within two consecutive months).

   Bipolar disorder is a mixture of major depressive episodes and manic episodes. Manic episodes are a distinct period of persistently elevated, expansive, or irritable mood lasting at least four days, and that is clearly different from the usual nondepressed mood. If numerous periods of depressive symptoms and numerous periods of manic symptoms occur, the individual may be diagnosed as having *cyclothymic disorder.*

depression—an emotional state of persistent dejection ranging from mild discouragement and gloominess to feelings of extreme despondency and despair.

Women who had experienced childhood abuse and/or adult abuse were studied over eight years by researchers who discovered that childhood and adult abuse were both independently related to chronic or recurrent depression in these women.[43] Women college undergraduates who reported exposure to abuse between their parents (parental partner abuse) during their childhood were described as having depression and low self-esteem.[44]

Hormonal Effects on Depression

The onset of depression during pregnancy, antepartum depression, and following the delivery of a child, postpartum depression, is common. The significant hormonal shifts that a woman undergoes during and after her pregnancy are major contributors to antepartum and postpartum depression. In addition, antepartum and postpartum depression can be made worse with the presence of major life stressors. Among financially impoverished inner-city women, antepartum depression was found among 27.6 percent and postpartum depression was found among 23.4 percent of these women.[45] These rates were about double those found for middle-class samples. African American and European American women did not differ in their rates of depression. The larger incidence of antepartum and postpartum depression in the impoverished inner-city women was most likely due to the stress of their financial plight.

Severe hormonal shifts associated with menopause can incite depression. A survey of working, postmenopausal women reported that at least 40 percent of those surveyed faced difficulties in the work environment due to their menopausal symptoms.[46] These included: weight gain, hot flashes, irritability, depression, bloating, and mood changes.

Normal hormonal changes may serve as triggers for psychiatric illness in genetically vulnerable women. Research with female twins determined that there is a genetic liability for the onset of major depression in women who experience stressful events.[47] Thus, the tendency to develop depression may be inherited. Major depressive disorder is 1.5 to 3 times more common among first-degree biological relatives of persons with this disorder than among the general population.

Positive Experiences Versus Depression

Women who have positive experiences can enhance their self-esteem and decrease depression. There has been confirmation of a negative relationship between depression and the sense of humor in that as humor increases, depression decreases.[48] Support has been found for a positive relationship between achieving the dream of life success and mental health for midlife women.[49] In addition, women who indicated low self-esteem and a negative evaluation of self showed marked improvements in esteem and self-evaluation over a seven-year period due to positive life changes such as increased quality of personal relationships and work status.[50]

Developmental Issues and Depression

There are no consistent gender differences in rates of depression among prepubescent children. However by mid-adolescence, ages 13 to 15 years, girls show significantly higher rates of depressive disorders and depressive symptoms than boys.[51] Major depressive disorder is twice as common in adolescent and adult females as in adolescent and adult males.[52] Although not overlooking the biological differences of males and females that become more prevalent during adolescence, additional possible explanations for the emerging differences in the rates of depression exist. First, girls enter early adolescence responding to frustration and distress with a style that is less effective and action-oriented than boys. Second, girls begin to face uncontrollable stressors in early adolescence to a greater extent than boys.[53] Data suggested that girls exhibit more passive and introspective coping styles that are associated with longer and more severe depressive symptoms; girls undergo biological changes that are less favored by society; and girls and women face more negative life events and social conditions such as sexual abuse and stronger parental and peer expectations.

Multicultural Issues of Depression and Suicide

Suicide rates vary by gender, age, race, and ethnicity. Men are more likely to commit suicide than women, with rates in the United States generally higher for white men and Reservation Native American (Indian) men. Elderly white men (65 years of age and older) and young, male Reservation Native Americans are particularly susceptible. By comparison, the suicide rate for male adolescents is lower, but there has been a steady increase in suicide rates among all youth in the United States aged 15 to 19 years since the 1950s.[54]

The relationship between depression and stressful life events seems to cut across cultures. A survey of community housewives in a Taiwanese city revealed that as stressful life events increased so did the level of depression.[55] Younger housewives reported more depressive symptoms than older housewives. Also, the presence of social support seemed to protect women from depression.

As a member of a minority group it can be difficult to adjust to the culture of the majority. Mexican American women in Kansas City who reported greater difficulties with acculturation also demonstrated higher incidences of depression.[56]

Gender-role socialization can also impact depression. Native American women who were more traditional and more domestic in their role definition showed higher depression, higher role conflict, lower self-esteem, and lower life satisfaction than women who were less traditional and less domestic.[57] A similar pattern was prevalent among working black women. The more feminine-oriented group of black women had significantly higher depression and lower self-esteem than the black women who were more androgynous, that is, women who were more balanced between feminine (domestic, traditional) and masculine (adventurous, less traditional) orienta-

tions.[58] A sample of working white women demonstrated less depression and higher self-esteem for women who were more androgynous than for women who were less androgynous.[59]

Depression is very prevalent among the elderly population, regardless of ethnicity. In 1992, adults in the United States who were over the age of 65 had a suicide rate of 16.5 per 100,000.[60] The rates increase substantially to 22.8 per 100,000 among people over 85 years of age. The occurrence of depression in the elderly is most associated with the presence of financial strain and poor physical health.[61] Social support counters the effect of these particular stressors and is a great buffer against depression in the elderly.

Youth suicide is a major concern for most countries. In 1987, the suicide rate for youth, aged 15 through 19 years, in the United States was 10.3 suicides per 100,000 resident population.[62] Adolescent suicide in the United States has continued to rise since 1987, and in 1995 was reported to be the third leading cause of death among persons 15 to 24 years of age.[63] The teenage suicide rate dramatically increased in New Zealand between 1970 and 1990.[64] Young women were equally as troubled as young men. Suicide attempts for New Zealand teenagers were highly related to: a high rate of depression, substance abuse, family dysfunction, and sexual abuse. This pattern is repeated across the world, including in the United States. (See Table 5.1.)

The following facts regarding death by suicide are provided by the Department of Health and Human Services:[65]

- Between 1980 and 1991 the age-adjusted rate for suicide, the eighth leading cause of death, remained stable at 11.4 deaths per 100,000 resident population.
- Suicide is more prevalent among men than women. In 1991, suicide rates were more than four times as high for white males (19.9 deaths per 100,000 population) as white females (4.8), and nearly seven times as high for black males (12.5) as black females (1.9).
- Between 1980 and 1991, age-adjusted suicide rates increased 13 percent for black males and 5 percent for white males primarily because of increases in suicide rates among the elderly. During the same period, suicide rates declined 16 percent for white females. For black females, suicide rates fluctuated between 1.9 and 2.5 deaths per 100,000 showing no consistent trend.

Table 5.1

Suicide Mortality Rates in the United States[66] (suicide rates per 100,000 resident population)		
	1992	1990–92 (Average)
White male	19.5	19.9
Black male	12.4	12.4
Native American male	*	19.4
Asian male	8.5	8.7
Hispanic male	12.2	12.4
White female	4.6	4.7
Black female	2.1	2.1
Native American female	*	3.8
Asian female	*	3.5
Hispanic female	*	2.3
Overall	11.1	11.3

*=Insufficient data.

Predictors of Suicide

In 1987, in the United States 30,783 people died of suicide.[67] The following have been determined to be predictors of attempted or successful suicide:[68]

- Previous suicide attempts
- Inadequate treatment
- Medical illness
- Family history of suicide or psychiatric disorder
- Exposure to suicidal behavior
- Family violence
- Availability of firearms in the home
- Stressful life circumstances such as separation or divorce, unemployment, or limited socioeconomic resources

Men and women differ in why and how they attempt suicide.[69] Women tend to be suicidal more often in response to interpersonal problems, whereas men tend to be suicidal more often in response to intrapsychic conflicts and to commit suicide in response to job loss and legal problems. Also, women tend to use different methods for suicide than those used by men. Men prefer aggressive methods such as hanging and shooting, whereas women prefer passive methods such as drugs and poisons. The most common methods for attempted suicides are minor lacerations (for example, wrist cutting) and pill ingestion, whereas the most common method for successful suicide is firearms.

THE COUNSELING OPTION

There might be times in your life when you or someone you know needs counseling to assist with a mental or emotional concern. A mental health counselor can be very effective at facilitating the recovery process either through therapy or by recommending available resources.

When shopping for a mental health professional it is wise to get a referral from someone who has knowledge about the capabilities and expertise of a particular counselor that might be helpful for you. This referral might come from a family member, a friend, a physician, a teacher, or a spiritual counselor. If a referral is not possible, the telephone yellow pages can suggest several possibilities, though the expertise and training of a counselor cannot be guaranteed this way.

In setting up your first appointment, feel free to request time to interview the counselor before agreeing to enter into the therapeutic relationship and ask that, until you make your decision, you not be required to pay a counseling fee. Many counselors will require a payment for the first meeting, so you might want to interview the counselor over the telephone before meeting with them. During your initial interview with the therapist, be sure to inquire about his or her educational background, professional training, experience, professional credentials, and approach to counseling. You have a right to know about the training, credentials, and counseling approach of any counselor that you are considering.

Mental health providers are required by most states to be licensed or certified by a health board in order to practice counseling. In addition, counselors who have been found guilty of a breach of ethics or illegal acts risk losing their license to practice. These controls and standards are in existence to help protect the consumer from abuse, neglect, and sexual or other exploitation by their therapist. Not all states in the United States require that counselors be licensed or certified by a state health board. Thus, it is especially important to explore the background and training of a counselor who is not credentialed by a state licensing or certification board.

EMOTIONS AND HEALTH

Sometimes people talk about good emotions and bad emotions, or healthy emotions and unhealthy emotions. However, it is not the emotion itself that is

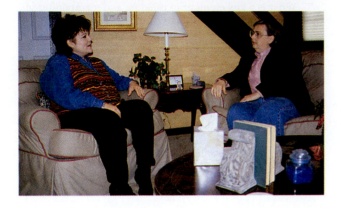

Counseling is a good option if you need more assistance than your friends or family can provide.

good or bad, nor is it necessarily the emotion that is healthy or unhealthy. Emotions are natural states that result from the perceived impact of an event or the memory of an event. Emotions serve as guideposts to help you understand just what kind of an impact something has on you. Emotions are designed to direct your behavior for life development and life survival. It is the choice of behavior that follows an emotion that can be judged as good or bad, appropriate or inappropriate, or healthy or unhealthy.

Keeping your emotions pinned up inside you can be very detrimental to your health. Suppressing your feelings can cause escalating tension in the body. Releasing your feelings and thoughts on a regular basis by talking to someone, laughing, or crying can help relieve the pressure that is building inside you. Without regular release, the pressure can rise to the point where you explode, and you say or do things that are harmful to yourself or to others.

Confiding in others appears to protect the body against damaging internal stresses and seems to have long-term health benefits.[70] Whenever possible, confide in friends or family members whom you trust. When this is not sufficient to get you through a stressful time, then seek out the services of a professional mental health provider. What you feel and think is important, and sharing your feelings and thoughts with someone else in confidence can be good for you.

CONCLUSION

Life is a challenge and it helps to have guidance from significant others, teachers, and role models. It also helps to have life skills that help you to cope with the demands that life presents. The greater the personal support system you have and the more life skills you learn and practice, then the higher the likelihood that more of your emotions will be happy ones instead of sad ones, or that the sad ones that you do have will not linger as long. However, remember that emotional health is not determined by how many happy feelings you have versus how many sad feelings. Both happy and sad feelings are normal and natural responses to life's challenges. If you have a good support system and well-developed life skills, then the many challenges that life presents can be more enjoyable and perhaps less harsh than they otherwise would be.

Chapter Summary

- Being aware of the various social influences that impact your development can enhance your potential life satisfaction.
- Assertiveness training is a life skill that can enhance self-confidence and result in improvements in relationships and performance.
- Effective listening is required to facilitate healthy communication.
- When conflicts or problems arise, effective problem solving is a useful tool to reach resolution. This involves a step-by-step process: defining the problem, generating solutions, evaluating solutions, making a decision, and implementing the decision.

- Building and maintaining a positive self-image is paramount to feeling good about yourself and achieving successes.
- Similar to self-image, self-esteem involves being realistic about who you think you should be, and loving and accepting who you already are.
- The journey through life will include the loss of loved ones along the way. The grief process is a normal response to loss.
- When life's challenges become too great, depression may arise. If you feel lost and alone, you need to reach out to others for support.
- Sometimes seeking out personal therapy is necessary to facilitate growth when you feel stuck in an uncomfortable emotional state.

Review Questions

1. Can you name some of the social and cultural influences that can impact the development of the self?
2. Can you name some situations in which one may need to be assertive?
3. What are the six basic types of assertive messages? Can you give examples?
4. What are the basic components of effective listening? Can you give examples?
5. What are some misconceptions about conflict and problem solving?
6. What are the six basic steps to problem solving? Can you describe what is involved with each of these steps?
7. What is a key element to building and maintaining self-image?
8. Can you define the three clinical conditions related to body-image dissatisfaction?
9. Can you define self-esteem?
10. What is the process of self-esteem enhancement?
11. What are the three phases of mourning and the five stages of the grief process?
12. Can you name and describe the various types of depression?
13. What are some common predictors of suicide?

Resources

Organizations and Hotlines

American Counseling Association (ACA)
5999 Stevenson Ave.
Alexandria, VA 22304-3300
Telephone: (703) 823-9800

American Psychological Association (APA)
750 1st St. NE
Washington, D.C. 20002-4242
Telephone: (202) 336-5500

American Association for Marriage and Family Therapy
1100 17th St. NW
10th Floor
Washington, D.C. 20036
Telephone: (202) 452-0109

Audiotapes

1. *Depression.* Duluth, MN, 1995, Whole Person Associates (Phone: 1-800-247-6789).

Videotapes

1. *Learning to Manage Anger: The Rethink Workout for Teens.* Champaign, IL, 1995, Research Press (Phone: 217-352-3273).
2. *The Practical Parenting Series.* Champaign, IL, 1995, Research Press (Phone: 217-352-3273).
3. *Anger Management for Parents.* Champaign, IL, 1995, Research Press (Phone: 217-352-3273).
4. *Facing Death.* Champaign, IL, 1995, Research Press (Phone: 217-352-3273).
5. *A Family in Grief.* Champaign, IL, 1995, Research Press (Phone: 217-352-3273).
6. Kilbourne, J. *Slim Hopes: Advertising and the Obsession with Thinness.* Northampton, MA, 1995, Media Education Foundation.

Websites

National Mental Health Association
http://www.nmha.org/

American Psychiatric Association
http://www.psych.org/

American Psychological Association
http://www.apa.org/

American Counseling Association
http://www.counseling.org/

Suggested Readings

Ahrons, C. 1994. *The good divorce.* Philadelphia: Harp.
Alberti, R. 1990. *Your perfect right: A guide to assertive living.* Obispo, Calif.: Impact Pub.
Alberti, R. 1994. *Making yourself heard: A guide to assertive relationships.* Obispo, Calif.: Impact Pub.
Anderson, P. 1991. *Affairs in order: A complete resource guide to death and dying.* New York: Macmillan.
Benziger, K. 1992. *Overcoming depression: A self-help workbook.* Westminster, Calif.: KBA Pub.
Burns, D. 1993. *Ten days to self-esteem!* New York: Morrow.
Butler, P. 1992. *Self-assertion for women.* San Francisco: Harper Collins.
Campbell, S. 1984. *Beyond the power struggle: Dealing with conflict in love and work.* Obispo, Calif.: Impact Pub.
Crary, E. 1984. *Kids can cooperate: A practical guide to teaching problem solving.* Seattle: Parenting Press.
Deits, B. 1992. *Life after loss: A personal guide dealing with death, divorce, job change and relocation.* Tuscon, Az.: Fisher Books.
Eberhardt, L. 1987. *Working with women's groups, volumes I and II.* Duluth, Minn.: Whole Person Associates.

Fay, A. 1994. *Prescription for a quality relationship.* Obispo, Calif.: Impact Pub.

Fisher, B. 1992. *Rebuilding when your relationship ends.* Obispo, Calif.: Impact Pub.

Guerra, N., A. Moore, and R. Slab. 1995. *Viewpoints: A guide to conflict resolution and decision making for adolescents.* Champaign, Ill.: Research Press.

Hundley, M. 1993. *Awaken to good mourning.* Arlington, Tex.: Crocker Associates.

Krementz, J. 1988. *How it feels when parents divorce.* New York: Knopf.

Lazarus, A., C. Lazarus, and A. Fay. 1993. *Don't believe it for a minute: Forty toxic ideas that are driving you crazy.* Obispo, Calif.: Impact Pub.

McKay, G., and D. Dinkmeyer. 1994. *How you feel is up to you: The power of emotional choice.* Obispo, Calif.: Impact Pub.

Neeld, E. 1990. *Seven choices: Taking the steps to new life after losing someone you love.* New York: Clarkson N. Potter.

Newman, L. 1991. *Somebody to love: A guide to loving the body you have.* Chicago: Third Side Press.

Palmer, P. 1994. *I wish I could hold your hand: A child's guide to grief and loss.* Obispo, Calif.: Impact Pub.

Palmer, P., and M. Froehner. 1989. *Teen esteem: A self-direction manual for young adults.* Obispo, Calif.: Impact Pub.

Preston, J. 1989. *You can beat depression: A guide to recovery.* Obispo, Calif.: Impact Pub.

Preston, J. 1993. *Growing beyond emotional pain: Action plans for healing.* Obispo, Calif.: Impact Pub.

Tubesing, D., and N. Tubesing. 1991. *Seeking your healthy balance.* Duluth, Minn.: Whole Person Associates.

Zerbe, K. 1995. *The body betrayed: A deeper understanding of women, eating disorders, and treatment.* Carlsbad, Calif.: Gurze Books.

References

1. Lange, J., and P. Jakubowski. 1976. *Responsible assertive behavior.* Champaign, Ill.: Research Press, pp. 7, 218–20.

2. Harrington, M. 1995. Who has it best? Women's labor force participation, perceptions of leisure and constraints to enjoyment of leisure. *Journal of Leisure Research* 27 (1): 4–24.

3. Hart, L., and L. Silka. 1994. Building self-efficacy through women-centered ropes course experiences. Special issue: Wilderness therapy for women: The power of adventure. *Women and Therapy* 15 (3–4): 111–27.

4. Aubrey, A., and M. MacLeod. 1994. So . . . What does rock climbing have to do with career planning? Special Issue: Wilderness therapy for women: The power of adventure. *Women and Therapy* 15 (3–4): 205–16.

5. Keisling, B., and M. Gynther. 1993. Male perceptions of female attractiveness: The effects of targets' personal attributes and subjects' degree of masculinity. *Journal of Clinical Psychology* 49 (2): 190–95.

6. Lange and Jakubowski, *Responsible assertive behavior.*

7. Jakubowski, P., and A. Lange. 1978. *The assertive option.* Champaign, Ill.: Research Press, pp. 157–69.

8. Dillard, J., and R. Reilly. 1988. *Systematic interviewing: Communication skills for professional effectiveness.* Columbus, Ohio: Merrill Pub.

9. Jakubowski and Lange, *The assertive option.*

10. Gordon, J. 1974. *Teacher effectiveness training.* New York: Wyden Books.

11. American Psychiatric Association. 1994. *Diagnostic and statistical manual of mental disorders, 4th edition.* Washington, D.C.: APA.

12. American Movie Channel (AMC). *The Hollywood fashion machine.* AMC television broadcast March 2, 1996.

13. Ibid.

14. Kilborne, J. 1995. *Slim hopes: Advertising and Obsession with Thinness,* video. Northampton, Mass.: Media Education Foundation.

15. Cohen, B. 1986. *The snowhite syndrome.* New York: Macmillan.

16. Wolf, N. 1991. *The beauty myth.* New York: Anchor/Doubleday.

17. Fallon, A. 1990. Culture in the mirror: Sociocultural determinants of body image. In T. Cash and T. Pruzinsky, *Body images: Development, deviance and change.* New York: Guilford.

18. Zimmerman, J. 1997. An image to heal. *Humanist* 57 (Jan/Feb) (1): 20.

19. Lee, A., and S. Lee. 1996. Disordered eating and its psychosocial correlates among Chinese adolescent females in Hong Kong. *International Journal of Eating Disorders,* 20 (2): 177–83.

20. Ben-Tovim, D. 1996. Is big still beautiful in Polynesia? *The Lancet* 348: 1047–48.

21. Akan, G., and C. Gril. 1995. Sociocultural influences on eating attitudes and behaviors, body image, and psychological functioning: A comparison of African-American, Asian-American, and Caucasian college

women. *International Journal of Eating Disorders* 18 (2): 181–87.

22. Furnham, A., and N. Greaves. 1994. Gender and locus of control correlates of body image dissatisfaction. *European Journal of Personality* 8 (3): 183–200.

23. Koff, E., J. Rierdan, and M. Stubbs. 1990. Gender, body image, and self-concept in early adolescence. *Journal of Early Adolescence* 10 (1): 56–68.

24. Cash, T., and A. Labarge. 1996. Development of the Appearance Schemas Inventory: A new cognitive body-image assessment. *Cognitive Therapy and Research* 20 (1): 37–50.

25. Probst, M., W. Vandereycken, H. Van Coppenolle, and G. Pieter. 1995. Body size estimation in eating disorder patients: Testing the video distortion method on a life-size screen. *Behaviour Therapy and Research* 33 (8): 985–90.

26. Ibid.

27. Sanford, L., and M. Donovan. 1988. *Women & self-esteem: Understanding and improving the way we think and feel about ourselves.* New York: Penguin Books, pp. 97 and 101.

28. Miller, L., L. Cooke, J. Tsang, and F. Morgan. 1992. Should I brag? Nature and impact of positive and boastful disclosures for women and men. *Human Communication Research* 18 (3): 364–99.

29. Woods, N., M. Lentz, E. Mitchell, and L. Oakley. 1994. Depressed mood and self-esteem in young Asian, Black, and White women in America. *Health Care for Women International* 15 (3): 243–62.

30. Hundley, M. 1993. *Awaken to good mourning.* Arlington, Tex.: Crocker Associates, p. 83.

31. Ibid.

32. Kubler-Ross, E. 1969. *On death and dying.* New York: Macmillan.

33. Wolfelt, A. D. 1997. *The journey through grief: Reflections on healing.* Fort Collins, Colo.: Center for Loss and Life Transition.

34. APA, *Diagnostic and statistical manual of mental disorders.*

35. Ibid.

36. Ibid.

37. Ibid.

38. Pajer, K. 1994. New strategies in the treatment of depression in women. 147th Annual Meeting of the American Psychiatric Association, Philadelphia, Penn.

39. Nolen-Hoeksema, S. 1990. *Sex differences in depression.* Stanford, Calif.: Stanford University Press.

40. Furnham, A., and N. Greaves. 1994. Gender and locus of control correlates of body image dissatisfaction. *European Journal of Personality* 8 (3): 183–200.

41. Brown, G., T. Harris, and C. Hepworth. 1995. Loss, humiliation and entrapment among women developing depression: A patient and non-patient comparison. *Psychological Medicine* 25 (1): 7–21.

42. Fox, K., and B. Gilbert. 1994. The interpersonal and psychological functioning of women who experienced childhood physical abuse, incest, and parental alcoholism. *Child Abuse and Neglect* 18 (10): 849–58.

43. Andrews, B. 1995. Bodily shame as a mediator between abusive experiences and depression. *Journal of Abnormal Psychology* 104 (2): 277–85.

44. Silvern, L., J. Karyl, L. Waelde, and W. Hodges. 1995. Retrospective reports of parental partner abuse: Relationships to depression, trauma symptoms and self-esteem among college students. *Journal of Family Violence* 10 (2): 177–202.

45. Hobfoll, M., C. Ritter, J. Lavin, M. Hulsizer, et al. 1995. Depression prevalence and incidence among inner-city pregnant and postpartum women. *Journal of Consulting and Clinical Psychology* 63 (3): 445–53.

46. High, R., and P. Marcellino. 1994. Menopausal women and the work environment. *Social Behavior and Personality* 22 (4): 347–53.

47. Kendler, K., R. Kessler, E. Walters, and C. MacLean. 1995. Stressful life events, genetic liability, and onset of an episode of major depression in women. *American Journal of Psychiatry* 152 (6): 833–42.

48. Thorson, J., and F. Powell. 1994. Depression and sense of humor. *Psychological Reports* 73 (3): 1473–74.

49. Drebing, C., W. Gooden, S. Drebing, and H. Van de Kemp. 1995. The dream in mid-life women: Its impact on mental health. *International Journal of Aging and Human Development* 40 (1): 73–87.

50. Andrews, B., and G. Brown. 1995. Stability and change in low self-esteem: The role of psychosocial factors. *Psychological Medicine* 25 (1): 23–31.

51. Nolen-Hoeksema, S. 1994. An interactive model for the emergence of gender differences in depression in adolescence. *Journal of Research on Adolescence* 4 (4): 519–34.

52. APA, *Diagnostic and statistical manual of mental disorders.*

53. Nolen-Hoeksema, An interactive model of gender differences in depression.

54. Centers for Disease Control. 1986. *Youth suicide in the United States, 1970–1980,* Atlanta, Ga., Division of Injury Epidemiology and Control.

55. Lu, L. 1994. Life events, social support and depression amongst Taiwanese housewives. *Counseling Psychology Quarterly* 7 (2): 221–26.

56. Masten, W., E. Penland, and E. Nayani. 1994. Depression and acculturation in Mexican-American women. *Psychological Reports* 75 (3): 1499–1503.

57. Napholz, L. 1995. Mental health and American Indian women's multiple roles. *American Indian and Alaska Native Mental Health Research* 6 (2): 57–75.

58. Napholz, L. 1994. Sex role orientation and psychological well-being among working Black women. *Journal of Black Psychology* 20 (4): 469–82.

59. Napholz, L. 1994. Indices of psychological well-being and sex role orientation among working women. *Health Care for Women International* 15 (4): 307–16.

60. U.S. Dept. of Health and Human Services. 1996. *Healthy People 2000: Midcourse Review and 1995 Revisions.* Boston: Jones & Bartlett.

61. Mendes-de-Leon, C., S. Rapp, and S. Kasl. 1994. Financial strain and symptoms of depression in a community sample of elderly men and women: A longitudinal study. *Journal of Aging and Health* 6 (4): 448–68.

62. Centers for Disease Control (CDC). 1987. *National Vital Statistics System.* Washington, D.C.: CDC.

63. U.S. Dept. of Health and Human Services, *Healthy People 2000.*

64. Disley, B. 1994. Suicide prevention initiatives: Youth suicide: The world wide picture. *Community Mental Health in New Zealand* 8 (2): 5–11.

65. National Center for Health Statistics. 1994. *Health United States 1993.* Hyattsville, Md.: DHHS Pub. No. (PHS) 94–1232.

66. National Center for Health Statistics. 1995. *Health United States 1994.* Hyattsville, Md.: July, DHHS Pub. No. (PHS) 94–1232.

67. National Center for Health Statistics. 1990. *Health United States 1989 and Prevention Profile.* Hyattsville, Md.: DHHS Pub. No. (PHS) 90–1232. U.S. Department of Health and Human Services.

68. Klerman, G. 1987. Clinical epidemiology of suicide. *Journal of Clinical Psychiatry* 48: 33–38.

69. Lester, D. 1988. *Why women kill themselves.* Springfield, Ill.: Charles C Thomas, pp. 8–9.

70. Pennebaker, J. 1990. *Opening up: The healing power of confiding in others.* New York: William Morrow.

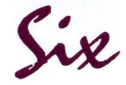

Managing the Stress of Life

■ chapter objectives

When you complete this chapter you will be able to:
- Describe the anatomy and physiology of stress.
- Identify the warning signs of too much stress.
- Summarize the different types of life stressors.
- Describe the impact of stress on women.
- Demonstrate effective coping strategies for stress management.

Nine to Five

Tumble out of bed and stumble to the kitchen.
Pour myself a cup of ambition.
Yawn and stretch and try to come to life.
Jump in the shower and the blood starts pumping
Out on the street the traffic starts jumping.
With folks like me on the job from nine to five.
Working nine to five.
What a way to make a living.
Barely getting by.
It's all taking and no giving.
They just use your mind.
And they never give you credit.
It's enough to drive you crazy if you let it . . .
    By Dolly Parton (Velvet Apple Music, 1980).

Too much to do and too little time to do it.

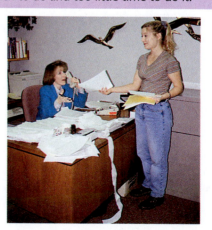

HEALTHY PEOPLE 2000 OBJECTIVES

- Reduce to less than 35 percent the proportion of people aged 18 and older who experienced adverse health effects from stress within the past year. 1995 progress toward goal: 60 percent
- Decrease to no more than 5 percent the proportion of people aged 18 and older who report experiencing significant levels of stress who do not take steps to reduce or control their stress. 1995 progress toward goal: -20 percent
- Increase to at least 40 percent the proportion of work sites employing 50 or more people that provide programs to reduce employee stress. 1995 progress toward goal: 80 percent

CONCEPTS OF STRESS

You, like most people, have a lifestyle that, in one way or another, and at some time or another, can create stress in your life. **Stress** is the body's response to demands. A **stressor** is the demand itself. Such demands can include everyday life events such as getting up, going to work or school, being at work or school, rushing home to fix dinner, dashing off to play a quick game of tennis, spending time with the family in the evening, and catching up on work at home before going to bed at night. Stress is not something you can ever completely get away from; however, it is something you can learn to understand and to manage. Figure 6.1 identifies the types of stressors we encounter.

FIGURE 6.1 Types of stressors.

Stressors can be grouped into five categories:[1]

- Social stressors—noise, crowding, etc.
- Psychological stressors—anxiety, worry, etc.
- Psychosocial stressors—loss of a job, death of a family member, spouse, or friend, etc.
- Biochemical stressors—heat, cold, injury, pollutants, poor nutrition, etc.
- Philosophical stressors—value system conflict, lack of purpose, lack of direction, etc.

Stress and Perception

The way in which you might respond to an event depends greatly on how you may perceive that event. Perceptions can vary greatly from person to person. Perceptions can be impacted by immediate potential consequences and by a cumulation of life experiences. For example, students who must take a final exam may each have different stress responses to the event depending upon their own expectations of self and/or the value of the event. (See *Her Story:* "Janet and Ellen.")

Where do the expectations you place on yourself and onto others come from? Many psychologists believe that expectations come from your social environment—the messages you receive from your

Her Story

Janet and Ellen

Janet was nervous about the final exam because it was the last thing that stood between her and maintaining a high grade of "A" in the class, which is what she expected of herself. Janet's nervousness about the test caused her to have test anxiety, which made it even more difficult to remember what she had studied. On the other hand, Ellen felt relief about taking the final exam because she would be satisfied with at least a "B" in the class and could have a lower grade on the final exam and still be able to achieve at least a "B" class average. Ellen was very relaxed when taking the exam and found it easy to recall the necessary information. Janet and Ellen each experienced different stress levels regarding the same event because each had different expectations of self and the value each of them placed on the event was not the same.

- Why do you think Janet and Ellen placed a different value on the exam and on the grade they wanted in the class?
- What recommendations might you have for Janet to help her deal with her anxiety?

stress—physiological and psychological state of arousal caused by the perceived presence of a challenging or threatening event.

stressors—factors or events, real or imagined, that elicit a state of stress.

Many students suffer with test anxiety.

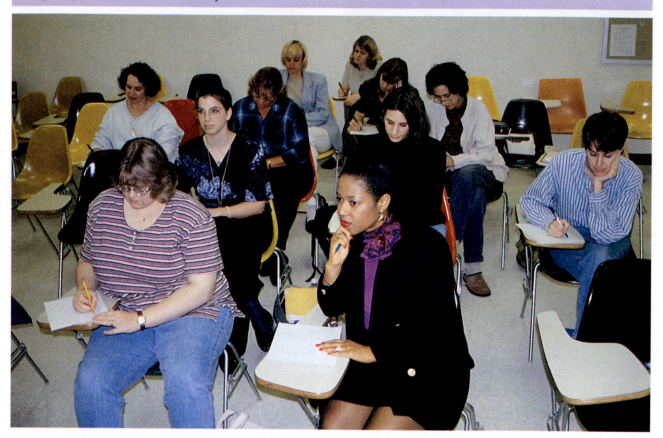

family, friends, and society that you integrate into your own belief and value system. These expectations can be less than, equal to, or exceed the demand of a particular situation. If your expectations of yourself are at a certain criteria for performance and you do not meet that criteria, then you will probably be greatly bothered by the failure to meet the criteria. The level at which you set the criteria for success is going to effect how much stress you experience in trying to meet or surpass that goal. This is why having realistic expectations of yourself is important in managing your stress level.

Look outside of yourself and beyond family members by examining the goals and ambitions of your peers and healthy role models. This will help you determine what is realistic and what is not. This is not meant to imply that you should not strive toward excellence; it only suggests that you should pick and choose specific areas to excel in and that you should not try to excel in every area of life; that could be too stressful and too exhausting.

In some situations, some amount of stress is necessary in order to motivate you to perform and strive to do your best. Too little stress, as well as too much stress, can impede performance. A moderate amount of stress can drive you to try harder and improve your current abilities. If you want to win the sports tournament or a grand prize at the state fair, then you have to work hard. Hard work involves stress.

The same kind of sensitivity to being realistic and self-aware may direct you to adjust the demands of a situation to your preferred stress level. Imagine that you were asked to perform the following tasks within the next week: write two papers, prepare a major presentation, have fifteen appointments, attend two weddings, and watch one of your best friends play in an all-weekend basketball tournament. How are you going to accomplish all of these tasks and still find time to do daily home chores, exercise, eat nutritionally, and find time to relax, much less sleep? It would be very difficult to maintain this kind of schedule and expect to stay healthy for very long.

In addition, you may not enjoy this high of a demand level; it may create much more stress in your life than you prefer. You might need to prioritize events and exercise assertiveness by saying "no" to some demands or by renegotiating completion dates. In addition, you might recruit some assistance for those tasks that you cannot complete alone within a realistic time span.

Positive Versus Negative Stress

Not all stress is bad. There is constructive stress and destructive stress. Whereas debilitating or excessive stress is often referred to as **distress,** constructive stress is called **eustress** (prefix *eu* from Greek meaning "good").[2] Stress arousal can be a positive motivating force that improves the quality of life. Initially, as stress increases so does health, performance, and general well-being. However, as stress continues to increase, an *optimal stress* level is obtained, and if stress continues beyond this point to *maximum stress,* then performance quickly declines and health begins to erode. Complete *Journal Activity:* "How Do You Handle Stress?" to determine how you handle stress.

THE STRESS RESPONSE

Fight-or-Flight Response

The **fight-or-flight response** is your body's natural response to a perceived danger.[3] The body goes on alert and various physiological changes occur that will allow you to survive the threat. For instance, imagine that you are walking through a beautiful mountain forest with luscious pine trees and a fresh breeze is blowing your hair. You are relaxed and allowing your mind to wander and enjoy the experience. You hear the sound of thunder overhead. You look up and suddenly you realize that the thunder is actually the sound of a large boulder falling down from the cliff above and heading for your path. Instantly your body begins to respond to the threat. Blood vessels constrict, forcing more blood toward your heart and lungs. Your heart begins to pound, sending blood to vital organs. Your lungs open up and your breathing gets faster. Your pupils dilate so you can see better. Adrenalin is sent into your system to give you a burst of strength. With all of this added metabolic help you are able to leap away from the giant rock as it explodes past you. In this

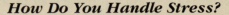

JOURNAL ACTIVITY

How Do You Handle Stress?

Think of some times in your life when you experienced stress from events in each of the five categories of stressors (see Fig. 6.1). Write about the experience and suggest ways to alter or manage those stressors. Altering a stressor is finding a way to change the event to be less stressful, that is, extending deadlines, getting assistance, and so on. Managing the stressor is finding a way to experience less stress during the stressor, that is, practicing relaxation exercises, eating healthy foods, and so on.

particular instance, you chose the "flight" response. And a wise choice it was, because you might not have been able to defeat the large boulder in a fight. When the perceived threat is past, your body will begin to return to its prearousal condition. It takes longer for your body's systems to return to a state of relaxation than it does to become aroused. So you may be a little shaky for several minutes or so, depending upon how often you replay the experience again in your mind.

The stress response created by a life-threatening event is easy to recognize. However, your body has the ability to respond to stressors in varying degrees according to how important an event is perceived or imagined to be by you. Just getting out of bed and rushing to work or school can elevate the stress response, although to a degree much less noticeable than when running from an avalanche of rock. The stress response helps you to maximize your performance and to survive danger. However, if your stress response is not turned off periodically, it can create wear and tear on your body's systems. Your body will begin to break down and illness can set in.

---

distress—stress that diminishes the quality of life; commonly associated with disease, illness, and maladaptation.

eustress (you stress)—stress that adds a positive, enhancing dimension to the quality of life.

fight-or-flight response—the body's innate response to stress either by confrontation or avoidance.

General Adaptation Syndrome

The **general adaptation syndrome (GAS)** is a specific pattern of responses that your body experiences as a reaction to life demands or threats.[4] The GAS has three stages: (1) alarm reaction, (2) stress resistance, and (3) stress exhaustion. In the alarm reaction stage, hormones are released that create the arousal response in your body necessary to respond to the demand being placed upon it from the environment. This is the initiation of the fight-or-flight response. The stress resistance stage is when your body tries to return to a state of internal balance that existed before the onset of the stress; this state is referred to as **homeostasis.** The persistent presentation of stressors throughout the day results in cumulative stress. As stressors continue to be presented and the stress response occurs followed by the body working to return to balance, your body eventually becomes exhausted. This is the stress exhaustion stage when parts of your body begin to break down.

You can learn to voluntarily control the stress response. Then you can give yourself the added burst when you need it, but also monitor the use of the stress response and turn it way down or even totally off frequently. You can conserve your stress response in the same way that you conserve electricity in your home. The less you use, the less you have to pay for later.

Anatomy and Physiology of Stress

An event in your life begins the journey to becoming a perceived stressor as a message to your cerebral cortex, the higher centers of the brain (see Fig. 6.2). The thalamus, the part of the brain that serves as the main relay center for sensory impulses to the cerebral cortex, sorts the information, makes a decision that the event is indeed of a stressful nature and, thus, a stressor is perceived. Next, another part of the brain, the **hypothalamus,** is stimulated. Once the hypothalamus is stimulated, two major response pathways are activated in the body: the endocrine system and the autonomic nervous system.

Endocrine System

The endocrine system is activated by the anterior section of your hypothalamus. The anterior portion of the hypothalamus gland releases a hormone called the corticotrophin-releasing factor (CRF). CRF stimulates the **pituitary gland** of the brain and it releases **adrenocorticotropic hormone (ACTH).** ACTH is continuously released into the body, via the bloodstream, in small amounts during the day. However, a mental or physical demand can cause up to twenty times this amount to be secreted within seconds after a perceived stressor. ACTH stimulates the **adrenal glands,** which are located on top of the kidney and secrete **corticoids.** The adrenal glands secrete mostly gluco-corticoids, primarily cortisol, and mineralo-corticoids, primarily aldosterone.

Aldosterone, transported by the blood, acts on the kidney to increase sodium absorption. This creates an increase in osmotic pressure that forces extracellular fluid into the blood, causing an increase in blood volume and an increase in blood pressure. Cortisol creates metabolic alterations in the body, increasing the **metabolic rate** in response to stress and decreasing the metabolic rate when stress is no longer perceived. The body attempts to get as much glucose into circulation as possible. Glucose is the body's most basic source of energy. If the stress response is maintained, glucose may become depleted and the body will then begin to draw off of the remaining energy reserves, fat deposits, and muscle tissue. As the body meets the demands and relief begins to occur, excess cortisol levels will act to shut down the production of CRF in the hypothalamus and the physiological stress response will begin to stop.

Autonomic Nervous System

The autonomic nervous system is activated by the posterior section of your hypothalamus. The autonomic nervous system (ANS) excites and inhibits various bodily functions. The ANS stimulates motor functions, blood sugar production, and inhibitory functions. The ANS stimulates the adrenal medulla, which then secretes the hormones **epinephrine** (adrenalin) and **norepinephrine** (adrenalin-like substances). Norepinephrine increases blood pressure, and the strength and frequency of the heartbeat. Epinephrine increases oxygen consumption, relaxes smooth muscles of the digestive system, increases carbohydrate metabolism, dilates arterials in the heart and skeletal muscles, accelerates heart rate, increases the volume of the blood, and decreases blood clotting time.

The shutdown of the digestive system during stress reduces the production of saliva, a fluid that contains digestive enzymes, and may result in a dry mouth. Also, decreased digestive activity can contribute to indigestion and stomachaches from poorly digested food.

DISTRESS AND THE BODY

Stress and "Dis-ease"

Prolonged stress can put your body at "dis-ease." The longer the body is under a strain, the more likely this dis-ease will lead to uncomfortable and sometimes disabling symptoms or disorders. Your body is not capable of maintaining high levels of stress or arousal for prolonged periods of time without its systems beginning to break down. The stress response in humans is better designed for short bursts of energy and strength to survive immediate and short-lived challenges or dangers. Your body can maintain greater health status if there are sufficient periods of nonarousal between the heightened arousal episodes. The stress-adaptation theory suggests that stress depletes your reserve capacity, thereby increasing your vulnerability to health problems.[5] This relates to the general adaptation syndrome mentioned earlier.

Stress-Related Disorders

Prolonged stress can lead to the development of a broad range of stress-related disorders in the individual, from the somewhat painful and annoying to life-threatening diseases. These stress-related disorders are called **psychosomatic disorders.** Just a few examples of these types of symptoms and disorders include: tension and migraine headaches; muscle pain specific to the neck, back, or shoulders; insomnia; anxiety attacks; depression; digestive disorders (ulcers, colitis); cardiovascular disorders (high blood pressure, heart arrhythmias); respiratory disorders (asthma, allergies); pancreatic disorders (diabetes); and cancer. One of your body's systems that is most vulnerable to the effects of prolonged stress is your immune system. Hormones released during the stress response, specifically adrenal hormones, can have a destructive effect on important immune system cells. Under prolonged periods of stress your immune system will become less capable of fighting off illness and disease, thus making you more prone to colds, flu, or bacterial infections. (See *FYI:* "Researchers Link Hormones of Stress with Disease.")

Stress Amenorrhea A stress symptom that is specific to women includes **stress amenorrhea.** Stress amenorrhea is when menstruation stops because of physical or mental stress.[7] Stress can also cause irregularity in the menstrual cycle; that is, time between periods can vary significantly and so can flow rates. Fasting, irregular eating habits, or too much exercise can also place enough stress on the body to cause menstrual irregularity or cessation. If you experience menstrual cessation or irregularity, you need to consult with your health-care provider, as you would with any other conditions of concern.

general adaptation syndrome—sequenced physiological response to the presence of a stressor; the alarm, resistance, and exhaustion stages of the stress response.

homeostasis (home ee oh **stay** sis)—the state of internal balance that the body tries to maintain.

hypothalamus—portion of the midbrain that provides a connection between the cerebral cortex and the pituitary gland.

pituitary gland—"master gland" of the endocrine system; the wide variety of hormones produced by the pituitary are sent to structures throughout the body.

adrenocorticotropic hormone (ACTH) (uh **dreen** oh kore tick oh **trope** ick)—hormone produced in the pituitary gland and transmitted to the cortex of the adrenal glands; stimulates production and release of corticoids.

adrenal glands—paired triangular endocrine glands located on the top of each kidney; site of epinephrine and corticoid production.

corticoids (**kore** tic koids)—hormones generated by the adrenal cortex that influence the body's control of glucose, protein, and fat metabolism.

metabolic rate—rate or intensity at which the body produces energy.

epinephrine (epp uh **neff** rin) and **norepinephrine**—powerful adrenal hormones whose presence in the bloodstream prepares the body for maximal energy production and skeletal muscle response.

psychosomatic disorders—physical illnesses generated by the effects of stress.

stress amenorrhea (a men ah **ree** ah)—cessation of the menstrual flow caused by stress.

FIGURE 6.2 The stress response: physiological reactions to a stressor.

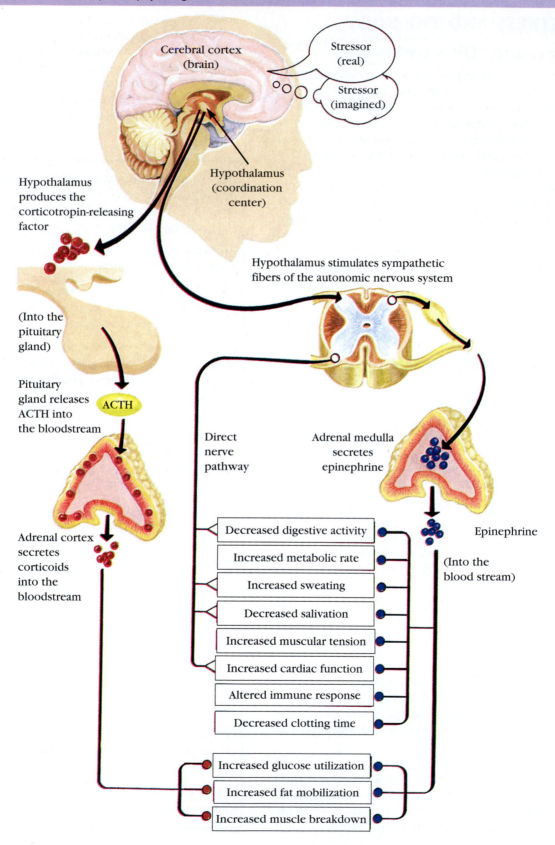

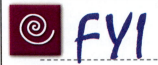

FYI

Researchers Link Hormones of Stress with Disease[6]

Stress and depression that send emergency hormones flowing into the bloodstream may help to cause brittle bones in women, infections, and even cancer. These hormones, such as cortisol, are good for you when you are in danger, but if these hormones become unregulated, as in being triggered daily from stress with little relief, then they will produce disease.

Migraine   Another stress symptom that is more specific to women is **migraine headaches.** At least 60 million people in North America will experience a migraine headache at one time or another during their lives.[8] Over the course of a lifetime, between 25 and 29 percent of all women will experience at least one migraine attack. Various factors can trigger a migraine and, usually, it takes one or more of these together to cause an attack. Common migraine triggers may include: stress, the letdown after a period of stress, glare and eyestrain, changes in the weather, sleep irregularities, certain medicines, tobacco or tobacco smoke, grinding or clenching your teeth, allergies, eating irregularly, fasting, and dietary factors. *Health Tips:* "Migraine, Medicine, and Food" summarizes additional migraine triggers to watch for.

It is important to note that both the frequency and intensity of migraine attacks worsen at those times in a woman's life that are associated with hormonal change: menstrual periods, mid-menstrual ovulation, and menopause. About 14 percent of female migraine sufferers only experience attacks associated with their periods. If you suffer from migraine headaches, it is a good idea to consult with your health-care provider to get an accurate diagnosis. See *Her Story:* "Kathryn" about someone who suffers from migraines.

STRESS AND LIFESTYLE

Major Life Events

Major life events can create significant stress in your life. When you have a financial crisis, a death in the family, a break off of a relationship, or so on, the

---

health tips

Migraine, Medicine, and Food

Medicines to avoid that may bring on a migraine attack:

- Oral contraceptives
- Stimulants
- Diuretics
- Blood vessel dilators
- Decongestants
- Antidepressants
- Asthma medications blood
- Certain pain killers

Foods to avoid that may bring on a migraine attack:

- Caffeine, commonly found in coffee, tea, and colas
- Common food additives, such as monosodium glutamate [MSG], common in meat tenderizers and Chinese food
- Alcohol
- Foods that contain tyramine, such as chocolate or cocoa, aged cheeses, vinegar, liver and kidney or other organ meats, sour cream, lima beans, nuts, citrus fruits, bananas, avocados, yogurt, and yeast extracts
- Substances that contain nitrates, such as smoked fish, bologna, pepperoni, bacon, frankfurters, corned beef, pastrami, canned ham, and sausages
- Aspartame, an artificial sweetener sold under the trade names Nutrasweet and Equal

---

pain of such an event and the adaptation required to adjust to the consequences generated by the event can present huge challenges for you. Several attempts to describe and measure the impact of such major life events have been made. However, the degree of stress experienced is dependent on how each individual uniquely perceives the event.

College Stress

It is difficult to specify the sources of stress for college students because the students represent many diverse backgrounds located at many different institutions.

---

migraine headaches—headaches created by prolonged constriction of the blood vessels; causes may vary.

Her Story

Kathryn

Kathryn experienced migraine headaches. She had them most of her life. She was going to graduate at the top of her college class in about two months and get married a week later. She was very busy maintaining her academic standing in school and planning her wedding. Her migraines were really getting in her way of being able to function. After an assessment it was determined that Kathryn had stress-induced migraine headaches. One common symptom of migraines is cold hands, measured as an exterior finger temperature less than 90°. In Kathryn's case, her finger temperature was consistently in the seventies, even though it was warm outside and comfortable in the room. Following eight sessions of relaxation training that incorporated some biofeedback therapy (to be discussed later in this chapter), Kathryn learned to raise and maintain a finger temperature above 90° even outside of the therapy setting. Her migraines disappeared and she was able to go on with her life with much less pain and discomfort.

- Do you know someone that suffers with migraines? What is it like for them?
- Have they tried stress management and relaxation exercises to help them with their migraine headaches?

It has been reported that up to 50 percent of the college students who seek counseling complain of difficulty studying or anxiety, tension, and depression due to poor grades, and fear of doing poorly in courses.[9]

Some of the more common factors related to college student stress include: adapting to a new environment, expectations of parents, meeting demands of faculty members, pressure to achieve good grades, rising costs of higher education, and pressure to find employment before and after graduation. For the first time in their lives, many college students must find their own way in structuring and managing time for coursework, jobs, socializing, recreation, and daily chores.

Undergraduate college women are more likely than men to report an unacceptable stress level.[10] To reduce stress, college women are more likely to indicate a need to limit commitments, exercise more, and worry less. Frequent reasons given by women in college for not reducing stress are lack of time and lack of self-discipline.

Daily Life Hassles

It is not just major life events that can effect your stress level. Those little daily life hassles can eat away at your composure and elevate your stress level by a significant amount. Hassles are irritants that can range from minor annoyances to fairly major difficulties. Contrary to hassles, some daily events can uplift your life by creating good feelings. Uplifting events can serve as sources of peace, joy, or satisfaction. Some hassles and uplifting events occur often, whereas others are relatively rare. It is often a combination of the presence or absence of hassles and uplifting events in your life that impacts your stress level and coping ability. Typical hassles are such things as misplacing or losing things, troublesome neighbors, the health of a family member, and having to wait in lines. Typical uplifting events are such things as being lucky, being rested, feeling healthy, and enjoying a hobby. Daily hassles prove to be a better predictor of the manifestations of stress symptoms than uplifting events, which are a deterrent to the manifestation of stress symptoms.[11] Thus, it seems that we may assign greater meaning to the hassles in life than we spend appreciating the uplifting events.

Complete *Assess Yourself!:* "Stress Checklist" to help determine your stress level.

IMPACT OF MULTIPLE ROLES

The demands on today's woman are extreme. They often involve any combination of the following: maintain a household, care for a family, and work in or outside of the home. A woman is expected to play multiple roles in her life, such as daughter, sibling, spouse, mother, boss, employee, pet owner, friend, neighbor, social volunteer, and hobbyist. Dedication to each of these various roles can create a major strain. It is often difficult for a woman to find time for herself, much less find time to relax, because of all the demands placed upon her. Society often views the woman as the "giver" of assistance rather than the "receiver" of assistance. Women may experience different levels and types of stress depending upon the particular role they play. In addition, high demands in combination with a sense of low control over how tasks are done makes a task more stressful.[13] Persons in nonprofessional positions, such as a typist, have high demands placed upon them, may find their jobs monotonous, and

Assess **Y O U R S E L F**

Stress Checklist[12]

Check the following symptoms you have experienced in the past three months. Then find your score to determine your level of stress.
____ 1. Worrying
____ 2. Feeling anxious or uneasy
____ 3. Going over the same thing in your mind
____ 4. Feeling pushed
____ 5. Unable to concentrate
____ 6. Cold hands or feet occasionally
____ 7. Tiredness at the end of the day
____ 8. Sore or stiff neck
____ 9. Occasional headaches (1 or 2 per month)
____10. Irritable
____11. Frequent headaches (more than 2 per month) or an occasional severe headache (at least 1 every 3 months)
____12. Indigestion or stomach problems
____13. Backaches
____14. Irregular sleeping pattern (either over or not sleeping)
____15. Prolonged feelings of depression or anxiety (more than 1 week)

Instructions for scoring and interpretation of the Stress Checklist:

Number of items checked:
1–5   Mild level of stress
6–10   Moderate level of stress
11–15   Severe level of stress

Interpretation:
(Note: The Stress Checklist is not a thorough assessment instrument for stress. It is designed to be used for the purpose of a quick health screening. It is also important to consider additional possible causes for the symptoms listed other than stress. Stress symptoms can be evaluated for severity by trained professionals.)
• *Mild Stress*—Changing your lifestyle or routine may help to reduce stress.

• *Moderate Stress*—Although changing your lifestyle or routine may help to reduce stress, sometimes a more thorough assessment of the stress symptoms may be necessary. Direct intervention may be needed. This might include activities such as stress management instruction or biofeedback therapy to help prevent and/or alleviate symptoms.
• *Severe stress*—More thorough assessment and immediate intervention may be needed. The type of intervention will depend upon the results of the more thorough assessment. Activities could include any or all of the following: a lifestyle modification to lessen the stress, stress management instruction, biofeedback therapy, physical and/or mental health counseling, or medication.

In which life area(s) does stress create the most impact for you? If you have checked two or more items in any one of the following areas, you may be considered as possibly having difficulties in that life area. Appropriate recommendations for each area are provided.
• *Excessive worry*—Items 1, 3, 4, and 10. Recommendation: Focus on worrying less; talk over your concerns with others whom you trust.
• *Depressed mood*—Items 5, 11, 14, and 15. Recommendation: Talk with someone about your stress and depression: a trusted friend, family member, or counselor.
• *Physical discomfort*—Items 2, 7, 9, and 12. Recommendation: Perhaps seek assistance from a physical or mental health provider about your physical discomfort.
• *Prolonged physical impact*—Items 6, 8, and 13. Recommendation: You should seek assistance from a physical or mental health provider about your physical condition.

may experience boredom, frustration, and even a decline in self-esteem. Consequently, they have higher overall stress levels than persons in professional positions, such as a teacher. Furthermore, women seem to cope better with stress than men; however, women seem to have more stress to handle.

Stressors are different for employed women with children than they are for full-time homemakers with children. As a result, they require different kinds of support to enable them to cope effectively with their chosen roles.[14] One example is the cost of child care for employed women, which is a huge financial stressor on most families. Employed women identify work, children, and household duties as the most frequent stressors, whereas nonemployed women identify children, finances, and self-concerns as stressors.

There are advantages and disadvantages to being either a woman not employed outside of the home or a woman employed outside of the home.[15] Each experiences stress, just in different ways. As a result of the different configurations of their work characteristics, women employed outside of the home and women not employed outside of the home experience, on average, similar levels of depressive symptoms. As compared to women employed outside of the home, full-time homemakers benefit from having less responsibility for things outside of their control. Women employed outside of their home appear to benefit from having less routine work than full-time homemakers.

Destructive Qualities of Stress

Stress can lead to violence. Women who experienced violence in their relationship from their male partner, described stress as a significant predictor of marital aggression within one year following their wedding.[16] In other words, the greater the stress level that was present in the lives of each of the partners the more violence was present in the relationship.

Stress is a common problem among women. From a sample of 1,000 British women who completed a survey, 79 percent indicated that they felt overly stressed.[17] The main manifestation was identified as increased irritability, this being most pronounced among working mothers with children under 16 years of age. Twenty-five percent of all women aged 15–24 years turned to smoking, and 23 percent of subjects aged 25–34 years turned to alcohol as means of relieving stress.

Stress, anxiety, and depression have been found to be among the most frequently reported health problems for women.[18] Significant factors contributing to these mental health problems include lower socioeconomic status, being an ethnic minority, being a member of a complex family structure, a lowered quality of family relationships, and intensity around participation in the labor market.

MULTICULTURAL ISSUES

Spiritual Beliefs

Cultural perspectives can impact health. Religious beliefs or, in the broader spectrum, spiritual beliefs can influence your frame of mind. Some beliefs emphasize a fatalistic philosophy—that one has no control over destiny. Other beliefs emphasize hope and a positive outlook on life—that one will reap positive rewards for efforts. Positive or hopeful attitudes seem to enhance health, whereas pessimistic or fearful attitudes can contribute to health deterioration.[19,20]

Ability to Acculturate

Degree of acculturation can impact health perspectives. Acculturation is how well an individual has adjusted to and become integrated into a community or country they have moved to. Being a newcomer in a foreign environment can be stressful just because you do not know very many people, have not built up a good support system yet, and cannot utilize new resources as well. For example, Mexican American women who are more acculturated to the "Westernized" culture (one with a more biomedical basis for health and well-being) have less belief in and reliance on traditional folk healing than Mexican American women with less acculturation. Thus, the acculturated women experience less stress as a result of feeling more in control over medical outcomes.[21] The less acculturated women expressed having a somewhat lower sense of control over their own health.

Racial Issues

Ethnicity can impact the degree of stressors or support an individual experiences. Race, for example, is a significant predictor of both levels of social support and occupational stress for women. African American women report lower levels of coworker support than do Caucasian women.[22] Women in Japan are suffering significant stress from that culture's current emphasis on overwork.[23] Putting in long hours to beat the competition can take its toll on the body and the emotions. Being a member of an ethnic minority group can be stressful as a result of the amount of bigotry and discrimination that still exists in the world today.

Age Factors

Stressors can be more specific to certain age groups. Women in their twenties suffer from the syndrome referred to as the "type E woman"—being everything to everybody.[24] These women are divided among three competing goals in life: they want a career, a relationship, and a family. Retired women workers experience significant financial stress even in the early years after retirement.[25] This is even more significant for unmarried retired women workers. Women not only enter old age poorer than men but become poorer with age as a consequence of widowhood, higher health care expenditures, and pay and pension inequities.[26]

FINANCIAL STRESS

The ever-rising costs of living and unhealthy economic trends have placed a burden of financial stress on women. Many women are required to seek employment, and often work at more than one job, in order to pay all of the bills. The mobility of our society almost requires that women own their own mode of transportation or pay for public transportation. Paying rent or mortgage payments takes a huge bite out of women's income. The rising cost of food impacts pocketbooks daily. Clothes get more expensive all of the time, and women are expected to wear a variety of colors and designs. They are not supposed to wear just one or two types of suits or outfits to work as many men can. Also, it is not very difficult to accrue high interest debts from using credit cards when cash is not available to purchase an attractive temptation of clothing or to put food on the dinner table. Also, more women shop as a means to relax than do men.[27] Accruing finance charges can stretch the limits of a paycheck and create additional stress in the lives of women.

The Impact of Technology

The advancement of technology has made it difficult to remain an active and informed participant in the community without a huge investment. If you are unavailable, people expect to be able to leave a message on an answering machine or with an answering service, or send you a letter via electronic mail or by fax. Access to television or radio programming is a vital link to staying informed about recent events so you can understand what in the world everyone else is talking about. Employers or college professors may expect you to meet shorter deadlines because of the availability of desktop computers and the accessibility to computerized information networks and sophisticated software. Staying involved with a "high tech" world is very expensive and very stressful.

The Workforce

Women's jobs receive lower pay, offer fewer opportunities for advancement, and have less gains from accumulated experience and authority.[28] Some women are not paid enough to "make ends meet" at the end of each month. Though some progress has been made over the years, the average wage earning for women is still significantly below that of men. Women employed full-time earn about two-thirds (71.52%) as much as men.[29] This is an economic disadvantage that may affect health.[30]

Women are more than twice as likely as men to work in part-time jobs: 26 percent of women compared to 10 percent of men in the civilian workforce.[31] These types of positions are even more segregated than full-time work, offer less training, fewer promotional opportunities, and fewer employment benefits.

Women executives were doing better in 1993 than in 1982 in terms of job opportunities and salaries, but they were also paying a heavier price in regard to home and on-the-job stress.[32] Women executives were significantly outnumbered by men in 1993 but they were at least receiving more money and more recognition than in 1982. The average salary of a senior female executive doubled by 1993 to $187,000 but women still only earned approximately two-thirds of what men in comparable positions earned. More than 90 percent report that a "glass ceiling" prevents women from reaching the top in any great numbers. More than half (58.8%) say they have been sexually harassed on the job, but their most likely response was to ignore the harassment. Women executives were more likely to be married and have children in 1993 than in 1982. They were also more likely to report feeling stressed and burned out, the result of juggling work and a disproportionate load of family obligations.

Women have made only slight progress over time in approaching the employment and weekly earnings of men in the category of full-time wage and salary earners aged 16 years and older. In 1983 women comprised only 40 percent of this workforce and in 1994 they comprised only 43 percent of this group. In 1983 the median weekly earnings of men was 121 percent of the overall U.S. median figure, but women only made 81 percent of the overall median figure and in 1994 men made 112 percent of the overall median figure whereas women only made 85 percent of the overall median figure.[33] (See Table 6.1.)

Many women are expected to be primary caregivers to their children and have a difficult time earning a wage while caring for their dependents. Of all the U.S. women who are mothers of children 5 years

Table 6.1

Employment and Earnings by Gender in 1993[34]
(based on persons 15 years of age and older)

MAJOR OCCUPATION	NUMBERS EMPLOYED (persons times 1,000)		MEDIAN EARNINGS (dollars per year)	
	Men	*Women*	*Men*	*Women*
Executive/Manager	7,873	5,503	42,722	28,876
Professional Specialty	6,597	5,521	45,136	31,906
Technical Support	1,481	1,533	35,048	26,324
Sales	5,807	3,514	32,327	18,743
Clerical	2,924	9,456	26,746	20,683
Crafted Repair	9,234	956	27,653	21,357
Machine Operator	3,664	1,955	23,378	15,379
Transportation	3,382	218	26,532	19,652
Handlers/Equipment Cleaners	2,005	397	17,556	14,826
Service Workers	4,205	4,165	20,860	13,126
Farming, Forestry, Fishing	1,702	237	15,655	10,581

of age and younger, 59 percent are in the labor force and 64 percent of them work full-time. Of all U.S. families, 13 percent are maintained by women who are the primary wage earners. In 9 percent of U.S. families, women are the sole wage earners.[35] Women who receive financial assistance through social service programs often are not able to provide for themselves and their dependents, and find the resources to invest in an education, training, or employment opportunity. Thus, these women are often not able to break from the cycle that keeps them dependent on social services, and limits their opportunities to engage in self-development or careers.

It is quite common that women in a relationship are likely to have a spouse or partner who is also working. However, this is often still not enough to eliminate or significantly reduce financial worries. When both partners are working, an added stress is placed on the relationship. It becomes difficult to find time to spend with family members, and the time that is spent often is not of very high quality, such as during family crises or hurried activities.

EMPLOYMENT AND HEALTH

Some women work because they want to. A career is often a way to discover additional personal significance and self-worth. Employed women are physically healthier than nonemployed women, and participation in the labor force improves health over time.[36,37,38,39] Accumulating evidence suggests that, when compared with not working for pay, employment improves health. Thus, we can expect that women's lower likelihood for employment will negatively affect their health.[40]

Working Against Stereotypes

Due to current social trends and to legislation that has opened opportunities in the workplace to women, such as Affirmative Action, more women are exercising their right to pursue careers. Some are even in fields that were once, and may still be, dominated by men. The pressure to perform and not fail is constant for many women in the workplace. The entrance into fields once dominated by men is still relatively new. Thus, women are heavily scrutinized by men and by other women to determine if they are truly capable of performing their duties on the job. The nature of this scrutiny is often unfair for women in that they must far exceed the expectations placed on men in the same job in order to demonstrate that they are capable.

The "equal pay for equal work" principle led to the passage of legislation that makes it illegal to pay any worker (usually a female or a minority group member) lower rates of pay than that paid to others (usually white males). Some employers still use evasion to avoid compliance by using a different title for a position held by women and ethnic minorities, despite only minor differences in assigned duties, to justify a lower rate of pay.[41]

Women who are competing with negative social stereotypes are often forced to become "super achievers." High and persistent achievement-oriented individuals are often referred to as "Type A" persons. Type A persons find it difficult to slow down and relax, often equating relaxation with laziness. Type A persons are more prone to developing and maintaining stress symptoms. Type A women have greater frequency of illness and higher blood pressure than non-Type A women.[42] This could be a direct link to the rising numbers of cardiovascular illnesses reported among women.

ENVIRONMENTAL STRESS

There are elements in the environment that can produce stress. Overcrowding in the home, in the neighborhood, or at work is a common cause of irritability and tension. Chemical toxins and pollutants can create stress on the body that affects physical and psychological well-being.[43] Even everyday items can be toxic to most people. Toxins that we come into contact with on a daily basis include: insecticides, house cleansers, and personal toiletries including shampoos and cosmetics. Just the odor from any of these chemicals can cause severe negative reactions in the body. The "closed building syndrome" refers to the escalation of airborne infectious illnesses and allergic reactions to pollutants because of recycled air. Closed-loop ventilation systems provide minimal access to fresh air and little opportunity for contaminated air to escape. Spending time in a high-rise office building, shopping mall, or commercial airplane could be risky because many of these facilities do not have sufficient circulation of fresh air. (See *Viewpoint:* "Tired or Toxic?")

Noise pollution is a common and frequent stressor. Women have been found to be more sensitive to high pitch noises, like the continuous machine noise from a computer. This noise generated high levels of irritability and stress for women, whereas it did not seem to bother men.[44] (See *FYI:* "Ergonomics.")

Just as some noise can create stress, so can certain sounds create a relaxing effect. Music with a soft, slow, flowing movement created by instruments, such as the piano, cello, harp, or violin, can sooth and calm the body and mind. Soothing sounds also occur naturally in the environment: rustling leaves on a tree; distant chirping of crickets, frogs, or birds; and water moving in a stream, from a waterfall, or ocean waves rolling onto the shore.

The concept of "safe neighborhood" is vital to consider in relation to stress levels. It is very difficult to relax when your life is endangered. There are nu-

---

Viewpoint

Tired or Toxic?

New research suggest that the environment has become so toxic that it is giving rise to new illnesses such as atypical immune system dysfunction and chronic fatigue syndrome. The medical community is slow to accept this proposition despite existing evidence. Many women with these disorders are considered hypochondriacs because of the hesitancy by some health providers to diagnose the toxic affects of pollution on the body. What do you think about the possible toxic effects on the body of pollutants in the environment?

---

merous instances for which a woman or her family and friends are at risk: from gunshots, bullets striking your home, or being hit by a stray bullet; the car breaking down on the side of the road; walking in an isolated area; and having to remember to lock yourself in at night, and even during the day. The high incidence of rape and other violence against women is evidence that women are not safe in this world. (See chapter 13.)

STRESS AND TRAUMA

Women who become victims frequently experience severe stress. The stress reaction can be immediate or delayed. It can be brief, or it may last for years. The stress reaction from trauma experiences can take on a variety of manifestations including heightened startle and fear responses, anxiety and panic attacks, distancing from friends and family, and avoidance of strangers or crowded places. Mental health counseling can be effective in facilitating the healing process for trauma victims. (See *FYI:* "Clinical Disorders Caused by Stress or Trauma" and *Her Story:* "Linda.")

COPING SKILLS FOR STRESS: PREVENTION, MANAGEMENT, AND TREATMENT

You Are What You Think

When an event occurs, you may make a judgment about that event that may impact how much stress you will or will not experience as a result of that

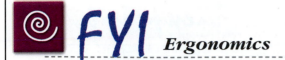

FYI *Ergonomics*

Ergonomics is the study of the problems of people adjusting to their environment. This science seeks to adapt working conditions to suit the worker. A working environment that does not suit the worker can place stress and strain on the mind and the body. Let's look at the example of the computer station. Many people develop back or neck aches due to the strain of sitting in front of a computer for long extended hours of work. Thus, through the study of postural positioning, new chairs were devised to help alleviate the strain on the body. These new "ergonomically correct" chairs range in design from an S-shaped chair that provides a padded knee rest, to a giant rubber ball chair that provides complete leg and knee support; each of these designs straightens the back, and pulls the shoulders back thus preventing back and neck strain. Typing at the computer keyboard for long periods of time can lead to the development of a very sore wrist, hand, or arm. This condition can be serious enough to be diagnosed as carpal tunnel syndrome. This condition was alleviated with the design of ergonomically correct keyboards, which do not require

such a wide reach to each key. Carpal tunnel syndrome can be treated via physical therapy or biofeedback therapy. Some people even have surgery for this condition, which is recommended only as a last resort. Now, let's examine the computer screen. The brightness of this screen can cause eye strain and severe headaches. To alleviate this problem some computers now have the ability to adjust the color and brightness of the screen. You can also purchase a tinted cover for your computer screen that will tone down the glare. Some computers can be very noisy. This noise can result in irritability and headaches for the user. Thus, computers are now designed to produce only minimal amounts of noise from the hard drive and the printer, so a quieter working atmosphere is created.

Take a look at your own working environment. Is there anything you can change that will make your work easier, more comfortable, and result in a happier and healthier place to work? How about your living environment? Can you make some adjustments in your home to create a safer and more pleasant place to live? ⌒

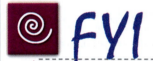

FYI *Clinical Disorders Caused by Stress or Trauma*[45]

- Panic attack—sudden onset of intense apprehension, fearfulness, or terror often associated with the feeling of impending doom. Symptoms include shortness of breath, palpitations, chest pain, or discomfort, choking or smothering sensations, and fear of "going crazy" or losing control.
- Agoraphobia—anxiety about, or avoidance of, places or situations from which escape might be difficult; the anxiety typically leads to an avoidance of a variety of situations such as being alone outside of the home, being in a crowd of people, traveling, and being in an elevator.
- Specific phobia—anxiety provoked by exposure to a specific object or situation.
- Social phobia—anxiety provoked by exposure to certain types of social or performance situations.
- Obsessive-compulsive disorder—characterized by obsessions that cause marked anxiety and/or by compulsions that serve to neutralize anxiety.

- Post-traumatic stress disorder (PTSD)—persons who are victims of assault frequently experience PTSD. An individual suffering from PTSD will reexperience the traumatic event over and over again through dreams, recurrent images, or flashbacks. The subject may try to avoid anything or anyone that reminds them of the event and will have persistent symptoms of increased arousal, such as difficulty sleeping, difficulty concentrating, irritability or outbursts of anger, an exaggerated startle response, and hyper vigilance (overly alert).
- Acute stress disorder—symptoms similar to PSTD but these occur within the first month after the trauma and are short lived.
- Generalized anxiety disorder (GAD)—persistent and excessive anxiety and worry for at least six months; individuals with GAD often worry about routine life circumstances such as job, finances, family, and daily chores and schedules. ⌒

Her Story

Linda

Linda was assaulted by a stranger with a knife. She survived the attack. Along with some deep cuts on her hands, she experienced significant emotional trauma. She exhibited all of the symptoms relevant to post-traumatic stress disorder. She was afraid to be alone, found crowds to be extremely anxiety provoking, and was startled by the smallest events, such as someone walking too close to her. After mental health counseling to help Linda recover from PTSD, treatment that also incorporated many relaxation techniques, Linda's symptoms were all either significantly reduced or eliminated.

- Do you know anyone who has ever had anxiety from experiencing a traumatic event?
- Were they able to overcome it completely?
- Did they seek assistance from a mental health provider?

JOURNAL ACTIVITY

Stop the Negative, Accentuate the Positive

Make a list of the self-defeating thoughts you say to yourself. Now take index cards and on each one write a positive self-suggestion to replace each self-defeating thought. Carry the cards with you during the day. Once a day repeat the positive affirmation to yourself. At first, you may want to focus on just one affirmation at a time to get used to the process. The more you practice a positive self-suggestion, the quicker you will change in the desired direction.

event. If you take time to examine this process, you can understand it better and use it to your advantage; this is known as the technique of cognitive appraisal. Cognitive appraisal is the process of categorizing an encounter with respect to its significance for well-being.[46] The two main evaluative issues of cognitive appraisal are "Am I in trouble or being benefited, now or in the future and in what way?" and "What, if anything, can be done about it?"

Because the amount of stress experienced is so dependent upon how a stress-eliciting event is perceived, one obvious technique for managing stress is to learn to alter your destructive thought patterns. There are numerous methods for altering negative patterns of thinking.[47,48] One important technique for altering negative self-suggestions is "thought stopping." Each time a negative thought comes to mind, you immediately say to yourself "stop." The command "stop" acts as a distractor and interrupts the flow of self-defeating thinking. Thought stopping can be followed by substitutions of positively reassuring or self-accepting statements. Positive affirmations are self-statements that accentuate positive feelings or actions. Affirmations can be applied to any area of life. Example affirmations might be "I am confident and strong," "I feel good about myself," "I am calm and relaxed," "I am a beautiful and worthwhile person,"

and so on. You may not believe the statements at first, but with continued daily practice you will eventually begin to act as if you believe the statement. Before long, you will begin to, consciously or unconsciously, create the feeling or behavior you desire. The power of self-suggestion, whether it be positive or negative, has a powerful influence on the state of your mind and body. Complete *Journal Activity:* "Stop the Negative, Accentuate the Positive" to help accomplish this behavior.

Stress and Nutrition

Maintaining a well-balanced and nutritious eating pattern is vital for maintaining health and well-being and for countering the ill effects of stress. Although comprehensive coverage of nutrition is provided in chapter 7, certain food substances that can contribute to stress by stimulating the sympathetic stress response are emphasized here.

Certain substances act as **vasoconstrictors,** in that they constrict the blood vessels of the body causing an elevation in blood pressure and heart rate.[49] They also create a temporary elevation in mood or energy level. Some of these stimulants are commonly present in our everyday life such as caffeine, found in coffee, tea, sodas, and some diet pills;

vasoconstrictors (vaz oh kun **strick** tors)—certain substances, such as some foods and medications, that cause the blood vessels to become narrow thereby increasing blood pressure in the body.

chocolate or cocoa; processed sugar; and nicotine, found in cigarettes. These substances tend to interfere with the ability to reduce stress and anxiety levels. When the effects of these stimulants wears off, the individual often experiences a "crash" period. The body is exhausted from the pressure placed on it during the period of physiological elevation. These substances create elevations in stress or anxiety levels, and they also lead to greater fatigue and exhaustion. There is sometimes a temptation to take more of these substances in order to re-elevate the energy or mood level. Thus, these substances not only increase the stress and anxiety level, but for many people, they can be a part of an extremely detrimental addictive cycle. Reductions in types and amounts of these substances from one's diet should be undertaken gradually. These substances can produce such a strong physiological response in the body that some withdrawal symptoms may be present. If withdrawal symptoms become too uncomfortable, then an individual should consult with a health-care provider for assistance in reducing and eliminating these substances from their diet.

Women under stress may crave foods high in fat and sugar. These foods can cause a person to feel lethargic. Stress can also lead to bouts of overeating or undereating. Special attention should be paid to one's eating patterns during stressful life periods.

Some vitamins are especially helpful for cushioning the blow of stress on the body. The vitamin B category is effective in countering stress and depression and many women take a form of Stress B Complex for these purposes. Ask your health-care provider about incorporating a regimen of healthy vitamins into your daily routine.

The intake of appropriate amounts of water is necessary to maintain a healthy body. Approximately 90 percent of your body is made up of water. When an individual is under stress, toxins seem to build up more in the body. Because water flushes the waste products from your body, an increase in water consumption during stressful periods may be advised.

Use of Herbs

Native healers from many continents have used herbs for healing practice since ancient times. The World Health Organization also recognizes the potential benefits to using natural herbal medicines.[50] Medicinal plants and herbs are important to the health of many communities; between 35,000 and 70,000 species have at one time or another been used for medical purposes, and international use of herbal medicines and natural products is steadily increasing. Today, healing herbs can be found in many local health food stores. Many herbs have healing and soothing effects on the nervous system.[51] In various combinations, the following herbs (plants and oils) can be used for relaxing baths: oatmeal, lime flowers, chamomile flowers, lavender, rosemary, thyme, and yarrow. Some herbal teas and tonics can also have a relaxing and soothing effect. It is important to consult a trained herbalist or herbal guide before utilizing these herbal baths, teas, or tonics. Also, if you have allergies, exercise caution in using these substances.

Aromatherapy is the use of the scent or aroma from essential oils produced from certain herbs that benefit the individual. The use of essential oils can enhance recovery from particular mental and physical ailments. Essential oils can be used in baths, massage, as room fragrances, or as inhalants. Essential oils effect the body through the olfactory system. The olfactory system, used in the sense of smell, has a direct link to the limbic system, the part of the brain that deals with emotions. Herbalists claim that the scent from certain oils can directly impact the brain, stimulating certain systems in the body that may facilitate healing.

Essential oils are very potent. It only takes a few drops of an essential oil in several ounces of a base oil for a massage, or a few drops of essential oil into bath water to get the desired effect. Several essential oils can be helpful in countering stress and anxiety disorders including: jasmine, eucalyptus, rosemary, lavender, chamomile, clary sage, rose, and ylang ylang.[52] An individual who wishes to utilize aromatherapy should consult an aromatherapist or aromatherapy guide.

Massage and Reflexology

Massage involves systematically stroking, kneading, and pressing the soft tissues of the entire body to induce a state of total relaxation.[53] Massage works mainly on the muscles, ligaments, and tendons and affects particularly the body's balance of blood and fluids. A most effective massage can be obtained by visiting a certified massage therapist. However, individuals can learn some simple techniques to share with one another at home using a massage guide.

Reflexology is the use of compression massage on designated areas on the hands and feet. Reflexology is based on the principle that there are areas, or

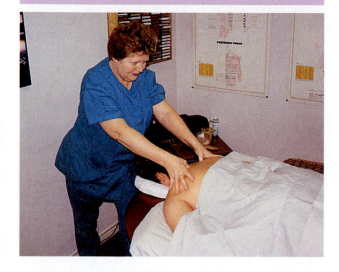

Massage therapy is good for helping the body to relax.

reflex points, on the feet and hands that correspond to each organ, gland, and structure in the body.[54] Reflexology is a means of helping the body attain balance in all its functions. It influences areas where weakened circulation has allowed waste matter to interfere with functioning. Through reflexology, the body is encouraged to renew itself so that all its processes are working in harmony. A basic understanding of human anatomy is vital for doing proper reflexology. Improper use of reflexology can be harmful, so it is recommended that you receive treatment from a trained reflexologist.

Acupressure and Acupuncture

Acupressure is a relaxing natural therapy that teaches the body to identify and release patterns of holding tension.[55] Acupressure has been used by Chinese healers for several centuries and is now in common practice in many cultures including the United States. Acupressure treatments consist of slow, gradual finger pressure applied to designated sites on the body. These sites correspond with neural receptor sites. Acupressure is sometimes used to support conventional medical treatment. It can be used to recover from shock or trauma. Acupressure is frequently used for relaxation, improved circulation, tension release, and pain control.

Acupuncture is a therapy related to acupressure. Acupuncture, which is also an ancient art that has been practiced for centuries in Asia, utilizes fine needles inserted into acupressure points to stimulate relaxation and healing. Consumers around the world utilize acupuncture; 90 percent of the pain clinics in the United Kingdom and 77 percent in Germany use acupuncture.[56]

Exercise

A regular exercise routine is a very effective approach to stress management. Exercise allows us to release pent-up anxiety and to stimulate and flush out the body's systems through movement. Exercise techniques are covered in a later chapter of this book. It is important to remember that simply taking the time to go for a walk can be an effective stress reducer.

Time Management

Managing one's time effectively can reduce stress. This often requires some planning, prioritizing, and structuring. High achievement-oriented persons may not have trouble with the planning and structuring part, but they often have difficulty with prioritizing. They feel the obligation to get everything done. It takes some discipline to accept the idea that sometimes not everything will get done. Weighing the most important tasks (such as time with family versus time at work, or time for self versus time with the family), putting them in the order of most importance, and then just doing the best you can and not worrying about the rest is a healthy and realistic attitude. (See *Journal Activity:* "Time Management.")

Body Awareness

Your body talks to you. It tells you when it is getting too stressed. When you do not listen to it or choose to ignore what it is telling you, then it will start "screaming" at you with various aches, pains, and disorders. A body "scream" can take many forms. Many of these are listed in earlier sections of this chapter as stress symptoms and disorders. The longer it takes the body to get your attention the more severe the manifestation of the body's "scream."

You can refine your listening skills and respond to the body's needs before it gets to the "screaming" stage. Focus on your forehead. Stay aware of when you create lines or wrinkles due to tightening the forehead (frontalis) muscles. You do not need to "scrunch" the forehead while concentrating or focusing and certainly not while worrying. Keep the forehead as smooth and relaxed as possible at all times.

Be aware of your jaw. When you are truly relaxed, there should be a slight space between your upper and lower teeth while your mouth is closed. Tension in the jaw (masseter) muscles will prevent this. If you have carried high levels of tension in your jaw for a long time, it may take awhile, sometimes several days, for it to completely relax.

Be aware of your neck and shoulders. As tension builds during the day, many people tend to start moving their shoulders gradually up toward their ears without even realizing it. Keep your shoulders down and relaxed. This will minimize the tension in those neck and shoulder (trapezius) muscles.

The few suggestions given regarding awareness refer directly to the body. However, a more relaxed body can also lead to a more relaxed mind and vice versa. The state of the body affects the mind and the state of the mind affects the body. They are interconnected. Attention to both the mind and the body will promote more holistic health.

Relaxation Exercises

Relaxation exercises are designed to calm the body, mind, and emotions.[57] Practiced daily, they can be most effective in managing stress. Most relaxation exercises last only about 15 minutes or less, so it is possible to incorporate at least one into your daily routine. Progressive relaxation is one of the most

commonly used relaxation techniques.[58] This technique involves alternately tensing and releasing the muscles, beginning with the feet and slowly working through each section of the body. This technique enhances awareness of tension and facilitates relaxation in each part of the body. Many people are not aware that they are as tense as they are until they engage in a relaxation exercise.

Autogenic phrases is another commonly used relaxation exercise.[59] These are self-statements designed to calm the body and mind. (See the examples in *Journal Activity:* "Relaxation Exercise.")

It is possible to set aside only a minute or so and receive substantial benefits using certain brief

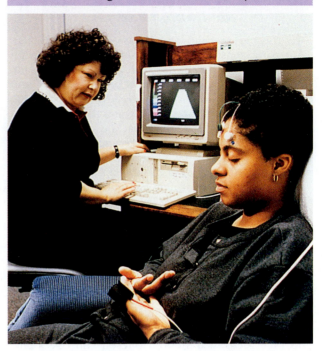

Biofeedback therapy is effective for stress-related disorders, learning disabilities, and chronic pain.

techniques. The "relaxation response" is a technique through which one learns to quiet the body and mind by using long, easy exhalations allowing the body to relax while sitting in a comfortable position.[60] Upon perceiving a stressful event, the "quieting reflex" is a set of specific responses, such as striving for a positive mental state, an "inner smile," and a deep exhalation with the tongue relaxed and the shoulders relaxed, which should be used immediately.[61] (See the example in *Journal Activity:* "Brief Relaxation Response.")

Biofeedback

Biofeedback is the use of electronic equipment to monitor the physiological state of the body while the individual learns techniques to voluntarily regulate the body's systems and reduce unwanted symptoms. Biofeedback for stress reduction is used with relaxation exercises. Biofeedback enhances the learning of techniques for reducing mental, emotional, and physical tension. With biofeedback equipment, an individual can immediately see the negative effects of stressful thoughts and feelings and the positive effects of relaxation techniques on the body. Immediate and accurate feedback about the effects of stress and relaxation on the body facilitates the learning of voluntary control over the autonomic nervous system. Biofeedback is a noninvasive and painless therapy. A few examples of some disorders or conditions that are effectively treated with biofeedback therapy include: migraine and tension headaches, high blood pressure, neck and back pain, irritable bowel syndrome, Raynaud's disease (chronic cold hands), phobias, panic and anxiety, jaw pain, teeth grinding, and other stress-related disorders.

There are many types of biofeedback. The modality used depends on the nature of the presenting problem.[62] Biofeedback is used to teach a person to voluntarily warm the hands and feet which lowers blood pressure; to relax muscle tension which reduces and eliminates pain; to facilitate healthy breathing for relaxation; and to alter brain wave patterns thereby allowing the individual to achieve and maintain a state of alert relaxation that is ideal for learning and performance. Brain wave biofeedback, or neurotherapy (neurofeedback), is frequently used to treat learning disabilities, attention deficit disorder, and addiction disorders. Biofeedback therapy is available from mental or physical health therapists who have received specific education and training in biofeedback techniques.

biofeedback—the use of electronic equipment to monitor the physiological state of the body while the individual learns techniques to regulate the body's systems and to reduce unwanted symptoms.

Meditation

Meditation is a common technique utilized to foster health and well-being. Meditation can facilitate feelings of personal balance and harmony, relaxation, and increased awareness of oneself and one's environment. Meditation can assist with the development of intuition, self-insight, and greater self-trust. An expansion of consciousness often occurs from meditation that replaces feelings of isolation, provides greater personal security, and creates a sensation of being in communion with the universe. (See *Journal Activity:* "Meditation Exercise.")

Meditation can be a guided exercise or can take the form of completely blanking one's mind to allow for spontaneous imagery or insight. Meditations designed for healing purposes may involve a focus on the body and its healing mechanisms. A healing meditation may also be more abstract such as to visualize a swim in healing waters or to be showered by a colorful rainbow that symbolically represents the chakras, hypothetically, the main energy centers in the body. Tai Chi is utilized as a meditation of "movement" that simultaneously aligns the body with mind and spirit. There exists a variety of schools or types of meditation.[64]

Numerous benefits can be gained by the individual from the practice of meditation: (1) meditations can bring about an increase in ego strength; (2) meditations can be applied to special problem areas and can be used to help explore a specific area and help "loosen" defenses (resistance to insight or change); (3) meditations assist with "centering," the quality of feeling at ease with oneself and with one's environment; (4) meditations facilitate growth by teaching the individual to regard his or her being as something of real value and to give serious attention to the totality of being; and (5) meditations assist with growing beyond the ability to function in everyday life while being relatively "pain-free."[65]

Yoga

Yoga involves the practice of body postures and poses to improve health by bringing the body into balance and reducing stress and tension. Hatha Yoga was developed in ancient India as a simple system of eight to ten poses that have evolved into the elaborate technique of today.[66] Yoga techniques range from very simple stretches to more complex twists and headstands. Yoga is an activity that can be used by persons of varying mobility and age.

Proper Breathing

Breath is life. Breathing is a variable rhythm that is linked to all metabolic functions.[67] Although breathing is automatic, it is affected by emotional and physiological demands on the body. Short, quick, and shallow breathing that originates mostly from the chest area is the least effective pattern for full oxygenation of red blood cells. In chest breathing, known as thoracic breathing, the rib cage spreads and the chest goes up. In spite of its appearance, this breathing mode results in very little air entering the lungs. This type of breathing is most common under stress.

Abdominal breathing, referred to as **diaphragmatic breathing,** is a healthy type of breathing. This is accomplished by alternately contracting the diaphragm and abdominal muscles that increases the space in the chest into which the lungs can expand to accept air.

Sometimes the individual is unaware of their breathing pattern. Breathing training should begin

Yoga is good for relaxation, and is a great fitness activity too.

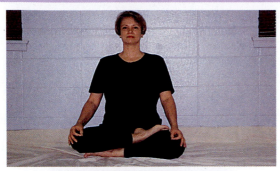

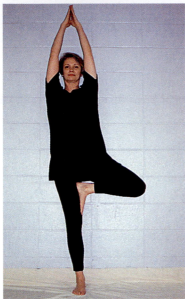

with heightened awareness of current breathing patterns and then practice to create longer, deeper, and fuller breaths. For fuller benefits, breathing should be initiated from the abdomen (diaphragm). Healthy breathing, or diaphragmatic breathing, involves first filling up the bottom of the lungs in the upper diaphragm area with air, and completing the task by filling up the top of the lungs in the chest area. Exhaling reverses this pattern. Healthy, relaxing breaths should be easy and unlabored. When sitting quietly, a woman's breathing rate should be about 14 to 15 breaths per minute or less (12 to 24 for men).

Her Story

Natalie

Natalie went to a stress management workshop and then never tried any of the techniques in her daily life. She said she was too busy. After talking with her for awhile she admitted that she had a low opinion of people who did not work hard all of the time; she thought they were lazy. So she resisted relaxing. Natalie realized that her misconceptions about herself and others were interfering with her own health and well-being. After a personal attitude adjustment, Natalie tried some of the techniques and was amazed at how better her life became. She had fewer emotional and physical discomforts and she could manage her busy schedule much better. She also reported having a more worry-free and relaxed attitude about life. She was enjoying life more now that she was managing her stress better.

- Do you know someone who finds excuses not to practice relaxation?
- Why do you suppose they put relaxation as such a low priority in their lives?
- Do you think that relaxation practice is important for your health?

CONCLUSION

Many people claim they have no time for stress management. This simply implies that they have no understanding of what stress management is. Stress management makes life easier, not harder. It does not entail more work. Instead, it is fun and relaxing. Think of it as a form of entertainment and recreation. If you claim to have no time for stress reduction or management, then you should consider the reasons why you are hesitant to relax. Now, go out and try some stress management for yourself. Remember, you are worth it. (See *Her Story:* "Natalie.")

diaphragmatic breathing (die a fruh **mat** ick)— healthy, relaxed breathing pattern that results in more complete and deeper breathing.

Chapter Summary

- **Stress** is the physical, mental, and emotional response to the presence of a perceived stressor.
- The primary anatomical areas that are involved in the stress response are the cerebral cortex, the hypothalamus, the adrenal glands, the hormone ACTH, corticoids, and adrenalin.
- Life stressors fall into five major categories: social, psychological, psychosocial, biochemical, and philosophical.
- The immediate stress response is the mobilization of the body for confrontation or avoidance of challenge; this is referred to as the fight-or-flight response.
- The general adaptation syndrome is the long-term response to stress and consists of three stages: alarm, resistance, and exhaustion.

- There is good stress and bad stress. Eustress is considered good stress because it is motivational stress, whereas distress is debilitating stress. When stress is too great, it can become distress.
- The effects of stress are cumulative; symptoms may begin as relatively minor body aches and pains, and gradually progress to more severe disorders and diseases. Major life events as well as daily hassles can produce stress.
- A variety of coping techniques can be easily learned and may prove to be beneficial in reducing stress.
- A positive attitude and taking time to play may protect some people from the potentially damaging effects of stressors.

Review Questions

1. What is stress and why do people perceive stressors differently?
2. What is optimal stress and what is the impact of going beyond this?
3. How does the stress response impact the endocrine system and the autonomic nervous system?
4. What are the three stages of the general adaptation syndrome?
5. What are some of the disorders or conditions that may result from prolonged stress?
6. Which stress-related disorders are more specific to women?
7. What types of stressors exist for women in various roles?
8. What types of stressors are more specific to multicultural issues?
9. What are some effective strategies for coping with stress?

Resources

Organizations and Hotlines

Association for Applied Psychophysiology and Biofeedback
10200 West 44th Avenue, Suite 304
Wheat Ridge, Colorado 80033
Telephone: (303) 420-2902

Audiotapes

1. *Worry Stoppers: Breathing and Imagery to Calm the Restless Mind.* Duluth, MN, 1995, Whole Person Associates (Phone: 800-247-6789).
2. *Calm Down: Relaxation and Imagery Skills for Managing Fear, Anxiety, Panic.* Duluth, MN, 1995, Whole Person Associates (Phone: 800-247-6789).
3. *Relax . . . Let Go . . . Relax.* Duluth, MN, 1982, Whole Person Associates (Phone: 800-247-6789).
4. *Take a Deep Breath.* Duluth, MN, 1992, Whole Person Associates (Phone: 800-247-6789).
5. *Stress R-E-L-E-A-S-E.* Duluth, MN, 1983, Whole Person Associates (Phone: 800-247-6789).
6. *Warm and Heavy.* Duluth, MN, 1994, Whole Person Associates (Phone: 800-247-6789).
7. *Countdown to Relaxation.* Duluth, MN, 1993, Whole Person Associates (Phone: 800-247-6789).
8. *Daydreams and Get-Aways.* Duluth, MN, 1993, Whole Person Associates (Phone: 800-247-6789).
9. *For People Coping with Headaches, Vols. I and II.* Image Paths, P.O. Box 5714, Cleveland, OH 44101 (Phone: 800-800-8661).

Videotapes

1. *Managing Job Stress.* Duluth, MN, 1995, Whole Person Associates (Phone: 800-247-6789).
2. *Healthy Stress.* Duluth, MN, 1995, Whole Person Associates (Phone: 800-247-6789).
3. *Stress Overload.* Duluth, MN, 1995, Whole Person Associates (Phone: 800-247-6789).
4. *Managing Stress, Anxiety, and Frustration.* Human Relations Media, Pleasantville, NY, 1980.

Websites

American Council for Headache Education
http://www.achnet.org/

Suggested Readings

Babior, S., and C. Goldman. 1995. *Overcoming panic, anxiety & phobias.* Duluth, Minn.: Whole Person Associates.

Charlesworth, E., and R. Nathan. 1987. *Stress management: A comprehensive guide to wellness.* New York: Ballantine Books.

Davis, M., E. Eshelman, and M. McKay. 1995. *The relaxation and stress reduction workbook.* 4th ed. Oakland, Calif.: New Harbinger.

Gawain, S. 1982. *Creative visualization.* New York: Bantam Books.

Lusk, J. 1992. *30 scripts for relaxation imagery & inner healing. Vols. I & II.* Duluth, Minn.: Whole Person Associates.

Mason, L. 1985. *Guide to stress reduction.* Berkeley, Calif.: Celestial Arts.

Peper, E., and C. Holt. 1993. *Creating wholeness: A self-healing workbook, using dynamic relaxation, images, and thoughts.* New York: Plenum.

Seaward, B. 1997. *Managing stress: Principles and strategies for health and wellbeing.* 2nd ed. Boston: Jones & Bartlett.

References

1. Curtis, J. D., and R. A. Detert. 1981. *How to relax: A holistic approach to stress management.* Mountainview, Calif.: Mayfield.
2. Selye, H. 1975. *Stress without distress.* New York: New American Library.
3. Cannon, W. 1932. *The wisdom of the body.* New York: Norton.
4. Selye, *Stress without distress.*
5. *Mosby's medical, nursing, and allied health dictionary.* 4th ed. 1994. St. Louis: Mosby-Year Book.
6. Associated Press. Researchers link hormones of stress with disease. *Denton Record Chronicle,* Denton, Tex., 17 November 1996, 3A.
7. *Mosby's medical, nursing, and allied health dictionary.*
8. Saper, J. 1993. *Reference book for migraine and headache,* Canada: Hume Medical Information Services.
9. Whitman, N., D. Spendlove, and C. Clark. 1984. *Student stress: Effects and solutions.* Washington, D.C.: ERIC Clearinghouse on Higher Education.
10. Campbell, R., L. Svenson, and G. Jarvis. 1992. Perceived level of stress among university undergraduate students in Edmonton, Canada. *Perceptual and Motor Skills,* 75 (2): 552-54.
11. Kanner, A., J. Coyne, C. Schaefer, and R. Lazarus. 1981. Comparison of two modes of stress management: Daily hassles and uplifts versus major life events. *Journal of Behavioral Medicine,* 4 (1): 1-39.
12. Chandler, C., and C. Kolander. 1997. Quick and effective stress screening. *Human Stress: Current Selected Research,* 5: 203-206.
13. Barko, N. 1983. Stress in professionals and nonprofessionals, men and women. *Innovation Abstracts,* 5 (9).
14. Canam, C. 1986. Perceived stressors and coping responses of employed and non-employed career women with pre-school children. *Canadian-Journal-of-Community-Mental-Health,* 5 (2): 49-59.
15. Lennon, M. 1994. Women, work, and well-being: The importance of work conditions. *Journal of Health and Social Behavior,* 35 (Sept.): 235-47.
16. MacEwen, K., and J. Barling. 1988. Multiple stressors, violence in the family of origin and marital aggression: A longitudinal investigation. *Journal of Family Violence,* 3 (1): 73-87.
17. Wheatley, D. 1991. Stress in women. *Stress and Medicine,* 7 (2): 73-74.
18. Walters, V. 1993. Stress, anxiety and depression: Women's accounts of their health problems. *Social Science and Medicine,* 36 (4): 393-402.
19. Siegel, B. 1986. *Love, medicine and miracles.* New York: Harper and Row.
20. Borysenko, J. 1988. *Minding the body, mending the mind.* New York: Bantam.
21. Castro, F., P. Furth, and H. Karlow. 1984. The health beliefs of Mexican, Mexican American and Anglo American women. *Hispanic Journal of Behavioral Sciences,* 6 (4): 365-83.

22. Snapp, M. 1992. Occupational stress, social support, and depression among black and white professional managerial women. *Women and Health,* 18: 41–79.

23. "Koroshi"—Overwork—Taking its toll on women in Japan. *WIN News,* Winter 1992, p. 61.

24. Francis, M., and C. Sacra. 1994. Stressed out? *Mademoiselle* (Sept.): 190–93.

25. Logue, B. 1991. Women at risk: Predictors of financial stress for retired women workers. *The Gerontologist,* 31 (5): 657–65.

26. Minkler, M., and R. Stone. 1985. The feminization of poverty and older women. *The Gerontologist,* 25: 351–57.

27. Survey. *Orange County Register,* October, 1994.

28. England, P., G. Farkas, B. Kilbourn, and T. Dou. 1988. Explaining occupational sex segregation and wages: Findings from a model with fixed effects. *American Sociological Review,* 53: 544–58.

29. U.S. Department of Commerce. *Statistical Abstracts of the United States,* Bureau of the Census, Washington, D.C. (Sept. 1995).

30. Bird, C., and M. Fremont. 1991. Gender, time use, and health. *Journal of Health and Social Behavior,* 32 (2): 114–29.

31. Part-time work, full-time work and occupational segregation. 1987. *Gender in the workplace,* edited by C. Brown and J. A. Pechman, pp. 217–38. Washington, D.C.: Brookings Institute.

32. Presley, B. 1993. Women pay more for success. *The New York Times* (July 4), sec. 003, p. F25.

33. U.S. Department of Commerce. *Statistical Abstracts of the U.S.*

34. Ibid.

35. Ibid.

36. Marcus, A., T. Zeeman, and C. Telesky. 1983. Sex differences in reports of illness and disability: A further test of the fixed role hypothesis. *Social Science and Medicine,* 17: 993–1002.

37. Nathanson, C. 1980. Social roles and health status among women: The significance of employment. *Social Science and Medicine,* 14a: 463–71.

38. Verbrugge, L. 1983. Multiple roles and physical health of men and women. *Journal of Health and Social Behavior,* 24: 16–30.

39. Waldron, I., and J. Jacobs. 1988. Effects of labor force participation on women's health: New evidence from a longitudinal study. *Journal of Occupational Medicine,* 30: 977–83.

40. Ross, C., and C. Bird. 1994. Sex stratification and health lifestyle: Consequences for men's and women's perceived health. *Journal of Health and Social Behavior,* 35 (June): 161–78.

41. Isaacson, L., and D. Brown. 1993. *Career Information, Career Counseling, and Career Development.* 5th ed. Boston: Allyn & Bacon.

42. Lawler, K., and L. Schmied. 1992. A prospective study of women's health: The effects of stress, hardiness, locus of control, Type A behavior, and physiological reactivity. *Women and Health,* 19 (1): 27–41.

43. Rogers, S. 1990. *Tired or toxic?: A blueprint for health.* Syracuse, N.Y.: Prestige.

44. Dow, C. 1988. Monitor tone generates stress in computer and VDT operators: A preliminary study. Presentation at the Annual Meeting of the Association for Education in Journalism and Mass Communications, Portland, Ore.

45. American Psychiatric Association. 1994. *Diagnostic and Statistical Manual of Mental Disorders,* 4th ed. (DSM-IV). Washington, D.C.: American Psychiatric Association.

46. Lazarus, R., and S. Folkman. 1984. *Stress, appraisal, and coping.* New York: Springer.

47. Chandler, C., and C. Kolander. 1988. Stop the negative, accentuate the positive. *Journal of School Health,* 58 (7): 295–97.

48. Peale, N. 1990. *The power of positive thinking.* New York: Doubleday.

49. Block, K., and M. Schwartz. 1995. Dietary considerations: Rationale, issues, substances, evaluation, and patient education. In *Biofeedback: A practitioner's guide.* 2nd ed. Edited by Mark Schwartz, Guilford, N.Y.

50. Zhang, X. 1996. Traditional medicine and WHO. *World health* (March-April): 4–5.

51. Mabey, R., M. McIntyre, P. Michael, G. Duff, and J. Stevens. 1988. *The new age herbalist: How to use herbs for healing, nutrition, body care, and relaxation.* New York: Macmillan.

52. Devereaux, C. 1993. *The aroma therapy kit: Essential oils and how to use them.* Boston: Charles E. Tuttle.

53. Lidell, L., S. Thomas, C. Cook, and A. Porter. 1984. *The book of massage: The complete step-by-step guide to Eastern and Western techniques.* New York: Simon and Schuster.

54. Bayly, D. 1988. *Reflexology today.* Rochester, Vt.: Healing Arts Press.

55. Bauer, C. 1991. *Acupressure for everybody.* New York: Henry Holt.

56. Zhang. Traditional medicine and WHO.

57. Davis, M., E. Eshelman, and M. McKay. 1995. *The relaxation and stress reduction workbook.* 4th ed. Oakland, Calif.: New Harbinger.

58. Jacobson, E. 1978. *You must relax.* New York: McGraw-Hill.

59. Luthe, W. 1969. *Autogenic training,* Vols. 1–3. New York: Grune & Stratton.

60. Benson, H. 1975. *The relaxation response.* New York: Avon.

61. Stroebel, C. 1978. *Quieting response training.* New York: BMA.

62. Schwartz, M. 1995. *Biofeedback: A practitioner's guide.* 2nd ed. New York: Guilford Press.

63. Gawain, S. 1986. *Living in the light.* Mill Valley, Calif.: Whatever Publishing.

64. Novak, J. 1989. *How to meditate.* Nevada City, Calif.: Crystal Clarity.

65. LeShan, L. 1974. *How to meditate.* New York: Bantam.

66. Folan, L. 1981. *Lilias, yoga, and your life.* New York: Collier Books.

67. Fried, R. 1990. *The breath connection: How to reduce psychosomatic and stress-related disorders with easy-to-do breathing exercises.* New York: Plenum Press.

Part Three

CONTEMPORARY LIFESTYLE AND SOCIAL ISSUES

CHAPTER SEVEN
Eating Well

CHAPTER EIGHT
Keeping Fit

CHAPTER NINE
Avoiding Tobacco Use

CHAPTER TEN
Using Alcohol Responsibly

CHAPTER ELEVEN
Using Other Psychoactive Drugs

CHAPTER TWELVE
Becoming a Wise Consumer

CHAPTER THIRTEEN
Preventing Abuse Against Women

Seven

Eating Well

■ chapter objectives

When you complete this chapter you will be able to:
- Describe the factors to consider when making food choices.
- Summarize the Dietary Guidelines for Americans.
- Explain the components of the Food Guide Pyramid and how the principles can be applied to meal planning.
- List and describe the nutrients needed for proper nutrition.
- Summarize the nutritional requirements for women that are associated with pregnancy, breast-feeding, and exercise.
- Describe the causes and treatments for eating disorders.
- Summarize some of the consumer issues related to good nutrition.

EATING WELL AND EATING WISELY

In America today, there is probably no single health topic that generates as much attention as that of nutrition. Every day the media report something related to what we should or should not eat. Research continues to define the relationships between the foods we eat and the quality of our lives. Yet with all the research that has been done, we still have many questions about food and nutrition that are waiting to be answered. There is good news, however. In a very general sense, we have determined that what we eat has a strong influence on our health status. Certainly, women can protect their health by what they *don't* do, such as avoiding cigarette smoke, ex-

cessive use of drugs and alcohol, etc. There are also things women *can* do to protect their health. Eating well is one of those things. Perhaps no other health practice has the greatest impact on our well-being than eating wisely.

As an adult woman, you are faced with many nutritional choices every day. You either plan your meals or select from a menu of some sort every time you eat, day in and day out. In our culture, eating is a ritual; something that is enjoyed and brings us pleasure. We do not eat to prevent starvation or to ensure that we survive. Our choices are not related to eating, but rather to the psychic pleasure and other factors associated with the meal. Take the *Assess Yourself:* "Determining Your Food Choices" that follows to determine the manner in which you make your food choices.

HEALTHY PEOPLE 2000 OBJECTIVES

- Reduce dietary fat intake to an average of 30 percent of calories or less and average saturated fat intake to less than 10 percent of calories among people aged 2 and older. 1995 progress toward goal: 38 percent
- Increase complex carbohydrate and fiber-containing foods in the diets of adults to five or more daily servings for vegetables (including legumes) and fruits, and to six or more daily servings for grain products. 1995 progress toward goal: unavailable
- Increase to at least 50 percent the proportion of overweight people aged 12 and older who have adopted some dietary practices combined with regular physical activity to attain the appropriate body weight. 1995 progress toward goal: –60 percent
- Increase calcium intake so at least 50 percent of youth aged 12 through 24 and 50 percent of pregnant and lactating women consume three or more servings daily of foods rich in calcium, and at least 50 percent

of people aged 25 and older consume two or more servings daily. 1995 progress toward goal: –30 percent (females aged 19–50: 0 percent)
- Decrease salt and sodium intake so at least 65 percent of home meal preparers prepare foods without adding salt, at least 80 percent of people avoid using salt at the table, and at least 40 percent of adults regularly purchase foods modified or lower in sodium. 1995 progress toward goal: unavailable
- Reduce iron deficiency to at least 3 percent among children aged 1 through 4 and among women of childbearing age. 1995 progress toward goal: unavailable
- Increase to at least 75 percent the proportion of mothers who breast-feed their babies in the early postpartum period and to at least 50 percent the proportion of women who continue breast-feeding until their babies are 5 to 6 months old. 1995 progress toward goal: 10 percent

Assess Y O U R S E L F

Determining Your Food Choices[1]

Look at each of the associated factors below. Consider how much each one of them influences your food choices. As you consider each one, think of it in the role it plays *most* of the time. Circle the number that best reflects your perception of the factor.

Factor	Not significant			Very significant		
Family influences	0	1	2	3	4	5
Weight control	0	1	2	3	4	5
Health	0	1	2	3	4	5
Nutrition knowledge	0	1	2	3	4	5
Convenience/time	0	1	2	3	4	5
Advertisements	0	1	2	3	4	5
Emotions/stress	0	1	2	3	4	5
Peers (friends, coworkers)	0	1	2	3	4	5
Customs/ethnic background	0	1	2	3	4	5
Physical activity level	0	1	2	3	4	5
Food costs	0	1	2	3	4	5

Interpretation: The factors that you scored as 4 or 5 are those factors that influence your food choices the most. Think about each one of those, and place a "+" or a "–" sign next to it, depending on whether you feel the factor is a positive or negative influence on your eating habits and your health. The first step in a mature dietary program is to evaluate the things you eat, and why you eat them. Is achieving good health a reason for your food choices? Should you make it a greater priority? It is only through thoughtful choices that your eating experiences can be rewarding for you.

GUIDELINES TO GOOD EATING

Just what should a woman be eating to stay healthy? Years of laboratory research and data collected from many segments of our population have revealed a number of things that can help us answer this question. Studies have given us a picture of what the typical American woman's diet includes. For example, did you know that the typical American consumes foods from which:

- 15 percent of the energy value comes from protein sources.
- 46 percent of our food energy comes from carbohydrates.
- 38 percent of our energy comes from fats in our diet.

Dietary Guidelines for Americans

Over the years, scientists have conducted a considerable amount of nutrition research. **Epidemiological** studies on human populations have given us some good data that describe the typical person's dietary profile, and how that diet might affect them. Using data from these studies, the United States government issued a set of *Dietary Guidelines for Americans* beginning in 1980. The guidelines have been revised every 5 years since then. The dietary guidelines offer suggestions for good eating based upon what the typical diet consists of and what a person's dietary needs are. The latest guidelines were released in January 1996.[2] The recommendations are as follows:

1. *Eat a variety of foods.* A woman's body needs more than 40 different nutrients to ensure good health. You may be familiar with some of them. How many different nutrients can you think of? Your nutrients should come from a variety of foods, not just a few selected food choices with an occasional vitamin and mineral supplement. Keep in mind that there is no single food that can supply all the nutrients in the amounts you need. For example, chicken contains protein, but no fiber. Cheese may have vitamin B12, but it has no vitamin C. (See *FYI:* "Variety Is Healthier.")

   Self-check and suggestion: Write down what you ate yesterday. Is there a variety of foods on your list? Does it appear that you have eaten foods from all the food groups represented on the food pyramid? (See p. 124.) Can you identify the nutritive value of the foods you ate? The U.S.

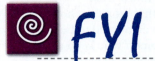

Variety Is Healthier[3]

A new study has confirmed that people who eat a variety of foods typically consumed less fat and more nutrients than those who eat a narrow range of favorite foods. These findings support earlier research that concluded that people who eat from all food groups live longer than those who eat foods from only a narrow range of selection.

Department of Agriculture recommends that a daily well-balanced diet* contains:

- *Fruits*—2 to 4 servings
- *Vegetables*—3 to 5 servings
- *Breads, cereals, rice, pasta*—6 to 11 servings
- *Milk products*—2 to 3 servings
- *Meat, poultry, fish, beans, eggs, nuts*—2 to 3 servings

2. *Balance the food you eat with physical activity.* We are a nation of overfat individuals. In fact, it would surprise us to learn that human beings in industrialized settings, and in terms of percent body fat, rank among the five fattest animals on earth.[4] Public health efforts over the past decade have attempted to reduce the percent of overweight people in our country, but to no avail. According to data from the third National Health and Nutrition Examination Survey (NHANES), 33 percent of all adults in America are overweight.[5] This condition is particularly overrepresented among women. Approximately 35 percent of white females and 60 percent of African American women are overweight or obese. At the present time, scientists have not been able to identify specifically what "healthy

*Note: Lower number of servings is for less active, smaller people; the larger size is for those who are more active.

epidemiological (epp ah dee **me** ah logical)— pertains to the study of the causes of death and/or illness.

weight" is, but we do know from epidemiological data that women who are overweight or underweight tend to be less healthy than those women who keep their weight within recommended ranges.

Self-check and suggestion: Are there a lot of oils or fats on or in the foods you eat? If so, consider the fact that fats are high in calories. You might consider reducing those types of foods, and increase those foods that are lower in calories and higher in nutrients. Also, be sure you engage in some form of exercise, and drink little or no alcohol.

3. *Choose a diet with plenty of grain products, vegetables, and fruits.* Research has revealed that typical American diets do not include enough foods from these food groups. Increasing the consumption of these foods can accomplish a number of things. Fruits, vegetables, and grains are generally low in fats, and are rich in vitamins and minerals. They also contain dietary fiber, especially if whole grain products are consumed.

Self-check and suggestion: Do you make a conscious effort to consume fiber? Can you identify high fiber foods? To increase your fiber intake try eating less processed foods, eating the skin on fruits and vegetables, and eat a variety of foods.

4. *Choose a diet low in fat, saturated fat, and cholesterol.* Although our nation's fat consumption is 4 percent lower overall than it was 20 years ago we are still consuming 8 percent more fat than we need for good health. High fat diets have been linked to higher incidence of heart disease and some forms of cancer, particularly breast cancer. More important, however, is the fact that dietary fat is more likely to contribute to obesity, which in turn is linked to other health concerns.

Self-check and suggestion: Do you know what percent of your diet comes from fat? Use the *Health Tips:* "Calculating Fat Intake" to calculate what your recommended fat intake should be.

You can reduce the amount of fat in your diet with slight modifications:

- Use less salad dressing. One tablespoon will provide 10–11 grams!
- Use fats sparingly when cooking.
- Check food labels for fat content.
- Trim fat from meat and remove skin from poultry.

- Switch to a lower-fat milk. If you drink whole milk, try drinking 2% milk instead.
- Use low-fat foods as substitutes for other fatty products, for example lite or fat-free salad dressing.

5. *Choose a diet moderate in sugars.* Studies regarding sugar use have not shown any relationship between sugar consumption and hyperactivity, hypoglycemia (low blood sugar), or diabetes.[6] There are harmful effects of excessive sugar consumption, however. Foods high in sugars tend to have fewer nutrients in

h e a l t h   t i p s

Calculating Fat Intake

Adult women need an average of 2,200 calories per day. This figure, of course, will vary depending upon activity level. To find out what *your* total fat intake should be, multiply your daily calories by .30 (30%) and divide that figure by 9 (the number of calories in a gram of fat). For example:

2,200 calories × .30 = 660 calories from fat.
660 calories ÷ 9 = 73 grams of fat

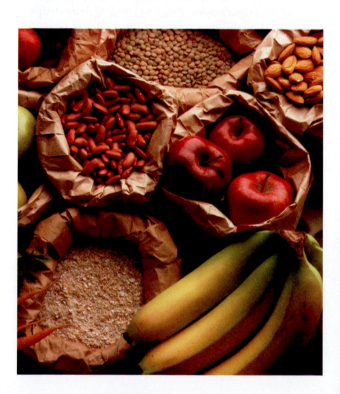

health tips

Removing Sugar from Your Teeth

Research indicates that you can reduce the amount of decay-causing acid created by sugar on your teeth after eating a sugar food if you eat fruit, cheese, peanuts, or use sugar-free gum.

them. The sugars will provide energy, but there is also the likelihood that the sugars will add additional calories that a woman may not need. Sugars can also be a contributing factor in the development of tooth decay. (See *Health Tips:* "Removing Sugar from Your Teeth.") Sugars come in many different forms. Food labels may list them as:

sucrose (table sugar)	fructose	honey
confectioner's sugar	corn syrup	maple syrup
dextrose	molasses	glucose

Self-check and suggestion: Do you read food labels when you shop and/or cook? Are you able to identify other sources of sugar in addition to table sugar?

6. *Choose a diet moderate in salt and sodium.* Most Americans consume more salt and sodium than they need. It is estimated that the average American consumes about 8,690 mg of sodium each day, most of which comes from table salt we add to our foods when we eat or prepare them. We have grown accustomed to salting our food to give it flavor. Actually we don't need that much salt in our diet. If a woman prepared only unprocessed foods and added no salt at all, she would get about 500 milligrams of sodium naturally from the food—more than enough to prevent any deficiency. There are approximately 10–15 percent of adults with high blood pressure that is exacerbated due to sodium sensitivity. Those adults would benefit from a low-sodium diet. It appears, however, that sodium per se does not cause hypertension. In fact, intakes of sodium as high as 3,300 mg per day do not pose a risk for developing hypertension.[7]

Self-check and suggestion: Do you:
Eat cured or processed meats such as ham, bacon, or lunchmeat? Eat cheese?
Add salt, salad dressings, or sauces to food?
Add salt to water when you cook vegetables or pasta?
Eat store-bought meals?
Eat salty snacks like potato chips, peanuts, popcorn, etc.?
Frequently eat at fast-food restaurants?

If you answer "yes" to most of these questions, your diet may be high in sodium. You might consider making a healthy adjustment to your eating habits by doing the following:

- Read labels of the foods you buy. Be sure to look for other sources of sodium, such as *sodium* citrate, mono*sodium* glutamate, celery *salt,* etc.
- Experiment with herbs and spices to add flavor to your food.
- Prepare your own salad dressings and sauces.
- Reduce the number of "shakes" you use to salt your food.

7. *If you drink alcoholic beverages, do so in moderation.* Each woman has to evaluate the role alcohol plays in her life. It is not necessary to consume alcoholic beverages. In fact, there is no real health value to alcohol consumption. Alcohol supplies calories, but does not contain any other nutrients. It is a drug that can be addicting. Alcohol contributes to five of the ten leading causes of death in the United States. In short, alcohol is one of the most preventable causes of death in this country. Alcohol consumption also contributes to a variety of vitamin disorders because the alcohol interferes with vitamin absorption. For example, it is believed that excessive alcohol consumption can lead to vitamin A deficiency by hastening its degradation in the liver.[8]

Food Guide Pyramid

Nutritionists have long advocated that our diets should be balanced. Being balanced meant that we would consume foods from a variety of sources to insure adequate intake of nutrients. Until the early 1950s, it was recommended that we consume foods from seven food groups—milk, dairy, vegetables, fruits, meat, bread, and cereal. After that time, the emphasis shifted to consuming foods from four food groups—milk and milk products, protein-rich foods, fruits and vegetables, and breads and cereals. In 1979, the U.S. Department of Agriculture (USDA) revised

FIGURE 7.1 The USDA Food Guide Pyramid.

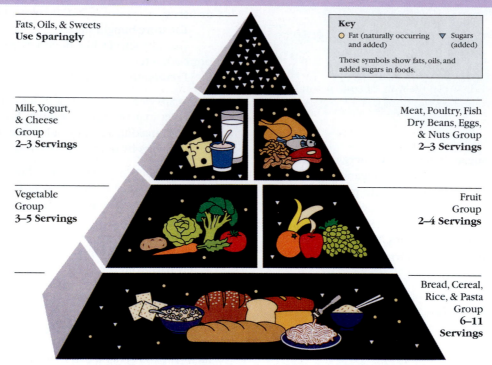

Fats, Oils, & Sweets
Use Sparingly

Key
○ Fat (naturally occurring and added)   ▽ Sugars (added)
These symbols show fats, oils, and added sugars in foods.

Milk, Yogurt, & Cheese Group
2–3 Servings

Meat, Poultry, Fish Dry Beans, Eggs, & Nuts Group
2–3 Servings

Vegetable Group
3–5 Servings

Fruit Group
2–4 Servings

Bread, Cereal, Rice, & Pasta Group
6–11 Servings

the names of the groups and added another, which was the "other" group. You may know it as the one that included all those foods that were considered to be "less healthy." This group included sweets, pastries, alcoholic beverages, fats, and oils. The consumer was advised to use foods sparingly from the "other" group.

Since 1992, the USDA has advocated the use of the Food Guide Pyramid in meal planning. The pyramid reflects the nutritional goals discussed earlier. Although the Food Guide Pyramid represents the five food groups that were used before its conception, it represents a pictorial way of presenting the five groups and the amount of each that should be represented in the daily diet. As you can see in Figure 7.1, the foundation of meal planning according to the Food Guide Pyramid would be the foods made from grains—bread, cereal, pasta, and rice. It also places less importance on the "meat group," putting meat sources higher up the pyramid for better health.

Recommended Dietary Allowance

The **Recommended Dietary Allowances** are standards set by the Food and Nutrition Board of the National Academy of Sciences. The RDAs have been around in some form since World War II. Originally they were identified as Recommended *Daily* Allowances, but the term *Dietary* is now used because it was difficult for individuals to consume all of the RDAs every day. The RDAs have been revisited and revised as needed by the Food and Nutrition Board every 5 years until 1989.

The RDAs were established as guidelines for *groups* of people, not individuals. The RDAs varied slightly from group to group. For example, an adult woman may need 180 micrograms of folacin, but a pregnant women needs 400 micrograms.[9] Folacin (or folic acid) is important for cell growth. A pregnant woman is not only growing her own new cells while the uterus grows and her blood supply doubles, she is responsible for providing the nutrients for her developing fetus. Currently there are RDAs for protein, all fat-soluble and seven water-soluble vitamins, and seven minerals. There are no RDAs for the other classifications of nutrients.

At its last meeting in 1993, the Food and Nutrition Board, after considerable scientific testimony, created **Dietary Reference Intakes** (DRIs) as a generic term to replace the RDAs. Dietary Reference

Intakes provide a better measure of nutritional intakes. They are composed of three reference values:

1. *Estimated Average Requirement.* The intake value of a particular nutrient that is adequate for 50 percent of an age- and gender-specific group. At this level of intake, 50 percent of the referenced group would not have met its needs.
2. *Recommended Dietary Allowance.* The intake levels that are sufficient to meet the nutritional needs of virtually all people in a particular reference group.
3. *Upper Intake Levels.* The maximum level of a daily nutrient that is unlikely to pose a health risk for any people in the particular reference group.[10]

The Food and Nutrition Board has established seven panels to investigate the following nutrient groups:

- Calcium, vitamin D, phosphorus, magnesium, and fluoride
- Folate and other B vitamins
- Antioxidants
- Macronutrients
- Trace elements
- Electrolytes and water
- Other food components (e.g., fiber, phytoesterogens)

In August 1997, the first of the panel reports was released on calcium.[11] The panel now suggests that women consume at least 1,000 mg of calcium per day; and 1,200 mg if they are over age 50. Further, the panel has moved away from the previous recommendation that pregnant and lactating women need more calcium. Additional panel reports are expected through 1998. All reports are scheduled to be completed and the DRIs released by the year 2000.[12]

NECESSARY NUTRIENTS

When we eat, we give little thought to the real purpose of food in our bodies. Generally we know we are hungry or that we are full. We tend to make our food choices based upon hunger and the availability of the foods we prefer to eat. Little thought is given to the role that food will play once it gets into our bodies. Once consumed, the food enters our digestive tract only to be broken down into nutrients that are absorbed into the bloodstream so they can be distributed to the body's cells. The nutrients come in many forms, each form serving specific roles in building body cells, providing energy for the body, and controlling body processes. Each class of nutrients will be discussed in the following sections.

Carbohydrates

Carbohydrates are energy sources for the body. Each gram of carbohydrate yields about four calories. Carbohydrates can be found in two forms: simple carbohydrates and complex carbohydrates. The simplest of the carbohydrates are the **monosaccharides**—the simple sugars. Glucose is a simple sugar found floating in our bloodstream and is the primary source of energy for the body cells. The liver converts sugars from other foods to form glucose. Glucose is the immediate energy source provided to the body during an intravenous feeding.

Fructose is a common sugar that comes mostly from fruit and honey. It is sometimes added to certain soft drinks. It goes straight to the liver after it enters the small intestine and is quickly metabolized. Galactose is a monosaccharide that is similar to glucose. It is not found in the food we eat, rather it occurs following digestion of lactose.

Disaccharides are also simple sugars but they are formed by the combination of two monosaccharides. The most common disaccharides are sucrose, maltose, and lactose. Sucrose is ordinary table sugar. It is made from sugar cane, sugar beets, maple sugar, or honey. Maltose is formed when grains are allowed to form malt. Lactose is a disaccharide found in milk products. As you may already have figured out, disaccharides

Recommended Dietary Allowances (RDA)—recommended nutrient intakes that meet the needs of people similar in age and sex; the RDAs represent adequate quantities for all healthy people, based on current scientific knowledge.

Dietary Reference Intakes—recently created generic term that refers to three types of reference values in the diets of particular age and gender groups.

monosaccharides—simple sugar molecules; examples include glucose, fructose, and galactose.

disaccharides (**die** sack a rides)—compound made up of two monosaccharides, or simple sugars; examples include sucrose, maltose, and lactose.

(See *FYI:* "Spaghetti by Any Other Name.")

FYI

Spaghetti by Any Other Name

The Italian noodles we eat are known as spaghetti. In Italian, this means "strings." Pasta, Italian for "paste" because it's made from dough and water, comes in many other forms too. Spaghetti, vermicelli, and linguine are all made from the same kind of dough. A cup of it contains only about 210 calories and only one gram of fat! ☺

will take longer to be useful to the body than glucose because they must be broken down to glucose before they can be used by the cells. Therefore, a woman who is competing in athletics would find fruit to be a more ready form of energy than a candy bar.

Complex carbohydrates are also known as starches. Whereas simple carbohydrates are known as monosaccharides and disaccharides, complex carbohydrates are **polysaccharides** because they are composed of numerous monosaccharide units. Some starches have as many as 3,000 glucose units.[13] Complex carbohydrates are found in foods containing grains, and certain vegetables like potatoes. (See *FYI:* "Spaghetti by Any Other Name.")

There is no Recommended Dietary Allowance for carbohydrate intake. If a woman does not consume enough carbohydrates to meet the energy requirements of her body, for example, during long-term periods of starvation, her muscles, heart, liver, and other vital organs will begin to break down into amino acids. Some of these amino acids will further convert to glucose to give energy to her body. Lack of carbohydrates will also interfere with fat metabolism resulting in the formation of **ketones.** Ketones disrupt the acid-base balance of the body, a condition known as ketosis. It is, therefore, important that a woman consume sufficient amounts of carbohydrates to prevent energy supply problems in her body. This can be accomplished by consuming 50–100 grams of carbohydrates each day. Three fruit servings, three slices of bread, or a little more than a cup of cereal will provide the needed amount of carbohydrates.[14]

Women should be aware of **nutrient density** when making carbohydrate food choices. Foods that are high in energy value, but contain few other nutrients, lack nutrient density. These "empty calorie"

foods do not contribute to a well-balanced diet. Soda pop and sugary candies are examples of empty calorie foods. Alcohol is another "food" substance that supplies the body with energy and nothing else.

Protein

Proteins serve very important functions in the body. Women use proteins to build and repair body tissue including the blood, to help regulate body processes, and to provide some fuel for body cells.[15] Proteins are made from amino acids joined together by chemical bonds. The proteins consumed from the food we eat are broken down into amino acids in the body, and become the proteins needed to accomplish the tasks just listed. The human body uses 20 or so different amino acids. Nine of these amino acids are called *essential* amino acids because they must be consumed in the foods we eat. The remaining amino acids are referred to as *nonessential* because they can be manufactured by the other amino acids we consume.

Proteins in our diet come from two main categories. *Complete protein* comes from animal tissue. It is called complete because the food contains all the amino acids necessary to either make protein or make other necessary amino acids in our bones. *Incomplete protein* sources are found in foods that come from plants. It is possible for a woman to gain the appropriate number of amino acids from combining one or more plant sources. For example, beans and rice each contain incomplete proteins, but when eaten together they complement each other by providing an amino acid from each that the other food lacks. Beans eaten with a flour tortilla would also provide all the essential amino acids.

How much protein does a woman need each day? There is no absolute answer to this question. Also, more importantly, a woman needs a sufficient number of *amino acids* rather than a particular amount of protein. Generally speaking, Americans do not have a problem getting enough protein in their diets. Men consume twice as much protein as is recommended, and women nearly one-and-a half times the needed amount.[16] This is due in large part to the American custom that meat is the center of "a balanced meal." There are disadvantages to consuming more protein than the body needs, especially if the woman is eating animal sources of protein. The body will only use the protein it needs and excretes those that are unneeded. The consumption of animal protein may also pose an increased risk for cardiovascular disease and cancer.[17]

Fats

Fat is the "f" word that creates much concern and anxiety among women who are interested in their health and/or physical appearance. It is perhaps the most talked about, but the least understood of all the nutrients. Fat is perceived as the villain among the food nutrients. It is linked with heart disease, cancer, and obesity. The concern may be somewhat valid because Americans have one of the fattiest diets in the world. In general, we consume more than 37 percent of our calories from fat.[18] We are continually trying to assess the relative risks and benefits from fat consumption. Though their diets are high in fat, the people on the island of Crete have very low rates of heart disease. This is because most of their dietary fat comes from olive oil, a monounsaturated fat that tends to reduce levels of LDL cholesterol and boost levels of HDL cholesterol. Eskimos also have high fat diets, but their levels of heart disease are also low due to their intake of fish rich in omega-3 fatty acids. These fatty acids are found in salmon and mackerel (as well as canola and soybean oil). These fatty acids lower both LDL and triglyceride levels in the blood.[19]

Dietary fats come in many forms. Collectively they are referred to as *lipids*. Lipids contain carbon, hydrogen, and oxygen atoms. The simplest form of lipids are the fatty acids. Fatty acids are joined together to form the fat molecule. Fats are a highly concentrated form of food energy, supplying nine calories per gram (compared to the 4 calories found in each gram of carbohydrate). Lipids are not soluble in water, but rather, they can be dissolved in compounds such as ether or benzene. Some lipids, like butter and lard, are solids at room temperature. Other lipids like cooking oil are liquid at room temperature. Whether or not a lipid is solid or liquid depends upon how many hydrogen atoms there are on the molecule. A *saturated fat* is composed of fatty acid molecules that contain all the hydrogen atoms they can carry. Butter, milk fat, lard, and meat fat are examples of saturated fats. Palm oil and coconut oil are also saturated fats. Unsaturated fatty acids are classified according to the number of pairs of hydrogen atoms that are missing. *Monounsaturated fats* like olive oil, peanut oil, and canola oil lack only one pair of hydrogen atoms. Corn oil, safflower oil, and sesame oils lack two or more pairs of hydrogen atoms and are therefore said to be polyunsaturated. Unsaturated fats are generally liquid at room temperature. (See *Viewpoint:* "Where Is the Hidden Fat?")

Not only are fats a source of energy in the body, they serve other purposes in our diet. Fats transport one of the essential fatty acids, linoleic acid, around the body. Fat-soluble vitamins, A, D, E, and K, are also carried by the fats in the bloodstream. To some degree, fats help contribute to our sense of fullness when we eat because fats take longer to leave the stomach than other nutrients.

Viewpoint

Where Is the Hidden Fat?

Because of all the concern about saturated fats, most fast food chains and food manufacturers have switched from using beef fats and tropical oils to vegetable oil. Vegetable oil is liquid. To give it a firmer consistency and reduce the likelihood of spoilage, food manufacturers pump hydrogen into the vegetable oil, producing a more hydrogenated oil. This oil is referred to as **trans fat** or *trans fatty acid*. Trans fat has been associated with increasing the LDL cholesterol levels in the blood, just as saturated fats will. Trans fat has also been associated with *lowering* HDL cholesterol. You can get an idea how much trans fat a food contains by reading the label. One clue is found in the list of ingredients. If you see something like "partially hydrogenated canola oil," you can count on that being a trans fat. If the label gives you the amount of other fats, such as saturated, polyunsaturated, and monounsaturated, add the figures for all the fats and subtract them from the amount of total fat stated on the label.

Select two packaged foods from your cupboard or look at two the next time you go shopping. Can you determine the amount of trans fat? Are you able to detect that there is a "hidden fat" in the products? Which of the two products contain the healthiest amount of fat?

---

polysaccharides—compounds composed of numerous saccharide units; complex carbohydrates.

ketones (**key** tones)—chemical by-products resulting from the incomplete breakdown of fats.

nutrient density—ratio of the nutrients in a particular food, and the amount of energy that food contains; a food has a favorable nutrient density if the nutrients are more abundant than the calories; soda pop, for example, has little nutrient density.

trans fat—the fatty acids formed when hydrogen is pumped into liquid vegetable oils to make them more firm.

Vitamins

Until the beginning of this century, scientists believed the only things necessary for a good diet were proteins, carbohydrates, and fats, but studies in the late 1800s were beginning to suggest that other elements in our foods were essential for health. The first of these elements to be identified was what we now know as vitamin B-1, whose chemical composition included an "amine"; thus the word "vitamine" was created meaning "an amine needed for life."[20]

Vitamins are trace nutrients that perform unique functions in the body. These nutrients enable the body to use carbohydrates, proteins, and fats to build and maintain the tissues in the body. Nutritionists call vitamins and minerals *trace nutrients* because a person does not have to consume large quantities of these nutrients in order for their associated functions to be carried out. In fact, we generally need less than a gram of the various vitamins and minerals each day. Too often the term *trace nutrients* is misunderstood. Some women believe they do not need to eat a lot of food in order to get sufficient amounts of vitamins or minerals. The reality is that vitamins and minerals exist in trace levels in foods also. Consuming less food results in insufficient levels of the vitamins and minerals.

There are 13 vitamins that are known to benefit human beings. Four of these vitamins (A, D, E, and K) are *fat soluble;* that is, they are absorbed into and carried through the body along with dietary fat. The other nine vitamins are water soluble. Because *water soluble* vitamins dissolve in water, women should keep in mind that large amounts of these vitamins can be lost during food preparation. For example, steaming or boiling broccoli until it is deep green and very soft will result in much of the vitamin C being left behind in the pan. For more information on vitamins see Tables 7.1 and 7.2.

Antioxidants   Three vitamins, vitamin C, vitamin E, and beta-carotene, are known as **antioxidants.** These compounds are believed to provide a defense against such diseases as cancer and heart disease. We have known for some time now that our body cells use oxygen to "burn" the fuels inside them. As with any burning process, an "exhaust" will be given off as a by-product. This waste product comes in the form of oxidants, or *free radicals.* It is believed that these free radicals combine easily with cholesterol to damage the blood vessels, or with other chemicals to create the carcinogenic effects of cancer formation. The role of antioxidants is a recent occurrence and

the medical community has reported mixed reviews about the efficacy of antioxidants. Physicians suggest that women should consume fruits and vegetables rich in these antioxidants to reduce the likelihood of certain cancers and heart disease. So far we do not have any single studies that conclusively demonstrate that taking these antioxidant vitamins in pill form will lead to a healthier life,[21] but it appears there is a protective effect if the antioxidants come from natural food sources. One recent investigation[22] has summarized the findings of numerous studies and concluded that vitamin E taken in doses of 100–200 IU for more than 6 years can reduce the risk of heart disease. At this point we can say that consuming the appropriate foods and taking supplements are not harmful, and are likely to be protective of our health.

Minerals

Like vitamins, minerals are needed in relatively small amounts. There are seven minerals included in the RDAs. Three minerals, calcium, magnesium, and phosphorus, are **macrominerals,** or major minerals. Four other minerals, iron, zinc, iodine, and selenium, are trace minerals. We obtain minerals from both plant and animal sources. Minerals obtained from animal sources possess a greater level of *bioavailability;* that is, they become more readily available to a woman's body once they are consumed. Plant sources tend to have compounds that bind up the minerals, thus reducing mineral bioavailability.[23]

Minerals serve a variety of purposes within the body. No doubt you are familiar with the role of calcium in developing bone, and iron that helps to build good red blood cells. But other minerals serve many other very important functions. A healthy water balance requires appropriate levels of sodium, potassium, calcium, and phosphorus. Sodium, potassium, and calcium influence the movement of nerve impulses, and iodine is a key ingredient in the hormone thyroxin. Refer to Table 7.3 for more information about the major minerals. Two minerals are of specific interest to women: calcium and iron. These will be discussed in the following sections.

---

antioxidants—compounds that reduce the destructive capacity of oxidizing compounds.

macrominerals—nutrients required in the body in amounts exceeding 100 mg/day.

Table 7.1

The Fat-Soluble Vitamins, Their Functions, Deficiency Conditions, and Food Sources

VITAMIN	MAJOR FUNCTIONS	DEFICIENCY SYMPTOMS	PEOPLE MOST AT RISK	DIETARY SOURCES	RDA	TOXICITY SYMPTOMS
Vitamin A (retinoids) and provitamin A (carotenoids)	Promote vision: light and color Promote growth Prevent drying of skin and eyes Promote resistance to bacterial infection	Night blindness Xerophthalmia (dry eye) Poor growth Dry skin (keratinization)	People in poverty, especially preschool children (still very rare in the United States)	Vitamin A Liver Fortified milk Provitamin A Sweet potatoes Spinach Greens Carrots Cantaloupe Apricots Broccoli	Females: 800 RE* (4,000 IU †) Males: 1,000 RE* (5,000 IU †)	Fetal malformations, hair loss, skin changes, pain in bones
D (chole- and ergocalciferol)	Facilitate absorption of calcium and phosphorus Maintain optimal calcification of bone	Rickets Osteomalacia	Breast-fed infants, elderly shut-ins	Vitamin D-fortified milk Fish oils Sardines Salmon	5 micrograms (200–400 IU)	Growth retardation, kidney damage, calcium deposits in soft tissue
E (tocopherois, tocotrienols)	Act as an antioxidant: prevent breakdown of vitamin A and unsaturated fatty acids	Hemolysis of red blood cells Nerve destruction	People with poor fat absorption (still very rare)	Vegetable oils Some greens Some fruits	Females: 8 milligrams Alpha-tocopherol equivalents Males: 10 milligrams Alpha-tocopherol equivalents	Muscle weakness, headaches, fatigue, nausea, inhibition of vitamin K metabolism
K (phyllo- and menaquinone)	Help form prothrombin and other factors for blood clotting	Hemorrhage	People taking antibiotics for months at a time (still quite rare)	Green vegetables Liver	60–80 micrograms	Anemia and jaundice

*Retinol equivalents.
†International units.

Table 7.2

The Water-Soluble Vitamins, Their Functions, Deficiency Conditions, and Food Sources

NAME	MAJOR FUNCTIONS	DEFICIENCY SYMPTOMS	PEOPLE MOST AT RISK	DIETARY SOURCES	RDA OR ESADDI	TOXICITY
Thiamin	Coenzyme involved with enzymes in carbohydrate metabolism; nerve function	Beriberi; nervous tingling, poor coordination, edema, heart changes, weakness	People with alcoholism, people in poverty	Sunflower seeds, pork, whole and enriched grains, dried beans, brewer's yeast	1.1–1.5 milligrams	None possible from food
Riboflavin	Coenzymes involved in energy metabolism	Inflammation of mouth and tongue, cracks at corners of the mouth, eye disorders	Possibly people on certain medications if no dairy products consumed	Milk, mushrooms, spinach, liver, enriched grains	1.2–1.7 milligrams	None reported
Niacin	Coenzymes involved in energy metabolism, fat synthesis, fat breakdown	Pellagra, diarrhea, dermatitis, dementia	People in severe poverty for which corn is dominant food, people with alcoholism	Mushrooms, bran, tuna, salmon, chicken, beef, liver, peanuts, enriched grains	15–19 milligrams	Flushing of skin at >100 milligrams
Pantothenic acid	Coenzyme involved in energy metabolism, fat synthesis, fat breakdown	Using an antagonist causes tingling in hands, fatigue, headache, nausea	People with alcoholism	Mushrooms, liver, broccoli, eggs; most foods have some	4–7 milligrams	None
Biotin	Coenzyme involved in glucose production, fat synthesis	Dermatitis, tongue soreness, anemia, depression	People with alcoholism	Cheese, egg yolks, cauliflower, peanut butter, liver	30–100 micrograms	Unknown
Vitamin B-6, pyridoxine and other forms	Coenzyme involved in protein metabolism, neurotransmitter synthesis, hemoglobin synthesis, many other functions	Headache, anemia, convulsions, nausea, vomiting, flaky skin, sore tongue	Adolescent and adult women, people on certain medications, people with alcoholism	Animal protein foods, spinach, broccoli, bananas, salmon, sunflower seeds	1.8–2 milligrams	Nerve destruction at doses >100 milligrams
Folate (folic acid)	Coenzyme involved in DNA synthesis	Megatoblastic anemia, inflammation of tongue, diarrhea, poor growth, mental disorders	People with alcoholism; pregnant women; people taking certain medications	Green leafy vegetables, orange juice, organ meats, sprouts, sunflower seeds	180–200 microgram	None, nonprescription vitamin dosage is controlled by FDA
Vitamin B-12 (cobalamins)	Coenzyme involved in folate metabolism, nerve function	Macrocytic anemia, poor nerve function	Elderly, because of poor absorption; vegans	Animal foods, especially organ meats, oysters, clams (B-12 not naturally in plant foods)	2 micrograms	None
Vitamin C (ascorbic acid)	Collagen synthesis, hormone synthesis, neurotransmitter synthesis	Scurvy: poor wound healing, pinpoint hemorrhages, bleeding gums, edema	People with alcoholism; elderly men living alone	Citrus fruits, strawberries, broccoli, greens	60 milligrams	Doses >1–2 grams cause diarrhea and can alter some diagnostic tests

Table 7.3

Water and the Major Minerals

NAME	MAJOR FUNCTIONS	DEFICIENCY SYMPTOMS	PEOPLE MOST AT RISK	RDA OR MINIMUM REQUIREMENT	NUTRIENT-DENSE DIETARY SOURCES	RESULTS OF TOXICITY
Water	Medium for chemical reactions, removal of waste products, perspiration to cool the body	Thirst, muscle weakness, poor endurance	Infants with a fever, elderly persons in nursing homes	1 milliliter per kcalorie expended*	As such and in foods	Probably occurs only in those with mental disorders: headache, blurred vision, convulsions
Sodium	A major ion of the extracellular fluid; nerve impulse transmission	Muscle cramps	People who severely restrict sodium to lower blood pressure (250–500 milligrams/day)	500 milligrams	Table salt, processed foods	High blood pressure in susceptible individuals
Potassium	A major ion of intracellular fluid; nerve impulse transmission	Irregular heart beat, loss of appetite, muscle cramps	People who use potassium-wasting diuretics or have poor diets, as seen in poverty and alcoholism	2000 milligrams	Spinach, squash, bananas, orange juice, other vegetables and fruits, milk	Slowing of the heart beat; seen in kidney failure
Chloride	A major ion of the extracellular fluid; acid production in stomach; nerve transmission	Convulsions in infants	No one, probably, when infant formula manufacturers control product quality adequately	700 milligrams	Table salt, some vegetables	High blood pressure in susceptible people when combined with sodium
Calcium	Bone and tooth strength; blood clotting; nerve impulse transmission; muscle contractions; cell regulation	Poor intake increases the risk for osteoporosis	Women in general, especially those who constantly restrict their energy intake and consume few dairy products	800 milligrams (age greater than 24 years)	Dairy products, canned fish, leafy vegetables, tofu, fortified orange juice	Very high intakes may cause kidney stones in susceptible people, poor mineral absorption in general
Phosphorus	Bone and tooth strength; part of various metabolic compounds; major ion of intracellular fluid	Probably none; poor bone maintenance is a possibility	Elderly persons consuming very nutrient-poor diets; possibly total vegetarians and people with alcoholism	800 milligrams (age greater than 24 years)	Dairy products, processed foods, fish, soft drinks	Hampers bone health in people with kidney failure; poor bone mineralization if calcium intakes are low
Magnesium	Bone strength; enzyme function; nerve and heart function	Weakness, muscle pain, poor heart function	Women in general, people on thiazide diuretics	Men: 350 milligrams Women: 280 milligrams	Wheat bran, green vegetables, nuts, chocolate	Causes weakness in people with kidney failure
Sulfur	Part of vitamins and amino acids; drug detoxification; acid-base balance	None have been described	No one who meets his or her protein needs	None	Protein foods	None likely

*Just an approximation; best to keep urine volume at level greater than 1 liter (4 cups).

Calcium About 99 percent of the calcium in a woman's body is found in bone. The remaining 1 percent is used to stimulate muscle contractions and nerve impulses, and to regulate blood clotting.[24] For the past decade, women have become increasingly more aware of their calcium needs. Medical research has uncovered a considerable amount of information about *osteoporosis,* an age-related condition characterized by demineralization of bone. In the United States, osteoporosis affects more than 25 million people over age 45.[25] The vast majority of these cases are among women. Historically, the medical community viewed osteoporosis as an inevitable problem of aging,[26] but we now know that osteoporosis is largely preventable.

Osteoporosis is perceived as a disease that afflicts old people. Research indicates, however that the quality of a woman's bones in old age, in the absence of risk factors, is related to what a women is able to do for herself. Genetics contributes about 80 percent toward osteoporosis formation.[27] The rest is related to diet and lifestyle. The development of bone mass density (BMD) is related to calcium intake over the woman's lifetime. Specifically, it appears that the greatest influence comes during childhood and the elderly years. The intake of calcium is very important in preventing osteoporosis, but there are other factors that affect bone mass.

- Excess alcohol consumption has a detrimental effect on BMD.
- Cigarette smoking has a deleterious effect on BMD. Smokers experience earlier menopause and accelerated rate of postmenopausal bone loss.
- Caffeine is related to increased urinary excretion of calcium.[28] (See *Health Tips:* "Coffee and Calcium Loss.")

So, a woman who has a family history of osteoporosis, drinks alcohol, smokes cigarettes, and consumes numerous cups of coffee each day is at great risk for osteoporosis. If she has a diet that is calcium poor, she is at even greater risk. Although dairy products are the best sources of calcium, there are other ways of getting calcium if the woman is lactose intolerant or if she does not like dairy products. (See *FYI:* "Calcium Sources" for suggestions for additional calcium sources.) Additional coverage of osteoporosis can be found in chapter 19.

Iron Humans need 10–12 mg of iron daily in order to manufacture **hemoglobin.** Hemoglobin is found

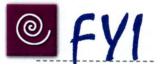

Calcium Sources

Women are often aware of their need for calcium, yet they think they must drink a lot of milk to obtain adequate amounts of calcium for their diets. Milk is not the sole source of dietary calcium, nor is it the best source. Consider some alternatives to make your diet rich in calcium. ∞

Food	Calcium (mg)
sardines (3 ozs.)	370
sesame seeds (¼ cup)	335
skim milk (1 cup)	300
dried figs (1 cup)	287
black-eyed peas (1 cup)	211
spinach (1 cup)	200
green beans (1 cup)	165
almonds (½ cup)	150

in our red blood cells and is responsible for transporting oxygen to, and carbon dioxide away, from the body cells. Iron also helps build certain enzymes and proteins in the body. Because of the blood loss associated with menstruation, women have a greater need for iron than men do. A woman may need as much as 15 mg per day, and even more if her menstrual flow is heavy.

A typical adult diet contains 5–7 mg of iron per 1000 calories.[29] Women consume about 2,000 calories per day. Therefore, it is necessary for a woman to carefully evaluate the foods she eats to assure sufficient iron consumption. There are two forms of iron found in our diet.[30] **Heme iron** is found in animal tissue (e.g., in red meat), and is more rapidly absorbed than **nonheme iron,** which is found in plant sources such as spinach and grains. The amount of dietary iron will vary depending on the types and amounts of the various iron-containing foods. Not all of the dietary iron will be absorbed by the body, however. Many diet-related factors tend to interfere with absorption. Zinc competes with iron for absorption. Caffeine has a negative effect on iron absorption whereas vitamin C has a positive effect on absorption. Substances called tannins found in tea interfere with iron absorption.

If a woman wants to have good iron levels, red meat should *not* be completely avoided. Foods rich in vitamin C should be consumed to take advantage of nonheme iron sources. During pregnancy, iron supplements are a must, because a woman will almost double her blood volume to accommodate the growing fetus.

Water Often overlooked as a nutrient, water is, without a doubt, our most important nutrient. Depending on our fat stores, we can live for extended periods of time without foods that supply vitamins, minerals, proteins, fats, and energy, but we can expect to live only a few days without water. Most of your body is composed of water—more than 60 percent of the body's weight. Water serves a number of very important functions in the body.

- Water helps to regulate the temperature of the body. Water in the blood collects heat generated by the body and transports it to the surface of the skin. Heat energy is taken from the body as perspiration evaporates.
- Water is necessary for many of the chemical reactions that take place in the body.
- Water serves as a vehicle for removing waste products from the body. Cellular by-products are picked up by the blood and transported to the kidneys for processing and excreting the by-products with the urine.

Thirst is regulated by the concentration of sodium in the blood. When water levels drop and the percent of sodium increases, the thirst sensation is triggered.[31] A woman needs to drink at least six cups of water each day. She will obtain an additional 4 cups from the foods she eats. It is advisable not to rely entirely on your thirst response, however. It is not unusual, especially in cool weather, to overlook the need for water. (See *FYI:* "Water.")

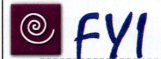

Water: The Overpriced Nutrient

Although the quality of our tap water is regulated by local law and the Environmental Protection Agency, many people are dissatisfied with water that comes from the faucet. Consequently, water has become our most overpriced nutrient. In 1992, American consumers downed an estimated 2.2 billion gallons of bottled water, paying more than 2.5 billion dollars.[32]

Phytochemicals Phytochemicals or phytonutrients are the nonnutritive substances in plant foods that otherwise act on the body's physiology in some positive way. More and more evidence is emerging that these components tend to have health-protective qualities.[33] Table 7.4 represents some of the phytochemicals and their functions.

There may be a time that phytonutrients may become classified as essential nutrients.

PREGNANCY AND BREAST-FEEDING

A woman's nutritional condition is always an important part of her life. Nutrition takes on even greater importance when she becomes pregnant. The changes that occur within her reproductive system are profound. These changes require more complex

hemoglobin—the iron-bearing molecules found in red blood cells that carry oxygen to, and carbon dioxide away from body cells.

heme iron (heem)—iron found in animal tissue in the form of hemoglobin and myoglobin.

nonheme iron—iron found in plant sources and tissues in animals other than heme iron tissues.

phytochemicals—nonnutrient substances found in plant foods that have a positive effect on the body's physiology; phytonutrients.

Table 7.4

Food Sources and Functions of Phytochemicals		
PHYTOCHEMICAL	FOOD SOURCE	ACTION
Carotenoids	yellow and orange fruits and vegetables, dark green leafy vegetables	an antioxidant
Allylic sulfides	garlic, onions, chives	induces detoxification enzymes; anticarcinogenic; cardiovascular protection
Phytosterols	green and yellow vegetables	block the uptake of cholesterol
Phytoesterogens	cereals, grains	prevention of diseases and conditions related to aging and menopause

and challenging adaptations to the way she eats. In addition to her own well-being, she is faced with the nutritional demands of the fetus. Many factors influence a successful pregnancy, but there is no single factor more important than nutrition.

Energy Needs During Pregnancy

On average, a pregnant woman will need to consume approximately 300 more calories per day than she did in her pre-pregnant condition. Some women get the impression that they are "eating for two" during their pregnancy. Such thinking leads to a greater weight gain than is necessary or healthy for the woman. The amount of weight that should be gained during pregnancy varies from woman to woman. There is no amount of weight gain that is perfect for every pregnant woman.

Research based on maternal weight gain associated with births of desired-weight infants indicates that a woman who is underweight should gain more weight (35–45 pounds) than an obese woman (16–20 pounds).[34] A normal weight woman should gain approximately 28 pounds during pregnancy. A weight gain over 45 pounds tends to be counterproductive.

Nutrient Requirements During Pregnancy

According to the RDAs, pregnant women need only 15 percent more calories, but up to 100 percent more nutrients than do women who are not pregnant. Ideally, a pregnant woman has to make intelligent food choices that allow her to increase the intake of important nutrients without increasing her caloric intake to the point that she gains more weight than is necessary. (See Table 7.5.)

Protein A woman will produce about two additional pounds of protein during her pregnancy. About one-fourth of this increase will go to developing her blood supply, and 50 percent of it will be used to manufacture fetal tissue. The average woman, on a 2,100 cal/day diet, normally needs about 45g of protein (a small roasted chicken breast). During her pregnancy, she will need to increase protein consumption to 75–100 g. The challenge will be in her ability to increase protein without increasing calories, particularly fat calories found in many meat sources.

Iron The most common nutrient deficiency among pregnant women is iron.[35] A woman tends to have low iron stores to begin with, but during pregnancy her iron needs increase dramatically. In addition to the iron needed to build her increasing number of red blood cells, the fetus will demand iron as well. It is extremely unlikely that a woman will be able to consume enough iron in the foods she eats—to do so would require about 20 slices of beef liver every day! It is therefore recommended that pregnant women take daily iron supplements. Research indicates that 30–60 mg is sufficient.[36]

Folacin Folacin (folic acid or folate) is another very important nutrient during pregnancy. Folacin is necessary for the formation of tissue. One can see how important this nutrient is, given the amount of tissue being generated by the mother and the fetus. Lack of dietary folate, particularly in the first trimester, is related to a number of birth defects. Folate deficiency has been associated with neural tube birth defects such as **spina bifida.** Neural tube malformations, which are defects of the brain and spinal cord in the embryo, represent the number one birth defect in the country today, affecting between one and two infants

Table 7.5

Recommended Dietary Allowances for Women (25 years old) During Pregnancy and Breast-Feeding

NUTRIENTS	PRE-PREGNANT	PREGNANT	LACTATING	SOURCES
Protein	50 g	60 g	65 g	meats, fish, poultry, grains, dairy products
Vitamin A	800 µg	800 µg	1,300 µg	fortified milk, deep yellow and orange fruits and vegetables, green vegetables
Vitamin D	10 µg	10 µg	10 µg	fortified milk, liver, eggs, codfish, sunlight
Vitamin E	8 mg	10 mg	12 mg	vegetables, oils, milk, eggs, codfish, grains
Vitamin K	65 µg	65 µg	65 µg	leafy green vegetables, pork, liver, yogurt, egg yolk, kelp, alfalfa
Vitamin C	60 mg	70 mg	95 mg	citrus fruits, tomatoes, green pepper, cantaloupe
Thiamin	1.1 mg	1.5 mg	1.6 mg	enriched grains
Riboflavin	1.3 mg	1.6 mg	1.8 mg	liver, milk and dairy products, enriched cereals, eggs
Niacin	15 mg	17 mg	20 mg	fish, liver, meat, poultry, eggs, enriched grains, milk
Vitamin B-6	1.6 mg	2.2 mg	2.1 mg	liver, chicken, potatoes, bananas, wheat germ, beef, egg yolk
Folate	180 µg	400 µg	280 µg	liver, spinach, asparagus, broccoli, grains, leafy vegetables
Vitamin B-12	2.0 µg	2.2 µg	2.6 µg	animal proteins
Calcium	800 mg (1200)*	1,200 mg	1,200 mg	dairy products
Phosphorus	800 mg	1,200 mg	1,200 mg	dairy products, grains, eggs, dried beans
Magnesium	280 mg	320 mg	355 mg	spinach, broccoli, almonds, oatmeal, wheat bran, cereals, brown rice, seeds, beans
Iron	15 mg	30 mg	15 mg	meats, eggs, grains

*Change as of August 1997.

out of every 1,000.[37] The importance of getting enough folacin in the first few weeks of pregnancy cannot be overemphasized. It is during this time period when neural tube defects begin to manifest themselves in the absence of sufficient levels of folacin. Determine your knowledge of sources of folacin by completing *Assess Yourself:* "Foods for Folacin."

Calcium Calcium is needed to support the mineralization of bone in the fetus. Much of the calcium required for this purpose is needed during the third trimester. It is important for a woman to increase the amount of calcium in her diet early in her pregnancy. If her diet is poor in calcium at the start of her pregnancy, and she makes no adjustments to improve calcium intake, calcium will be automatically removed from her own bones so that blood levels of calcium can be maintained for the fetus.[38] Along with dairy products and fortified orange juice, other sources of calcium are included in *FYI:* "Calcium Sources" on

p. 132. If the woman doesn't like these kinds of foods, she is advised to take calcium supplements.

Vitamin and Mineral Supplements Many pregnant women, in an effort to help the growing fetus, will routinely take a complete vitamin/mineral supplement during pregnancy. This practice is not recommended if a woman's diet is good at the start of her pregnancy. The only nutrients that require supplementation are iron, folacin, and calcium (especially if the woman does not drink milk). All other nutrients will be obtained from the slight increases she will make in her food consumption. A woman should take particular care not to consume high

spina bifida—congenital birth defect in which the spine fails to enclose the spinal cord; usually occurs within the first month of pregnancy.

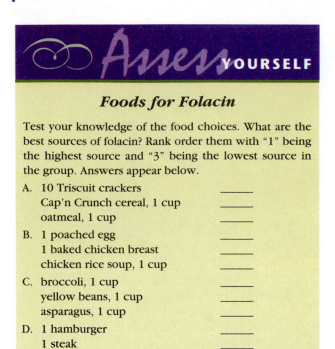

Assess YOURSELF

Foods for Folacin

Test your knowledge of the food choices. What are the best sources of folacin? Rank order them with "1" being the highest source and "3" being the lowest source in the group. Answers appear below.

A. 10 Triscuit crackers   _____
    Cap'n Crunch cereal, 1 cup   _____
    oatmeal, 1 cup   _____

B. 1 poached egg   _____
    1 baked chicken breast   _____
    chicken rice soup, 1 cup   _____

C. broccoli, 1 cup   _____
    yellow beans, 1 cup   _____
    asparagus, 1 cup   _____

D. 1 hamburger   _____
    1 steak   _____
    ham, 1 cup   _____

Answers: A. 3,1,2   B. 1,3,2   C. 3,1,2   D. All three low

doses of vitamins during pregnancy, especially vitamins B-6, B-12, and C. Excessive amounts of these vitamins will create **rebound deficiencies.** The high amounts of vitamins place the fetus's excretion mechanisms into high gear during pregnancy. This high rate of excretion continues after delivery thus excreting the small amounts of vitamins that the infant receives.[39]

Breast-Feeding

After a woman delivers her baby, she will have to decide whether or not she wants to breast-feed. Her options will be to breast-feed or use an infant formula. Cow's milk is not recommended until the infant reaches 1 year of age. The protein in cow's milk is much too difficult for a newborn to digest, and the newborn's kidneys are not developed enough to process the high mineral content of cow's milk.[40]

A woman's nutrient needs during breast-feeding are similar to those needs she had during her pregnancy. Proportionally, she will continue to require more nutrients than calories. She should continue with a nutrient-dense diet, and supplement with vitamins as needed. Her calcium intake deserves special attention. If she fails to consume enough calcium in her diet, she can experience calcium loss from her

bones in order to meet the needs of the infant.[41] It will also be important for the woman to drink fluids after she nurses. If she fails to drink enough fluids, her milk production will diminish.

A breast-feeding woman should be aware that the things she takes into her body will make their way into her milk supply. Alcohol can be delivered to the infant via breast-feeding, as can caffeine from coffee. If the mother's diet is high in saturated fats, so will be the infant's. A woman is advised to be careful about the quality of her diet if she expects to have a healthy baby.

PHYSICAL ACTIVITY

Fitness activities will have an effect on a woman's nutritional needs. The degree to which her needs are affected will depend upon her activity level. A woman can consider herself to be *mostly inactive* if she has some form of continuous activity less than 3 days per week; *moderately active* if she engages in 20 minutes of sustained activity 3 days per week (such as golf, dancing, skiing, aerobics), or *active* if she is involved in sustained activity for 20 minutes or more at least 5 days per week (such as cycling, jogging, cross-country skiing, or walking for 45 minutes). If she is a competitive athlete or happens to engage in vigorous activity for an hour or more at least 5 days per week, she could classify herself as *highly active.* As you might expect, the higher the activity level, the greater the attention she will need to give to her diet.

Caloric Intake

Your energy requirements will vary according to your activity level. Energy consumption is a function of the intensity of the activity and the length of time you engage in that activity. For example, if you classify yourself as moderately active and you weigh 110 pounds, you will use about 200 calories for an hour's worth of the activity. If you are highly active, you might burn about 500 calories in an hour. If you are involved in some form of activity, your body will tell you if you are meeting your energy needs. If you are exercising and you notice a weight loss, you are not meeting your energy demands. If you are not using your exercise regimen to intentionally lose weight, you will need to increase slightly your caloric intake. Ideally, your energy intake should match your energy expenditure.

Nutrients

It is generally believed that there is no need to increase the amount of nutrients beyond the RDAs as a person becomes physically active.[42] Exercise increases the athlete's need for more energy and water, not for more protein, vitamins, or minerals. There are, however, some aspects of nutrition and athletic performance for women that deserve special mention. They will be discussed next.

Iron deficiency has been an area of interest for some time. Investigations have revealed that iron levels are not significantly different among female athletes versus nonathletes. Those studies that report differences attribute them to poor diet rather than to physical activity.[43] Also, one of the confounding factors in measuring iron levels is the menstrual cycle, which can influence the level of iron in the blood. Vegetarian athletes or those athletes who do not eat red meat are especially vulnerable to low iron levels.[44] It is strongly recommended that women who are active or highly active should be sure to get at least 15 mg of iron daily, either from their diet or through supplementation.

Calcium intake is another area that has been studied among female athletes. It appears that female athletes may not be getting all the calcium they need. Many female athletes, particularly those who are concerned with being thin, have been observed with calcium intake levels that are below RDA levels.[45,46] If calcium levels are low, and the woman develops amenorrhea, she is likely to experience demineralization of her bones, which in turn will increase her potential for leg injuries or stress fractures.

If you are physically active and follow a vegetarian diet, you should be aware of potential problems. Vegetarians, because of high fiber intake, tend to lose estrogen. A vegetarian diet may also increase the likelihood of altering a woman's menstrual cycle, particularly if the diet is low in fat, low in protein, and high in fiber.[47]

VEGETARIANISM

About 3 percent of the U.S. population practices some type of vegetarianism,[48] which is about a 30 percent increase since 1970. Part of the increase is related to a relatively new form of vegetarianism, *semi-vegetarianism,* whereby a person excludes only red meat from the diet. The more traditional forms of vegetarian diets include:

- Vegan—excludes meat, fish, poultry, eggs, and dairy products
- Lactovegetarian—excludes meat, fish, poultry, and eggs
- Lacto-ovo-vegetarian—excludes meat, fish, or poultry

There are advantages and disadvantages to following a vegetarian regimen.[49] First and foremost, nutritional health is dependent upon balance, variety, and moderation in the diet. Whether the diet is **omnivorous,** or vegetarian, attention needs to be paid to achieving the RDAs. Women considering vegetarian diets should learn about the benefits and risks before starting a vegetarian diet. (See *Her Story:* "Tara.")

Benefits of Vegetarianism

Research indicates that vegetarians tend to:

- Be leaner than nonvegetarians. This is mostly because vegetarians are more health conscious and more physically active.
- Have lower levels of serum cholesterol. It is lowest among vegans than among lactovegetarians or nonvegetarians.
- Have lower blood pressure. This is due largely to leaner body mass than the effects of diet.
- Have less colon cancer. Diets high in animal tissue and animal fat tend to increase the risk of colon cancer.

Concerns of Vegetarianism

If a vegetarian encounters nutritional problems, it may be in the form of:

- *Iron deficiency.* Iron levels are reportedly lower among lacto-ovo-vegetarians, and more so for women than men.
- *Insufficient levels of calcium.* Because dairy products are the best source of calcium, this nutrient can be erroneously omitted from the diet.

rebound deficiencies—high doses of vitamins administered to a woman during her pregnancy resulting in her fetus over-excreting excess vitamins; causes the newborn to continue excreting after birth.

omnivorous (uhm **niv** or us)—consuming foods from both plant and meat sources.

Her Story

Tara

Tara has been trying to control her weight, but she is also interested in maintaining good health. For the past few weeks, she has been thinking more and more about becoming a vegetarian. She feels that if she doesn't eat meat, she can save a lot of calories. Besides, she is leaning toward the fact that she might not like the idea of animals being slaughtered.

A few of her classmates are vegetarians. Tara believes that vegetarianism is not that difficult. On the one hand, she can just stop eating meat, but on the other hand, she is not sure exactly how to get enough of the right foods in her diet. Tara has come to you as her friend and wants to talk with you about her decision to change.

- What would your response be to the questions she is likely to ask?
- Can vegetarians be more healthy than those people who eat meat and vegetables?
- If Tara takes meat out of her diet, what nutrients might she lose?
- What vegetables could she eat to gain those lost nutrients?

- *Vitamin D deficiency.* Strict vegetarians may have insufficient levels of this vitamin due to the absence of milk products. Milk is about the only food fortified with vitamin D to aid calcium absorption.[50]
- **Vitamin B-12 deficiency.* Pernicious anemia develops in the absence of vitamin B-12.[51] In fact, women can pass this deficiency on to their infants through breast-feeding.[52]

If you have an interest in following a vegetarian dietary regimen, there are certain principles you should follow for optimal health.

- No single plant food contains all essential amino acids. Vegans must combine foods with incomplete proteins to form meals throughout the day that become complete with the essential amino acids—for example, eating whole grain cereal with milk, peanut butter with wheat bread.
- Animal foods contain zinc, calcium, and iron.[53] Attention should be paid to consuming other plant foods that contain these nutrients.
- Be aware that the iron in plant foods is not as well absorbed as the iron from meat sources. Be

careful, too, about consuming too many grain, bran, and soy products. These foods contain phytates that inhibit the absorption of iron, calcium, and zinc.[54]

The bottom line is that vegetarianism requires intelligent planning of meals, a working knowledge of how foods interact with one another, and knowledge of the factors that influence nutrient uptake.

NUTRITION AND THE CONSUMER

We are constantly confronted with food products that claim to do amazing things. There are claims that special foods can maintain our youth, cure or prevent cancer, and supply us with an endless supply of energy. Labels on special food products and dietary supplements are usually the means by which such products deliver their claims. Understanding terminology such as "health foods," "organic," and "natural," knowing which sources of information are reliable and trustworthy, and interpreting food labels can improve a woman's ability to become a healthier consumer.

What are *health foods?* Obviously, by the term, they are foods that are meant to be beneficial to one's health! Where do we find health foods? In reality, we find them at every store that sells food, not just stores named "Health Food Stores," which is a misleading designation. When eaten in variety and moderation, and according to guidelines described in the Food Guide Pyramid, all foods can be healthy. Stare, Aronson, and Barrett, state:

> The term is merely a gimmick used to boost sales. . . . Some foods . . . popular as health foods are rich in nutrients, but no food has unique health-promoting properties. All foods can contribute to health when eaten as part of a variety and balanced diet. The problem with so-called health foods is that they are promoted with false claims and usually are overpriced.[55]

Table 7.6 lists products commonly promoted as health foods.

Additives

Many women are concerned about the amount of additives found in their foods. We tend to think of food additives as chemicals that are unnatural and added to our foods unnecessarily. The truth is that food additives play very important roles in the food we consume. Food additives are used in foods for five principle reasons:

Table 7.6

Are the "Health" Food Claims True?

PRODUCT	CLAIMS	TRUTH
Alfalfa	Contains nutrients not found in other foods	Less than in common vegetables
	Contains all essential amino acids	Untrue
Aloe vera	Cure or alleviate asthma, glaucoma, arthritis, hemorrhoids, or anemia	Unsubstantiated
	Promotes skin softening and moisturizing	Probably true
Bone meal	Provides a rich source of fiber	Yes, but poorly absorbed by the body
Carob	Used in products as a chocolate substitute; lower in fat and caffeine-free	Yes; however, has similar calorie content
Coenzyme Q^{10}	Prevents aging and increases enzyme levels in body tissue	No evidence; however, may help reduce formation of atherosclerotic formation
Fish-oil capsules	Lower blood-cholesterol and reduce heart disease	Amounts to eat are unknown; need to eat fish twice each week
Garlic	Purifies the blood, reduces high blood pressure, prevents cancer, etc.	Has lowered blood-cholesterol, but other beneficial claims are preliminary; and causes bad breath, heart burn, and may inhibit blood clotting
Goat's milk	Provides a highly nutritious cow's milk substitute	No more nutritious than cow's milk
	Effective against arthritis and cancer	Untrue
		Unpasteurized goat's milk can contain pathogens that cause disease
Granola	"Natural" and contains high amounts of nutrients	High in price, sugar, fats, and calories
RNA/DNA supplements	Rejuvenate old cells, improve memory, and prevent aging skin	Inactivated by the digestive process

1. *To maintain product consistency.* Anti-caking agents help products like salt flow freely. Emulsifiers prevent products from separating.
2. *To improve or maintain nutritional value.* For instance, vitamin D is added to milk to help reduce the incidence of malnutrition. Vitamin D is necessary for the appropriate uptake of calcium into bones.
3. *To reduce spoilage.* Preservatives will prevent spoilage caused by mold, bacteria, and fungi.
4. *To provide leavening or control alkalinity.* Leavening agents are added to help baked goods rise during cooking.
5. *To enhance flavor or provide a desired color.*

Knowing that additives are placed in foods to maintain quality is one thing. However, concern that "unnatural chemicals" are added to our food is something else. The fear is that chemicals will harm us. Consider the ingredients in the following foods:

Product A: acetone, methyl acetate, furan, butanol, methyfuran, isoprene, methyl butanol, caffeine, essential oils, methanol, acetaldehyde, methyl formate, ethanol, dimethyl sulfide, and propionaldehyde.

Product B: actomycin, myogen, nucleoproteins, peptides, amino acids, myoglobin, lipids, linoleic acid, oleic acid, lecithin, cholesterol, sucrose, ATP, glucose, collagen, elastin, creatine, pytoligneous acid, sodium chloride, sodium nitrate, sodium nitrite, and sodium phosphate.

What do you think about these two products? Do you feel you could safely consume either of them over extended periods of time? Would you feel better knowing that product A is coffee, and product B is cured ham? The media and special interest groups have attempted to color our food supply as harmful, but the truth is that all foods we consume are made of chemicals. Calcium propionate is a common food additive. Although it may sound unnatural, it is actually a compound found naturally in swiss cheese! It is added to food to prevent bacterial growth.

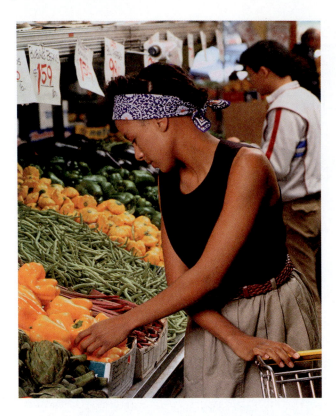

Food additives are carefully regulated by the FDA and are permitted only after extensive testing. If an additive is shown to produce cancer, for example, it cannot be used—even if the additive causes cancer only when consumed in very high doses. Using it would violate the Delaney Clause in the 1958 Food Additives Amendment.[56] It is safe to say that food additives are far more protective than harmful. It would be impossible to feed everyone in this country without food additives. Diets high in fat and alcohol actually pose greater risks to health than any of the chemicals found in our food supply.

Organic Foods

"Organic foods" claim to be produced, grown, and processed without use of commercial chemicals such as fertilizers, pesticides, or synthetics such as color or flavor. Are they healthier, more nutrient rich, or better appearing? Not necessarily! Produce that is grown, processed, and sold by reputable producers have equivalent nutrient values. Longitudinal studies reveal insignificant differences in nutrient content of organically grown crops and those using standard agricultural methods.[57] The difference actually appears to be only in the price of organic foods and regular foods. Studies reveal that organic foods may cost twice as

JOURNAL ACTIVITY

Organic vs. Standard-Grown Foods

Visit markets that sell organic foods and compare their claims, price, and appearance with foods that have been grown and processed via standard agriculture methods? What are your findings? Do you receive more nutrient benefits from organic foods? How do you know? Make a chart of five foods and compare costs between the two groups. Are organic foods easy to find? How do you know foods labeled as organic are indeed organic? Do you have to travel to a special store to purchase organic foods? What were the claims of the store clerk about these foods? What is your decision about these two types of foods?

much as other foods.[58,59] So if you choose to purchase organic foods, be aware that you may be spending an unnecessary amount of money on foods that cannot match their claims. Complete *Journal Activity:* "Organic vs. Standard-Grown Foods" to help you determine whether organic foods are a wise choice for you.

Natural Foods

Foods containing no food additives and requiring only minor processing during growth and marketing procedures are labeled as "natural" foods. Why is this important? Proponents believe that natural food is replete with increased nutrition—more so than other "unnatural" foods—and that consuming any preservatives or additives is not good for your health and well-being. What is important to remember is that foods labeled natural usually are higher priced, and they do not provide any more nutrients than fresh foods eaten in a varied and complete diet. The most widely used additives are sugar, salt, and corn syrup—all of which are natural foods.

Take the short *Assess Yourself:* "What Do You Know About the Foods You Eat?" to determine what you know about some of the foods you eat.

Knowledge, understanding, and application of this information helps us become more confident, wiser, and healthier consumers. So does finding reliable assistance when we have consumer-related nutritional questions or concerns. The agencies and organizations listed at the end of this chapter provide a number of sources to obtain nutritional information. Registered dietitians in hospitals, public health departments, or clinical settings are very knowledgeable and will answer consumer-related nutrition

Assess Y O U R S E L F

What Do You Know About the Foods You Eat?

Circle the answers you think are correct and then check your answers below.

1. The skins of fruits and vegetables are a significant source of nutrients and fiber, but pesticides may make them less healthy. From which of the following should you always trim the peel?
   a. carrots
   b. cucumbers
   c. pears
   d. apples
2. Which of the following foods should be avoided if mold appears?
   a. yogurt
   b. peanut butter
   c. individual cheese slices
   d. all of the above

3. How soon after a meal should leftovers be refrigerated?
   a. within ½ hour
   b. within 1 hour
   c. within 2 hours
   d. within 3 hours

Answers:

1. *A*—Peel apples and cucumbers only if they have been waxed.
2. *D*—If you can safely remove at least one inch of the food along with the mold, it may be safe to eat the food. It may not be possible to completely remove all mold from products like those above.
3. *C*—Prepared foods can safely sit at room temperature for up to 2 hours before needing refrigeration.

---

questions. Health educators, nurses, and physicians also provide reliable sources. Articles reviewed and approved by experts in their specific professions and found in professional journals and magazines are also valuable and reliable sources of information.

Food Labeling

When you purchase or use prepared foods, do you take the time to read the labels? If so, what do you look for? Brand names, ingredients, fat content, calories? Like all consumers, you are probably interested in specific things about the product. Reading food labels has become easier because there must now be consistency in information and terminology that describe the contents of food products. As a result of the 1990 Nutritional Labeling and Education Act and regulatory actions by the FDA and the U.S. Department of Agriculture, consumers can better determine the food products that meet their individual nutritional needs. David Kessler, M.D., former Commissioner of Food and Drug Administration stated that, "The new food label is an unusual opportunity to help millions of Americans make informed, healthier food choices."[60]

In 1994, food manufacturers were required to place labels on their products that offered more complete, accurate, and useful nutritional information. Anyone who shops is now able to make comparisons among all foods found in grocery stores everywhere. Nutritional labels on packages contain the following mandatory dietary information: total calories, calories from fat, total fat, saturated fat, cholesterol, sodium, total carbohydrates, dietary fiber, sugars, protein, vitamins A and C, calcium, and iron.[61] Other dietary components as specified by the FDA, can be voluntarily placed on the label. The daily value, which is the daily nutrient intake level recommended by nutrition authorities, is stated in percentages and reveals how much of a day's ideal total of a particular nutrient a consumer is receiving if she is consuming a 2,000 calorie per day diet. This quickly allows a woman to see how a packaged food product meets her nutritional needs. Serving sizes are standardized and reflect the amount of food usually consumed. Nutritional claim terminology such as "light" and "low-fat" are now standardized. Food manufacturers must meet these standards to use these terms to market their product.

Label Terminology Terms and their meanings are continually being revised. For you as the consumer to better comprehend what you are buying, understanding nutritional terms is essential. With new food label regulations, food manufacturers are required to use standardized terms when describing nutrient content of foods. Descriptors such as "less," "high-fiber," "low-fat," "free," "light," "lite," or "reduced-calories"

FIGURE 7.2 Common food label terminology.

The following are terms with brief explanations found on food product packaging.

Fat

Fat-free: less than 0.5 grams (g)
Low-fat: 3 g or less fat than found in the full-calorie product

Saturated Fat

Saturated fat free: less than 0.5 g and less than 0.5 g trans fatty acid per serving
   (Trans fatty acid is found in solid vegetable fat products, like margarine. The FDA suggest that levels of trans fatty acid be limited in products which claim to be "saturated fat free.")
Low saturated fat: 1 g or less per serving and not more than 15 percent of calories coming from saturated fatty acids
Reduced or less saturated fat: at least 25 percent less each serving than the reference food (the same product that had the original level of fat).

Calories

Calorie-free: Fewer than 5 calories each serving
Low-calorie: 40 or fewer calories per serving
Reduced or fewer calories: at least 25 percent fewer calories per serving than the full-calorie food

Calories and Fat

Light (two meanings):
(1) One-third fewer calories or half the fat of the full-calorie food. (If food is comprised of 59 percent or more of calories from fat, the reduction has to be 50 percent of fat.)
(2) A "low-calorie," or "low-fat" food where the sodium amount has been reduced by 50 percent of the full-calorie food.
"Light in sodium" means that the food product has 50 percent or less sodium than the full-calorie food.

Sugar

Sugar-free: less than 0.5 g per serving
No added sugar, without added sugar, not sugar added:
   Has no sugar or ingredients containing sugars, such as fruit or fruit juice added during process or packing.
   Has no ingredients made with added sugars, such as jellies or fruit juice.
   (If a label states, "sugar free" or "no sugar added," this applies only to a reduction in calories related to sugar, not to calories from fat, protein, or other carbohydrates.)
Reduced sugar: at least 25 percent less sugar than the full-calorie food

Fiber

Note: Any food claiming increased fiber content must also meet the definition for "low-fat" or the amount of total fat per serving must appear next to the claim.
High-fiber: 5 g or more per serving
Good-source of fiber: 2.5 g to 4.9 g per serving
More or added fiber: at least 2.5 g more per serving than the full-calorie food

must meet requirements that have been established by the FDA. For meat, poultry, and fish, the terms for "lean" and "extra lean" apply to the fat content of these products and must meet the established percentages for fat and lean content. Figure 7.2 provides a review of the meanings for these terms that will increase your understanding of nutritional content of food products.

Food labels have two distinct sections: a principal display panel (PDP) and an information panel.

The PDP is usually the front of the product and must contain the name of the product (not the name of the company), for example, "tuna packed in vegetable oil," and the net quantity of the product. The PDP may also be where the manufacturer states certain claims, such as "low fat," "fortified," etc.

The information panel is the part of the label that is of greatest interest to consumers. Figure 7.3 is an example of a typical food label. The cate-

FIGURE 7.3 How to read the new food label.

Serving size

Is your serving the same size as the one on the label? If you eat double the serving size listed, you need to double the nutrient and calorie values. If you eat one-half the serving size shown here, cut the nutrient and calorie in half.

Calories

Are you overweight? Cut back a little on calories! Look here to see how a serving of the food adds to your daily total. A 5'4", 138-lb. active woman needs about 2,200 colories each day. A 5'10", 174-lb. active man needs about 2,900. How about you?

Total carbohydrate

When you cut down on fat, you can eat more carbohydrates. Carbohydrates are in foods like bread, potatoes, fruits and vegetables. Choose these often! They give you nutrients and energy.

Dietary fiber

Grandmother called it "roughage," but her advice to eat more is still up-to-date! That goes for both soluble and insoluble kinds of dietary fiber. Fruits, vegetables, whole-grain foods, beans, and peas are all good sources and can help reduce the risk of heart disease and cancer.

Protein

Most Americans get more protein than they need. Where there is animal protein there is also fat and cholesterol. Eat small servings of lean meat, fish, and poultry. Use skim or low-fat milk, yogurt, and cheese. Try vegetable proteins like beans, grains, and cereals.

Vitamins & minerals

Your goal here is 100 percent of each for the day. Don't count on one food to do it all. Let a combination of foods add up to a winning score.

Nutrition Facts

Serving Size 1/2 cup (114g)
Servings Per Container 4

Amount Per Serving

Calories 90   Calories from Fat 30

	% Daily Value*
Total Fat 3g	5%
Saturated Fat 0g	0%
Cholesterol 0g	0%
Sodium 300g	13%
Total Carbohydrates 13g	4%
Dietary Fiber 3g	12%
Sugars 3g	
Protein 3g	

Vitamin A	80%	Vitamin C	60%
Calcium	4%	Iron	4%

*Percent Daily Values are based on a 2,000 calorie diet. Your daily values may be higher or lower depending on your calorie needs:

	Calories	2,000	2,500
Total Fat	Less than	65g	80g
Sat Fat	Less than	20g	25g
Cholesterol	Less than	300mg	300mg
Sodium	Less than	2,400mg	2,400mg
Total Carbohydrate		300g	375g
Fiber		25g	30g

Calories per gram:

Fat 9   •   Carbohydrate 4   •   Protein 4

More nutrients may be listed on some labels.

Total fat

Aim low: Most people need to cut back on fat! Too much fat may contribute to heart disease and cancer. Try to limit your calories from fat. For a healthy heart, choose foods with a big difference between the total number of calories and the number of calories from fat.

Saturated fat

A new kind of fat? No—saturated fat is part of the total fat in food. It is listed separately because it's the key player in raising blood cholesterol and your risk of heart disease. Eat less!

Cholesterol

Too much cholesterol—a second cousin to fat—can lead to heart disease. Challenge yourself to eat less than 300 mg each day.

Sodium

You call it "salt," the label calls it "sodium." Either way, it may add up to high blood pressure in some people. So, keep your sodium intake low—2,400 to 3,000 mg or less each day.*

*The AHA recommends no more than 3,000 mg sodium per day for healthy adults.

Daily value

Feel like you're drowning in numbers? Let the Daily Value be your guide. Daily Values are listed for people who eat 2,000 or 2,500 calories each day. If you eat more, your personal daily value may be higher than what's listed on the label. If you eat less, your personal daily value may be lower.

For fat, saturated fat, cholesterol and sodium, choose foods with a low % Daily Value. For total carbohydrate, dietary fiber, vitamins and minerals, your daily value goal is to reach 100% of each.

g = grams (About 28 g = 1 ounce)
mg = milligrams (1,000 mg = 1 g)

---

gories you see are those that are currently required by the U.S. Food and Drug Administration. All labels must indicate: serving size and amounts per serving for total calories, calories from fat, total fat, saturated fat, cholesterol, sodium, total carbohydrates, dietary fiber, sugars, protein, vitamin A, vitamin C, calcium, and iron. Other options such as "potassium" or "calories from saturated fat" can also be listed. Some of the vitamins and minerals are not listed on package labels because consensus from the public health community indicates that deficiencies of those substances are not likely to exist in a person's diet.

Table 7.7 compares the nutritional concerns of consumers when food shopping between 1983 and 1995. Note the dramatic increase in concern about fat content.

MANAGING WEIGHT THROUGH NUTRITION

There are few personal health topics that have attracted the interests of the medical community as much as weight management. According to epidemi-

ological data, women as a group, are fatter now than they have ever been in our nation's history, and the percentage of overweight African American and Mexican women is greater than among white women.[63] At any given time, 50 percent of American women are trying to lose weight, and are spending billions of dollars to do so. Statistics like these are interesting, but what does all this mean to you? How much should you weigh? What is the best way to keep weight off?

Underweight, Overweight, and Obesity

For quite some time, healthy weight has been described in the Metropolitan Life Insurance Company's Height and Weight Tables. (See Table 7.8.) The tables specify a height-weight range that is considered to be ideal for a particular age and gender. Although the tables have been helpful guides for many years, we now know that they are not the best way to determine ideal weight because the tables fail to consider the percent body fat and how the fat is distributed. For example, we might compare two women who each weigh 120 pounds. If

Table 7.7

Consumers' Nutritional Concerns[62]

A survey by the Food Marketing Institute compared the concerns of 950 food shoppers in 1983 and 1995. (Note the dramatic increase in the concern about fat content.)

1983		1995	
Chemical additives	27%	Fat content	65%
Vitamin and mineral content	24%	Salt content	20%
"No preservatives"	22%	Cholesterol	18%
Sugar content	21%	Sugar content	15%
Salt content	18%	Calories	13%
"Natural" (unprocessed)	12%	"No preservatives"	11%
Fat content	9%	Chemical additives	10%
Calories	6%	Vitamin and mineral content	8%
Cholesterol	5%	"Natural" (unprocessed)	5%

Table 7.8

1983 Metropolitan Life Insurance Height and Weight Table

HEIGHT	SMALL FRAME	MEDIUM FRAME	LARGE FRAME
		Weight in pounds	
Men*			
5'2"	128–134	131–141	138–150
5'3"	130–136	133–143	140–153
5'4"	132–138	135–145	142–156
5'5"	134–140	137–148	144–160
5'6"	136–142	139–151	146–164
5'7"	138–145	142–154	149–168
5'8"	140–148	145–157	152–172
5'9"	142–151	148–160	155–176
5'10"	144–154	151–163	158–180
5'11"	146–157	154–166	161–184
6'0"	149–160	157–170	164–188
6'1"	152–164	160–174	168–192
6'2"	155–168	164–178	172–197
6'3"	158–172	167–182	176–202
6'4"	162–176	171–187	181–207
Women†			
4'10"	102–111	109–121	118–131
4'11"	103–113	111–123	120–134
5'0"	104–115	113–126	122–137
5'1"	106–118	115–129	125–140
5'2"	108–121	118–132	128–143
5'3"	111–124	121–135	131–147
5'4"	114–127	124–138	134–151
5'5"	117–130	127–141	137–155
5'6"	120–133	130–144	140–159
5'7"	123–136	133–147	143–163
5'8"	126–139	136–150	146–167
5'9"	129–142	139–153	149–170
5'10"	132–145	142–156	152–173
5'11"	135–148	145–159	155–176
6'0"	138–151	148–162	158–179

*Weights at ages 25 to 59, based on lowest mortality. Weight in pounds according to frame (in indoor clothing weighing 5 lb, shoes with 1" heels).

†Weights at ages 25 to 59, based on lowest mortality. Weight in pounds according to frame (in indoor clothing weighing 3 lb, shoes with 1" heels).

one of the women is quite athletic, she will have a greater percentage of muscle mass. Muscle tissue has a greater density than fat tissue, so the athlete will not appear as heavy as the nonathlete.

Of interest is a woman's body composition, or how much fat she possesses compared to how much lean mass (muscle, organs, bone, skin) she has. The Metropolitan Tables are based on death and illness data collected from an insured population. The Tables represent the most healthful weight ranges. The farther above the ideal ranges that a woman is, the greater her health risk. There is also a slight health risk for a woman who might be 25 percent or more *below* the ideal.

Measurement techniques that look closely at the actual amount of fat found on the body are described in the discussion of body composition in chapter 8.

Approximately 22 percent of men and 24 percent of women in the United States are classified as obese.[64] Obese individuals weigh more than 20 percent over their desirable weight or have more than 30 percent body fat. We know more about the consequences of obesity than we do about the causes. There seem to be the conflicting explanations between nature (genetic and biological causes) and nurture (those factors in the environment) as the causes of obesity. The answer lies somewhere between the two theories. As with any other human condition, it is difficult to determine the exact and singular cause. Research has linked obesity to genetic, biochemical, metabolic, psychological, and physiological factors.

Researchers continue to study the genetic causes of obesity. Recent studies have uncovered a "fat gene" in mice and it is suspected that this gene has a human counterpart.[65] Studies of identical twins separated at birth were found to have height and weight profiles similar to their natural parents.[66] Scientists have also isolated a specific gene, that if it undergoes mutation, interferes with the body's ability to burn fat.[67]

The dietary factors related to obesity are easier to understand than the genetic. For example, children learn to eat to satisfy hunger, but they may also become conditioned to eat for the relief of boredom, to please their parents, or as a means to relieve stress.[68] The result is that the child does not respond well to hunger cues, but more so to the psychological and emotional signals associated with eating. Research indicates that access to highly preferred foods may lead to overweight and obesity in women.[69] Fast foods are also suspected of contributing to obesity. Fast-food outlets tend to offer high-fat, high-calorie foods, and Americans are consuming more of these products than ever before.

Obesity itself is not a life-threatening condition. However, it is a known risk factor for diabetes, heart disease, high blood pressure, gallbladder disease, arthritis, and some forms of cancer.[70] In addition, obese people have a more difficult time recovering from surgery. The health-care costs associated with obesity are estimated to be around $70 billion dollars a year.[71]

Weight Loss

If the causes of obesity are so many, so are the ways of controlling it. Fifty million Americans are dieting at any given point in time[72] and spending more than 32 billion dollars a year trying to lose weight. All of that money goes toward programs that are advertised as easy and successful, but the winners in the long run are the companies advertising their programs, and not the women purchasing such programs.

Dieting vs. Balanced Food Intake

The major problem a woman faces when she goes on a diet is that she will eventually go *off* the diet. Herein lies the problem associated with weight loss. After realizing that she may weigh more than she feels she should, or failing to fit into clothes that she once wore very comfortably, a woman looks for ways to lose weight. The pattern becomes one in which she follows some weight loss regimen until her weight gets to be where she would like it to be. She goes off her weight loss regimen returning to her previous eating habits until she gains the weight back. Then the cycle starts all over again. Dieting in this fashion leads to a weight loss–weight gain cycle known as "yo-yo" dieting. For years, data have revealed that two things happen when a woman engages in yo-yo dieting. Once weight is lost and regained, subsequent weight loss attempts will take longer to remove the weight. Moreover, after the weight is lost and the woman goes off her diet, the lost weight comes back more rapidly than it did on previous occasions.[73] Recent studies have disclosed some contradictions with these findings. It appears that women with a history of yo-yo dieting generally burn calories as fast as other people do.[74] This form of weight management has been associated with poor health, especially with increased mortality risk.[75] Concerns surrounding the efficacy of yo-yo dieting still remain. The practice is not recommended because dieting in this fashion does not produce a weight management lifestyle for a woman.

The key to any "diet" is not to have to go on one to begin with. Regulating your weight is something you must start when you are young. It involves a life-long commitment to a lifestyle that balances the intake of calories with your caloric expenditure. Did you know that after your early twenties, you will require fewer calories as you age? Your **basal metabolic rate,** the amount of energy you need to maintain your body functions, will decline about 2 percent each decade after age 30.[76] If you consume a 2000 calorie diet now, and 10 years from now you are eating the same way, you can expect to gain weight. Expect that you will need about 40 less calories per day per decade as you age. This will be especially important if your activity level drops off. So you can also see the value of maintaining a physically active lifestyle in addition to monitoring your caloric intake.

The goal of any weight loss program is to have a woman burn more calories than she consumes in order to lose weight. Once she reaches a comfortable weight, the goal then becomes that of burning the calories she consumes so her weight is maintained. Keep the following points in mind to be successful with your weight management goals.

- One pound of fat equals 3,500 calories. In order to burn one pound of fat, a woman must either consume 3,500 fewer calories or perform some kind of physical activity that would use 3,500 calories more than she has consumed. Conversely, if a woman eats 3,500 calories more than she burns through activity, she will gain a pound of fat.
- Exercise is crucial to a weight management program. In fact, research has shown that, over the long term, exercise alone will contribute more to weight management than a regimen of caloric restriction and dieting.[77]
- Proper weight management is a lifetime-lifestyle commitment. It is not something that should be undertaken because you want to fit into a particular bathing suit this summer, or because you finally realize that you are 30 pounds over your ideal weight.
- There is no fast way to weight loss. Rapid weight loss is unhealthy, not to mention that there is often a "rebound effect" causing a woman to gain the lost weight back about as fast as she lost it, and then some. Weight loss programs that advertise quick and effortless weight loss are no good.
- Fad diets and weight loss programs are not the answer to weight management. Fad diets

generally expect the woman to consume some special nutrient. One diet program claimed success if you ate an abundance of protein, whereas another claimed you should not eat any carbohydrates. You may remember the "Beverly Hills Diet." The dieter was to consume large amounts of fruits, especially pineapple. Weight loss programs generally expect you to buy certain products to help you lose weight. The bottom line is that none of these programs really work. They may be good in the very short term, but their lack of behavioral change and support cause participants to eventually fail because they cannot continue the expected regimen. The dieter can then be left with considerable damage to both her self-esteem and her bank account.

- Weight management through medications does not work. The medical community has attempted to use certain drug regimens to combat obesity. These regimens do not work for the long term. Tolerance develops over time, and the drugs will only be effective for 4 to 6 months.[78] In addition, a number of adverse side effects may come with drug therapy, ranging from depression to hypertension. (Also see *FYI:* "Phen/Fen and Heart Defects.") Perhaps the most significant reason for avoiding drug therapy is that it results in the avoidance of responsibility. The dieter expects a "magic bullet" to take care of the "weakness" within the person who eats too much and exercises too little.

EATING DISORDERS

For reasons that continue to remain unclear, some people, mainly young women, become afflicted with life-threatening eating disorders. These disorders are known as **bulimia nervosa** and **anorexia nervosa.** Bulimia is the most common eating disorder, affecting 4 to 5 percent of female college students. Anorexia is reported in 1 percent of young females.[80] Both of these disorders have psychological causes. If left untreated, they can lead to severe health problems and can even be life-threatening. In 1988, the National Center on Health Statistics reported 67 deaths attributed to anorexia.[81] It should be noted that many women can suffer from both disorders at the same time: about 50 percent of anorectic patients display bulimia as well.[82]

The starvation that takes place with these conditions contributes to a myriad of health problems. The

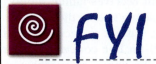

Phen/Fen and Heart Defects[79]

In July 1997, physicians from the Mayo Clinic reported cardiac problems observed in women who had used Fenfluramine and Phentermine (Fen/Phen), two appetite suppressant drugs. Data collected from twenty-four women who had been on the medication regimen for an average of one year revealed heart irregularities (for example, alterations in heart valves and changes in blood pressure) that were not present when the women began the Fen/Phen regimen. Further study is expected to determine the validity and health effects of these findings.

body responds by slowing or stopping specific bodily processes. The reduction of fat causes body temperature to fall. Blood pressure falls and the breathing rate slows down. The thyroid gland fails to function properly. In severe cases, the loss of muscle mass that occurs after all fat has been metabolized can compromise the function of the heart.[83] The skin becomes dry and hair gets brittle. The entire chemistry of the body eventually changes to the point that heart failure occurs.[84]

Anorexia Nervosa

Generally, anorexia begins in the teen years, but it can occur at any age. Anorectics lose the ability to see their body image correctly. A young women who weighs 80 pounds may still describe herself as overweight. She may hold this view as she continues to waste away and even die from the condition. The *Diagnostic and Statistical Method of Mental Disorders, Volume IV,*[85] described the diagnostic criteria for anorexia nervosa as:

1. Refusal to maintain body weight at a minimal normal weight for age and height.
2. Intense fear of gaining weight or becoming fat, even though underweight.
3. Distortion in the way in which one's body weight, size, or shape is viewed.
4. In women, the absence of at least three consecutive menstrual cycles when these would otherwise be expected to occur.

Treatment begins with early medical help; something that is easier said than done. Anorexics will deny that a problem exists. Generally, it is only through the

collective and loving support of friends and family that the anorectic enters treatment. The first step in treatment is to restore a healthful food intake. Eating takes place in a clinical setting to insure that the patient is indeed consuming the food given to her. Even in the clinic, it is not uncommon for clients to hide food in and under furniture or try to find other ways to avoid eating. Psychological therapy is also used to help the patient gain a sense of control over her life. To heal, the patient must reject the sense of accomplishment that accompanies the dramatic weight loss.[86] With proper care, an anorectic can recover from her condition in less than 6 years.

Bulimia Nervosa

Bulimia is at least two to three times more common than anorexia. Some studies indicate that it is continuing to increase.[87] Bulimia, literally translated, means "ox-hunger" because it is characterized by large feasts or binges. Women with bulimia tend to be at a more normal weight than anorectics. The reason is that bulimics *do* eat, and they eat a lot. The episodes are followed by purging exercises, either by vomiting or using laxatives. Approximately 80 percent of bulimics report vomiting daily.[88] The foods chosen for binging episodes are generally high-calorie junk foods, particularly sweets.

Like anorexia, bulimia is a psychological disorder, described in *Diagnostic and Statistical Manual of Mental Disorders, Volume IV,* as:

1. Recurrent episodes of binge eating (that is, rapid consumption of large amounts of food in a discrete period of time).
2. Feeling that the patient has no control over eating behavior during binges.
3. Regular episodes of self-induced vomiting, use of laxatives or diuretics, or vigorous exercise to prevent weight gain.

basal metabolic rate—the minimal amount of energy expended to keep a resting person alive.

bulimia nervosa—psychologically imposed eating disorder characterized by compulsive overeating that is followed by vomiting.

anorexia nervosa—psychologically imposed eating disorder characterized by starvation and distorted body image.

4. A minimum of two binge episodes a week for three months.
5. A persistent concern with body shape and weight.

Bulimics are affected with a number of serious health problems. The use of laxatives eventually creates a dependency upon them for normal bowel function. The constant vomiting causes their teeth to erode and their salivary glands to enlarge due to the effects of acidic stomach fluids that pass through the mouth.

Therapy for bulimia, like that for anorexia nervosa, requires early intervention and a team approach in which the patient receives family support along with help from counseling and medical personnel. Counseling focuses the patient to accept herself as a person and not dwell on her concern for her body weight.[89] Eventually she comes to accept conditions such as depression and self-doubt as normal concerns that we all experience from time to time. The goal of nutritional counseling is to help her establish regular eating habits. Often a food diary is used to help accomplish this. ∞

Chapter Summary

- A multitude of factors, such as family, knowledge, and emotions, influence the daily food choices we make.
- A typical American's energy values are derived from a number of sources.
- Dietary guidelines that assist American women in developing positive eating habits include the following: eat a variety of foods; balance food you consume with physical activity; select a diet with plenty of grain products, vegetables, and fruits; and choose a diet low in fat, saturated fat, and cholesterol; select a diet that is moderate in sugar, salt, and sodium; and if you drink, do so in moderation.
- The Food Guide Pyramid provides a visual account of the variety and amount of foods that should be consumed to ensure a balanced, healthy diet.
- The six major nutrients—carbohydrates, protein, fats, vitamins, minerals, and water—provide the chemicals our bodies need for energy, building and repairing tissue, and functioning effectively.
- Food additives pose no threat to our well-being.
- Special conditions such as pregnancy, exercise, or chronic disease often result in the need for special foods or increased amounts of certain nutrients.
- Being overweight may not mean that a woman is overfat; however, there are serious health consequences as a result of being overfat.
- The most effective way to lose weight is to monitor caloric consumption and maintain a physically active lifestyle.
- Anorexia nervosa and bulimia are eating disorders that are psychological in nature but appear as nutrition-related issues.
- Good nutrition consumer skills can be an important asset when selecting food products that are both beneficial and assist with weight management.

Review Questions

1. What are the U.S. government's seven recommended dietary guidelines?
2. What are the Recommended Dietary Allowances and the current changes that are taking place with respect to their values?
3. What is the role of carbohydrates in the body, and what are the most healthful sources to choose from?
4. What is meant by the term "nutrient density"?
5. What are the sources of the water-soluble vitamins?
6. Other than milk, what are significant sources of calcium in the diet?
7. What are the specific nutritional needs that a woman has during pregnancy?
8. What are the specific cautions a woman must recognize if she chooses to follow a vegetarian diet?
9. What changes take place in a woman's nutrient needs during exercise?
10. What are the main things required by law to appear on the information panel of a food label?
11. What are the health problems associated with eating disorders?
12. List and explain the various ways of measuring the amount of fat a woman has in her body.

Resources

Organizations and Hotlines

American Anorexia/Bulimia Association
418 East 76th Street
New York, NY 10021
Telephone: (212) 734-1114

The American Dietetic Association
216 W. Jackson Boulevard
Chicago, IL 60606
Telephone: (312) 899-0040

American Institute of Nutrition
9650 Rockville Pike
Bethesda, MD 20814-3998
Telephone: (301) 530-7050

Food and Drug Administration
Office of Consumer Affairs
Department of Health and Human Services
5600 Fishers Lane
Rockville, MD 20857
Telephone: (301) 443-3170

Food and Nutrition Information Center
Agricultural Research Service, USDA
National Agricultural Library, Room 304
10301 Baltimore
Beltsville, MD 20705-2351
Telephone: (301) 504-5719

Jean Meyer USDA Human Nutrition Center on Aging
Tufts University
Boston, MA 02111
Telephone: (617) 556-3334

National Dairy Council
6300 N. River Road
Rosemont, IL 60018-6233
Telephone: (708) 803-2000

Nutrition Information Center
515 East 71st Street S 904
New York, NY 10021
Telephone: (212) 746-1617

Overeaters Anonymous
P.O. Box 44020
Rio Rancho, NM 87174
Telephone: (505) 891-2664

Society for Nutrition Education
2001 Kilebrew Drive, Suite 340
Minneapolis, MN 55425-1882
Telephone: (612) 854-0035

Videotapes

A Matter of Fat (1993), Films for the Humanities, Box 2053, Princeton, NJ 08543-2053.

*Eat and Be Healthy** (1994), Milner Fenwick, Inc., 2125 Greensprings Drive, Timonium, MD 21093

*Lean and Easy: Preparing Meals with Less Fat and More Taste** (1994), American Dietetic Association, 216 W. Jackson Boulevard, Chicago, IL 60606

*The New Lean Life Foods** (1995), Nutrivisuals, PO Box 1367, Shingle Springs, CA 95682

*Weight Management: Steps for Lasting Success** (1995), Mosby Great Performance, 14964 NW Greenbriar Parkway, Beaverton, OR 97006

CD Rom/Software

Nutrition for Women 3.5 for Windows
NutriGenie
P.O. Box 8226
Stanford, CA 94309

Websites

American Cancer Society
http://cancer.org

Ask NOAH About Nutrition
http://www.noah.cuny.edu:8080/nutrition/nutrition.html

Eating Disorders
http://www.nimh.nih.gov/publicat/eatdis.htm

Eye on Women: Eating Disorders
http://www.eyeonwomen.com/eating.htm

Internet Resources on Nutrition
http://refserver.lib.vt.edu/refhtml/subjects/hnf2.html

NutriGenie
http://members.aol.com/nutrigenie/index.html

Yahoo: Nutrition
http://www.yahoo.com/Health/Nutrition/

Suggested Readings

Fletcher, A. M. 1994. *Thin for life.* Shelburne, Vt.: Chapters Publishing.

Gleim, G. W. 1993. Exercise is not an effective weight loss modality in women. *Journal of the American College of Nutrition,* 12 (August): 363-67.

Green, R. 1995. *Diary of a fat housewife.* New York: Warner Books.

Harvard Medical School. 1997. Health beat: Measuring antioxidants. *Harvard Health Letter,* 22 (January): 2.

Rinzler, C. R. 1997. *Nutrition for Dummies.* Chicago: IDG Books.

U.S. Department of Agriculture and U.S. Department of Health and Human Services. 1995. *Nutrition and your health: Dietary guidelines for Americans.* Home and Garden Bulletin no. 232, U.S. Government Printing Office.

*It may be possible to obtain this material from the National Agricultural Library via interlibrary loan. Check with your university interlibrary loan office.

References

1. Wardlaw, G. M., P. M. Insel, and M. F. Seyler. 1997. *Contemporary nutrition: Issues and insights.* St. Louis: Mosby.

2. U.S. Department of Agriculture and U.S. Department of Health and Human Services. 1996. *Dietary guidelines for Americans.* U.S. Government Printing Office: Home and Garden Bulletin no. 232.

3. Drewnowski, A., S. A. Henderson, A. Driscoll, and B. J. Rolls. 1997. The dietary variety score: Assessing diet quality in healthy young and older adults. *Journal of American Dietetics Association,* 97 (March): 266–71.

4. Weck, I. 1996. The dangerous burden of obesity. *FDA Consumer* (November): 16–19.

5. Kuczmarski, R. J., C. L. Johnson, K. M. Flegal, and S. M. Campbell. 1994. *Journal of the American Medical Association,* 272: 205–11.

6. Consumers Union. 1991. The sugar bugaboo. *Consumer Report on Health,* 42–44.

7. Consumers Union. 1990. Too much salt? *Consumer Reports* (January): 48–50.

8. Wardlaw et al., *Contemporary nutrition.*

9. Gershoff, S. 1996. *The Tufts University guide to total nutrition.* New York: Harper Perennial.

10. Connolly, H. M. et al. 1997. Valvular heart disease associated with fenfluramine-phentermine. *CNN Interactive.* Http://www.cnn.com/HEALTH/9707/08/fenphen.report, July.

11. Stolberg, S. G. 1997. Brand-new recipe for healthy bones adds calcium. *New York Times,* 1+.

12. Connolly et al., Valvular heart disease.

13. Wardlaw et al., *Contemporary nutrition.*

14. Ibid.

15. Carpenter, K. J. 1992. Protein requirements of adults from an evolutionary perspective. *Journal of Clinical Nutrition,* 55: 913.

16. Consumers Union. 1994. Do we eat too much protein? *Consumer Reports on Health* (January): 1–3.

17. Ibid.

18. Health Letter Associates. 1993. The new thinking about fats. *University of California at Berkeley Wellness Letter* (September): 4–6.

19. Mayfield, E. 1994. *Reprint from FDA consumer* (November): 1–5.

20. Gershoff, *The Tufts University guide to total nutrition.*

21. Harvard Medical School. 1996. Antioxidants disappointment and hope. *Harvard Health Letter,* 21, (October): 1.

22. Jha, P., M. Flaather, E. Lonn, M. Farkouh, and S. Yussuf. 1995. The antioxidant vitamins and cardiovascular disease: A critical review of epidemiologic and clinic trial data. *Annals of Internal Medicine,* 123: 860–72.

23. Wardlaw et al., *Contemporary nutrition.*

24. Brown, J. E. 1991. *Every woman's guide to nutrition.* Minneapolis: University of Minnesota Press.

25. Wardlaw, G. M. 1993. Putting osteoporosis in perspective. *Journal of the American Dietetic Association* 93: 1000–6.

26. Brown, *Every woman's guide to nutrition.*

27. Wardlaw, Putting osteoporosis in perspective.

28. Ibid.

29. Wardlaw et al., *Contemporary nutrition.*

30. Harvard Medical School. 1996. Vegetarian diets. *Harvard Womens Health Watch,* 21 (January): 2–3.

31. Gershoff, *The Tufts University guide to total nutrition.*

32. Tufts University. 1993. A decade in the life. *Tufts University Diet and Nutrition Newsletter* (March): 3–6.

33. Bloch, A. and C. A. Thomson. 1995. Position of the American Dietetic Association: Phytochemicals and functional foods. *Journal of the American Dietetics Assoc.,* 95 (April): 493–96.

34. Brown, *Every woman's guide to nutrition.*

35. Ibid.

36. Gershoff, *The Tufts University Guide to Total Nutrition.*

37. Williams, R. D. 1994. FDA proposes folic acid fortification. *FDA Consumer* (May): 11–14.

38. Brown, *Every Woman's Guide to Nutrition.*

39. Ibid.

40. Wardlaw et al., *Contemporary nutrition.*

41. Brown, *Every woman's guide to nutrition.*

42. Prentice, W. 1997. *Fitness for college and life.* St. Louis: Mosby.

43. Ruud, J. S. and A. C. Grandjean. 1994. Nutritional concerns of female athletes. In I. Wolinsky and J. Hickson (eds.) *Nutrition in Exercise and Sport,* Boca Raton, Fla.: CRC Press.

44. Murray, R. G. and J. J. B. Anderson. 1994. Introduction to exercise and sport. In I. Wolinsky and J. Hickson (eds.) *Nutrition in Exercise and Sport.* Boca Raton, Fla.: CRC Press.

45. Ruud and Grandjean, Nutritional concerns of female athletes.

46. Murray and Anderson, Introduction to exercise and sport.

47. Ruud and Grandjean, Nutritional concerns of female athletes.

48. Brown, *Every woman's guide to nutrition.*

49. Dingott, S. and J. Dwyer. 1991. Benefits and risks of vegetarian diets. *Nutrition Forum* (November/December): 45–47.

50. Gershoff, *The Tufts University guide to total nutrition.*

51. Ibid.
52. Dingott and Dwyer, Benefits and risks of vegetarian diets.
53. Ibid.
54. Ibid.
55. Stare, F. J., V. Aronson, and S. Barrett. 1991. *Your guide to good nutrition.* Buffalo, N.Y.: Prometheus Books.
56. Wardlaw et al., *Contemporary nutrition.*
57. Herbert, V. and S. Barrett. 1981. *Vitamins and "health" foods: The great American hustle.* Philadelphia, Pa.: George F. Stickley Co.
58. Newsome, R. 1990. *Food Technology,* 44: 123–30.
59. Traiger, W. W. and D. S. Cohen. 1983. *New York City Department of Consumer Affairs Health Food Stores Investigation.* New York: The Department.
60. Kurtzweil, P. 1993. Good reading for good eating. *FDA Consumer* (May): 7–13.
61. Kurtzweil, P. 1993. Nutrition fats to help consumers eat smart. *FDA Consumer* (May): 22–27.
62. American Institute for Cancer Research. 1996. *American Institute for Cancer Research Newsletter.* (Winter): 3.
63. National Institute of Diabetes, and Digestive, and Kidney Disorders. 1996. *NIDDK Homepage, NIH Pub 96-4158* http://www.niddk.nih.gov/ObStats/ Obstats.htm.
64. Brown, *Every woman's guide to nutrition.*
65. Pelleymounter, M. A., M. J. Cullen, M. B. Baker, R. Hecht, D. Winters, T. Boone, and F. Collins. 1995. Effects of the obese gene product on body weight regulation on ob/ob mice. *Science,* 260: 540–43.
66. Gershoff, *The Tufts University guide to total nutrition.*
67. Walston, J., K. Silver, C. Bogardus, W. Knowler, et al. 1995. Time of onset of non-insulin-dependent diabetes mellitus and genetic variation of the beta3-andrenergic-receptor gene. *New England Journal of Medicine* 333: 343–47.
68. Murray and Anderson, *Introduction to exercises and sport.*
69. Brown, *Every woman's guide to nutrition.*
70. NIDDK Homepage.
71. Consumers Union. 1993. Losing weight: What works, what doesn't. *Consumer Reports* (June): 347–52.
72. Ibid.
73. Brownell, K. 1988. Yo-Yo dieting. *Psychology Today,* 20+.
74. Consumers Union. 1997. Hope for yo-yo dieters. *Consumer Reports on Health,* 9 (August): 89.
75. University of Texas Health Notes. 1991. *University of Texas Health Sciences Center Lifetime Health Letter* 3: 1.
76. Wardlaw et al., *Contemporary nutrition.*
77. Eller, D. 1997. The best way to lose weight. *Health* (May/June): 34–36.
78. Anonymous. 1996. Long-term pharmacotherapy in the management of obesity. *JAMA* 276 (December): 1907–15.
79. Connolly et al., Valvular heart disease associated with fenfluramine-phentermine.
80. Ruud and Grandjean, Nutritional concerns of female athletes.
81. Farley, D. 1992. Eating disorders require medical attention. *FDA Consumer* (March): 27–29.
82. Harvard Medical School. 1992. Eating disorders—Part 1. *The Harvard Mental Health Letter* (December): 1–4.
83. Gershoff, *The Tufts University guide to total nutrition.*
84. Farley, Eating disorders require medical attention.
85. American Psychological Association. 1994. *Diagnostic and statistical manual of mental disorders.* Washington, D.C.: American Psychological Association.
86. Wardlaw et al., *Contemporary nutrition.*
87. Harvard Medical School, Eating disorders—Part 1.
88. Brown, *Every woman's guide to nutrition.*
89. Wardlaw et al., *Contemporary nutrition.*

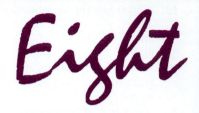

Keeping Fit

■ chapter objectives

When you complete this chapter you will be able to:
- Describe the physical, psychological, and social benefits of fitness activities.
- Distinguish between the four health-related components of fitness and explain the specifics of each component.
- Explain the importance of warm-up and cool-down activities.
- Describe the methods to assess physical fitness levels.
- Identify ways to make fitness programs successful.
- Develop a comprehensive fitness program using the four health-related components of fitness.
- Identify special considerations for exercise during pregnancy and menstruation.
- Explain the dangers involved in compulsive exercising.
- Describe the advantages of weight maintenance through fitness workouts.

BENEFITS OF FITNESS

One doesn't have to venture far to observe people of every age, size, and culture engaging in walking, biking, or running their way toward improved physical condition. Today we are more aware of the increased role that fitness plays in enhancing each dimension of our health. It could be considered both a miracle drug and a fountain of youth that is *free* for the taking! Fitness not only plays a part in reducing the risks of developing heart disease and stroke, diabetes, and osteoporosis, but actually promotes the development of positive attitudes, increased energy, and well-being in general.

Is there some recreational activity you enjoy, such as tennis, racquetball, or swimming? If your fitness level were better, could you enjoy the activity more? Do you have enough energy to take care of daily responsibilities? Is stress a major part of your lifestyle, with no end in sight? Women need to ask themselves if fatigue, minor aches, or lack of stamina is experienced on a regular basis. Improvement in each of these areas is possible by engaging in a regular and well-developed fitness program.

Physiological benefits are well documented in hundreds of research studies conducted over many years. Often the physical benefits, such as weight loss or disease prevention, are the initial reason for

HEALTHY PEOPLE 2000 OBJECTIVES

- Reduce overweight to a prevalence of no more than 20 percent among people aged 20 and older, and no more than 15 percent among adolescents aged 12 through 19. 1995 progress toward goal: –133 percent
- Increase to at least 30 percent the proportion of people aged 6 and older who engage regularly, preferably daily, in light to moderate physical activity for at least 30 minutes per day. 1995 progress toward goal: 24 percent
- Increase to at least 40 percent the proportion of people aged 6 and older who regularly perform physical activities that enhance and maintain muscular strength, muscular endurance, and flexibility. 1995 progress toward goal: 18 percent

Table 8.1

Fitness and Disease

Cardiovascular disease	Aerobic exercise (walking, jumping rope, cross-country/downhill skiing, swimming) strengthens and tones the heart muscle, improves blood circulation, helps control hypertension, lowers cholesterol, increases levels of high-density lipoproteins (HDLs), increases the number of red blood cells, and reduces weight that lessens the risk of heart disease caused by obesity.
Osteoporosis	Aerobic as well as weight-bearing exercises helps to strengthen bones and prevents bone-density loss in women; helps to strengthen and tone muscle, increases muscle mass needed to support the skeletal system; and reduces risks of fracture. In older women, exercise can improve strength, flexibility, and balance that can reduce the chance of falls and fractures.
Arthritis	Exercises for range of motion (stretching), as well as water aerobics, walking, biking, and swimming, can help joints maintain strength and flexibility, and may relieve some pain.
Diabetes	After physician approval, light aerobic exercises and moderate use of weights can lower blood sugar and help the body use insulin more efficiently; helps with weight management.[1]
Breast cancer	Exercise and sport activity among women in their reproductive years lowers the risk of developing breast cancer before menopause.*

Note: Women who participated in physical activity an average of 3.8 hours or more per week reduced their risk of breast cancer by 50 percent; those who participated for 1 to 3 hours per week reduced their risk by 30 percent.[2]

engaging in fitness activities, but the multitude of additional benefits a woman gains is usually the reason for continuing the program. A fitness program can produce a number of positive outcomes that result in prevention of the diseases that cause illness and death in women. (See Table 8.1.)

Psychological benefits gained from participating in a regular fitness program can be somewhat subjective and may vary from research study to study. The International Society of Sport Psychology (ISSP) released a position paper in 1992 that summarized a number of the psychological benefits that can result from fitness activity participation. These benefits are not limited to any age or either sex, and may be achieved by all participants.

Included in this report were the following: lessened feeling of depression and anxiety; improved mood; tension and stress relief; improvement in self-image and self-confidence; relief from premenstrual tension; clearer thinking and improved alertness; positive coping strategies in daily responsibilities; more energy; and increased enjoyment of exercise and social contacts.[3] The degree and extent to which these benefits are attained will vary depending upon the participant and her dedication to a regular fitness activity.

Social benefits are certainly a part of the attractive package a fitness program can provide. These offer an opportunity to be a part of groups and organizations in which women not only enjoy the company of others, but gain a multitude of health benefits in the process. Health clubs offer a choice of activities, and often new friendships with similar interests can be made. Community recreational programs often develop activity-related programs such as biking clubs; hiking, walking, or running groups; and tennis leagues in which one can find associates with mutual interests and lifestyles. Women can also associate with individuals having similar goals and interests by participating in special activities such as yoga, tai chi, meditation, and self-defense. (See *FYI:* "Martial Arts as

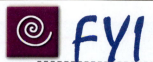

Martial Arts as an Alternative Fitness Activity

Martial arts are becoming increasingly more popular with American women, not only as a means of knowing how to defend one's self, but also as a different mode of exercise. Among the varied forms of martial arts, *tai chi* (pronounced tie-jee) appears to be an activity that the majority of women can engage in to achieve health benefits by using slow, graceful, and low-impact movements. The benefits of tai chi include gaining strength, increasing flexibility, enhancing balance, inducing relaxation, and improving posture.[4] Tai chi needs no special facility, clothing, or equipment. You may need to enroll in tai chi classes taught by a certified instructor to learn accurate movements and reap the full benefits that this alternative activity has to offer.

an Alternative Fitness Activity.") The social benefits abound when participating in fitness-related activities whether in small or large group settings.

Achieving any one of these fitness benefits is a positive addition to our lifestyle. However, the good news is that we usually achieve many of them! Regardless of "why" you decide to participate in a fitness regimen, whether it is to reduce weight, relieve stress, or prevent bone loss, a woman still reaps a variety of the benefits. Fitness activities that improve your physical, psychological, and social well-being are worth your time, energy, and money.

HEALTH-RELATED COMPONENTS OF FITNESS

Research firmly supports the concept of health promotion and disease prevention as a result of involvement in a regular fitness program. However, the fitness program must consist of several components. Do you have a friend who has no problem lifting, pushing, or carrying objects, yet is out of breath after walking two flights of stairs? Well, your friend has developed one component of fitness (strength), but is lacking in another (endurance). A well-designed and comprehensive physical fitness program consists of four **health-related components of fitness:** cardiorespiratory endurance, flexibility, muscular

strength and endurance, and body composition. Other components of fitness can also be an important part of a fitness program. However, these components, agility, balance, power, and speed, are performance-related fitness components and not included in the scope of this book, but can be found and discussed thoroughly in most fitness texts. In creating your own personal fitness program, the four health-related components of fitness need to be included. A brief explanation of each component follows.

Cardiorespiratory Endurance

Cardiorespiratory fitness is considered to be the most important component of a physical fitness program because it affects vital organs of the body: the heart, lungs, and arterial system. These are the systems that deliver life-giving oxygen to every cell in the body; the health and fitness of these body organs are essential to the basic life-support of our bodies. **Cardiorespiratory endurance** is the ability to perform physical activities for long periods of time while oxygen is supplied to the various tissues of the body.[5]

Activities that produce this outcome, called **aerobic activities,** include cycling, swimming, jumping rope, cross-country skiing, walking, running, aerobic dancing. roller blading, and jogging. Each of these calls for the use of large muscles and repetitive movements over a sustained period of time.

Principles of Conditioning To benefit from participation in cardiorespiratory endurance activities, you need to include the following principles of conditioning:

- *Intensity*—This is "how hard" you should engage in the aerobic activity. Intensity is determined by the number of times the heart beats (its pace) in one minute during any given activity. To determine one's level of intensity, you must learn to calculate your target heart rate and then measure it during the activity. (See *Assess Yourself:* "Calculate Your Target Heart Rate.")
- *Duration*—This is how many minutes you should spend in the aerobic phase of your fitness program. For minimal improvement, you should work continuously in the aerobic phase for 20 minutes at your target heart rate (THR). As your fitness level improves, increase the minutes engaged in activity at your THR per workout period. You will find that as you increase the duration of your workout, your cardiorespiratory endurance will improve.

Assess Y O U R S E L F

Calculate Your Target Heart Rate

To determine intensity during the aerobic phase of the physical activity workout, follow these simple instructions:

1. Measure your pulse rate at either the radial artery (on the thumb side of the wrist) or the carotid artery (found in the neck groove by the "Eve's" apple).
2. Use your index and middle finger to locate the pulse; do not press hard on these arteries or you will get an inaccurate measure.
3. Count your pulse for 15 seconds and multiply this by four in order to find your one-minute pulse rate. During the workout, count your pulse for 10 seconds and multiply this by six, that also gives you the one-minute pulse rate.
4. To determine your target heart beat (the intensity in which you want to exercise to attain benefits), complete the following calculation:
   a. Find your maximal heart rate (MHR) by subtracting your age from 220. (For example, 220 minus 20 equals 200.)
   b. You will now have your personal MHR.
   c. Now multiply your MHR by 60, 70, and 80 percent to determine the target heart rate (THR) that is less intense, moderately intense, or highly intense for you. Select one of these percentages depending on your initial physical condition, then increase the THR to 70 percent or 80 percent (or even 90 percent) as you become more fit.

Examples:

200	200	200
$\times.60$	$\times.70$	$\times.80$
120 beats/min	140 beats/min	160 beats/min

   d. As you increase your fitness level, you may want to increase your THR in order to continue to improve your physical fitness.

• *Frequency*—This is "how often" you should engage in an aerobic workout. A minimum is considered to be three aerobic activity sessions per week; at this rate you will see slight improvement. The rate of 5 days per week provides greater and steadier improvement. It is not recommended to work out 7 days a week, but to "rest" at least 1 day so that the body can repair itself and soreness, if any, can subside.

Flexibility

Flexibility allows an individual to use the full range of motion at a joint that improves performance in fitness and recreational activities, and helps to reduce and prevent injuries and soreness. Flexibility has a genetic base; genetics determines how elastic the muscles and connective tissues will be and therefore makes individuals more or less flexible. Can you increase your flexibility? Absolutely! At any age, flexibility can be greatly increased by using a variety of stretching exercises before and after fitness activities.

There are many stretching techniques that are helpful to improve one's flexibility. Following are four types of stretching techniques, with their specific benefits.[6]

• **Static stretching,** the safest way to stretch, involves stretching a specific muscle, usually for 15–60 seconds, until tension is felt. It is believed that this activity will eventually produce a semipermanent change in muscle and tissue length (See Fig. 8.1.)

---

health-related components of fitness— cardiorespiratory endurance, muscular strength and endurance, flexibility, and body composition.

cardiorespiratory endurance—the ability to perform physical activities for long periods of time while oxygen is supplied to various tissues of the body.

aerobic activity—physical activities that require the heart and lungs to supply the increased demand of oxygen throughout the body.

flexibility—the range of motion of a joint.

static stretching—stretching of muscles in a slow and gentle manner, and then held in that position for several seconds.

FIGURE 8.1 Static stretch.

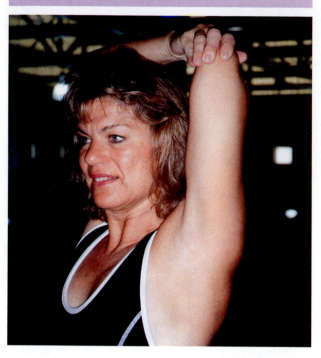

FIGURE 8.2 Isolated stretch.

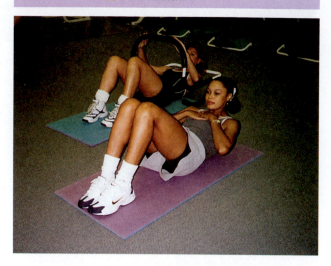

FIGURE 8.3 PNF stretch.

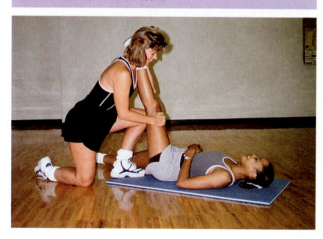

- Active isolated stretching involves the same muscles as in the static stretch, but the position is only held for 1–2 seconds and repeated eight to ten times. The positive aspects of this type of stretch is that the individual does not force the muscle to stay contracted and the muscle is relaxed between the stretch. (See Fig. 8.2.)
- Proprioceptive neuromuscular facilitation (**PNF**) is often done with the help of a partner who helps the exerciser to contract, release, and then stretch a particular muscle or muscle group. When a muscle is contracted and released, the resistance is less and you will be able to stretch the muscle farther. (See Fig. 8.3.)
- **Ballistic** or dynamic **stretching** is done by slowly moving into a particular stretch position, and followed by a bouncing motion. This type of stretching, formerly used as the standard method of stretching, is believed to place too much pressure on muscles and connective tissues and is not recommended by exercise physiologists. See *Health Tips:* "Tips for Safe and Effective Stretching" for proper stretching techniques.

Passive stretching occurs when an external pressure, such as another person, assists in the movement of the joint that stretches the muscle. Active stretching consists of moving the joint and stretching the muscles as a result of the contraction of the opposing muscle, which is the muscle on the opposite side of the area being stretched.

Lack of flexibility reduces one's quality of life by limiting the enjoyable activities one can engage in as well as restricting the ability to carry out responsibilities. For example, Mary Jane, age 45, was restricted in her ability to play tennis with friends due to injuries to her skeletal system and subsequent weakening of the connective tissues. Additionally, the lack of doing any flexibility exercises resulted in further

Tips for Safe and Effective Stretching

- Prior to stretching, engage in a moderate activity, such as walking briskly, to initiate warming of muscles and joints.
- Stretch beyond your normal range, slightly beyond comfort, but not to the point of pain. (Pain is an indication that something is wrong and that injury has or may occur in that area.)
- Hold the position for approximately 30 seconds, release, rest for 30 to 60 seconds, and stretch again. Try to make the stretch longer during successive stretches.
- Perform all stretches on both sides of the body.
- Increase intensity and duration of the stretching movements over several months.
- Use caution when stretching back and neck areas to avoid compressing the vertebrae and discs.
- Do not hold your breath during stretching; breathe as normally as possible.
- For maximum benefits, stretch five to six times per week; for minimal benefits, stretch three times per week.

Increasing muscle strength can be achieved by participating in weight-bearing exercise such as free weights (barbells), weight machines, (such as Nautilus), or performing exercises such as push-ups or pull-ups. Classification of weight-training exercises includes isometric exercise, isotonic exercise, and isokinetic exercise. **Isometric** weight training applies force without movement such as applying force in the muscle and holding the force (such as tightening the buttocks while sitting at your desk). A form of **isotonic** weight training uses force with movement, such as use of a barbell; both the muscle and the weight move. Isotonic exercise is used more often because it better develops and utilizes strength in varied activities. Another type of weight training that can improve muscular strength is **isokinetic** weight training, an exertion of force (such as your leg) at a constant speed against an equal force exerted by a special strength-training machine. Although this type of exercise develops strength and endurance, strength-training machines are usually located in fitness facilities to which you must be a member, or the machinery is too expensive to purchase. (See Fig. 8.4.)

You may need the help of an exercise professional in order to develop a strength- and endurance-

weakening of connective tissues to her skeletal system. As a teacher, Mary Jane found that she had difficulty writing on the board and putting up classroom displays. Worse yet, she found it difficult to lift, carry, and play with her new grandchild. Upon consultation, Mary Jane's physician suggested a variety of stretching exercises to be done four to five times per week as well as simple muscular strengthening activities. Mary Jane noticed an improvement after about six weeks and is determined to continue these activities in order to keep her connective tissue flexible and her muscles strengthened.

Muscular Strength and Endurance

Muscular strength is the ability of a muscle to generate force against some type of resistance; **muscular endurance** is the ability to continue to generate a force over a period of time or for a number of repetitions. As a result of muscular strength and endurance, a woman can improve her performance in physical activities, reduce the possibility of injury, improve physical appearance, and improve the ratio of lean body mass to fatty tissue.

PNF—contraction and relaxation of a muscle prior to stretching it; allows for longer stretches and faster development of joint flexibility.

ballistic stretching—stretching of a muscle by repeated bouncing, jerking, or swinging.

muscular strength—ability of a muscle to generate force against a resistance.

muscular endurance—ability of a muscle to generate force over a period of time.

isometric—exercise that increases muscle tension by applying pressure against stable resistance; accomplished by opposing different muscles.

isotonic—muscle contraction in which force is generated while the muscle changes in length.

isokinetic—exercise in which muscular force is exerted at a constant speed against an equal force that is exerted by a strength training machine.

FIGURE 8.4 (*A*) isometric exercise. (*B*) isotonic exercise. (*C*) isokinetic exercise.

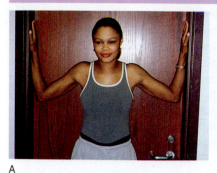

A

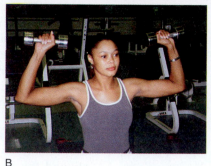

B

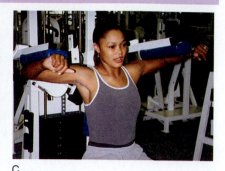

C

training program that benefits all muscle groups. All areas of the body—calves, thighs, buttocks, abdomen, lower and upper back, arms, shoulders, and neck—should be included in a strength-enhancing workout. Determine your current level of fitness and the appropriate avenue needed to improve your strength and endurance. For example, lift approximately 80 percent of your maximum capacity to improve your strength. Choose less weight but increase repetitions to improve your endurance.

Workouts to improve muscular strength and endurance should be done 2–4 days each week with rest between days to allow for recovery. However, you can train more than 4 days per week, if desired, by working out different muscle groups on different days. For example, work the lower body muscles (legs, buttocks) one day, the upper body muscles (upper back, arms, shoulders) on the next day, and then return to lower body on the third day. As you lift weights, select eight to ten exercises that focus on the muscle groups you want to develop. Perform eight to twelve repetitions for each exercise, called sets, with weights that are heavy enough to create muscle fatigue. Be sure to include a warm-up stretch and a cool-down stretch with each weight-training session.

Body Composition

Women with good to optimal body composition tend to be more active, healthier, and feel better about themselves. **Body composition** is comprised of two components: lean body mass that includes the muscles, bones, teeth, connective tissue, and organ tissue, and fat tissue that includes *essential fat* and *nonessential fat*. Essential fat, which makes up ap-

Table 8.2

Classifications of Percent Body Fat in Women[7]

PERCENTAGES OF FAT	CATEGORIES
Under 8%	Excessively lean
8–17%	Lean
18–25%	Average
26–32%	Moderately overweight
Over 32%	Obese

proximately 12 percent of total body fat in women, is just what the term implies—it is fatty tissue that is essential to normal, healthy functioning of the body. This particular type of fat is a component of our brain, nerves, mammary glands, and other important organs in the body and is necessary for proper body functioning. Nonessential, or storage, fat is located just below the skin within fat cells (adipose tissue) and around major organs. Although it offers cushioning for important body organs and stores energy for future needs, too much nonessential fat can be unhealthy and unsightly.

Measurement of body composition (discussed on page 161) provides a better analysis of one's "body weight" than simply stepping on a scale and looking at the numbers. This measurement provides the weight for all the components of our body. The percentage of a woman's body weight that is comprised of fat, called percent body fat, is more important because too much fat is negatively associated with one's health status. Table 8.2 shows the range of percent body fat for women.

Putting Together a Physical Activity Program

The major components of a physical fitness program are included in the following example. Additionally, suggestions are provided for making your workout work better for you.

WARM-UP PHASE

- Spend 10–15 minutes in the warm-up phase.
- Move slowly into an activity that is similar to what your aerobic activity will be (for example, walk, do slow dance movements, etc.) for about 5 minutes. This will start to cause an increase in heart rate.
- Following this, use long stretching movements that stretch the muscles and take the joints through their full range of motion for 5–10 minutes. Stretch all areas and joints of the body: neck, shoulder, arms, trunk, hips, legs, thighs, calves, knees, and ankles.

WORKOUT PHASE

- Spend 20–60 minutes, depending on your fitness level.
- Include endurance activities, flexibility movements, muscular strength, and endurance activities.

- Remember to watch for the intensity, duration, and frequency of the activities you do (a minimum of 60 percent of your heart target heart rate for 20 minutes at least three times per week).
- Check your target heart rate; decrease or increase the intensity accordingly.
- Slow down and/or rest as needed.
- Remember that "no pain, no gain" is not a true statement.

COOL-DOWN PHASE

- Ease into a reduced intensity level of activity.
- Spend 5–10 minutes reducing the heart rate and "coming down" from your workout.
- Slow your movements, and stretch each area of the body as well as all your joints.
- Do relaxing forms of activity to slow down your body.
- Check your heart rate. It should be reduced from the intense level of your workout.

OTHER EXERCISE CONSIDERATIONS

A *warm-up* before engaging in the endurance component of a fitness program better prepares the body for a more effective workout and helps to reduce injury during the fitness activity.

As an individual begins the brief warm-up period, (usually 5–10 minutes) the increase in the body temperature produces a number of beneficial outcomes: An increased amount of oxygen is delivered to the muscles and an increased ability of hemoglobin in red blood cells releases oxygen at higher temperatures. Because of improved muscle contractability and elasticity, there are faster, stronger contractions and improved muscle relaxation. Increased nerve impulses result in improved coordination and, due to an adjustment in hormone production, fat becomes more available to be used for body fuel.[8] The warm-up period enables the person's body to receive sufficient blood and oxygen and prepares the muscle groups for more strenuous endurance activities.

The *cool-down* phase is similar to the warm-up period and just as important. The major intent of the

cool-down phase of the workout is to bring blood back to the heart for reoxygenation so that blood can supply essential oxygen to the brain, heart, and other major body organs, and not pool in major muscle groups. Additionally, during cool-down, the heart rate and breathing rate begin to return to normal and the body begins to cool. It aids the body in moving from an active state to a resting state. Engaging in a 5- to 10-minute cool-down stretching routine will reduce the probability of sore muscles and injury.

PERSONAL FITNESS PROGRAMMING

Having learned about the important components of a comprehensive fitness program, you can formulate a personal fitness program to meet your individual needs and interests. (See *Health Tips:* "Putting Together a Physical Activity Program.")

body composition—the amount of lean and fat tissue in the body.

The Centers for Disease Control (CDC) and other agencies recommend focusing on the frequency of physical activity rather than intense exertion. According to the CDC, women should accumulate 30 minutes or more at least 5 days each week by engaging in physical activity that involves body movements and energy expenditure. A well-designed and regular fitness program is desirable and will yield positive results. However, some activity is better than no activity, and many women who do not participate in *exercise* programs can still realize positive benefits by accumulating 30 minutes of physical activity (gardening, vacuuming, or walking) per day over a 5-day period each week.

Fitness Assessments

Deciding to participate in a fitness program is a major step, but designing a personal fitness program is quite another. It may call for some professional assistance, especially in the assessment area.

Fitness assessments are designed to determine an individual's physical fitness condition as it relates to cardiorespiratory endurance, muscular strength and endurance, flexibility, and body composition. The following assessments can assist you in determining your fitness level before engaging in a physical activity program.

1. *Cardiorespiratory endurance.* One easy and dependable method of determining your cardiorespiratory endurance capacity is to take the 3-minute step test. You will only need a stopwatch and a sturdy bench, block, or stepping tool that is 12 inches high. It will be easier and more accurate if you have a partner who monitors your time and counts your pulse upon completing the step test. You will start the stopwatch and begin your bench-stepping at the same time. As you proceed, be sure you place both feet on the bench and then both feet on the ground to the rhythm of 24 complete steps per minute for 3 minutes. It may be advantageous to say to yourself, "Up, up—down, down" as you step. Immediately upon completing the 3 minutes, sit down and have your partner count your pulse for 1 minute. The number of heart beats counted in 1 minute is your score. Compare it to Table 8.3.[9]

2. *Muscular strength and endurance.* To assess muscular strength and endurance, complete the following two activities:

Table 8.3

Scoring Standards for Women (Heart Rate for One Minute)					
AGE	18–29	30–39	40–49	50–59	60+
Excellent	< 80	< 84	< 88	< 92	< 95
Good	80–110	85–115	88–118	92–123	95–127
Average	> 110	> 115	> 118	> 123	> 127

a. Modified push-ups: Lie face down on a mat and with your knees bent and your upper body supported by your arms. Your back and arms need to be straight. Lower your upper body until your chest is abut 3 inches off the floor. Then return to the starting position. Count the number of push-ups you can perform within 1 minute. Refer to Table 8.4 to determine your strength level.

b. Abdominal muscle strength: Lie flat on your back, cross your arms at the chest, and bend your knees at a 90° angle with your feet flat on floor about 18" from the buttocks. If necessary, have someone hold your feet in place while you raise your head and chest off the floor or mat for 1 minute. Count the

Table 8.4

Test Standards for Modified Push-ups for Women[5]

	FITNESS CATEGORIES						
Age	Superior	Excellent	Very Good	Good	Average	Poor	Very Poor
15–29	>49	46–48	34–45	17–33	10–16	6–9	0–5
30–39	>38	34–37	25–33	12–24	8–11	4–7	0–3
40–49	>33	29–32	20–28	8–19	6–7	3–5	0–2
50–59	>26	22–25	15–21	6–14	4–5	2–3	0–1
60–69	>20	16–19	5–15	3–4	2–3	1–2	0

Table 8.5

Test Standards for Sit-ups for Women[5]

	FITNESS CATEGORIES						
Age	Very Poor	Poor	Average	Good	Very Good	Excellent	Superior
17–29	0–14	14–28	29–32	33–35	36–42	43–47	47+
30–39*	0–11	11–22	23–28	29–34	35–40	41–45	45+
40–49	0–9	9–18	19–23	24–30	31–34	35–40	40+
50–59	0–6	6–12	13–17	18–24	25–30	31–35	35+
60–69	0–5	5–10	11–14	15–20	21–25	26–30	30+

*Over age 30 values are estimated.

number of curl-ups you can do in 1 minute and compare this with Table 8.5, *Suggestion:* keep your chin tucked in and sit up until your elbows touch your thighs.

3. *Flexibility.* Two ways to measure flexibility include:
   a. *Shoulder flexibility*—Raise your left arm above your head and then bend it at the elbow and reach down your back as far as possible; at the same time, take your right arm and bend it behind your back and try to touch the fingers together from both arms. Finger overlap reflects fairly good flexibility; reverse the position and try to touch fingers again. You are usually more flexible on one side than the other.
   b. *Sit and reach*—Using a box that is 8–12 inches high with a measuring stick taped on top and extending 6 inches in front of it, sit on the floor with legs outstretched and feet flat against the box. Slowly stretch your fingers across the ruler to determine how far you can reach. Make three attempts to stretch across the ruler. Be sure you warm up first! Compare your results with Table 8.6.

Table 8.6

Sit and Reach Scoring for Women

Excellent	> 13 inches
Good	9–13 inches
Fair	4–9 inches
Poor	< 4 inches

4. *Body composition.* Rather than "weighing in" each day to determine body weight, a much better measure is to determine healthy body weight by calculating body composition and comparing lean tissue to fat tissue. Two methods of doing this are by skin-fold measurement and by calculating body mass index (BMI).
   a. *Skin-fold measurement.* Using **calipers,** the thickness of skin measured at certain sites on the body can be applied to a formula and the percentage of fat can be determined. (See Fig. 8.5.) These skin-fold measurements have been compared to laboratory techniques that research studies have shown to be an accurate measure to determine body composition.

FIGURE 8.5 Body fat determination using skinfold calipers.

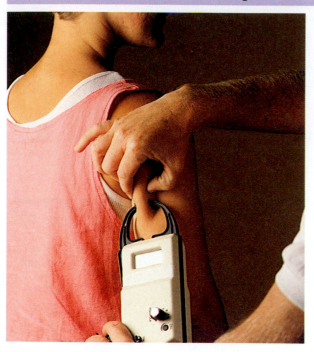

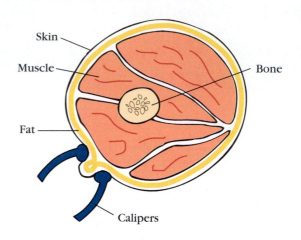

b.   Another means by which to calculate body composition is with electrical empedance equipment that measures the electrical resistance of small currents directed through the human body. Electrodes are attached to the body, then to a small machine attached to a computer. The electrical current is harmless and painless and the feedback regarding body composition is very rapid. Hydrostatic weighing, considered the "gold standard" of calculating body composition, measures the relative amount of fat and lean body mass while the person is submerged under water. Through the use of a special scale, a woman's underwater body weight is compared to her body weight out of the water and then calculations are made to determine percentage of body fat.

c.   **Body mass index (BMI)** is a method of expressing the relationship of body weight (expressed in kilograms) to height (expressed in meters) for both men and women. Although the BMI does not determine body composition, it is quite accurate in determining healthy body weight. (See Fig. 8.6 and Table 8.7.)

FIGURE 8.6 Calculating BMI.

To determine your body mass index (BMI):

1. Divide your weight in pounds by 2.2 to convert it to kilograms.

$$A = \text{weight (kg)} = \text{your weight (lb)} \div 2.2$$

2. Multiply your height in inches by 2.54 and divide by 100 to convert height to meters.

$$B = \text{height (m)} = \text{your height (inches)} \times 2.54 \div 100$$

3. Multiply B by B to get your height (in meters) squared.

$$C = \text{height (m)} \times \text{height (m)}$$

4. Divide A by C to determine BMI.

$$BMI = \text{weight (kg)} \div \text{height}^2 \text{ (m)}$$

Example: 176-lb person, 72 inches tall (6 feet) tall

1. $A = 176 \div 2.2 = 80$

2. $B = \dfrac{72 \times 2.54}{100} = \dfrac{182.88}{100} = 1.83$

3. $C = 1.83 \times 1.83 = 3.35$

4. $BMI = \dfrac{80}{3.35} = 23.88$

Table 8.7

Desirable Body Mass Index in Relation to Age	
AGE-GROUP (YEARS)	**BMI (KG/M²)**
19–24	19–24
25–34	20–25
35–44	21–26
45–54	22–27
55–65	23–28
>65	24–29

DESIGN YOUR PERSONAL FITNESS PROGRAM

Knowing the benefits from and the "how-to" of fitness workouts is one thing. We usually have a motivating factor (such as a wedding, spring break, or more energy) for beginning the program. However, keeping the program successful enough to stay with it creates a need for additional information and know-how!

Getting Started

How do you "get into" a fitness program that includes the necessary components, meets your needs, and safely helps you achieve the benefits you want to see? In order to answer this question, consider the following as an entry into a fitness program that can provide healthy and satisfactory rewards.

Should you get a physical checkup? Ask yourself the following questions in order to determine if you should see a physician before embarking on your potential change of lifestyle program.

- Do I have any medical condition that might need special attention before starting a fitness program, such as heart problems, chest pains or pressure, dizziness or fainting spells, or high blood pressure?
- Have I experienced any shortness of breath after any type of exertion?
- Are my joints painful or my muscles overly sore following activity?
- Has my mother, father, brother, sister, or grandparents had a heart attack before age 50?
- Have I had a recent physical exam, other than for an ailment (such as flu, cold, or other communicable disease)?

- Do I have any serious problems with my menstrual cycle?
- Am I bothered by breathing problems as a result of asthma or allergies?

If you answered "yes" to any of these questions, you should see your physician; if not, you are probably ready to engage in a sensible, fun, and comprehensive fitness program.

Another aspect of starting a fitness program is to assess your present physical condition to determine where you need to begin your program. The assessments found on pages 160–162 can assist you in this aspect of starting a fitness program.

The next step involves writing a personal contract about what you want to achieve as well as how and when you will carry out your plan. A contract will not only assist you in getting started, but will help you stay involved as well as achieve progress toward your objectives. *Journal Activity:* "My Personal Fitness Contract" provides an example of how to develop a fitness program contract.

Pacing yourself in the initial phase of your fitness program will allow you to build your fitness level gradually and avoid injury as well as burnout. Consider the information in the *Health Tips:* "Putting Together a Physical Activity Program" on page 159 and use this information to begin at the lower part of your Target Heart Rate (around the 60% range). Over a period of weeks increase the intensity, duration, and perhaps frequency. After a month or so, you may want to change your routine as well as some of your goals. Consider a different environment, perhaps from an indoor facility like a health club, to activities that take you outside and into a park or track facility providing weather permits.

In summary, check with your physician, if necessary, then assess your current fitness level, develop a contract, and remember your personal goals of being

calipers (**kal** ah pers)—device that measures the thickness of skinfolds taken at different sites on the body; the data is used to determine an individual's percent body fat.

body mass index (BMI)—numerical expression of body weight based on height and weight in determining healthy body weight.

My Personal Fitness Contract

A. My physical fitness program will begin on _____ (date) and accomplish the following goals:

    1.

    2.

    3.

    4.

B. The activities that I will use to meet these goals include:

	Activity	Day	Time	Intensity Level
1.				
2.				
3.				
4.				

C. As I accomplish each goal listed in Part A, I will reward myself by:

	Goal	Date	Reward
1.			
2.			
3.			
4.			

D. The following will help me to achieve each goal:

    1. For support, my personal helper is:

    _____ (signature)   _____ (date)

    2. Monitoring tools and assessments include:

        a.

        b.

        c.

    3. Additional daily activities include:

        a.

        b.

        c.

E. Possible future fitness goals include:

    1.

    2.

    3.

_____   _____
(your signature)   (date)

involved in a fitness program, (e.g., losing weight, looking good, shaping up, or preventing disease). Be sure you include the steps that assist you in staying with your program: making a commitment, finding a partner, setting a schedule, checking your progress, varying your routine, and rewarding yourself.

Staying Involved

Starting a fitness program is usually easy to do because we often have some knowledge of the benefits or have an impetus to begin a program. However, staying with the fitness program is often more of a challenge. Sometimes we don't have a structured program, or we engage in the wrong program for our personal needs, or perhaps we start at the wrong level and then proceed too fast or too slow. Usually, once our motivational factor has been achieved (such as losing weight, toning muscles, etc.) our activity regimen often lessens or may stop altogether. What can you do to stay involved in a fitness program?

Dr. Jon Robison has developed a six-step program to promote adherence to fitness programs for clients at his preventative medicine center. These steps include writing a contract, charting your progress, working out with others, making it enjoyable, dealing with the details, and staying with it.[10]

Following is a brief description of each of these suggestions:

1. Develop a personal contract to reach an obtainable weekly or monthly fitness goal. Be specific about what you want to do, when and how you will achieve this goal, and the reward (such as money) for attaining the goal. Have a support person sign the contract each time a goal is reached. Additionally, if you do not reach the goal, take away money from your reward.

2. Keep track of your progress by knowing your starting physical levels and charting your progress each time you engage in a fitness activity. Dr. Robison suggests giving yourself a "star" each time you participate and achieve your goal. Place the "star" or sticker on an area where you can see the progress on a regular basis.

3. Exercising with others holds you accountable to yourself and to at least one other person or group of people. Attempt to find others at school or work who have similar fitness interests and goals who you can share your activity time with. We are all likely to have days when we just

don't want to be active, but when others are counting on us, we tend to respond to the extra pressure. If necessary, place more pressure on yourself to be active by telling others your goals.

4. An enjoyable fitness activity is more likely to be done. If you hate to run, don't run; if you hate to swim, don't swim! The best exercise is the one you like, whether it's walking, gardening, or a vigorous game of racquetball. Fitness activities should not feel like self-punishment, but more like a special time you give yourself. Not only should the activity be enjoyable, but reward yourself with some self-indulgence after the week's activities: a favorite movie, a massage, or a new CD!!

5. Plan for your fitness activity by taking care of the details. After deciding what activity fits you, determine where and when to work out, what clothing, shoes, and equipment is needed, the time of day that is best for you and your partners, and a contingency plan for unforeseen changes (weather or facility problems). Taking care of the details helps to eliminate excuses for not participating and lessens the perception of inconvenience.

6. Staying with the program seems to be easier said than done with most exercisers. Researchers contend that if you can stay with a fitness program for six months, the odds are you'll still be exercising after a year. It is important to see yourself as an active woman, rather than someone who is temporarily involved in a fitness program just to achieve a specific goal (for example, just to lose five or ten pounds). This mind set usually happens after six months of being involved in a fitness activity. Just keep on plugging. After a few months, you will feel "unnatural" if you are not exercising.

Avoiding Injuries

Women who participate in sports and other fitness activities need to be aware of and take precaution to avoid injuries that hinder or suspend the continuation of their fitness program. Engaging in exercise too frequently or too intensely can often result in a variety of injuries that are usually preventable. In general, most fitness-related injuries can be avoided simply by a warm-up and a cool-down stretching routine before and after every workout and by varying your fitness activities.

What are some of the more common injuries that women sustain during fitness activities and what can be done about them? One of the more common and serious injuries is a tear of the **anterior cruciate ligament (ACL),** which is a major support structure of the knee. This injury occurs more often in active women than in active men and is usually an injury caused by overuse. If you experience swelling and pain of the knee, you should see a physician. This type of injury calls for rehabilitation exercises under the guidance of a physical therapist. Sometimes surgery is necessary. Another type of knee injury is called **patellofemoral knee pain,** which can result from a number of causes (e.g., repetitive jumping, improper stretching, or joint surface degeneration). Symptoms include inflammation with swelling, tenderness, and pain during movement.

Shin splints are recognized because of the pain that occurs in the shins and is usually caused by too much activity performed on hard surfaces such as gym floors or hard-surfaced roads. This may occur because of strains in the muscles that move the ankle and foot at the attachment points in the shin. Arch supports, either over-the-counter or, if needed, custom-made by a sports podiatrist, will usually cure the problem. It may be necessary to reduce or temporarily discontinue your fitness activity until the injury is healed.

Lower back pain can result from weak back or abdominal muscles, especially if you begin exercising with too much intensity or too frequently. Preventing lower back pain can be accomplished in a number of ways: First, try reducing strenuous activity to a level that your body can safely accommodate. Secondly, improve your back muscles by carefully engaging in abdominal- and back-strengthening exercises. However, if back pain persists, see a physician for an evaluation of the problem.

Persistent inflammation and pain near the tip of the shoulder is called shoulder impingement, and is caused by a continual forceful overhead motion of the shoulder. Activities such as serving a tennis ball, swimming, weight lifting, or throwing can cause this injury. Strengthening the shoulder muscles with light weight-bearing exercises or eliminating activities that strain this area can help with this injury.

The simple **RICE** plan (rest, ice, compression, and elevation) can be most useful for temporary relief. *Rest* the injured area and apply an *ice* pack, usually 20 minutes on the injury and 20 minutes removed from the injury. *Compress* the injured area with an elastic bandage and then *elevate* it several times a day. RICE should reduce pain and swelling of the injured area. If there is not improvement within a week, then it is time to see a physician.[11]

JOINING A FITNESS CLUB

Would you like to learn about fitness clubs and fitness equipment? A special January 1996 issue of *Consumer Reports*[12] features a number of articles that detail information regarding workout machines, health clubs, developing your own program, and what to look for in a health club contract. *FYI:* "Whether to Join a Fitness Club" can be used in determining whether a fitness club is right for you.

SPECIAL CONSIDERATIONS
Exercise and the Menstrual Cycle

History tells us that women went to bed during their menstrual period. In more recent years, menstruating women were told not to swim, not to participate in activity classes, and were even excused from participation on sports teams. Today this concept has changed. It is recognized that this normal biological event usually presents no problems to women who participate in active events. One's personal menstrual factors may restrict a woman from being physically active during this monthly event.

However, a number of symptoms may interfere with a woman's participation in physical activities. Varying degrees of pain and cramping, which may be accompanied by pain in the lower back or legs, can curtail one's ability and desire to be physically active during the menstrual period. Painful menstrual periods, called **dysmenorrhea,** can be so severe that some women are incapacitated for several days. Certainly women with this type of pain should seek and follow the advice of their physician.

Premenstrual syndrome (PMS) affects some women and is characterized by feelings of irritability, depression, bloating, headaches, tender breasts, and possible weight gain. Although most women who experience PMS can maintain normal functioning, some may need a variety of treatments and professional medical help. As a result in the monthly hormonal changes, a woman's motivation to continue her fitness activities may subside. Yet, engaging in a reduced intensity level activity has been shown to reduce the symptoms of PMS and produce a feeling of well-being.

Amenorrhea, the cessation of the menstrual period, is related to overexercising, which can be the case with long-distance running, cycling, gymnastics, or swimming. When a woman's body fat drops below 12 percent, which often occurs in highly fit female athletes, irregular or absent menstrual periods often are the result.

If discomfort during the menstrual period is a problem for you, consider reducing the frequency, duration, and intensity of your fitness activity, rather than eliminating it. Pamper yourself after a workout by enjoying a soothing, warm shower, time in a hot tub, or briefly relaxing to pleasant music. It is also beneficial during the menstrual period to incorporate relaxing activities that promote a good night's sleep.

Exercise and Pregnancy

Pregnancy may be compared to preparing and running a marathon as far as the physical stress it can have on a woman's body. Therefore, a woman needs to prepare her muscles, increase her stamina, and boost the immune system in case of infection as she moves toward the big finish line: the birthing process. If a woman is exercising prior to pregnancy, then it is usually healthy to continue during pregnancy, with her physician's approval, perhaps with some modifications.

What are the benefits of exercising during pregnancy? A study from the Case Western Reserve School of Medicine in Cleveland compared exercising and nonexercising women between the ages of 28–43. Initial comparisons were very similar, but

anterior cruciate ligament (ACL) (**crew** she ate)—support structure of the knee that can be injured due to overuse in fitness activities.

patellofemoral knee pain—an injury to the knee that is characterized by nonspecific pain under the kneecap.

shin splints—strains of the muscle that move the foot and ankle at their attachment point to the shin; can result in a stress fracture to the long bone in the leg.

RICE—rest, ice, compress, elevate; temporary care of a minor injury that does not need a physician's attention.

dysmenorrhea (dis **men** oh rhea)—painful menstrual periods characterized by severe cramps, possible headaches, lower back and/or leg pain; occasionally incapacitating pain.

after 15 weeks the researchers found that weight gain was less in the exercising group. At the time of delivery, the pregnant women who exercised had gained between 31–33 pounds compared to 39–42 pounds gained by those who did not exercise. Additionally, those who exercised gained 4 1/2 pounds less body fat, spent one-third less time in labor, and were less likely to have a cesarean section.[13]

Pregnant women who exercise are also less likely to have hemorrhoids, low-back pain, fatigue, and develop varicose veins. Exercising throughout pregnancy can reduce the likelihood of having a cesarean section by 25 percent, and may even reduce labor time by an average of two hours.[14]

The cardiovascular system must circulate about 30 percent more blood during the 267+ days of pregnancy. Exercise can aid in increased and more efficient circulation. Exercise can reduce the likelihood of the feet and legs swelling. Controlling weight gain, avoiding low-back pain and improving the efficiency of the cardiorespiratory system can lead to an important psychological benefit during pregnancy. Exercise can give pregnant women a measure of control over their ever-expanding bodies and enhance their chances to feel good, look good, and have a positive self-image.

In 1994, the American College of Obstetricians and Gynecologists (ACOG)[15] revised its exercise guidelines for pregnant women. This organization suggests that women should not exercise if they are at risk for: induced hypertension, preterm membrane rupture, and persistent second- and third-trimester bleeding. Additionally, women who have an incomplete cervix, have experienced fetal growth retardation, or experienced premature labor during a previous or current pregnancy should not exercise while pregnant.

However, women who have none of these risks are encouraged to exercise in moderation, with the supervision of their physician. ACOG offers the following suggestions to help pregnant women exercise safely: monitor your heart rate during exercise and do not allow it to go over 140 beats per minute; do not exercise at a strenuous level for more than 15 minutes; avoid twisting, jarring, jumping, and rapid change-of-direction motions; drink plenty of liquids throughout the workout period; do not exercise during hot, humid weather to avoid overheating; and after the fourth month, avoid exercises that require lying on the back to perform. (See *Viewpoint:* "Should I Continue My Usual Exercise Level During Pregnancy?")

You may want to use less strenuous exercises, which follow, during pregnancy to achieve potential positive results. Your fitness level before becoming pregnant will dictate to a major degree the intensity, frequency, and duration of your exercise program. (*Warning:* These exercises should not be performed without your physician's approval! Do not exercise during pregnancy without the consent of your physician.)

- Swimming—one of the best exercises for pregnant women because swimming in a prone position promotes optimum blood flow. The water acts as a support cushion for both mother and the fetus. The pressure of the water also encourages water loss, and does not place extra strain on joints and ligaments for women in their third trimester.
- Walking—maintaining a heart rate of under 140 beats per minute for approximately 15 minutes at least three times per week. If you have exercised before pregnancy, you may increase the duration up to 30 minutes with physician approval. Supportive shoes and a pleasant and safe area in which to walk are additional benefits of this exercise.
- At-home exercises can include:[16]
- *Torso twist:* Sit on a stool holding a broomstick across the shoulders and slowly twist the shoulders eight to ten times from one side to the other.
- *Hamstring toning:* Use a 5-pound weight around each ankle and hold a chair or the wall for balance. Bend the weighted leg at the knee and pull the ankle up toward the buttocks. Do this eight to ten times for each leg.
- *Strengthening arm muscles:* Hold a 1–2-pound dumbbell in each hand and stand with feet about shoulder width apart. Slightly bending at the waist, move the dumbbells forward, then backward, making small circles; do eight to ten times for each arm. (See Fig. 8.7.)

COMPULSIVE EXERCISE

Too often, women incorporate health-diminishing behaviors into their lifestyles to attain an ideal image—an image that is usually dictated through external influences. Whereas too little exercise will not produce positive results, too much can be detrimental to your health. Ironically, exercise can be overused by women to reach an unnatural and unhealthy thin appearance. It is possible to exercise too much, too often. When we have a distorted view of ourselves (a perception of oneself that does not match society's or the media's portrayal of the opti-

Viewpoint

Should I Continue My Usual Exercise Level During Pregnancy?

Janene has been involved in an intense aerobic exercise routine throughout college. She married and became pregnant during her senior year. The energy, stress relief, and weight management that her aerobic running produced was something Janene wanted to continue to experience. She consulted her physician who suggested a reduction in the frequency and intensity of her workout and changing the running to a walking program. Janene is not happy with that idea and discussed this suggestion with the members of her running club, many of whom were knowledgeable in the area of exercise physiology. Their opinion was that because Janene had been in excellent aerobic condition before the pregnancy, she would not have problems maintaining her previous fitness activities. Consider the following:

- The fetus is in a "built-in" safe environment, surrounded by amniotic fluid that serves as a shock absorber.
- Exercise causes an increase in body temperature that results in an increase of temperature in the fetal environment that may not be safe for the fetus.
- A reduced sense of balance and coordination following the seventh month may increase the chances for accidents during activity.
- Aerobic activity such as bouncing, running, and step aerobics should not be undertaken during the third trimester.
- The heart rate should not exceed 140 beats per minute or less, depending on one's fitness level.
- After the fourth month of pregnancy, exercises requiring lying flat on the back should be avoided.

What would you recommend that Janene do about her level of fitness and her fitness activities during her pregnancy?

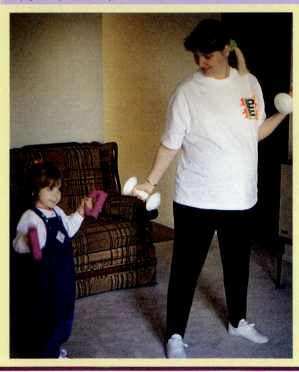

FIGURE 8.7 Exercise during pregnancy can be enjoyed by all family members.

---

mal body), we tend to adopt measures, regardless of the health consequences, to achieve this ideal. As a result we can become an appearance junkie and a fitness zealot, according to Judith Rodin, psychology professor at Yale University, who believes that how our body looks has become a significant part of our self-worth.[17] **Compulsive exercising** is the need to engage in fitness activities beyond the normal standards for good health, and despite potentially negative consequences.

Despite injury, neglect of other responsibilities, or inconvenience, a woman with a negative addiction to exercise will continue at an intensity that is considered excessive. Polivy and Clendenen[18] pro-

vided an excellent review of research that has been conducted related to compulsive exercising and negative outcomes. There is an apparent correlation between addictive behavior and self-concept, depression, stress, and eating disorders. Researchers still cannot understand the factors that lead to addiction to exercise.

compulsive exercise—a compelling emotional drive to exercise excessively to achieve an ideal but unrealistic image, rather than for health improvement.

What is the margin between gaining the benefits of a comprehensive fitness program and overdoing it? An exercise level equivalent to running 20 hours a week for 6 months appears to cause a stress response in our bodies. Feeling challenged, the body goes on the defensive and a number of negative physiological responses occur.[19]

- Reproductive hormones such as estrogen, progesterone, gonadotropin-releasing hormone, leutinizing hormone, and follicle-stimulating hormone decrease, and cortisol, a hormone that regulates a number of body functions, increases. This new mix of hormones can have serious effects on the body.
- The menstrual cycle and fertility can be effected due to excessive exercise. Ovulation and menstruation can stop or diminish.
- Increased production of cortisol, which can suppress the immune system, causes an increased susceptibility to infections.
- Excessive exercising can cause a decline in mood as well as in the ability to reason and concentrate.
- An energy imbalance develops caused by increased amounts of cortisol levels in the body that can lead to the loss of lean body mass and fat cells. This can result in a form of malnutrition and fatigue.
- Increased levels of cortisol and decreased levels of estrogen robs bone of minerals, and can cause a reduction in bone density. Young female athletes may never reach their peak bone mass and older women may increase the acceleration of bone loss.
- Increased numbers of injuries develop because of overuse of the body. These result in knee, joint, and bone problems.

Ironically, many of the very physical and psychological benefits that we gain from a well-designed and moderate fitness program are the ones we harm when we exercise to excess. Compulsive or addictive exercise patterns harm the health of a woman and eradicate any benefits that are intended to be gained through fitness activities. Professional medical help is usually needed to deal with compulsive behavior of any type. When it may be life-threatening as excessive exercising can be, especially in combination with eating disorders, it is imperative that a woman have professional assistance. (See *Her Story:* "Averica.")

MANAGING WEIGHT THROUGH EXERCISE

Why do we all expect to look as if our bodies are ready for the fashion runway, when in reality, most of us can never achieve that physique? Nor is it necessarily healthy to achieve that look! Certainly, our concept of the ideal female body has changed over the decades. A research study out of Helsinki gathered department-store mannequins that spanned the decades between 1920 and the present. The researchers worked out theoretical body fat percentages to determine body composition and size. Between 1920 and 1950, the mannequins representing women of those eras looked more like "real," robust women. However, after 1950, the mannequins tended to become taller and thinner; hip size went from about 34 inches to 31 inches, yet the average hip size of women today is about 37 inches.[20] Another study found that between 1959 and 1979, the idealized female physique, as portrayed in popular "male" magazines and by contestants in beauty contests, grew taller and thinner. Although a trend continues toward thin as the ideal image, this ideal is contradicted by reality; the reality is that the average college-aged female is becoming heavier.

Females tend to have an extrinsic reason for wanting to lose weight, whether through dieting, exercising, or both. For example, a recent survey found that 96 percent of women, compared to 11 percent of men, who were interviewed wanted to lose weight in order to look better. Fifty-one percent of men in this study said they would like to lose weight to improve their health, but only 9 percent of women had the same reason for losing weight.[21]

Maintaining proper weight for a woman's body type and activity level can be achieved by participating in a comprehensive exercise program. You need to expend at least the number of calories you ingest with your food intake each day so that caloric balance can be achieved. Study after study assert the advantages of fitness activities in weight management and body composition. In a recent study, a total of 142 men and women were divided into two groups; both ate the same types and amounts of food, but only one group engaged in an exercise program. After 1 year, the diet and exercise group had not only lost more weight, but also had lost more pounds of fat. In another study involving police and other public officials in a northern city, all participants were put on a low-calorie diet and half of the partici-

Her Story

Averica

Averica, while loving and admiring her sisters, also felt less attractive and less popular than both of them. She worked hard at proving herself at everything she tried. Discovering that she excelled in her physical education classes, Averica began to spend more and more time and effort at running and swimming activities. She increased her distance, her intensity level, and the amount of time she spent running during the weekdays. But, it was during the weekends on which she really ran long distances. Her mother was concerned about this intense drive that Averica had to continually be so physically active. Her mother noticed a decline in Averica's weight, and an increase in the number of colds and other minor infections that she continually contracted. But of greatest concern was the loss of Averica's monthly menstrual period. Her mother asked Averica to reduce the time she spent running and swimming. When Averica did this, she was irritable, restless, and unable to sleep, and she resented her mother for interfering with the activities in which she did so well. Averica decided to return to her former level of activities, and then sustained a knee injury. Upon seeing a physician for the injury, the doctor recognized signs that indicated the compulsive nature of Averica's running. The physician recommended a counselor who specialized in sport-related therapies. Averica, with the encouragement of her mother, is presently in counseling to find a way to engage in a running program without physically harming herself. She is working on the emotional issues that pushed her to exercise compulsively in the first place.

- What are the detrimental health-related concerns that resulted from Averica's compulsive exercise habits?
- What other negative consequences could result from compulsive exercising?
- If you know of someone who exercises in a compulsive way, what physical, emotional, and social consequences do you see?

pants also engaged in 90 minutes of fitness activities three times each week. Two months later, all participants had lost weight. However, a follow-up interview 3 years later found that the diet-only group had regained almost all of their weight, but the exercisers who remained active maintained almost all of their initial weight loss.[22]

More than half of all ingested calories are used to keep our bodies and minds functioning. This is the basal metabolism rate as discussed in chapter 7. As we engage in fitness activities, not only do we expend additional calories at the time of the activity, but exercise increases our basal metabolic rate even after the activity is over. Usually exercise alone (without dieting) will produce a weight loss; but, even if you don't lose weight, it often helps you become thinner. The reason? A pound of muscle tissue will take up less space in our body than a pound of fat tissue. Building muscle and losing fat can cause a loss of inches without even losing a pound. The result is looking better and feeling better.

As with many other health-related behaviors, knowing is not doing. We have presented information in this chapter that will help you develop a comprehensive and effective fitness program. That's the easy part. Engaging in the program, and more importantly, staying with it will be the challenge. Look at the suggestions for success with your fitness program in *Health Tips:* "Make Exercise Fun!" Establish your goals, make a commitment, find yourself a partner, and begin to realize all the positive results from this type of program. And good luck! ∞

health tips

Make Exercise Fun!

Take the "work" out of workout and make exercise an enjoyable experience rather than an essential but unpleasant part of your day. As one excellent speaker attests, we are never too old for recess! So how do we make exercise fun? Here are a few suggestions.[23]

- Select fitness activities that are fun: dancing, hiking, biking, sports, and active games.
- Develop hobbies that keep you moving: gardening, building, bird watching, and participation in active organizations.
- Be creative while exercising: listen to music, talk to your exercise partner, or even make plans for the coming week.
- Vary your exercise routine with whom, what, when, and where you exercise, as well as varying the intensity of your activity.
- Give yourself fun and nonfattening rewards.

Chapter Summary

- Participating in a comprehensive fitness program provides a multitude of physiological, psychological, and social benefits.
- A comprehensive physical fitness program consists of four major components: cardiorespiratory fitness, flexibility, muscular strength and endurance, and body composition.
- When developing a fitness program, special considerations such as warming-up and cooling-down should be included as essential components.
- Developing an exercise program to meet your individual fitness needs includes assessments conducted to determine your cardiorespiratory endurance, flexibility, muscular strength and endurance, and body composition.
- Determining what you want to achieve from your fitness program, developing a personal contract with a built-in incentive, and taking measures to stay involved will help your program to be more successful.
- Injuries related to knees and joints, shin splints, back pain, and inflammation can often be prevented through use of proper equipment, effective stretching, and a commonsense approach to personal workouts. Treatment of these injuries can be helped by using the RICE method (rest, ice, compression, and elevation).
- Exercising during pregnancy can be beneficial for women and their babies, but only when done under the supervision of a physician.
- Addiction to exercise can be detrimental to a woman's well-being. Professional counseling may be needed for recovery from this compulsion.
- One of the most effective weight methods is participation in a comprehensive fitness program.

Review Questions

1. In what ways does a physical fitness program benefit someone physically, psychologically, and socially?
2. What are the components of a comprehensive physical fitness program?
3. What are the differences between isometric, isotonic, and isokinetic weight training?
4. Why is it important to include the warm-up and cool-down phases of a workout session?
5. What are the methods that can help to make your fitness program successful? What are some strategies for staying involved with your program?
6. What are four types of physical fitness injuries? What are the methods to avoid or reduce injuries?
7. What are the benefits and precautions a woman should consider if she chooses to exercise during pregnancy?
8. What are the potential negative consequences of compulsive eating?
9. Why is exercise a positive and effective method of managing weight?

Resources

Organizations and Hotlines

American Volkssport Association
Walking events sponsored by chapters throughout the country
Telephone: (800) 830–WALK

Women's Sport Foundation
342 Madison Ave.
Suite 728
New York, NY 10017
Telephone: (800) 227–3988

President's Council on Physical Fitness & Sport
450 5th St. NW
Suite 7103
Washington, DC 20001
Telephone: (202) 272-3430

Videotapes

T'ai Chi: For Health and Fitness. Parade Video, 1993, (Phone: 800-272-4214).

Websites

National Council on Women's Health:
http://www.womens-health.com/
Dance Directory:
http://www.cyberspace.com/candehey/dance.html
American Volkssport Association:
http://www.nworld.com/~walking
Fitness Issues: http://www.inect.co.uk.nsmi/
Fitness Links to the Internet:
http://www.fitnesslink.com/links.htm
Fitness World: http://www.fitness world.
com/fitnews/news.html

Suggested Readings

Bailey, C. 1994. *Smart exercise: Burning fat, getting fit.* New York: Houghton Mifflin.

Fahey, T. D., and G. Hutchinson. 1992. *Weight training for women.* Mountain View, CA: Mayfield.

Fenton, M., and S. Bauer. 1995. *The 90-day fitness walking program.* New York: Perigee Book.

Hooten, Clair. 1996. *T'ai chi for beginners.* The Berkley Publishing Group, 1-800-788-6262.

Myers, C. 1992. *A complete guide to the complete exercise.* New York: Random House.

Shangold, M. M., ed. 1994. *Women and exercise: Physiology and sports medicine,* 2nd ed. F. A. Davis Company, 1-800-323-3555 or E-mail orders @fadavis.com

References

1. Exercise and women's health. 1995. *National Women's Health Report,* 17 (1):1-3, 7.
2. Bernstein, H. et al. 1994. Physical exercise and reduced risk of breast cancer in young women. *The Journal of the National Cancer Institute,* 86, 1403-8.
3. International Society of Sport Psychology. 1992. Physical activity and psychological benefit: A position statement. *International Journal of Sport Psychology,* 23, 186-91.
4. Meditation in motion: Ta'i chi and beyond. 1994. *University of California at Berkeley Wellness Letter,* 5 (5) (February) 3.
5. Prentice, W. 1997. *Fitness for college and life.* St. Louis: Mosby-Year Book, Inc.
6. Sullivan, D. 1995. Stretching the truth. *Women's Sports and Fitness,* 17, 56-60.
7. Fahey, T. D., P. M. Insel, and W. T. Roth. 1997. *Fit & well: Core concepts and lab in physical fitness and wellness.* Mountain View, CA: Mayfield Publishing Company.
8. Laffenburger, S. K. 1992. Efficient warm-ups: Creating a warm-up that works. *Journal of Physical Education, Recreation and Dance,* 63 (4): 21-25.
9. Payne, W., and D. Hahn. 1995. *Understanding your health.* St. Louis: Mosby-Yearbook, Inc.
10. Sharp, D. 1994. The quitter's exercise plan. *Health,* 8 (3): 68-71, 75, 76.
11. Prentice, W. 1997. *Fitness for college and life.* St. Louis: Mosby-Year Book, Inc.
12. Special. 1996. How to exercise. *Consumer Reports,* 61 (1): 14-30.
13. Beim, A. 1995. Exercise during pregnancy. *American Health,* 14, 44.
14. Moms in Motion. 1997. URL: *http://www/ctcb.com*
15. ACOG Technical Bulletin. 1994. Exercise during pregnancy and the postpartum period. *ACOG Technical Bulletin: An Educational Aid to Obstetrician-Gynecologists,* 189.
16. Longstreet, D. 1992. Expecting the best. *American Health,* 11, 89.
17. Rodin, J. 1992. Body mania. *Psychology Today,* 56-60.
18. Polivy, J., and V. Clendenen. 1993. Exercise and compulsive. Paper presented at the *Annual Convention of the American Psychological Association,* 12 (Toronto, Ontario, August).
19. Overdoing it. 1996. *Harvard Women's Health Watch,* 111 (12) (August): 6.
20. The new American body. 1993. *University of California at Berkeley Wellness Letter,* 10 (3) (December): 1-2.
21. Vital statistics. 1996. *Health,* 10 (4) (July/August): 18.
22. Losing weight. 1993. What works, what doesn't. *Consumer Reports* (June): 347-52.
23. How to make exercise fun. 1997. *Consumer Reports on Health,* 9 (4): 37, 39-40.

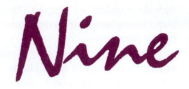

Nine

Avoiding Tobacco Use

■ chapter objectives

When you complete this chapter you will be able to:
- Explain why smoking-related deaths are the most preventable causes of death to women in this country.
- Describe the role women have historically played in the use of tobacco.
- Identify the substances in tobacco and the role each plays in the development of smoking-related diseases.
- Describe the available methods that can be used to stop smoking.
- Explain the relationship between the use of tobacco and the effects on reproduction in women.
- Explain the importance of a smoke-free environment in the home, the workplace, and in recreational facilities.
- Describe the physiological effects of caffeine upon the well-being of women.
- Describe the interaction between caffeine and pregnancy.

The chains of habit are too weak to be felt until they are too strong to be broken.

Samuel Johnson

TOBACCO: LOOKING BACK

More deaths could be prevented if individuals stopped using tobacco than by changing of any other lifestyle behavior. Despite the overwhelming amount of research linking tobacco use to *morbidity* (illness) and *mortality* (death), more than 3,000 young persons begin smoking every day.[1] As this chapter was being written, a historic ruling by a federal judge in North Carolina was rendered that gave the Food and Drug Administration (FDA) a measure of control over tobacco. The FDA can restrict and regulate access to tobacco products and control the labeling on tobacco packaging. However, the advertising of various forms of tobacco cannot be regulated by the FDA. The federal government, to some degree, has been reluctant to place major constraints on tobacco products because of the possible economic impact on the production, manufacturing, and selling of this product. Yet, as you will read in the remainder of this chapter, the substances found in tobacco cause serious health consequences, resulting in high costs in terms of poor health and an increased need for health care. Both the home and workplace are negatively impacted.

The history of the United States and the use of tobacco are intertwined. When Columbus discovered

HEALTHY PEOPLE 2000 OBJECTIVES

- Increase abstinence from tobacco use by pregnant women to at least 90 percent and increase abstinence from alcohol, cocaine, and marijuana by pregnant women by at least 20 percent. 1995 progress toward goal: 15 percent
- Reduce cigarette smoking to a prevalence of no more than 12 percent among women of reproductive age. 1995 progress toward goal: 0 percent
- Reduce cigarette smoking to a prevalence of no more than 10 percent among pregnant women. 1995 progress toward goal: 0 percent
- Reduce cigarette smoking to a prevalence of no more than 10 percent among women who use oral contraceptives. 1995 progress toward goal: 0 percent
- Increase smoking cessation during pregnancy so that at least 60 percent of women who are cigarette smokers at the time they become pregnant quit smoking early in pregnancy and maintain abstinence for the remainder of their pregnancy. 1995 progress toward goal: –40 percent

America, he also discovered Indians smoking pipes containing leaves and stems. Following his second trip, Columbus returned to Spain taking this substance, tobacco, with him. The smoking of tobacco, called "drinking," eventually became widespread throughout Europe and Asia. History notes that the English Queen Charlotte, wife of King George III (1760–1820), was highly addicted to powdered tobacco, called snuff, and as a result was nicknamed "Snuffy Charlotte."[2]

Tobacco, possibly named for a province in Mexico, was used medicinally for over 300 years, between A.D. 1500 and A.D.1800, to treat ailments such as colds, headaches, and of all things, coughs. However, physicians and researchers ultimately determined that tobacco was not the wonder drug it was purported to be. In the United States, the substance ceased to be used medicinally in the late 1800s. Today it is a drug that is used only recreationally because of the advertised image and activities associated with the use of tobacco and, more importantly, because of the serious health-related consequences that result from exposure to the various substances in tobacco.

WOMEN AND TOBACCO
Prevalence of Tobacco Use

Between 1974–1992, the percentage of American women smokers over the age of 18 decreased from 33 percent to 25 percent, except in the 18- to 24-year-old age group. However, the *number* of female smokers, because of a larger population, continues to increase. Presently, there are 46 million smokers in the United States, and approximately 22 million of them are female.[3] One-half of all long-term smokers will die because they choose to smoke tobacco. One-quarter will die in middle age (35–69). On average, this is a loss of 20 to 25 years of normal life expectancy. One-quarter will die in old age (70+), losing 5 to 10 years of normal life expectancy.[4] Female *death* rates attributable to smoking were about 14,000 in 1965, rising to over 240,000 in 1995. If current trends continue, death from smoking-related illnesses will occur in women more than men sometime between 2005 and 2010.[5] Worldwide, tobacco-related annual deaths in industrialized countries are expected to double in the next 30 years. Consequently, by the year 2020, more than one million adult women will die each year due to illnesses attributable to tobacco use.[6]

Each of the following conditions plays a significant role in the probability that a woman will die prematurely from the use of tobacco: the earlier the age at which a women starts to smoke, the longer she smokes, the more she inhales, and the higher the level of tar and nicotine in the tobacco product. (See Fig. 9.1.)

Why Women Smoke

Media influence is pervasive, compelling, and influential. There are over 1,000 television stations, 8,000 radio stations, 1,700 daily newspapers, and thousands of magazines and billboards all of which reach millions of women on a daily, even hourly basis.[7] Many thousands of these media avenues promote the concept that smoking relates to a desired image and lifestyle, fun times, attraction to others, athleticism, and quiet moments in beautiful surroundings. Mass media has certainly been utilized by the tobacco companies to zealously promote their product. In fact, cigarettes are one of the most widely advertised consumer products in this country even though this commodity has been banned from television and radio advertising since 1971. In 1992, the tobacco

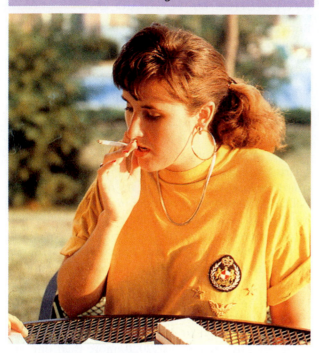

FIGURE 9.1 Unfortunately, the number of young women smokers is increasing.

industry spent $5.23 billion advertising various tobacco products, up from $3.13 billion in 1985.[8]

The idea of women using smoking tobacco was introduced into the advertisement media in 1919. However, to portray the practice in a more acceptable manner, the woman was Asian in appearance and smoking a foreign brand of cigarette. You can imagine why this type of portrayal was perhaps necessary when you learn that in 1908, it was illegal for women in New York City to smoke in public, and in the 1920s women lost jobs if they were smokers. When smoking among women became lawful, public opinion in regard to this practice was very closed, as revealed by this quote from a 1927 book:

> Smoking by women and even young girls must be considered from a far different standpoint than smoking by men, for not only is the female organism by virtue of its much more frail structure and its more delicate tissues much less able to resist the poisonous action of tobacco than that of men, and thus, like many a delicate flower, apt to fade and wither more quickly in consequence, but the fecundity of woman is greatly impaired by it . . . authorities cannot be expected to look on unmoved while a generation of sterile

women, rendered incapable of fulfilling their sublime function of motherhood, is being produced on account of the immoderate smoking of foolish young girls.[9]

Considering this attitude toward women's strength and purpose, is it any wonder that women were attracted to a product (a drug in this instance) that portrayed an image of freedom and choice? Through their advertisements, the tobacco industry captured some of women's energy, perhaps unrest, and certainly their desire to make some of their own decisions. Using slogans, pictures, and scenarios, cigarette manufacturers promoted the idea of freedom, choice, and appeal. Female movie stars, music, and eventually television stars, who were all portrayed as desirable, attractive, modern, and sexy were seen using tobacco—they "modeled" the woman who other women wanted to be. The women in tobacco advertisements personified confidence, a positive self-image, and appeal to others. Why not use a product that produces all of those benefits? The billions of dollars the tobacco industry has spent in promoting their products through the years has influenced women to embrace tobacco use and in the process, negatively affected their environment, their health, and even the well-being of their children.

Other factors also influence women to use tobacco. As unbelievable as it may be, some women are unaware of the health risks that result from smoking tobacco; as you read the remainder of this chapter you will have a better understanding of these risks. Parental smoking influences children to adopt this behavior; children whose parents smoke (especially if *both* parents smoke) are much more likely to become smokers themselves. We are certainly influenced by our peers; almost 90 percent of teens who smoke have friends who also smoke, and young women who smoke are more likely to have boyfriends who are also smokers. Additionally, if "your group" is comprised of numerous smokers, there is a much greater chance that you will also become a smoker. For example, associating with coworkers who smoke and friends who smoke at clubs and parties, or engaging in an activity at which participants smoke, such as bowling, may increase your chances of smoking. The environment in which we work and recreate plays a part in the choice to use tobacco. Take *Assess Yourself:* "Could You Become a Smoker?" to determine which factors could influence you to become a smoker.

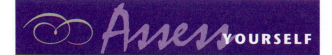

SUBSTANCES IN TOBACCO

Over 4,000 chemical compounds are found in tobacco smoke; 2,550 of which come from tobacco plants and 1,450 derive from additives, pesticides, and a multitude of other compounds.[10] Approximately 60 of these are **carcinogenic** or cancer-causing compounds including tar, carbon monoxide, hydrogen cyanide, ammonia, formaldehyde, benzene, and nicotine.[11] Various compounds in tobacco smoke, such as carbon monoxide, are so potent that continual exposure would be lethal. Radioactive materials, usually from the soil in which tobacco is grown, are also present in tobacco smoke. A two-pack-a-day smoker is exposed to enough compounds during a one-year time period that the exposure is equal to radiation from 250 to 300 chest X rays a year.[12]

A more in-depth look at three major tobacco components—nicotine, poisonous gases, and particulate matter (tar)—will provide a better understanding of this drug. Each component has its unique set of consequences leading to serious illnesses and possible death.

Nicotine is a highly physically and psychologically addicting stimulant substance that has an accelerating effect on the central nervous system (CNS). The immediate stimulation effect, produced by the release of adrenaline from the adrenal glands, causes an increase in heart rate, respiratory rate, oxygen consumption, and rise in the blood pressure due to the constriction of peripheral blood vessels and bronchial tubes. As adrenaline increases the heart rate, there is an increased need for oxygen *by* the heart, but not an increased supply of oxygen *to* the heart, which can create serious consequences. Increased electrical activity of the CNS can induce arrhythmia; increased platelet adhesives can lead to possible blood clotting. As you might imagine, the body's immediate response to nicotine can seriously affect the entire cardiovascular system.

Once inhaled, nicotine enters the respiratory system and reaches the brain in a number of seconds. An incredible 90 percent of the nicotine that reaches the alveoli is absorbed into the bloodstream. Of the total amount of nicotine that enters the body, approximately 10 percent leaves the body chemically unchanged; the remaining 90 percent is metabolized by the liver and excreted in urine.

Over 270 *poisonous gases* are present in tobacco smoke, including carbon monoxide, nitrogen, carbon dioxide, hydrogen, and cyanide. Carbon monoxide, one of the best known gases in tobacco smoke, increases the heart rate, elevates blood pressure, and impairs visual acuity. Carbon monoxide combines with oxygen to form *carboxyhemoglobin.* As a result, instead of oxygen being delivered to vital cells, tissues, and organs, a poisonous gas arrives and robs the body of life-giving oxygen. The blood of women who smoke today can have carbon monoxide levels far above the standards allowed for industry by the U.S. Air Quality Act.

carcinogenic (kar **sin** oh jen ick)—the ability to cause the development of cancer.

nicotine—physically and psychologically addictive stimulate substance found in tobacco.

Particulate matter or **tar** is a mixture of ingredients that are inhaled into the lungs and that inhibit effective functioning of the respiratory system. Image your lungs coated with a sticky, black substance that contains carcinogens. Small particles of tar and gases move to air sacs in the lungs, called **alveoli,** and larger particles remain on the various passages that lead to the lungs. Smoking one pack of cigarettes a day will cause an accumulation of 4 oz of tar within the lungs in one year's time.[13]

Tar, as well as gases, create another serious concern in the lungs. **Cilia,** hairlike structures that line the bronchi, help to clear the lungs by sweeping debris, dust, and particles out of lung passages then are expelled through coughing or sputum. However, gases and particulate matter deposited by smoking damage the cilia, sometimes permanently, and disables the cilia from functioning to rid the lungs of tar and other debris. Therefore, the carcinogenic-laden tar stays in contact with respiratory tract lining, which possibly lead to changes in cellular structure and to formation of cancerous tumors.

ADVERSE HEALTH EFFECTS

Smoking generates serious health problems for women just as it does for men, and long-term use of tobacco will cause various ill effects to become more discernible.

Bronchiectasis is a condition that develops within the bronchial tree and results in irreversible dilatation and destruction of the bronchial walls. Inflammation of airways and alveoli results in scarring and loss of elasticity in the airways of the lungs. Chronic bronchitis, characterized by long-term and persistent severe coughing, spitting, and excessive secretion of mucus, is a precursor to bronchiectasis. Smoking cigarettes causes the development of bronchitis or exacerbates the inflammation. This inflammation of the airways causes the passages to squeeze shut during exhalation, preventing the lungs from emptying completely.

Emphysema, a form of chronic obstructive lung disease (COLD), is a condition that can result from having chronic bronchitis. As airways lose their elasticity and trap unexpired air and toxins, the alveoli are destroyed and, thus, tear as a result of the pressure of inflation. Loss of alveoli will reduce the amount of surface area for gas exchange. This disease causes chronic shortness of breath due to the difficulty in exhaling and poor distribution of inhaled air

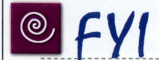

The Reality of Emphysema

Try this activity to have some realistic feeling of how the lack of the ability to breathe affects a woman physically, emotionally, and socially. Cut a small straw into about a 3-inch section. Place it between your lips, hold your nostrils closed and with lips closed tightly around the straw, breathe only through the straw for one minute. (*Note:* If you are unable to do this for one minute, stop any time you feel the need.) As you struggle to breathe enough through the straw, think of these questions:

What do you feel is your most immediate physical need?
Do you feel any dizziness?
Is there a feeling of panic or wanting to gasp for breath?
Could you walk up a flight of stairs breathing through the straw?
With this limited air supply could you engage in any recreational activity you enjoy? (tennis, jogging, biking, swimming)
Would you be able to enjoy all the aspects of social or intimate relationships?
In what other ways would difficulty in breathing affect your lifestyle?

Although the advertising media associates smoking with youth, vitality, and healthy appearance, the reality is the absolute opposite. Emphysema is only one disease that results from the use of tobacco; the only way to avoid the limitations that this disease creates is to not smoke. ∞

in lungs. As a result, the heart must work harder to exchange and deliver oxygen-ladened blood throughout the body. (See *FYI:* "The Reality of Emphysema" to learn more about emphysema.)

Women who are smokers have a greater potential for developing heart disease and stroke than women who do not smoke. In fact, smoking is one of the major, if not *the* major risk factor for the development of diseases of the cardiovascular system including hypertension, atherosclerosis, coronary heart disease, and aortic aneurysms. Smoking is linked to changes in blood chemistry. Cigarette smoking contributes to low levels of high-density lipoproteins (HDLs), which are considered to be beneficial components of the blood, and with an increase in low-density lipoproteins (LDLs). These two changes can lead to a buildup of plaque within the arterial system. The use of tobacco interferes with the production of red blood cells, reduces the blood's ability to clot, which can increase the possibility of hemorrhage during accidents or childbirth. Tobacco is a *vasoconstrictor,* and as such, can cause constriction of the coronary arteries. This condition is potentially dangerous because coronary arteries are the primary source of blood supply to the heart muscle, therefore, the reduction of blood supply to heart muscle tissue, even briefly, can at least damage the heart and at worst be fatal. Another detrimental effect of constricted blood vessels, combined with an increased heart rate, is the increase in blood pressure. The arterial system, therefore, endures more wear and tear as the heart works to force blood through smaller vessels creating high blood pressure. Smokers are more susceptible to cerebral infarction, or "stroke," due to the above mentioned factors.

Taking oral contraceptives and smoking cigarettes increases the risk of heart attack, stroke, and blood clots in women over age 25. In fact, a woman is four times more likely to have a *fatal* heart attack if she smokes and uses oral contraceptives than if she only engages in smoking.[14] The very serious likelihood of having a heart attack or stroke if you smoke and take birth control pills prompted the Food and Drug Administration to mandate that all oral contraceptives must include labeling that reads, "Women who use oral contraceptives should not smoke."[15] Therefore, it is highly recommended that if you take birth control pills that you do not smoke.

There is a strong relationship between cigarette smoking and the development of the vast majority of cancers at sites located throughout the body. Smoking is associated with cancers of the larynx, pharynx, lungs, stomach, uterus, and kidney. Additionally, 75 percent of esophageal cancer, between 30 percent and 40 percent of bladder cancers, 85 percent of lung cancers, and 20 percent to 30 percent of cervical cancer are caused by smoking tobacco.[16]

Smoking cigarettes accounts for 30 percent of all cancer deaths.[17] Lung cancer deaths in women—56,000 annually—have replaced the 46,000 annual breast cancer deaths, as the leading cause of cancer death in women.[18] Due to the continual exposure of body cells and tissues to carcinogens in tobacco smoke, women greatly increase the probability of developing many types of cancers if they choose to smoke. (See *Her Story:* "Sarah.")

Have you heard the comment that women experience weight gain once they quit smoking? There is an explanation for this. Nicotine decreases the strength of hunger contractions in the stomach (e.g., inhaling the smoke of one cigarette can reduce "hunger pains" for almost an hour), increases blood sugar level, and deadens taste buds. As an oral habit, smokers associate hand-to-mouth activity with pleasure (or relief from anxiety); therefore, when smoking stops, hand-to-mouth objects (food) substitutes for the former hand-to-mouth smoking behavior. With smoking cessation, the sense of taste and smell increase; therefore, food becomes more appealing. One research study[19] involving several hundred men and women ex-smokers found that the average female smoker gained 8.4 pounds following cessation of smoking compared to 6.1 pounds for the male. Interestingly enough, in conducting the study, the researchers discovered that the average smoker weighed less than nonsmokers. The amount of weight gain depends on the individual and her willingness to engage in behaviors that reduce the possibility of weight gain following smoking cessation. (See *Health Tips:* "Avoiding Weight Gain After Smoking Cessation" for suggestions to avoid weight gain.)

There are far better ways to control eating than to engage in a behavior that is harmful and possibly lethal. Imagine this—a woman would need to gain between 50 and 100 pounds before she could come close to the equivalent health risks associated with tobacco smoking.

Other Physical Consequences

In addition to the health conditions described above, there are other health effects related to tobacco smoking. Research in many of these problem areas is ongoing. Cataract formation in the eyes of women

---

tar—sticky, black particulate matter in tobacco smoke.

alveoli (al **vee** oh lie)—thin, saclike structures in the lungs in which gas exchange takes place between oxygen and blood.

cilia (**sill** ee uh)—small, hairlike structures that produce motion to help clear the lungs.

emphysema (em fuh **see** muh)—chronic shortness of breath.

Her Story

Sarah

Sarah and her best friend, Betty, would sneak cigarettes from Sarah's mother's purse when they were very young. They pretended to smoke like her and the beautiful women she saw in her Saturday afternoon movie outings. In high school, Sarah smoked for real and developed an addiction to tobacco that she carried with her throughout college, marriage, and two pregnancies.

As Sarah "welcomed" her fortieth year, she began to experience a persistent cough, and one respiratory infection after another. Her lack of energy, which she attributed to possible early menopause, curtailed her activity with her tennis group. She became frightened when she saw blood in her sputum. After a number of visits to her physician, she was advised to see her gynecologist. Then she went to see one medical specialist after another: a cardiologist, a respiratory therapist, and finally a pulmonary specialist who put Sarah through a series of tests that revealed shadows on her lungs. She was sent to an oncologist's office where, after X rays and **computerized tomography scans (CT scans),** she was diagnosed with lung cancer.

Not believing this could happen to her, Sarah sought the medical opinions of two other oncologists who confirmed the diagnosis of lung cancer. Anger, then rage filled Sarah's hours and days. Not to her, not to Sarah

with the supportive, loving husband and family, the intelligent and well-liked children, the new house near friends and her tennis club! Yes, Sarah. Sarah of the 24-year smoking habit; the "I can quit when I want, Sarah."

Reality hit with the onset of her treatments: First, she received radiation to shrink the tumors, then surgery to remove all possible cancerous tissue, and then the series of chemotherapy treatment and the accompanying side effects. Amazingly, through all of this, Sarah still wanted a cigarette—she had a massive craving for nicotine and found the withdrawal from it one of the more difficult parts of the entire process.

Sarah's story does not end happily. She lost her battle against lung cancer 3 years after the original diagnosis. She lost the life she shared in her nice neighborhood with her loving husband and exceptional children. Sarah did quit smoking, but unfortunately she also quit everything else she loved and enjoyed.

- What suggestions do you have to prevent Sarah's tragedy from happening to other women?
- Have you ever thought that "this won't happen to me," and then lit up a cigarette and smoked anyway?
- What are your feelings about Sarah after reading her case study?

health tips

Avoiding Weight Gain After Smoking Cessation

If you are a former smoker and want to control the possibility of weight gain, consider the following suggestions. You may even want to incorporate these suggestions into your lifestyle as a matter of improving your overall good health habits.

- Have low-fat, nutritious snacks easily accessible to help satisfy the hand-to-mouth habit.
- Keep a straw or other harmless object handy to chew on or use with your hands.
- Enlist the help of a significant other and try new active activities together.
- Walk, jog, bike, swim, etc., at least 3 times per week.
- Include in your diet your very favorite food (in moderation) at least once each week.
- Reward yourself at designated intervals for remaining smoke-free.

has been researched; although the exact relationship between smoking and cataract formation is not known, research has indicated that ex-smokers after years of not smoking, remained at risk for developing cataract.[20] Correlations in research studies have linked adult-onset leukemia (AOL) and smoking. It is estimated that 14 percent of AOL cases have been associated with smoking tobacco.[21] In one study, measurement of bone density was made on postmenopausal identical twins, only one of whom smoked. Loss of bone density (e.g., osteoporosis) was studied by looking at smoking and nonsmoking twins. The twins who smoked developed greater loss in bone density than the twins who were not smokers. Additionally, postmenopausal women who smoke have a greater degree of bone loss than nonsmoking postmenopausal women.[22] Female smokers often develop deeper facial wrinkles, sometimes called "smoker's face," at a faster rate than females who do not smoke. A possible explanation of this phenomenon may be the reduced amount of blood flow to the skin because of constricted blood vessels.

Research in a multitude of areas continues; however, it seems clearly evident that women who smoke tobacco harm their bodies in many ways and increase their likelihood of premature death. As a result of using tobacco, it is estimated that 40 percent will die prematurely of diseases that would not have developed had smoking not occurred.[23]

ADDICTION

Tobacco users develop a strong physical and psychological dependence on the product. A pack-a-day smoker has at least 50,000 hits of nicotine in a year; therefore, addiction and tolerance develop somewhat rapidly. Various studies have investigated the relationship between tobacco and addiction and results indicate that between one-third and one-half of all individuals who experiment with smoking become addicted. It was ascertained that a large majority of people who smoke at least 100 cigarettes will ultimately become habitual smokers.[24] The above becomes highly significant when compared to cocaine, a drug considered to be highly addictive. It appears that less than one-fifth of all cocaine experimenters become addicted to cocaine. Does everyone who uses tobacco become addicted? No, in rare instances, 5–10 percent of individuals who smoke do not develop an addiction and do not experience withdrawal symptoms with smoking cessation.

Over 90 percent of women who smoke develop a dependence on the nicotine, the major addicting agent in tobacco. Most women experience withdrawal symptoms, such as irritability, lack of concentration, sleep disorders, anxiety, hunger, headache, and craving for nicotine, if they stop smoking. A woman's body cells adapt to a certain level of nicotine and the smoker is compelled to maintain that level. The half-life of nicotine, which is the time required for the body to eliminate one half of the original drug dose, is about 100 minutes;[25] regular smokers seek to replenish nicotine as its level begins to drop following the initial peak concentration level.

Overcoming addiction is difficult, not only because of the physical and psychological dependency, but also because withdrawal symptoms are uncomfortable. Lifestyle rituals that accompany habitual smoking can also be difficult to change. Enjoying the morning cup of coffee, calling a friend, having a drink, riding in the car, or relaxing with a book may all be ritualistically tied to smoking a cigarette. Practices such as these bond the smoker to the substance and thus add to the difficulty of breaking the bonds

Viewpoint

What Rights Does the Smoker Have?

As research continues to show that involuntary smoking is dangerous to women who breathe the chemical-laden smoke, more and more businesses, institutions, and schools are establishing a tobacco-free environment. Individuals spend up to 80 percent of their time indoors, which can lead to problems for smokers as well as nonsmokers. Designating smoking areas may not always protect the nonsmoker.

However, the individual who makes the choice to smoke does have a right to make that choice. Considering the rights of both smokers and nonsmokers creates a dilemma for businesses, institutions, as well as the personal environment of women in the home.

Consider the following questions and discuss the predicaments created by the situation:

- Does the person who smokes have a right to have a place to smoke?
- What can business and industry do to address the needs of both groups?
- If the employer mandates a nonsmoking environment, should they pay for the assistance that the smoker may need in order to stop smoking?
- Where do individual rights and public rights begin and end in this situation?

between tobacco and user. (See *Viewpoint:* "What Rights Does the Smoker Have?")

ENVIRONMENTAL TOBACCO SMOKE

Environmental tobacco smoke (ETS), also referred to as *passive* or *involuntary* smoke, is inhaled from the surroundings in which we live and work. This smoke is discharged from the lighted end of the cigarette, called **side-stream smoke,** and accounts for about

computerized tomography (CT) scan (toe **mog** ruff ee)—an X-ray beam that rotates around the body; provides a series of X rays of a particular area of the body from various angles.

side-stream smoke—smoke from the lit end of the cigarette; contains more tar, nicotine, and carbon monoxide than mainstream smoke.

85 percent of the smoke in a room. Side-stream smoke has two times as much tar and nicotine, three times as much carbon monoxide, and three times as much ammonia and benzopyrene as is found in **main-stream smoke,** which is the smoke drawn through the cigarette and inhaled and exhaled by the smoker. Side-stream smoke produces pollutants that, upon inhalation, lead to the creation of **free radicals** in the human body. Free radicals are very toxic chemicals that cause damage to body cells and can lead to numerous ailments such as cancer.

The actual negative consequences from passive smoke is determined by the number of smokers in the room, as well as the number of cigarettes, ventilation, and amount of continual exposure. Studies involving passive smoke often consider the exposure to tobacco in terms of *pack years,* determined by the number of cigarette packs per day smoked by an individual, usually the spouse, multiplied by number of years the nonsmoking partner was exposed. In early 1990s, passive smoke was determined to present definite health risks to anyone who is exposed to it, especially on a long-term basis, such as smokers in home or at the workplace. A study of 1,906 women was recently conducted by medical center researchers determining their exposure to side-stream smoke and the development of lung cancer. Of these women, 653 developed lung cancer. It was determined that women married to smokers were 30 percent more likely to develop lung cancer than those married to nonsmokers.[26] Exposure to side-stream smoke was measured in environments outside the home. Passive smoke in the workplace produced a 39 percent increased risk of developing lung cancer and women who were exposed to passive smoke for 2 hours a week for over 6 months in social settings had a 50 percent greater risk of developing lung cancer than nonexposed women. Women, exposed to smoke both as a child and an adult, had almost twice the risk of developing lung cancer than women exposed only during the adult years.[27]

Effects on Adults

Passive smoke has been shown to create three times a greater chance for nonsmoking women married to smokers to have a heart attack than nonsmoking women who were married to nonsmoking

partners. Similar results have been shown in regard to lung cancer.[28] Passive smoke research comparing smoking/nonsmoking partners revealed additional health-related consequences. Exposure to passive smoke is linked to an increased risk of developing cervical cancer, increased risk of having low-birth-weight babies,[29] and depletion of certain vitamins, such as vitamin C.[30]

Effects on Children

Children of smokers experience detrimental health effects from breathing air containing cigarette smoke. The more smoke a child is exposed to, the greater the health problems will be for the child. Passive smoke increases the possibility of respiratory infections such as colds, bronchitis, and pneumonia, especially during the first 2 years of life. As children get older, they may develop a chronic cough and reduced lung function. The Environmental Protection Agency (EPA) stated that passive smoke impairs the respiratory health of thousands of young children, increases the incidence of middle ear disease, and both worsens asthmatic conditions and causes new cases of asthma.[31] In addition to the physical consequences, the child of a smoker is more likely, themselves, to become a smoker and begin smoking at a young age.

Now that you have read about the effects of tobacco smoke, complete *Journal Activity:* "A Bill of Rights."

SMOKING AND PREGNANCY

Women who smoke while pregnant harm their baby in numerous ways, especially if they smoke throughout the gestation period. Negative consequences related to maternal smoking can be caused by nicotine's ability to constrict fetal blood vessels and breathing movements, and by carbon monoxide reducing the oxygen supply to fetal blood. Additionally, the ability of the fetus to metabolize vitamins is reduced. An increased risk of ectopic pregnancy has been shown to be related to maternal cigarette smoking during the time of conception,[32] as well as almost two times the increased risk of spontaneous abortion (miscarriage). A research study, conducted by Lieberman et al.,[33] found that maternal smoking during pregnancy, especially during the third trimester, produced reduced-weight babies. A dose-related response has been found between smoking and infant birth weight: The more the female smokes during pregnancy, the greater the infant weight reduction. Smoking-related low-birth-weight babies and the requisite consequences are 100 percent preventable—don't smoke during pregnancy! Although the weight loss may be regained rapidly following birth, children born to smoking mothers show that they often will be shorter, have reduced reading and mathematical skills, exhibit hyperactivity, and have lessened social adjustment abilities than children born to nonsmoking mothers. If mothers of newborns continue to smoke while breast-feeding, studies reveal decreased breast-milk volume and reduced infant growth rate.[34] As a result, the health and well-being of the newborn is placed in jeopardy. (See Fig. 9.2.)

Infants born to women who smoke while they are pregnant have an increased likelihood of dying of **sudden infant death syndrome (SIDS).** This devastating death of an infant is generally unexplainable because the cause of death usually cannot be determined in a postmortem examination. This finding may be related to an environment in which the pregnant woman is exposed too often to passive smoke or due to the infant's exposure to environmental tobacco smoke. Studies have shown that two-thirds of women who quit smoking during pregnancy begin smoking once the baby is born.[35] Estimations are that 41 percent of all U.S. children between the ages of 2 months and 3 years live in an environment in which there is at least one smoker.[36]

During delivery, smoking mothers have an increased chance of hemorrhaging, an increased

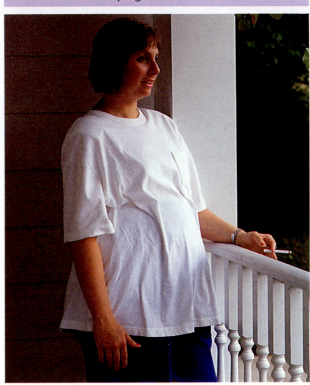

FIGURE 9.2 Pregnant women should avoid smoking as well as exposure to smoke to protect the health of the developing fetus.

chance of delivering a stillborn infant or an infant that only lives for a brief period of time. Hospital stays are often longer for a smoking mother and her baby. Following delivery, smoking mothers heal slower and often must spend more time caring for newborns who have more difficulties with feeding, digestion, sleeping, and restlessness.

main-stream smoke—smoke drawn through the cigarette, and inhaled and exhaled by the smoker.

free radicals—toxic chemicals in the body that cause damage to body cells and can lead to serious illnesses such as cancer.

sudden infant death syndrome (SIDS)—sudden and unexpected death of an apparently normal and healthy infant that occurs during sleep, and with no physical or autopsy evidence of disease.

The bottom line is that there are serious health consequences for babies born to women who smoke during and after pregnancy. And there are also detrimental effects experienced by women who smoke during pregnancy.

SMOKING CESSATION

Why do women decide to quit smoking? Warnings of imminent health problems, becoming pregnant, having children, or working in a smoke-free environment can each provide the impetus to stop smoking. Smoking has become restricted in such areas as public buildings, domestic air flights, restaurants, and schools; the inconvenience of finding a place in which a person is allowed to smoke may lead to cessation of the habit. Most women quit several times before they are able to completely eliminate the habit. Overall, 70–80 percent of smokers who quit often relapse within 3 months.[37] Therefore, smokers must be persistent in their attempts to stop. The benefits far outweigh the morbidity and mortality associated with smoking. Women may often need assistance in their attempts at smoking cessation and a number of methods are available to assist women who want to quit.

Behavioral Changes

There appears to be no easy or right way to quit smoking and those who have made the attempt, usually many times, will attest to that fact. Smoking cessation appears to be most successful for women who really want to quit and consider all the beneficial reasons to quit and barriers that could make cessation unlikely. *FYI:* "Smoking Cessation" provides suggestions to consider when deciding to quit. *Health Tips:* "Tips for Successful Smoking Cessation" provides suggestion for the most effective type of cessation.

Even though many women successfully quit on their own, smoking cessation programs that provide counseling and support groups may be more successful for women who smoke 25 or more cigarettes a day. The formal smoking cessation programs vary in their success rate, but the 1-year quit rate is between 20–35 percent for most programs.[39] Be reminded that women usually stop smoking a number of times before they quit for good. Research reveals that smoking cessation successes are more likely when a woman had a readiness to quit and believes that she will be successful.

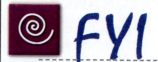

FYI

Smoking Cessation

- *You* must stop smoking because *you* want to, not because a husband or child wants you to.
- Seriously consider the medical reasons to stop smoking.
- Remember that your smoking habit is becoming more and more socially unacceptable.
- Social outcomes will be positive—no more tobacco-reeking clothes, breath, etc., and no more negative remarks about smoking.
- Public opinion reveals that women who don't smoke are considered more attractive than women who do smoke.
- Financially, you are better-off not smoking; more money is available for fun activities, and may even reduce your insurance rates.

health tips

Tips for Successful Smoking Cessation[38]

- Ask a family member or friend to help you stop smoking.
- Remember that nicotine withdrawal symptoms will pass after a few days.
- Do pleasant relaxation techniques during and after smoking cessation.
- Participate in fun and enjoyable activities during the times when you crave a cigarette.
- Exercise and eat healthy low-calorie and low-fat snacks to combat possible weight gain.
- Remember, if you slip and have a cigarette, immediately begin your smoking cessation program again.

Nicotine Replacement Devices

In recent years, the Food and Drug Administration (FDA) approved products that can aid in smoking cessation. Nicotine chewing gum, containing 2 milligrams (mg) of nicotine was approved in 1984, and in 1991, a 4-mg dosage was approved. A newer product, the transdermal nicotine patch, was approved in 1992 and acts as a conduit to deliver nicotine to the

Table 9.1

Transdermal Nicotine Patches		
BRAND NAME	DOSAGE	TYPE
Nicoderm	21 mg	24-hour
Habitrol	14 mg	
	7 mg	
Prostep	22 mg	24-hour
	11 mg	
Nicotrol	15 mg	Worn only while awake
	10 mg	
	5 mg	

Viewpoint

What Do You Think about OTC Smoking Cessation Aids?

The manufacturer of nicotine chewing gum, Nicorette, wants to change the product from prescription to non-prescription status. However, the FDA would need to consider Nicorette's own addiction potential because it contains nicotine. After reading the information about prescription smoking cessation aids, what do you think about making these products available over the counter?

bloodstream. There are four brands of nicotine patches: Nicoderm, Habitrol, Prostep, and Nicotrol. Each resembles a band-aid and must be changed daily. Table 9.1 lists the dosages and types of nicotines available.

The chewing gum and the patch are intended to be an aid while the smoker is involved in a comprehensive **smoking-cessation program.** The dosage of nicotine found in these products is intended to reduce unpleasant effects associated with nicotine withdrawal while the smoker is weaned away from smoking and eliminating exposure to other harmful chemicals in tobacco.

Physicians set important guidelines a smoker must follow while utilizing both the nicotine chewing gum and the patch. A very important guideline is that a woman must *not* smoke while using either product. When using nicotine chewing gum, the number of pieces of gum allowed per day is limited. When a smoker craves a cigarette, she is to place a piece of gum in the mouth and chew very slowly. Chewing slowly is important because it enables the smoker to properly release nicotine into the system and reduce unpleasant, and sometimes serious, side effects. Nicotine chewing gum users intermittently chew the gum and "park" the gum between the cheek and gums. A peppery taste or tingling sensation signals the smoker when to chew and when to "park" the gum. After about 2–3 months the smoker is usually ready to reduce the use of the gum and eventually move toward use of "sugarless" gum without nicotine.

The transdermal nicotine patch "delivers" nicotine to the bloodstream automatically, either over a 24-hour period or while the smoker is awake. A physician will determine what brand to prescribe and milligrams of nicotine that will be supplied to the smoker. Usually smokers start with a higher dosage of nicotine and after 1–2 months reduce the dosage, followed by another reduction within 2–4 weeks. The intent is to eventually eliminate all reliance on nicotine. However, as with the nicotine chewing gum, patches are intended to be one component in a comprehensive approach to smoking cessation.

Side effects exist from use of nicotine gum and patches, but are usually minimal. For example, if the gum is chewed too fast, especially in the first few days of use, side effects can include mouth sores, headaches, heart palpitations, and excess saliva. With the patch, the most common side effect is skin irritation in the area where the patch is placed, usually in a hairless, clean dry spot on the upper part of the body. However, placing the patch periodically at different spots can usually eliminate this problem.

Women who use these products must be aware of serious consequences if they continue to smoke while using nicotine substitutes. Nicotine overdose symptoms include tremors, respiratory failure, low blood pressure, and fainting due to weariness. If any of these symptoms appear, the smoker should immediately contact a physician. (See *Viewpoint:* "What Do You Think about OTC Smoking Cessation Aids?")

smoking-cessation program—a program to quit smoking that includes behavioral modification techniques, group support, program meetings, and occasionally includes nicotine substitutes.

Table 9.2

Short- and Long-Term Benefits of Smoking Cessation

As soon as 20 minutes after your last cigarette, your body will begin to benefit from not smoking. These benefits will continue as long as you do not smoke. However, you will lose each of these benefits if you smoke only one cigarette a day.[42]

TIME	BENEFIT
20 minutes	Reduced blood pressure and pulse rate; body temperature becomes normal
8 hours	Normal carbon monoxide levels in blood; blood oxygen level increases to normal
24 hours	Chance of heart attack decreases
48 hours	Senses of smell and taste improve; nerve endings start regrowing
2 weeks to 3 months	Blood circulation improves; easier to engage in activities because lung function increases to 30 percent
1 to 9 months	Decrease in coughing, shortness of breath, fatigue; cilia regrow in lungs allowing cleansing of lungs of dust and mucus; reduced chance of infection; increased energy
1 year	Risk of coronary heart disease is half that of a smoker's
5 years	Lung cancer death rate for former one-pack-a-day smoker decreases by almost half; stroke risk is reduced to that of a nonsmoker 5–15 years after quitting; risk of cancer of throat, esophagus, and mouth is half that of a smoker's
10 years	Lung cancer death rate similar to that of nonsmokers; precancerous cells are replaced; decreased risk of developing cancer of the mouth, throat, esophagus, bladder, kidney, and pancreas
15 years	Risk of coronary heart disease is that of a nonsmoker

Studies conducted at smoking cessation clinics reveal that smoking cessation rates increase among individuals who use either the nicotine gum or patches and engage in group-counseling sessions. Interestingly enough, use of the patch appears to be most valuable to smokers who are most nicotine dependent, yet for smokers who did not totally cease smoking, the majority reduced the number of cigarettes per day.

BENEFITS OF SMOKING CESSATION

Quitting smoking makes a big difference—and quickly. Food begins to smell and taste better, and the smoker also smells better. The cough disappears and energy begins to return. Women who have stopped smoking are sick less often, miss fewer days at work and play, and have fewer complaints about their general health. Quitting smoking also saves money; the average smoker spends about $1,000 per year on cigarettes[40] and there are many more fun things to do with that money than watch it go up in smoke.

Incentives for smoking cessation can be enhanced when women realize that within a few minutes their health can be positively affected. Table 9.2 summarizes the short- and long-term benefits that can be gained when a woman quits smoking.[41]

How to Stop Smoking!

Obviously if you need to know how to stop, it is too late to prevent the initial use of tobacco. The American Cancer Society (ACS) has a variety of highly effective materials that individuals and groups can use to make the "Smart Move" and stop this life-destroying habit. ACS suggest:

- developing a plan,
- changing smoking-related habits and commit yourself, and
- staying tobacco-free.[43]

Looking at each of these suggestions in more detail and following the steps suggested increases the smoker's understanding and chances of stopping this addiction.

In developing a plan to quit smoking, it is essential to determine the triggers that result in use of tobacco, meaning the links between an event and smoking a cigarette. Discovering when and where you light up and what you are doing prior to lighting a cigarette can be a key component for successful smoking cessation. When the trigger occurs, find something else to do instead of smoking. Suggestions are: take a walk, chew on a straw, have a glass of water, call someone, and chew sugarless gum.

Plan a "stop day" and complete and sign a "Stop Smoking Contract." Ask a friend to sign it as a means of

health tips

How to Stay Smoke-Free[44]

- Remember that if you are sleepier or more short-tempered than usual, this will pass.
- Try to exercise more.
- Keep a positive attitude by recalling all the good things about quitting: the health benefits for you and your family, feeling better about yourself, setting a good example, and having more vitality and energy.
- Eat regular meals.
- Start a money jar with your savings by not buying cigarettes.
- Talk to others about quitting; enlist their help in your smoking cessation efforts.
- Don't be discouraged if you slip and smoke! You may quit several times before you quit for good. Quit again.

support. Throw all cigarettes and related items away from your home, your car, and any other place where you may be tempted to smoke. You will feel a strong desire to smoke, but use the "Four D" technique to quell this feeling: delay, deep breathing, drink water, and do something else. Other suggestions include keeping objects such as gum, straws, low-calorie snacks near when you need/want something in your mouth; utilize nicotine chewing gum or patches, if needed; announce that you are no longer going to smoke; place "No Smoking" signs in important places; and treat yourself with something special when you stop.

Quitting smoking is one thing; remaining smoke-free may be more difficult. Some negative feelings may result within the first few days to weeks during withdrawal from nicotine. It is important to remember that these are normal and that they will go away. Find something else to do to cope with stressful situations other than falling back to a former bad habit—smoking! Include moderate exercise and nutritious, low-calorie food in your cessation program to avoid any possible weight gain. (See *Health Tips:* "How to Stay Smoke-free.") Continue to remember all the very important reasons not to smoke. In fact, write them down often. Feel proud because, by quitting, you have done a wonderfully healthy thing for yourself, for others, and for the future. Your life and the life of people around you will be healthier and of higher quality.

Obviously from the information regarding tobacco, it is clear that there are no positive effects from smoking tobacco, but there is an array of detri-

mental consequences. Prevention of this substance is essential because tobacco ingredients are highly addictive and smoking is difficult to quit. Because the vast majority of smokers start smoking before 18 years of age, educational systems must play a major part in prevention education. Schools and colleges should develop and enforce policies that prohibit tobacco use on the premises. Prevention education, beginning in kindergarten through grade 12, should include short- and long-term negative physiological, social, and financial consequences, as well as peer influence and refusal skills. Teachers need to be specifically trained to provide tobacco and other drug education, and families and the community need to be a part of tobacco use prevention effort.

CAFFEINE

A variety of beverages containing caffeine have become some of the more popular drinks of the 1990s. Teas of many types are served with meals or combined with a serene environment to provide a quiet, refreshing stress break. Cappuccino, latte, expresso, and cafe mocha are all flavorful specialty coffees that have gained widespread popularity, sometimes as a replacement for a high-calorie and fat-laden dessert. Nationwide, there are currently 4,500 coffee houses brewing varieties of caffeine drinks. This is a huge increase over 1989, when there were only 200 coffee houses in business in this country. The Specialty Coffee Association of America states that the number of coffee bars is expected to reach 10,000 by 1999.[45] Because there is an association of coffee and other caffeinated beverages with smoking, coverage of caffeine follows.

What Is Caffeine?

Caffeine is among a family of chemical compounds called **methylxanthines,** which stimulate particular neurotransmitters in the central nervous system. Found in over 60 plants and trees, caffeine has a long history of use in many drinks such as colas, tea, coffee, and cocoa, as well as over-the-counter drugs.

---

methylxanthines (meth ul **zan** theens)—family of chemical compounds that function as mild central nervous system (CNS) stimulants; includes caffeine.

Legend has it that a third century goat herder noticed his flock become more lively and animated with chewing berries from a particular plant. Monks, seeing the effects on the flock, began using the berries for a brew that helped them stay awake during evening prayers.[46]

Various types of coffee beans produce varying taste and deliver different levels of caffeine. For example, high-quality arabica beans, which are often used in specialty coffees, have a stronger taste and less caffeine than robusta beans, which often are used in national name brand coffees. The amount of caffeine in a drink is measured in milligrams and the potency will vary according to the type of coffee bean used in the drink and the way the beverage is brewed.

Caffeine, taken into the body in a water-soluble form, is absorbed into the bloodstream principally through the small intestine. Taking about 30 minutes for initial effects, peak effects on the CNS are felt within 2 hours following ingestion. Along with all other organs of the body, caffeine is distributed to the brain. It may also be passed into the placenta and to the fetus of any woman who is pregnant.[47]

Effects of Caffeine

Why is the use of products containing caffeine so prevalent? Perhaps it is due to the wide variety of possible stimulating effects caffeine produces. Among other reasons, millions of women use this drug to wake up and feel more energized each morning. It has been demonstrated to increase alertness, produce quicker reaction time, and reduce drowsiness. Coffee or colas are often the beverages college women drink to help "pull an all-nighter." This is because studies have shown that caffeine can improve reading speed, produce better results on math and verbal tests, and increase the capacity for sustained intellectual activities. However, if one desires to sleep, caffeine, even in small amounts, can cause sleep disturbances and increase the amount of time it takes to go to sleep.

Some of the research on caffeine's effects are inconsistent. For example, some studies indicate that this drug may *not* improve verbal or math abilities, nor short-term memory. Caffeine purportedly enhances athletic performance by helping the body metabolize fats for use as energy, saving glycogen for long-term energy. Drinking caffeine also appears to delay exhaustion in athletes following exertion. Yet, other studies basically refute these findings because caffeine causes little or no benefits in enhanced performance.

Caffeine Products

Coffee was not always the popular beverage that it is in today's society. It has fallen in and out of favor with humans living throughout the world. English women, in 1674, published an anti-coffee pamphlet entitled, "The Women's Petition Against Coffee," because it was believed that men who drank too much coffee were less lustful and more unfruitful.[48] Not true!

Coffee consumption was on the increase for years, however, there has been a downward trend since World War II. In 1993, about 10 pounds per person was ingested in this country.[49] Coffee intake appears to be on the rise once again.

Coffee is a stimulant and is used by millions of people to begin their day with a jolt! Coffee, in instant form, was introduced in the late 1800s and gained popularity during World War II. Instant coffee is less flavorful, but more convenient in today's busy world. As women continue to take on more time-consuming responsibilities, a quicker avenue to an enjoyable product is most appealing. A healthier product appears to be appealing, as well, as evidence by current widespread use of decaffeinated coffee. Americans today are consuming more decaffeinated coffee and less coffee with caffeine than ever before.

Tea in its early history was used medicinally but later came to be used more as a drink for social occasions. Pound for pound, tea has more caffeine than coffee, yet more cups of tea (about 200) are produced from a pound of dry tea leaves than cups of coffee (about 50–60) are made from a pound of coffee.[50] Therefore, less caffeine is found in an average cup of tea compared to an average cup of coffee. The caffeine content in a 5 oz. cup of tea can range from 18 mg to 107 mg, depending on the brand and the type of brew. As with coffee, flavored teas, instant tea, and herbal teas (some with artificial sweeteners) have gained greater popularity at home and in restaurants in this country than ever before.

Colas today contain less than 6 mg of caffeine for each ounce of cola. These types of beverages, both caffeinated and decaffeinated, are consumed increasingly worldwide. The history of colas is basically the history of the Coca-Cola Company, and most cola products are a replication of this product. Colas are considered to be refreshing, stimulating, and in sync with today's active lifestyle. Caffeine is an added ingredient in colas, whereas it is found naturally in coffee, tea, and chocolate. Although sugar-free and caffeine-free cola products are available and widely consumed, the well-known classic cola with sugar and caffeine is still the most widely sold. In the United States, the consumption of all colas averages approximately 47 gallons per person, per year.[51]

Chocolate was introduced in Europe before coffee or tea and its use grew slowly because the method of preparing it was not widely known. One of the women of history, Maria Theresa of France, wife of Louis XIV, thoroughly enjoyed chocolate and was instrumental in the promotion of its consumption. From chocolate bean, ground chocolate kernels, chocolate liquor, or cocoa butter to the Nestle milk chocolate of today, this substance has become one of the most widely consumed forms of caffeine. Caffeine in chocolate, though not as strong as caffeine in coffee, has similar physical effects. A cup of chocolate milk has about 4 mg of caffeine whereas caffeine in more dense baking chocolate ranges from 5 mg to 35 mg per ounce.

A number of over-the-counter (OTC) drugs containing caffeine produce a stimulating effect and suppress the appetite. They also may act as a stimulus for elimination of body fluids, called a diuretic. Products such as No Doz, Midol, Aqua-ban, and cold remedies have from 30 mg to 200 mg of caffeine as an active ingredient. Although one product alone may not impact greatly on daily caffeine consumption, women often ingest beverages, food, and OTC drugs each containing varying amounts of caffeine, which, when added together, can cause a number of unwanted physiological effects.

Now complete *Journal Activity:* "Your Caffeine Consumption" to determine your daily caffeine intake.

Effects of Caffeine on Health

Consumption of this psychoactive drug is widespread and acceptable, therefore research studies regarding caffeine use are numerous, varied, and to a large degree inconclusive. Data have been collected researching caffeine and its relationship to cancer, osteoporosis, pregnancy, benign breast disease, heart disease, nutrient absorption, cholesterol, gastrointestinal problems, and others. Let's consider the results of some of the studies as they pertain to women.

Osteoporosis is a loss of bone mass, especially in postmenopausal women, which can result in broken bones and fractures. A study reported by Bergman[52] found that women who consumed less than the Recommended Dietary Allowance (RDA) levels of calcium and who had a moderate intake of caffeine had decreased serum calcium levels and increased bone tissue turnover. In this same report, researchers

---

JOURNAL ACTIVITY

Your Caffeine Consumption

Over a 3-day period of time, record all intake of foods, drugs, and drinks you consume that contain caffeine. Determine your daily intake of milligrams of caffeine. The average daily intake of caffeine for a woman is 420 mg per day, about the equivalent of 4 to 5 cups of coffee. How does your consumption compare to this?

---

found a negative correlation between caffeine intake and dairy product intake, which magnifies the possibility of bone loss if a woman consumes low-calcium beverages in place of high-calcium beverages. The problem with loss of bone mass in women may not be due to consumption of caffeine-containing beverages, but drinking caffeine products instead of calcium-containing beverages. Women who do not consume calcium-rich foods throughout their life will increase their risk of osteoporosis, whether they drink caffeine or not.[53]

Pregnancy and caffeine intake have been the subject of numerous studies and the results are still not clear. A recent study cited in the Berkeley Wellness Letter[54] reported that pregnant women who drank 1.5 to 3 cups of coffee a day doubled the risk of miscarriage, and women who drank more than 3 cups per day during pregnancy, tripled the risk. A decrease in the birth weight of the fetus can occur due to slower growth during the fetal stage related to presence of caffeine in the mother. Additional studies conclude that females who consume caffeine reduce their chance of conceiving and increase the risk of miscarriage even if caffeine is ingested a month prior to conception. High levels of caffeine intake (300 mg or more per day) are potentially dangerous during pregnancy. Research is inconclusive about whether lower levels of caffeine consumption is safe. Because of this inconclusiveness, women should reduce or eliminate caffeine consumption if pregnant, or if considering becoming pregnant.

Fibrocystic breast disease consists of benign lumps that form in the woman's breast. Although these lumps are sometimes tender and painful, they are not cancerous. A plethora of research studies have found no relationship between caffeine intake and fibrocystic breast disease. However, some physicians advise women with benign breast lumps to eliminate caffeine consumption or at least consume it moderately. However, there is little scientific evidence that suggests that elimination of caffeine from the diet will improve conditions associated with fibrocystic breast disease.

Absorption of nutrients may be inhibited, not by caffeine, but by other substances in coffee, such as polyphenols. Important minerals, particularly calcium and iron, may not be utilized properly by the body as a result of drinking too many cups of caffeinated drinks each day. Because women are prone to develop osteoporosis, this information should create an awareness to be moderate in the consumption of caffeine-containing products.

Caffeinism

Caffeinism is the result of continual and excessive use of caffeine products, and may lead to a number of uncomfortable consequences. Women can develop a dependency and a tolerance to caffeine and, upon cessation of use, may experience headaches, nausea, irritability, depression, heart palpitations, insomnia, and reduced attention span. Although these symptoms are uncomfortable, they are short-lived and can usually be avoided by reducing caffeine consumption gradually.

Caffeine Research

As we have seen, caffeine research is largely inconclusive. Why is this so? Consider these variables: Each woman is biochemically different and the response to caffeine varies with each person; tolerance to caffeine may not be taken into account because studies often fail to isolate caffeine consumers from noncaffeine consumers; and the lifestyle of the research population may not be taken into account. For example, excessive coffee drinkers are sometimes more likely to smoke, have a high-fat diet, and not engage in exercise; therefore, negative health problems may be due to other lifestyle habits and not caffeine consumption.

It appears that moderate use of caffeine-containing products produces no major detrimental effect. However, as with many other issues, it is best to check with your physician if there is a concern.   ⚭

---

caffeinism (caff een ism)—chronic consumption of high levels of caffeine.

Chapter Summary

- Use of highly addictive tobacco products is a very serious health behavior among American women, and deaths related to tobacco use continue to increase.
- A number of factors influence women to begin and continue smoking. These include: media advertising, modeling parental and peer smoking habits, and the work and recreation environments.
- A number of substances in tobacco are toxic in the human body and cause morbidity and mortality in women. Types of morbidity include: heart diseases, cancers, disease of the respiratory system, osteoporosis, and aging skin.
- Environmental tobacco smoke (ETS) produces an environment laden with toxic chemicals and when breathed on a regular basis will cause a number of very serious diseases in women and children.
- Pregnant women should not smoke because of the serious detrimental effects, not only to the woman,

but especially to the developing fetus. Young children exposed to ETS will suffer a number of negative consequences.
- Cessation of smoking is difficult because of the highly addictive nature of the substances in tobacco. However, there are a number of smoking cessation programs, prescriptive aids, and behavioral changes that can be beneficial in this endeavor.
- The benefits of smoking cessation are numerous, both for your physical and financial health.
- Caffeine is found in many popular and widely used products and the health effects are still being researched.
- Caffeinated products such as colas, coffee, tea, and chocolate are sold all over the world and produce a number of concerns for the health of women.
- Women can develop a dependence upon caffeine.

Review Questions

1. What are mortality and morbidity? How has the number of women who smoke effected these rates in recent years?
2. How many women are current smokers? Has there been an increase or a decrease in the use of smoking tobacco among women? Why or why not?
3. What are four factors that influence women to smoke?
4. What effects do nicotine, carbon monoxide, and tar have on the body?
5. What are three diseases that result from smoking tobacco? How has smoking contributed to the development of these diseases?
6. What component in tobacco causes addition? What types of addiction patterns occur because of tobacco use?
7. What are the effects that environmental tobacco smoke has on the health of women and children who are exposed to it?
8. What are the risks for the fetus and for infants born to mothers who smoke during pregnancy?
9. What methods can be used to assist with smoking cessation?
10. In what ways can the Food and Drug Administration regulate tobacco use in the United States?
11. What are the benefits of quitting smoking? What is the length of time before a smoker can expect to experience these benefits?
12. In what ways can women's use of caffeine interfere with reproduction?
13. Does caffeine increase the risk of developing breast cancer? Why or why not?
14. What are the physiological and behavioral effects associated with the consumption of excessive caffeine?
15. What is the difference between the amount of caffeine found in a 12 oz. can of Coca-Cola, one cup of brewed coffee, a bar of chocolate candy, and a cup of brewed tea?
16. What are the indications that a woman has developed a dependence upon caffeine and what can be done to reverse the effects?

Resources

Organizations and Hotlines

American Cancer Society
1599 Clifton Road, NE
Atlanta, GA 30329
Telephone: (800) ACS-2345

American Lung Association
1740 Broadway
New York, NY 10019-4374
Telephone: (800) LUNG-USA or (212) 315-8700

ASH (Action on Smoking and Health)
2013 H St. NW
Washington, DC
Telephone: (202) 659-4310

Council for Tobacco Research
900 Third Ave.
New York, NY 10022
Telephone: (212) 421-8885

Drug Alcohol Tobacco Education (DATE)
3426 Bridgeland Drive
Bridgeton, MO 63044
Telephone: (314) 739-1121

Office of Smoking and Health (OSH)
3005 Rhodes Building (Kroger Center)
Chamblee, GA 30341-3724
Telephone: (404) 488-5705

Tobacco Institute
1875 I St., NW
Washington, DC 20006
Telephone: (202) 457-4800

Women's Health Initiatives
U.S. Department of Health and Human Services
Public Health Services
National Institutes of Health
Federal Building, Room 6A09
Bethesda, MD 20892
Telephone: (800) 54-WOMEN (800) 549-6636

Websites

Health Information Resources
http://nhic-nt.health.org/cgi-shl/...m&
Descriptor=FEDERAL+CLEARINGHOUSE

National Women's Resource Center
http://www.nwrc.org/

Tobacco BBS
http://www.tobacco.orh/

Women's Health Initiative
http://wellweb.com/survey/whi.HTM

Suggested Readings

Photo-Talk about Tobacco: Look Who's Getting Burned. 1992 brochure (8 pages) on tobacco and prevention (English & Spanish). Available at: Tobacco Education, Clearinghouse of California ETR Associates, PO Box 1830, Santa Cruz, CA 1-800-321-4407

Report of the Tobacco Policy Research Group on Marketing and Promotions Targeted at African Americans, Latinos, and Women. Tobacco Control Source I.D.: 1(suppl):S24–S30, 1992. Available from: Dr. Robert G. Robinson, Fox Chase Cancer Center, 510 Township Line Road, Cheltenham, PA 19012

References

1. American Cancer Society. 1994. Effective tobacco reduction strategies. *The Advocate* V (1).
2. Ray, O., and C. Ksir. 1996. *Drugs, society and human behavior.* St. Louis, MO: Mosby. 1996.
3. Brownlee, S., S. V. Roberts, M. Cooper, E. Goode, K. Hetter, and A. Wright. 1994. *U.S. News & World Report* 116, 32–36, 38.
4. Tobacco and women's health. (URL: http://www.health-net.com/tobac.htm.)
5. Lopez, A., and R. Peto. 1992. Tobacco mortality present and future. *Tobacco Alert: World Health Organization,* 9–10.
6. Chollat-Traquet, C. 1992. Women and tobacco. *8th World Conference on Tobacco & Health.* Buenos Aires: World Health Organization.
7. Erickson, A. C., J. W. McKenna, and R. M. Romano. 1990. Past lessons and new lessons of the mass media in reducing tobacco consumption. *Public Health Reports,* 105 (3): 239–44.
8. Siren's song of cigarette advertising. In *The Bryan/College Station Eagle,* Bryan, Tex., 13 August 1995, D2.
9. Lorand, A. 1927. *Life shortening habits and rejuvenation.* Philadelphia: FA Davis.
10. Burns, D. M. 1991. Cigarettes and cigarette smoking. *Clinics in Chest Medicine,* 12, 631–42.
11. Environmental tobacco smoke. (URL: http://mox.perl.com/smoking/ets.html.)
12. Evans, G. D. 1993. Cigarette smoke=radiation hazards. *Pediatrics,* 92, 464.
13. Pinger, R., W. Payne, D. Hahn, and E. Hahn. 1995. *Issues for today: Drugs.* St. Louis: Mosby.
14. Hatcher, R. E. A. 1992. *Contraceptive technology, 1992–1993.* New York: Irvington Publishers.
15. Pruitt, B., and J. J. Stein. 1994. *Healthstyles: Decisions for living well.* New York: Saunders College Publishing.
16. Doweiko, H. 1996. *Concepts of chemical dependency.* Boston: Brooks/Cole.
17. Ibid.
18. Bartecchi, C., T. MacKenzie, and R. Schrier. 1994. The human cost of tobacco use. *The New England Journal of Medicine,* 330 (13): 907–12.
19. Williamson, D., J. Madans, R. Anda, J. C. Kleinman, G. A. Giovino, and T. Byers. 1991. Smoking cessation and severity of weight gain in a national cohort. *The New England Journal of Medicine,* 324, 739–45.
20. Hankinson, S., W. C. Willet, G. A. Colditz, J. M. Seddon, B. Rosner, F. E. Speizer, and M. J. Stamper. 1992. A prospective study of cigarette smoking and risk of cataract surgery in women. *Journal of the American Medical Association,* 268, 994–98.
21. Doweiko, *Concepts of chemical dependency.*
22. Hopper, J. S., and E. Seeman. 1994. The bone density of female twins discordant for tobacco use. *The New England Journal of Medicine,* 330, 387–92.
23. Doweiko, *Concepts of chemical dependency.*
24. Ibid.
25. Rustin, T. 1992. *Review of nicotine and its treatment.* LaCrosse, Wisc.: Symposium at St. Francis Hospital.
26. Cancer, P.S.A.L. (URL: http://medic.med.uth.tmc.edu/ptnt/00000279.htm.)
27. Ibid.
28. Brownson, R., M. C. R. Alavanja, E. T. Hock, and T. S. Loy. 1992. Passive smoking and lung cancer in nonsmoking women. *American Journal of Public Health,* 82 (11): 1525–30.
29. Pinger et al., *Issues for today.*
30. Secondhand smoke, firsthand vitamin loss. 1994. In *Tufts University Diet & Nutrition Letter* 12 (4): 1.
31. Pinger et al., *Issues for today.*
32. Coste, J., N. Job-Spira, and H. Fernandez. 1991. Increased risk of ectopic pregnancy with maternal cigarette smoking. *American Journal of Public Health,* 81 (2): 199–201.
33. Lieberman, E., I. Gremy, J. Lang, and A. Cohen. 1994. Low birthweight at term and the timing of fetal exposure. *American Journal of Public Health,* 84 (7): 1127–31.
34. Vio, F., G. Salazar, and C. Infante. 1991. Smoking during pregnancy and lactation and its effect on breast milk volume. *American Journal of Clinical Nutrition,* 54, 1011–16.
35. Waller, K. (URL: http://www.arph.org/clinical/index.html.)

36. Ibid.
37. Christen, A., and J. A. Christen. 1994. Why is cigarette smoking so addicting? An overview of smoking as a chemical and process addiction. *Health Values,* 18 (1): 17–24.
38. Psyching up to quit. 1990. In *Lifetime Health Letter 5.* University of Texas, Health Science Center at Houston.
39. Ibid.
40. Smoking: Facts and quitting tips for black Americans. 1992. Pamphlet no. 92–3405. U.S. Dept. of Health and Human Services. Washington, DC: National Cancer Institute.
41. American Cancer Society. 1992. When smokers quit. *The Advocate,* IV (1): 1.
42. Ibid.
43. American Cancer Society. 1988. Smart move. Pamphlet no. 2515–LE.
44. Psyching up to quit.
45. For coffee drinkers, a shift in the daily grind. 1994. In *Tufts University Diet & Nutrition Letter.* 12 (5): 4–6.
46. Blonz, E. 1995. The buzz about caffeine. *Better Homes and Gardens,* 73, 50.
47. Pinger et al., *Issues for today.*
48. Ray and Ksir, *Drugs, society and human behavior.*
49. Ibid.
50. Ibid.
51. Ibid.
52. Bergman, E., M. L. Erickson, and J. C. Boyungs. 1992. Caffeine knowledge, attitudes, and consumption in adult women. *Journal of Nutrition Education,* 24, 179–84.
53. Coffee breaks. 1994. In *University of California at Berkeley Wellness Letter,* 10 (7): 1–2.
54. Coffee: grounds for concern. 1994. In *University of California Berkeley Wellness Letter,* 10 (6): 4–5.

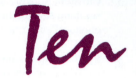

Using Alcohol Responsibly

■ chapter objectives

When you complete this chapter you will be able to:

- Explain the unique relationship between women, especially college women, and their use of alcohol.
- Identify and describe the various types of alcohol.
- Identify some of the negative effects that the abuse of alcohol can produce upon the physical, behavioral, psychological, and societal aspects as well as upon relationships in the lives of women.
- Describe the serious consequences between the use of alcohol during pregnancy and the negative effects upon the fetus and infant.
- Explain the process of addiction and alcoholism in women.
- Identify the appropriate resources to assist alcoholic women and their families.
- Suggest guidelines that can be used by colleges and universities to reduce alcohol abuse among college women.

WOMEN AND ALCOHOL

Alcohol, an intoxicating, but toxic chemical, has been consumed by humans for thousands of years. Early writings about alcohol use are found in Hebrew script, Egyptian tablets, and Chinese laws in which the use of wine was either allowed or disallowed over 41 times between 1100 B.C. and A.D. 1400.[1] Used for many purposes and reasons, alcohol is a drug of choice for present-day Americans who spend over $65 billion a year on alcoholic beverages of all varieties.

Societal attitudes regarding women's use of alcohol have been inconsistent and ambivalent. Roman laws did not allow women to drink alcoholic beverages because it was thought to make women aggressive and promiscuous; the Talmud denounced the overconsumption of alcohol by women, stating:

> One cup of wine is good for a woman;
> Two are degrading;
> Three induce her to act like an immoral woman;
> And four cause her to lose all self-respect and sense of shame.[2]

However, in ancient Babylon, women were temple priestesses who brewed beer. In Greco-Roman cults, women were a part of ceremonies in which alcohol was consumed. Through the centuries, alcoholic beverages were used medicinally and ceremoniously, but usually not in recreational circumstances as it is presently used. In early America, women played a significant role in the control of alcohol use as participants of the temperance movement, which was an attempt to "temper" or curtail the use of hard liquor (distilled spirits).

The Women's Christian Temperance Union was formed in the late 1800s in Cleveland, Ohio and women such as Carrie Nation, Mary H. Hunt, and Frances Willard were actively involved with this movement. In fact, Carrie Nation, with fevered activities, was arrested more than 30 times. Rather than advocating temperance, these women promoted complete prohibition—no sale or consumption of alcohol. In 1920 prohibition became law as the Eighteenth Amendment to the Constitution prohibiting the manufacture, sale, and transportation of the substance was passed. However, this law was difficult to enforce as even former abstainers began to drink as a rebellious act; personal freedom was lost and alcohol use became a "smart thing" to do. Alcohol was manufactured and provided outside the law and bootlegging became big business. By 1931 the Commission of Law Enforcement branded prohibition as a failure and in 1933, after 13 years of attempting to enforce prohibition, the Twenty-first Amendment was passed that repealed the Eighteenth Amendment. Today, alcohol is a legal substance with certain restrictions and is regulated by state governments.

Alcohol: The Beverage

Wine, beer, and distilled spirits contain **ethyl alcohol** or ethanol, a clear, somewhat tasteless, toxic liquid that initially causes a slight burning sensation when ingested and creates an intoxicating effect. It is a beverage produced through a process called **fermentation,** a chemical reaction between a mixture of yeast, sugar, and water. An average serving of wine (about 3½ oz.), distilled spirits (1-oz. shot), and beer (12-oz. mug) each contain approximately one-half ounce of pure ethyl alcohol and therefore produce similar effects on blood alcohol levels.

The alcohol content of a beverage varies in the percentage of alcohol contained in it. Beer has about 4 percent alcohol content unless the beverage is

HEALTHY PEOPLE 2000 OBJECTIVES

- Reduce the proportion of high school seniors and college students engaging in recent occasions of heavy drinking of alcoholic beverages to no more than 28 percent of high school seniors and 32 percent of college students. 1995 progress toward goal: high school seniors: 100 percent; college students: 20 percent
- Reduce the incidence of fetal alcohol syndrome to no more than 0.12 per 1,000 live births. 1995 progress toward goal: –450 percent

labeled low-alcohol beer, which is about 1.5 percent alcohol content. Wine has about a 12 percent alcohol content; however, fortified wine, such as port, contains 18 percent alcohol. Champagne is about 12 percent and wine coolers are approximately 6 percent alcohol. The percentage of ethyl alcohol in distilled spirits (gin, rum, or scotch, for example) is stated in terms of **proof,** usually ranging from 80–190. In distilled spirits, proof is twice the percentage of alcohol by concentration (e.g., 100 proof would be 50 percent pure ethyl alcohol). The remaining ingredients in distilled spirits consist of *congeners,* which are by-products of distillation such as other alcohol, oils, and organic matter and other liquids that influence the taste and color of the beverage. (See *FYI:* "What Is a Hangover?")

Alcohol, although providing calories in a person's diet, is not a good source of nutrition. A fluid ounce of distilled spirits will yield about 100 calories and twelve ounces of beer about 150 calories. The nutrient density, however, is virtually nonexistent.

ethyl alcohol—a clear, somewhat tasteless liquid found in various types of beverages that produce intoxication; ethanol.

fermentation—process by which sugars are converted into grain alcohol through the action of yeast.

proof—measurement of ethyl alcohol content found in beverages; stated in terms of percentages.

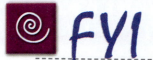

What Is a Hangover?

Have you ever heard someone say, "I'll never drink again, I feel like I have the drum section of a marching band in my head." They probably were experiencing a hangover caused by overindulging in alcoholic beverages. Hangovers are believed to be the symptoms of withdrawal from alcohol, and may include a headache, nausea, diarrhea, thirst, anxiety, depression, and general discomfort. Hangovers are not only caused by overconsumption of pure ethyl alcohol, but also are believed to be caused by congeners. Congeners, which are products of fermentation and the preparation process, provide the variety of taste, color, and smell in alcoholic beverages. What helps stop the distress associated with a hangover? A cold shower, another drink, coffee? Unfortunately, the "cure" is not quite that simple. Usually a pain killer for the headache and an antacid for the nausea will provide some relief. However, rest and time are the only "treatments" that will eventually eliminate the hangover. Perhaps you should decide if there is any "good time" for alcohol overconsumption, worth the resulting misery of a hangover, and the loss of a day in your life often needed to recover.   ☜

FIGURE 10.1 BAC is the level of alcohol contained in a person's blood volume. For example, a woman with a BAC of 0.10 percent has one part of alcohol for every 1,000 parts of blood. This BAC is considered legally drunk in all states. However, a BAC as low as 0.05 percent can impair function enough to cause a serious accident.

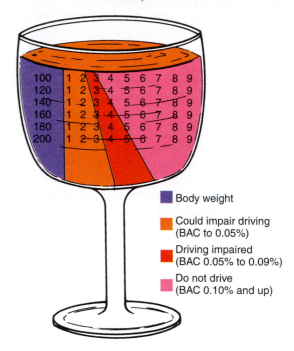

Number of drinks
in 2-hour period
($1\frac{1}{2}$-oz 86-proof liquor
or 12-oz beer)

■ Body weight

■ Could impair driving
(BAC to 0.05%)

■ Driving impaired
(BAC 0.05% to 0.09%)

■ Do not drive
(BAC 0.10% and up)

These beverages contain no vitamins, minerals, fat, or protein, and only a small amount of carbohydrates. This is an example of what is meant by "empty calories," meaning calories consumed from a food source lacking important nutrients.[3] As people have become more calorie-conscious, "light or lite" beer and wine have been introduced. The calorie content of these beverages has been reduced, but not the alcohol content.

Alcohol is a simple chemical and does not need to be digested to move into the bloodstream. Following ingestion, 5 percent of alcohol leaves the body through sweat, urine, or breath unchanged by any chemical reaction. For the remaining 95 percent to be removed from the body, it must be metabolized, or chemically changed. To do this the body begins to break down ingested alcohol as soon as it reaches the liver through a process called **oxidation.**

Absorption of alcohol takes place through the stomach in which about 20 percent is absorbed directly into the bloodstream, and from the small intestine in which 80 percent is absorbed and moves into the bloodstream and to all parts of the body. The absorption of alcohol in the body is determined by a number of factors. These include:

- Number of drinks consumed. The greater the number of alcoholic beverages consumed by a female, the faster the alcohol will be absorbed into the blood stream.
- Strength of alcoholic beverage. Beverages with higher concentrations of alcohol will increase the blood alcohol concentration (BAC). (See Fig. 10.1.)
- Other beverages. Alcohol mixed with fruit juices or plain water will be absorbed at a slower rate; "straight" alcohol or alcohol mixed with carbonated beverages will be absorbed at a faster rate.

Table 10.1

Types of Alcohol	
Ethyl (Ethanol)	Alcohol beverages
	Over-the-counter drugs
Methyl (Methanol)	Antifreeze, solvents
Isopropyl	Disinfectant rubbing alcohol
Butyl	Industrial and medical applications found in anesthesia

- Foods in the stomach. Foods with higher fat content will slow absorption because there is less stomach area exposed and protein in the food retains the alcohol.
- Emotional factors. Absorption of alcohol into the bloodstream can be affected by such factors as emotions (jealousy, anger, fear), illness, stress, and expectations.
- Blood chemistry. Each of us are biochemical individuals; absorption may be quickened or slowed due to an individual's blood chemistry.

Three additional types of alcohol are *methanol, isopropyl,* and *butyl,* each of which are toxic to human beings. (See Table 10.1.) Methyl alcohol, also called "wood alcohol," is an ingredient in such products as turpentine, solvents, and antifreeze. Isopropyl, a clear, colorless, bitter liquid, is a disinfectant used in rubbing alcohol; butyl alcohol, obtained from petroleum, is used in industrial and medication applications and may be found in anesthesia. None of these should be ingested by women because doing so could cause serious illness or death.

Why Liquor Is Quicker for Women

The absorption of alcohol in the body influences to an extent the physical and behavioral effects experienced by the person ingesting it. An enzyme, **alcohol dehydrogenase (ADH),** in the liver and in the stomach (gastric) lining, helps to break down the alcohol before it enters the bloodstream. The ADH activity in the stomach is lower in women than in men. As a result, about 30 percent more alcohol enters the female bloodstream, thus causing more alcohol to reach the female brain at a faster rate and creating an intoxicating effect; therefore, higher blood alcohol concentration (BAC) is reached by women at a faster rate than for men. Over years of drinking, as frequency and consumption of alcohol increases, the liver starts to fail, hence producing less ADH, causing the effectiveness of this enzyme to be impaired. Con-

sequently, women will absorb almost all alcohol consumed without breaking it down, and the effect will be similar to alcohol being intravenously injected.

Drinking equivalent amounts of ethyl alcohol per pound of body weight will produce a higher peak of alcohol level for women than for men. This may be due to the higher percentage of body water in men (55–65 percent) than in women (45–55 percent), causing alcohol to be less diluted in women than in men. Ethyl alcohol is highly water- and fat-soluble. Because women have more body fat than men of the same weight and because alcohol is not easily diffused rapidly into body fat, females will have a higher amount of alcohol concentration in the blood than men. Considering each of these factors, a woman's ability to perform certain tasks (e.g., driving, speaking, decision making) will be impaired at a faster rate than a man's.

During the premenstrual stage of the menstrual cycle, alcohol will be absorbed more quickly into the bloodstream. However, with fluid retention during the premenstrual cycle, alcohol in the blood will be more diluted and will have a reduced effect on the central nervous system. For a 130-pound woman who is in the premenstrual part of her cycle, 3 alcoholic drinks in an hour will produce the feelings of giddiness, happiness, and perhaps impulsive and clumsy actions. The same amount of alcohol over the same time period during the middle of the menstrual cycle may or can generate reduced attention span, uncontrolled laughter, and sometimes inappropriate behaviors.[4]

WOMEN AND ALCOHOL: A UNIQUE RELATIONSHIP

In the past, women have used alcohol medicinally to reduce menstrual cramps, lessen pain associated with childbirth, and for fortification while breastfeeding.[5] It has been used in recreational settings to promote the "time away" environment and as a

oxidation (ox ah **day** shun)—any process in which the oxygen content of a compound is increased.

alcohol dehydrogenase (ADH) (dee **hi** dro **jen** ase)—an enzyme in the liver that metabolizes almost all of the alcohol consumed by an individual.

Table 10.2

Drinking Classifications

CLASSIFICATION	ALCOHOL-RELATED BEHAVIOR
Abstainers	Do not drink or drink less often than once a year.
Light drinkers	Per drinking occasion, may drink once a month in small to medium amounts or drink small amounts no more than three or four times a month.
Moderate drinkers	Per drinking occasion, drink small amounts at least once a week or drink medium amounts three to four times a month or large amounts no more than once a month.
Moderate/heavy drinkers	Per drinking occasion, drink medium amounts at least once a week or large amounts three to four times a month.
Heavy drinkers	Per drinking occasion, drink large amounts at least once a week.

NOTE: Small amounts = One drink or less per drinking occasion

Medium amounts = Two to four drinks per drinking occasion

Large amounts = Five or more drinks per drinking occasion

One drink = 12 fluid oz. of beer, 4 fluid oz. of wine, or 1 fluid oz. of distilled spirits

Table 10.3

What's the Difference in Drinking Preferences?[6]

ALCOHOL USE	WOMEN	MEN
Frequency	Less often	More often
Consumption amounts	Smaller amounts	Greater amounts
Beverage preference	Spirits, beer, and wine	Beer, spirits, and wine
Drinking locations	Restaurants, clubs	At games, dorms, and concerts
Drinking companions	Mixed groups	Male groups
Intoxication levels	Usually not to get drunk	Drink to get drunk
Effects of drinking problems	On academics, and relationships	Creates more problems (accidents, and difficulties with family and school)

"social lubricant" to ease social interactions. As the discussion of alcohol continues, Table 10.2 helps to explain the various classifications of alcohol consumers. This should provide you with what is meant by small, moderate, and heavy use of alcohol and foster a better perspective for alcohol use and its consequences.

Are there special concerns for use of this chemical by women? How much is too much? Alcohol, a depressant *psychoactive drug,* produces a number of unique qualities that are of special interest and concern for women. For example, a daily glass of wine with dinner can add as much as 10 pounds of body fat a year; it can increase the risk of developing breast cancer and osteoporosis. Women who drink large amounts of alcohol are more likely than men to develop cirrhosis of the liver and other alcohol-related diseases. In fact, the overall rate of premature death related to alcohol abuse is 50–100 percent higher for women than for men and can reduce a woman's lifespan by as much as 15 years. This would yield a life expectancy of only 63 years. Heavy female drinkers, more than men, are more susceptible to depression and suicide attempts. Overconsumption of alcohol is less socially acceptable for women than for men. Society often considers women who drink too much more likely to engage in sexual activity. (Compare the differences between men's and women's drinking preferences during the college years in Table 10.3.)

Alcohol Consumption

Approximately two-thirds of the adult population drink alcoholic beverages; however, according to the 1992 National Institute on Drug Abuse's college survey[7] over 88 percent of college students drank alcohol at the beginning of this decade. People who

JOURNAL ACTIVITY

Alcohol Consumption Record

If you make the choice to drink, it is a wise idea to monitor your consumption. Below is a chart you can use to determine when, where, with whom, and how much you are drinking. If you find that you are experiencing problems as a result of alcohol consumption, it is important to seek professional help. The information recorded on this chart can be beneficial to your success.

Date	Time	Where	With Whom	Number of Drinks

choose to drink have varied drinking patterns and consumption levels. Only 20 percent of all alcohol beverages are consumed by approximately 70 percent of the drinking public. The remaining 80 percent of alcohol is consumed by 30 percent of people who drink and they can be categorized as heavy drinkers, or even alcoholics. This information was explained in an interesting and understandable way by Kinney and Leaton:

Ten beers shared among ten individuals who follow adult drinking patterns would likely be divided in this way:

3 persons abstain—representing the one-third who choose not to drink

5 persons share 2 beers—70 percent of drinkers drink 20 percent of the alcohol

2 persons share 8 beers—30 percent of drinkers drink 80 percent of the alcohol. Of these 2 drinkers, one drinks 2 beers, and the other drinks 6 beers.[8]

College-Aged Women and Alcohol

Today, more than in the past, college females are more often engaging in violations of university policies and experiencing greater negative health, aca-

demic, and social consequences. Why? Alcohol is a factor. Although the percentage of college women (34 percent) who say they drink has remained constant, college women are now drinking more often and more excessively than they did in the past.[9] Studies reveal that more women have increased their alcohol intake at one sitting, and more are drinking for the purpose of "getting drunk." In 1979, 10 percent of college females reported drinking for the purpose of getting drunk, and today, more than 35 percent drink for the same purpose. A study at Columbia University revealed that 90 percent of all reported campus rapes occurred when alcohol had been used by either the rapist, or the victim or both. Additionally, 60 percent of college women who had a sexually transmitted disease were drunk at the time of infection. Interestingly, alcohol use increases with increased education and income. Twenty percent of women with at least some college education are moderate to heavy drinkers, compared to 8 percent of women who do not have a high school education and drink alcohol.[10] (See *Her Story:* "Jessica.")

With the knowledge that abuse of alcohol certainly has serious consequences for some, women still feel the need to overconsume a chemical that can be a destructive force in their lives. Why is this the case? If you choose to drink, for what reasons do

you drink? How do your reasons compare with those of other college women? They include:

- To relieve stress and anxiety
- To feel more sociable
- To decrease inhibitions
- For the "high" that results
- To be part of the group
- To lessen sexual inhibitions
- To escape
- To relieve worrying
- To become less self-conscious
- To reduce depression

Colleges and universities are taking a closer look at the serious consequences that result from overconsumption of alcohol on campuses. *FYI:* "Reducing Alcohol Abuse on Campus" lists a number of measures that are being adopted on numerous campuses to curb the use of alcohol and the resulting consequences.

Health Tips: "Drinking Alcohol Responsibly" provides suggestions you can use as guidelines for drinking alcohol responsibly.

Associated Effects

Have you ever experienced negative consequences as the result of alcohol abuse? Overconsumption of alcohol can produce immediate and long-term negative physical, behavioral, psychological, social, and relational consequences. Although many of these negative outcomes are the result of chronic alcohol abuse, undesirable consequences can also result from occasional overconsumption of alcohol.

Hormonal Effects Physical effects resulting from alcohol consumption, especially long-term abuse of alcohol, can be serious and in some instances life threatening. Serious consequences, for example, include the impairment of proper functioning of essential hormones, briefly defined as chemical messengers that control and coordinate the operation of all tissues and organs. Hormone impairment results in a number of significant and severe medical consequences. One significant hormonal consequence of alcohol abuse causes low blood sugar levels, called hypoglycemia, and prevents an effective hormonal response to this condition.

Chronic heavy alcohol consumption can hamper a female's reproductive hormone functioning leading to a number of serious repercussions. For example, breast development, distribution of body hair, regulation of the menstrual cycle, and disruption of a pregnancy can be the results of impaired hormone functioning caused by alcohol abuse. Long-term consequences include serious hormonal deficiencies, sexual dysfunction, and infertility. Chronic heavy drinking in college-aged women can lead to menstruation cessation, menstrual cycle irregularities, failure to ovulate, and infertility. During pregnancy alcohol use can increase the likelihood of spontaneous abortion (miscarriage). Studies indicate a relationship between female alcoholism and sexual dysfunction, especially **anorgasmia.** The majority of female reproductive irregularities were found in studies of alcoholic women; however, a number of problems were also found in women who drank approximately 3 drinks per day.

Women, in general, are at increased risk for developing calcium-deficiency disorders, especially osteoporosis. However, alcohol consumption exacerbates this problem by causing hormone imbalances that reduce calcium absorption, excretion, and distribution. As a result calcium and bone metabolism are impaired. Additionally, acute alcohol intake prevents proper utilization of calcium and causes an increase in urinary calcium excretion. Because chronic drinking can disturb vitamin D metabolism, there is an increased risk of osteoporosis due to inadequate absorption of dietary calcium.

Studies have revealed a distinct link between alcohol intake and breast cancer. One recent study indicated that daily consumption of one ounce of pure ethyl alcohol (about two drinks), produced higher levels of estrogen in the body than when no alcohol was consumed. Increased production of estrogen has been linked to developing breast cancer. Another study found that even moderate alcohol ingestion was associated with a 50 percent increase in the risk for development of breast cancer.[11] To help explain this, if the risk for a female developing breast cancer

is 1 in 10, the risk for a female drinker would be 1.5 in 10. In other words, 10 out of 100 nondrinkers might get breast cancer, whereas 15 out of 100 drinkers may develop breast cancer.

On a more positive note, postmenopausal women who ingested alcohol in moderation (3–6 drinks per week) raised their estrogen levels and reduced the risk of developing cardiovascular diseases. This was accomplished without significantly reducing bone quality or increasing the risk of liver disease or breast cancer.

The effect of alcohol on hormone levels in women are important to know. For example, what effects do hormone levels and alcohol have on the progression of diseases such as osteoporosis and heart diseases and the development of alcohol-induced liver disease in postmenopausal women who are heavier drinkers?[12] Additional concerns related to alcohol and medications containing hormones include the possibility of impairment of reproductive functioning, suppression of the immune system, the development of cancer,[13] adverse effects on the menstrual cycle, and potential for early menopause.[14]

Medications containing estrogen, such as birth control pills or hormone replacement drugs, affect a woman's reaction to alcohol. Drinking alcohol in moderate amounts increases the estrogen levels in postmenopausal women. Approximately 1 in 4 postmenopausal women are involved in hormone replacement therapy, which lowers their risk for osteoporosis and heart disease and possibly increases their risk of developing breast cancer; research studies determined that 1–2 ounces of vodka tripled estrogen levels in women.[15] Studies suggest that any benefits derived from increased estrogen levels is maximal when alcohol intake averages *no more* than one drink a day.[16] (See *FYI:* "Are There Any Benefits to Drinking Alcohol?")

What should you do? Consultation with a physician should help you weigh the benefits versus the risks of taking medications with estrogen. Consider your family medical history related to cancer, heart disease, and osteoporosis, and your lifestyle as it relates to alcohol consumption, exercise, diet, and other health promotion or health risk behaviors. (See Table 10.4.)

anorgasmia (an or **gaz** me ya)—condition resulting in an inability to experience orgasm; also called orgasmic dysfunction.

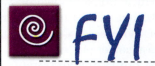

Are There Any Benefits to Drinking Alcohol?

Although the use and abuse of alcohol results in many negative consequences, studies have also determined that there are also a number of benefits from the *moderate* use of alcohol. Remember, moderate use of alcohol for women is one, or at the most, two drinks per day. (Refer back to Table 10.2.) These benefits include:

- Decreased risk of heart attack.
- Increases of high-density lipoprotein (HDL), the "good cholesterol."
- Decreased risk of coronary artery disease.
- Decreased anxiety.
- Relaxation.
- Increased ease during social situations.
- Increased life expectancy.

Although these benefits have been reported in professional literature, it must also be noted that there are additional methods by which you can gain these benefits without using a potentially addicting and toxic drug. This is one of the many lifestyle decisions we must make by considering all potential alternatives and consequences.

Dieting One interesting study revealed that college females who were dieting were more likely to drink alcohol than females who were not dieting.[17] In fact there was a strong relationship between the impulsiveness of dieting and the serious consumption of alcohol. The study revealed that females who were not dieting consumed less alcohol than females who were dieting. Additionally, dieting females who also drank alcohol experienced more harmful consequences, such as blackouts, unintended sex, and sexually transmitted diseases than nondrinking dieters. Another interesting aspect of this study was that females who stopped dieting did not decrease their intake of alcohol.

Disease When compared to men, women with alcohol-related problems are disabled more frequently and for longer periods of time. Alcohol-related liver damage in women develops after shorter periods of alcohol use and lower levels of consumption than with men. Studies have shown that alcohol-related diseases in women were comparable to that of men, even when the women had been drinking to excess for a significantly shorter period of time than men (14.2 years vs. 20.2 years). Such diseases and disorders as hypertension, obesity, malnutrition, fatty liver, and anemia developed in a briefer period of time for alcohol-abusing women.[18]

Table 10.4

The Physical Consequences of Alcohol Abuse	
Reproductive system	Early menopause, amenorrhea, infertility, miscarriage, fetal alcohol syndrome.
Sexuality	Reduced physiological arousal, decreased orgasmic intensity, sexual dysfunction.
Endocrine system	Increased possibility of osteoporosis, nutritional and metabolic disorders, poor absorption, and utilization of essential nutrients.
Cardiovascular system	Hypertension, cardiomyopathy, dysrhythmias, coronary artery disease; slows manufacture of red blood cells; degenerates blood clotting ability.
Liver	Chemical imbalance: liver fat accumulation, blood sugar imbalance, and altered protein production. Inflammation: impaired circulation, scar tissue formation, and alcohol-related hepatitis. Cirrhosis: poor circulation, kidney failure, and possibly death.
Digestive system	Oral: promotes possibility of cancer of the mouth, tongue, and throat. Esophagus: impaired swallowing. Stomach: irritation, gastritis, and ulceration. Pancreas: inflammation. Digestion: impaired absorption, and possible malnutrition. Nausea: diarrhea and vomiting.

Ethnicity Death rates associated with alcohol-related causes in 1990 was 2.8 per 100,000 for Caucasian females and 7.7 per 100,000 for African American females. The alcohol-induced death rate for African American women is higher than for women in the total population.[19]

Use of alcohol is more prevalent among Caucasian women than among women of other ethnic origins. Among moderate to heavy drinkers, 11 percent are African American women, 9 percent are Hispanic, 6 percent are Asian women; and 17 percent are Caucasian women.

Researchers have found an increase in alcohol consumption among Mexican American women with each successive generation, following their immigration to the United States. These changes in drinking patterns are thought to be part of an acculturation process in which these women adopt the behaviors and attitudes of women in the general population.[20,21]

Behavioral Effects Although long-term chronic alcohol abuse can cause a variety of negative physical consequences, a number of severe behavioral consequences can result from short-term or binge drinking. Alcohol-related behavior pertains not only to what women themselves do, but also what women may allow others to do to them. Because alcohol reduces a woman's inhibitions, or concerns about "what may happen if," she is more likely to act upon the immediate circumstances rather than considering the consequences of her actions. Steele called this social and behavioral "myopia" or nearsightedness because females are less mindful of long-term consequences, and concentrate more on the present.[22] Examples include making a decision to leave a party or club or have sexual relations with some person she just met, driving after drinking, picking up a hitchhiker, or being verbally abusive to friends or family. Each of these situations can have long-term serious consequences because they may lead to negative societal and relationship-related consequences. In each instance, a woman would probably make a different decision if she was not disinhibited by alcohol consumption.

A number of research studies investigated the long-term behavioral effects of alcohol abuse in regard to women. One study determined that women who abuse alcohol often develop impaired ability to function in the social world, asocial behavior, and antisocial behavior.[23] Indicators of impaired social world functioning include such effects as financial irresponsibility, unusual accidents such as falling down stairs, impulsiveness, dysfunctional relationships, and poor parenting skills. Asocial behavior indicators include poor communication skills, irresponsibility regarding appointments or commitments, relinquishing former hobbies or activities, and even discarding friendships. Shoplifting and stealing from family or friends were cited as indicators of antisocial behavior of female alcohol abusers.

Psychological effects related to alcohol abuse can be serious. Women may experience anxiety, guilt, and stress; exhibit disinhibitions, aggressiveness, and other strong emotions; or have strong dependency needs. Women may become suspicious of others, grow defensive, or even demonstrate obsessive-compulsive behaviors such as being a "super student" or compulsively perfectionistic. Compared to male drinkers, female drinkers who chronically abuse alcohol are more likely to experience bouts of depression.

Society often has a double standard related to women and men regarding alcohol consumption. Consider the following perceptions as reported in an article in *Alcohol Health & Research World.*[24] Drinking appears to imply permissiveness by a woman when related to rape situations. In fact, both men and women are less likely to perceive an occurrence of forced intercourse as rape when the victim and perpetrator had been drinking together. Following a sexual assault, the victim and the perpetrator are more likely to date again if both had been drinking at the time of the rape. You may be angered by these perceptions, but ask yourself these questions: What term(s) and statements are used to describe a female in a social setting (party, club) if she is drinking too much and is loud and overfriendly? Are the same words used to describe a man behaving in the same manner? What are the judgments of character and morals in each of these situations? When it comes to the use and abuse of alcohol by men and women, is there a double standard?

Social Effects Social consequences related to alcohol use and abuse are many. Alcohol often fosters relaxing effects that enable women to feel more confident, relaxed, and less inhibited in social situations. Although this may be perceived as a positive result of alcohol consumption, certainly being able to experience these qualities in social settings without the use of an intoxicating beverage would be an important skill to possess. In some instances abuse of alcohol can occur in social environments to the point at which such abuse becomes detrimental to our social well-being and to society at large. Negative situations can range from arguments to violent acts, loss of a job to career destruction, bill delinquency to financial ruin, minor home accidents to deadly vehicular collisions, or lousy dates to dysfunctional relationships. Alcohol can be seriously detrimental to our personal, familial, and professional quality of life.

Economic Effects Economic issues related to alcohol consumption reveals the financial burden and costs to society. Alcohol consumption cost you $479.00 last year, and that's only if you did *not* buy any. The cost related to alcohol abuse and dependence in the United States was estimated at $136.3 billion for 1990, and for 1995, it was $150 billion.[25] Fueling these costs were incidents related to crime, violence, accidents, suicide, and employment such as lost work time, lower productivity, and higher health-care costs. Alcohol and crime seem to have a kinship to one another because criminals often have problems with alcohol abuse. Studies have determined that in the majority of crimes, such as assault, robbery, homicide, or rape, alcohol was a factor. Prisoners frequently are alcoholics or have other drug problems. Abuse of alcohol by either the perpetrator, the victim, or both is a factor in 67 percent of all homicides. In fact, about 50 percent of murder victims had, themselves, been drinking at the time they were murdered. When incidences of rape occur, 50 percent of the time the rapist is intoxicated and 30 percent of the time the victim was also intoxicated.[26] The four leading causes of accidental deaths in this country are: (1) accidents, (2) falls, (3) drownings, and (4) fires and burns and alcohol is known to be a significant contributing factor to each. *FYI:* "Alcohol-Related Accidents" lists percentages of alcohol-related accidents.

Women who commit suicide often have abused alcohol prior to the act. Additionally, among all people who commit suicide, 20–36 percent of these individuals have been drinking prior to the suicide and/or have an alcohol problem. Suicides tend to be more impulsive and more violent when alcohol is involved.

Effects on Relationships Relationship failure can be related to the abuse of alcohol in the partnership or family. Conflicts often arise from the consequences associated with the time, money, and energy spent on alcohol consumption. Because alcohol

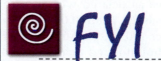

Alcohol-Related Accidents[27]

- 50 percent of fatal traffic crashes are alcohol related; a drunk driver is eight times more likely to have a fatal crash than a nondrinking driver
- 17–53 percent of fatal falls are alcohol related (about 13,000 deaths per year)
- 21–77 percent of nonfatal falls are alcohol related
- 38 percent of all drownings occur because of alcohol abuse; more than one-third of all boaters drink alcohol while on the water
- 6,000 deaths are the results of fires and burns; half of burn victims have a BAC of more than 0.10

affects a person's ability to think rationally and respond appropriately, spouses, children, other family members, or friends can be neglected, abused, or abandoned. Nurturing, intimate relationships of all types often degenerate as a result of excessive alcohol consumption. Social occasions with friends, holidays or vacations with families, and special times such as birthdays or anniversaries can be sabotaged because of alcohol abuse.

Most people will admit that their thinking ability becomes distorted when drinking alcohol. Drinking by both men and women greatly increases the chance that sexual relations will occur. When this sexual encounter is forced on a woman by her date or an acquaintance, while he and/or she are under the influence of alcohol, it is called date or acquaintance rape. Approximately 90 percent of campus rapes are alcohol related and usually result in long-lasting negative consequences.[28] A number of factors contribute to the increased likelihood of experiencing acquaintance/date rape while drinking alcohol: the decision-making abilities of both men and women are impaired; a man may be more aggressive, more insistent if under the influence; a woman may be fearful of angering her date by saying no or unable to refuse due to loss of consciousness. *Health Tips:* "Alcohol and Dating" can aid you in avoiding situations involving alcohol and potentially dangerous relationship behaviors.

For a more detailed discussion of alcohol and acquaintance rape, see chapter 13.

health tips

Alcohol and Dating: Safety Skills[29]

Drinking alcohol lessens your ability to be safe in many situations, including your intimate relationships with men. Remember the following tips to improve your safety when drinking alcohol while on a date. Remember the phrase: RAPE!

R ealize what situations can place you in danger of being a victim of a rape.

A void and manage conflicts with partners and intimates, and ask female friends for help.

P erceive clearly what others are doing, saying, or where they are going.

E stablish and communicate your desires and limits about sex.

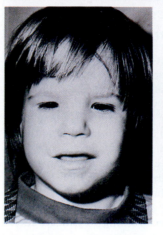
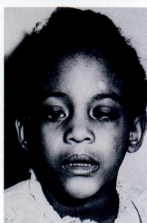

FIGURE 10.2 Widely spaced eyes are a facial characteristic of children with fetal alcohol syndrome. It can also be accompanied by abnormalities in the brain and other internal organs.

Alcohol and Pregnancy

Would you, as a mother, get your baby drunk after she was born? Would you deliberately attempt to sabotage your baby's opportunity to have a healthy productive life? Of course not! However, women who use alcohol, as well as other drugs, during pregnancy place their unborn child, and themselves, at risk for a reduced quality of life and reduced life expectancy. As a result of alcohol use during pregnancy women may impair their personal health and increase the risk of the infant developing multiple problems related to **fetal alcohol syndrome (FAS).** Pregnant women who consume alcohol are at greater risk for miscarriages.

Scientists suspected a correlation between alcohol use and pregnancy complications as early as 1899, but it was not until 1973 that FAS was officially described in medical literature. FAS is a completely preventable cluster of birth defects including irreversible mental and physical disabilities. (See Fig. 10.2.) These may develop as a result of expecting mothers consuming excessive amounts of alcohol during pregnancy. Characteristics of FAS include, but are not limited to, the following:

- Prenatal and postnatal growth deficiency. Additionally most of these children do not attain normal size throughout their lives.
- Central nervous system dysfunction. Many are jittery, poorly coordinated, and have short attention spans and behavioral problems.

- A pattern of deformed facial circumstances such as flat face (the zone between the eyes and mouth), narrow eyes, short nose, thin upper lip, no upper lip crease, or underdeveloped jaws.
- Major organ system malformations such as heart defects.

FAS is considered the leading cause of developmental disabilities and birth defects in the United States and each FAS child has one thing in common: a mother who consumed too much alcohol while pregnant. This serious alcohol-related syndrome has increased four-fold between 1980 and 1990 due to continual and excessive use of alcohol by women. Peter Jennings on an evening news program stated that in 1995, over 35 percent of all pregnant women reported being frequent drinkers during their pregnancy.[30]

What does research reveal about the relationship between pregnancy and alcohol use? Alcohol crosses the placental barrier and causes glucose and oxygen deficit to the fetal brain. The fetus may be more severely affected than the adult female because the fetus is unable to break down the alcohol as fast and

> **fetal alcohol syndrome (FAS)**—completely preventable cluster of birth defects including irreversible mental and physical disabilities and a characteristic set of facial abnormalities; occurs when women consume alcohol during pregnancy.

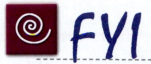

Native American Women and Fetal Alcohol Syndrome

Approximately 90 percent of Native American adults use or abuse alcohol, or are in recovery from alcohol abuse. Forty percent of Native American women drink alcohol during pregnancy, which places their babies at risk for developing FAS or FAE. FAS affects about 1 of every 100 Native American infants born in the Northern Plains of the United States, and FAE affects 1 of 50 infants. Within two to three generations, every Native American household will have one adult spouse who is an offspring of a fetal alcohol birth unless these circumstances change. Presently, there are groups of Native American women who are working to educate their peers and improve this very serious situation. One of these, the Native American Community Board in South Dakota, promotes legislation and education in an effort to reduce the use of alcohol during pregnancy.[32]

Viewpoint

What Should Be Done?

With all the information now available concerning fetal alcohol syndrome, what should be the legal consequences for women who consume alcohol during pregnancy and, as a result, have children with FAS? Does a woman have the right to choose unhealthy behaviors while pregnant with another human being? Should she be allowed to have more children and risk causing severe birth defects among them? Does the "right" to abort and the "right" to harm the fetus during pregnancy have any moral and legal ramifications? What is your opinion about this issue?

---

efficiently as the adult. The fetus is most vulnerable during the first trimester of pregnancy. How much alcohol consumption do physicians and researchers recommend for pregnant females? *NONE!* Correct: not any! Research hasn't established a "safe" level of alcohol use during pregnancy; therefore, there is no way to know if the fetus will be affected by any alcohol consumption during pregnancy. Even women who drink "moderately" may have infants with **fetal alcohol effects (FAE),** a variety of less severe birth defects including below level IQ, learning disabilities, hyperactivity, short attention span, and often similar physical malformations as FAS. Unfortunately, too many women do not appear to get the message. Studies have determined that between 20–73 percent of women consume alcohol while pregnant.[31] (See *FYI:* "Native American Women and Fetal Alcohol Syndrome" and *Viewpoint:* "What Should Be Done?")

Aren't you glad your mother took care of herself while she was pregnant with you? Do the same for your own children and return this morally and ethically correct courtesy should you ever become pregnant.

Research concerning male abuse of alcohol and resulting birth defects has not been clearly documented. Studies have shown some correlation between the father's drinking during the month prior to

conception and reduced birthweight of the infant.[33] Additionally, alcohol-related research using male rats have indicated that paternal exposure to alcohol prior to mating has shown an adverse effect on normal development and behavior of their offspring. A possible explanation is that alcohol may be a direct gonadal toxicant and may be harmful to sperm production.[34] Although research is inconclusive to some degree, it does indicate that paternal alcohol use must be researched in order to create a complete picture in regard to alcohol abuse and fetal consequences.

The National Center for Education on Maternal and Child Health in Arlington, Virginia, promotes the collaboration of state agencies such as maternal and child health bureau services, substance abuse services, and child welfare to address prevention and treatment for the abuse of alcohol and other drugs by pregnant women. The document, "Finding Common Ground: A Call for Collaboration . . ."[35] describes the methods by which state agencies can develop collaborative programming to work with women who use alcohol and other drugs during pregnancy.

ADDICTION AND DEPENDENCY

Addiction to alcohol, or any other drug, is a compulsive, uncontrollable dependence on a substance, habit, or practice to such a degree that cessation causes severe emotional, mental, or physiological reactions.[36] Components of addiction include tolerance, physical dependence, and psychological dependence.

Dependency: What Is It?

Pharmacologically, alcohol is a depressant drug. With long-term continual use, it is capable of creating a physical and psychological dependence. **Physical dependency** means that body cells have come to depend on the presence of this depressant to maintain **homeostasis** (or balance). Once physically dependent, if the body is deprived of alcohol, an addict will experience **withdrawal symptoms.** Withdrawal symptoms can be extremely uncomfortable at best, and fatal in the worst situation. (See *FYI:* "Stages of Withdrawal from Alcohol.") Fatalities may be as high as 1 in 7. During the initial phase of withdrawal, called **detoxification,** ridding the body of alcohol, women who have abused alcohol for a number of years may need to be hospitalized. Medically, withdrawal from alcohol is more severe and more likely to be fatal than is withdrawal from narcotic drugs. Experienced drinkers may appear to "hold their liquor." However, when measured, their BAC will be in proportion to their body weight, the amount of alcohol ingested, and the condition of their liver.

Delirium tremens (DTs) are usually experienced in Stage 3 of alcohol withdrawal and found mostly in serious cases of alcohol dependency. Although they often are manifested with shaking hands and jerky movements, the "DTs" also produce vivid hallucinations and nausea. Withdrawal symptoms such as insomnia, panic attacks, irregular breathing, abnormal blood pressure, and/or anxiety may last for weeks and the woman can feel an intense craving for alcohol. After-care programs, discussed later, are important at this time to prevent the woman from returning to use of alcohol.

Psychological dependence, a learned process affecting the behavior of a long-term drinker, occurs when the drinker strongly desires, or craves, the feeling alcohol provides. Like the mother of a newborn infant who learns to function with less sleep, alcohol drinkers learn to function with the effects of alcohol. Learning what to expect from alcohol intake in varying circumstances, the woman learns to control her behavior and act accordingly. Psychological tolerance deceives a woman into believing she can perform certain tasks under the influence of alcohol. In reality,

fetal alcohol effects (FAE)—a limited number of the characteristic birth defects associated with fetal alcohol syndrome such as below normal IQ, learning disabilities, hyperactivity, short attention span, and often similar physical malformations as with FAS; completely preventable.

addiction—compulsive, uncontrollable dependence on a substance, habit, or practice; withdrawal causes severe mental, emotional, or physiological reactions.

physical dependency—body cells dependent upon a chemical substance in order to maintain homeostasis.

homeostasis (home ee oh **stay** sis)—relative balance in the internal environment of the body; naturally maintained by adaptive responses that promote healthy survival.

withdrawal symptoms—unpleasant symptoms such as tremors, insomnia, and seizures when drug use is discontinued.

detoxification—a period of time when an addict does not drink to rid the body of alcohol and its toxic chemicals.

delirium tremens (DTs) (da **leer** ee um **trem** ins)—a psychotic condition resulting from withdrawal from chronic alcohol abuse and causing uncontrollable tremors, confusion, and vivid hallucinations.

psychological dependence—dependence upon the feeling produced by the presence of the drug in the body; an emotional or psychological desire to continue using the drug; habituation.

FYI

Stages of Withdrawal from Alcohol[37]

Stage 1	Tremors, excessively rapid heartbeat, hypertension, heavy sweating, loss of appetite, and insomnia
Stage 2	Hallucinations (auditory, visual, tactile, or a combination of these), and rarely, odors
Stage 3	Delusions, disorientation, delirium (sometimes intermittent in nature), and usually followed by amnesia
Stage 4	Seizure activity

she will not be able to determine to what extent the alcohol affects her abilities. Even if she looks and acts sober, it does not mean that she is capable of skilled performance such as driving a car, using sharp instruments, or operating mechanical devices. Because of the psychological feelings (e.g., temporary escape, mood swings, relaxation, euphoria) sometimes resulting from the use of alcohol, the ability to recover from this type of dependency may be more difficult to achieve than recovery from physical dependency.

ALCOHOLISM

> When a woman is unconscious about her starvation, about the consequences of using death-dealing vehicles and substances, she is dancing, she is dancing. Whether these are such things as chronic negative thinking, poor relationships, abusive situations, drugs, or alcohol—they are like the red shoes: hard to pry a person away from once they've taken hold.[38]

Demographics

Addiction to alcohol crosses all gender, economic, political, and social boundaries and generally is a well-established pattern of abuse by the time a male reaches his mid-to-late thirties or early forties, whereas women, if they develop alcoholism, generally do so at a later age and develop complications more easily and at a faster rate than males. **Alcoholism** is a chronic, progressive, and potentially fatal disease characterized by tolerance, and physical and psychological dependency; genetic, environmental, and psychosocial factors contribute to its development and progression. This disease is a direct or indirect result of ingesting alcohol and varies in the time it takes to develop. For some women the development can be somewhat rapid, for others alcoholism may be years in the making and shortens life expectancy by an estimated 10 to 15 years.

A myth about alcoholism is that a person would have to be drinking or drunk all the time to be considered an alcoholic. However, patterns of alcohol abuse vary. Regular daily intake of large amounts of alcohol, regular heavy drinking that is limited to weekends, or long periods of not drinking interspersed with binge drinking that can last from days to several weeks can each be typical of alcoholic drinking patterns. Another myth regarding alcoholism is that an alcoholic can resume drinking after they have remained sober for a number of years. Although some researchers have tried to prove this is the case, no one in recovery from alcoholism would

Her Story

Amanda

Amanda, a 22-year-old mother of one and a community college nursing major, maintained above average grades. She rarely missed class and was a responsible parent Sunday through Thursday nights. However, after class was done each Friday, she took Alissa, her two-year-old daughter, to stay with her grandmother. Amanda spent the remainder of the weekend drinking with friends and out of control: partying, driving while drunk, engaging in sexual activity, and disregarding any responsibilities related to school or her daughter. Amanda refuses to stop spending her weekends in a drunken stupor and feels that as long as she is taking care of her responsibilities during the week, she can do as she pleases on the weekends.

- Is Amanda an alcoholic?
- Is she creating present or future problems as a result of continual alcohol overconsumption?
- What consequences could result from her continual abuse of an addicting, toxic substance?
- Does she meet some of the criteria in the definition of alcoholism?

agree. Once a woman has developed the disease of alcoholism, she will always have the disease. Now, she may not always be a drinking alcoholic, but she will be unable to ever control her drinking again; therefore, abstaining from any drinking is imperative. (Read *Her Story:* "Amanda" to see what you think.)

Is Alcoholism a Disease?

There is an ongoing controversy about whether alcoholism is truly a "disease" or if it is a willful use of a harmful and intoxicating substance. The American Medical Association classifies it as a disease, as does *Alcoholics Anonymous,* a 1.5 million member organization whose "only requirement for membership is the desire to stop drinking." However, some professionals and researchers believe individuals should be responsible for their behavior under all circumstances and that it is wrong to "hide" behind the facade of disease to excuse any violent, antisocial, or illegal behavior because of alcohol abuse.

The cause of alcoholism is basically unknown, but studies have discovered that some of the following circumstances are revealed in the background of alcoholic women:

Her Story

Donetta

As she looks back at her descent into the disease of alcoholism, Donetta could trace indicators of escalating alcohol consumption. Early in the process, she experienced increased personal fears, anxieties, and negative emotions. She ignored or avoided responsibilities such as children, bills, and her job. She remembers drinking alone and secretively, using alcohol as a crutch to "make it through" a particular situation or task.

Donetta and her husband argued about her drinking, then she would promise to drink less, behave better, and meet her responsibilities. She felt uncomfortable in environments in which alcohol was not available and began to avoid friends and family members who did not drink. At first **blackouts** were rare, then occurred more often. She didn't remember what she did or said while she was drinking. This progression took a number of years to develop, but Donetta was lucky. She lost her job, her husband, and any financial means of support. Lucky? Yes, she "hit the bottom" before she lost her life. Donetta decided to seek help and move into recovery.

- What could have been done early during Donetta's descent into alcoholism to intervene, and perhaps have stopped her addictive process?
- What is meant by a blackout?

- Parent or parents are alcoholic, which could mean that they have a genetic susceptibility or environmental influence to alcohol abuse; at least 60 percent of all alcoholics have at least one alcoholic parent.
- Childhood abuse, of which almost half is the result of alcohol abuse. It may contribute to the abuse of a child and as a result of this experience, the abused child may become an alcoholic.
- Excessive drinking as teens establishes the habit and social patterns, or even dependence.
- Social factors such as disappearance of the extended family, mobility of families, slackened family ties, and decline of religious affiliations.

Indicators of Alcoholism

If someone were to ask you about the signs that may indicate alcohol was becoming a problem or that signs of alcoholism were prevalent, would you know what they are? A progression of drinking alcohol more frequently and in larger amounts yielding ever expanding negative consequences is indicative of alcoholism. *Her Story:* "Donetta" illustrates this progression in a very personal way.

How to Help

If someone you care about has a number of these indicators and continues to drink, what can you do? To better help the person(s) you care about and yourself through this serious situation, do the following:

- Learn the facts about alcohol and alcoholism, and find factual and unbiased resources.
- Develop a factual attitude rather than an emotional attitude toward the person and their drinking; avoid ridicule, criticism, and disgust.
- Don't use home remedies such as lecturing, hiding the liquor, soliciting promises the drinker won't or can't keep, saying, "if you loved me . . . ," or using an "holier than thou attitude."
- Find assistance for yourself and, if possible, the alcoholic such as your family doctor, minister, counselors, county agencies, and support groups (AA and Al-Anon).
- Talk with people who understand the illness, not just to friends and family.
- Allow the alcoholic to be responsible for her own behavior and the consequences of her drinking.
- Expect relapses and difficult days after recovery begins, immediate recovery will not happen.
- When protection from situations in which alcohol is present is not possible, she has to learn to say "no, thanks" on her own.

alcoholism—a chronic, progressive, and potentially fatal disease characterized by tolerance, and physical and psychological dependency; genetic, environmental, and psychosocial factors contribute to its development and progression.

blackouts—temporary loss of consciousness and memory; yet interaction and function may occur.

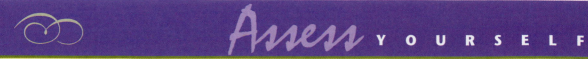

Assess **Y O U R S E L F**

Do You Have a Drinking Problem?

Use the following questions to determine if alcohol is a problem in your life. Check "yes" if the statement is true or "no" if the statement is not true about your drinking behaviors and patterns. Add each of your "yes" and "no" answers, and then consult the suggestions at the end of this survey.

Yes	No	Question
____	____	1. Do you drink more than three times a week?
____	____	2. Do you drink more than three drinks each time?
____	____	3. When everyone else is drinking, do you feel you should be drinking also?
____	____	4. Do you think it is acceptable for people to get drunk once in a while?
____	____	5. Do you find it difficult to say "no" when someone offers you an alcoholic drink even when you don't really want it?

Suggestions: If you answered "yes" more than "no" to these questions, it would be a good idea not only to reduce the amount and frequency of drinking if you can, but also to talk with a counselor who specializes in alcohol treatment.

Then complete *Assess Yourself:* "Do You Have a Drinking Problem?," above, to determine if you have a problem with alcohol. If you suspect a friend or relative has a problem, encourage them to take the assessment too.

A Family Disease

Growing up in a family in which alcohol was abused by one or both parents can produce lifelong negative consequences. Which would be a more difficult plight to endure: to be the daughter of alcoholic parents, to be the wife of an alcoholic, to be the mother of an alcoholic and having to see your child deal with alcoholism, or to be an alcoholic yourself? Each is hurtful, and many women experience all four circumstances. The physical and financial toll of alcoholism can to some degree be objectively calculated. However, the human loss to individuals, their families, communities, and society is incalculable. It is estimated that for every alcoholic, another four people are directly affected. The ripple effects from those four people then extends on to numerous others.

Codependency   Preoccupation with a particular individual and her or his problems to the point of self-neglect is an example of **codependency.** Eventually, the codependent's relationship with all others is affected. This results from prolonged association with the alcoholic, and the practice of oppressive "rules" that prevent the open expression of feelings, concerns, and problems. These rules, often developed subconsciously, include such things as: it's not okay to talk about a problem; it's not okay to talk about feelings; do as I say, not as I do; don't rock the boat; it's not okay to play or be playful; be the best, but don't enjoy it!! Codependent women often take care of their family's needs and wants. They tend to: worry a lot; check on people; lose sleep over family problems; abandon their routine due to upset feelings about somebody or something; try to catch people in acts of misbehavior; control family members' behavior; think they know what is best for others; and try to control events and people through helplessness, guilt, coercion, threats, advice giving, manipulation, and/or domination. Codependency is unhealthy because the individual tends to allow her physical, emotional, social, and mental quality of life to be dependent upon the quality of life of other people. Therefore, she feels as if she has little control over her own well-being. She is likely to develop stress-related disorders such as migraines, ulcers, arthritis, even heart disease and cancer. Women with codependent traits can obtain help through individual or family counseling with the alcoholic and other family members, involvement in twelve-step programs such as Al-anon and Co-dependency Anonymous, and by reading the plethora of self-help material related to codependency and alcoholism.

Adult Children of Alcoholics   *Adult children of alcoholics (ACOAs)* grow up in a group of related people in which one or more members are continually unmanageable or stressful conditions, such as alcoholism, continually create a dysfunctional environment. The family is the most significant social unit in our society and is responsible for the development of habits and beliefs that influence members' decision throughout the life span. Yet, children in the dysfunctional family do not often have role models that exhibit good habits or profess beliefs that help children develop important systems that can enhance their life. The dysfunctional home environment places *children of alcoholics (COAs)* at risk for early alcohol and drug dependence, underachievement or unhealthy overachievement, inappropriate classroom or social behaviors, lying, delinquency, unhealthy relationships with peers and adults, and emotional distress that can manifest itself in withdrawal, depression, or suicide attempts. As COAs become adult COAs, unless they receive help, many of them continue to have these risk factors. Three rules, although not written, are learned by COAs: don't talk or tell (don't discuss the problem; pretend it doesn't exist); don't trust (nothing is consistent or predictable); and don't feel (numb out the anger and the pain; it hurts too much to feel). These rules lead to some serious consequences for ACOAs. It sets the stage for shame and doubt, isolation, distrust of self and others, and uncertainty or numbing of feelings. Thus, there is no pain, but also, there is no joy.

Effects of Growing Up in an Alcoholic Family

Surviving difficult family circumstances often means that family members develop coping mechanisms and roles that help them momentarily deal with the chaos of living in an alcoholic family. Four roles, identified by treatment providers, COAs often develop to help them cope with problems related to parental alcoholism include: the hero, the scapegoat, the lost child, and the mascot. The hero is the superkid, caretaker, the "type E" female: everything to everybody; she is the cheerleader, honor student, and president of the class. Often irresponsible, disruptive, or antisocial, the scapegoat may become defiant and delinquent; she is vulnerable to unwholesome peer groups and drug abuse. The lost child (the loner) has her own private world of reading, television, computer, music, or any other refuge she can find that enables her to escape from the family chaos; she is at risk for unhealthy practices, early natural death, or suicide. Seemingly carefree, funny, center of attention, the mascot (or clown) deals with the dysfunctional family by denial of the problem. She diverts attention away from the painful family situation by offering comic relief; she is at risk for phys-

ical and emotional problems and drug abuse. These roles help children (and often adults) survive the dysfunctional family situation. Their development may be thwarted without help, and these coping roles may prevent them from leading fulfilling lives outside the family system. Many of these behaviors do not serve them well, when as adults, they use the behaviors on the job or interacting with family or friends. ACOAs must be taught the four Cs of a dysfunctional family: You didn't *cause* it, you can't *control* it, you can't *cure* it, you *can help yourself.*

Fortunately, as alcoholics are being assisted in overcoming their disease and dysfunctions, the family members can also be assisted in overcoming risk factors generated by growing up in an alcoholic family. Twelve-step programs, such as Al-anon, ACOA meetings, Co-dependency Anonymous groups, as well as individual and group therapy have been successful in overcoming negative behaviors associated with alcoholic families, and moving ahead to productive and positive lives. Schools also have developed support programs for COAs that include such activities as building self-esteem, establishing consistency, providing a safe environment for expressing feelings openly, and learning to trust. This is an attempt to reduce risk factors that could lead to development of alcohol and drug abuse among children of alcoholics and build protective factors that are traits or conditions intended to assist COAs in the development of healthy and productive lifestyles. (See *Journal Activity:* "Who and What Does Alcohol Affect?")

WHAT CAN BE DONE?

No one approach seems to be successful of recovery from alcoholism on their own. Seemingly, greater success is found by utilizing a combination of treatment approaches. It is important to remember that the alcoholic will rarely move to "treat" themselves and may need assistance in seeking help. However, no one can force another adult into treatment unless the legal system intercedes and this is only after some crime has been committed because of alcohol abuse.

> **codependency**—a preoccupation with a particular individual and her or his problems to the point of self-neglect. This results from prolonged association with an alcoholic who has an oppressive set of rules that prevent the open expression of feelings, concerns, and problems.

JOURNAL ACTIVITY

Who and What Does Alcohol Affect?

As you read the various events listed below, determine the area of greatest impact on one of the following: (a) the drinker (health effect), (b) the family (social effect), (c) or society (economic effect). Write the effect next to each event and explain why and what you believe the effects are. *(Hint: it may affect more than one area!)*

Event	Who or what?	Why?
1. Court system		
2. Auto death while DUI		
3. Increased welfare costs		
4. Injuring oneself in a fall		
5. Job loss		
6. Divorce		
7. Cirrhosis of the liver		
8. Neglect of one's children		
9. Heart disease		
10. Decreased work productivity		
11. Spousal abuse		
12. Passing out or vomiting at a party		
13. Increased medical costs		
14. Sexually transmitted diseases		
15. Abusing a child		
16. Depression		
17. Fighting at a sporting event		
18. Killing someone when driving drunk		

Resources

Locating resources for the alcoholic and yourself is an important first step toward resolving this problem. Who, what, where, how, and how much are all questions that need to have answers prior to movement toward assisting the alcoholic.

Intervention

Intervention is a process by which the alcoholic is confronted by a person or persons each describing the "facts" associated with their concern for the alcoholic's drinking problem. Individuals close to the alcoholic (e.g., child, parent, sibling, spouse, friends, employer) can share in this calm, yet truthful process that is intended to assure the alcoholic of their concern for her, but also assertively express the situation as it is. If the intervention is successful, the alcoholic should be willing to move into inpatient or outpatient treatment. Betty Ford states that when her family intervened because of her abuse of prescription drugs and alcohol, she became angry and hurt. But, as she listened, she heard the love that came through their comments to her and she realized they loved her too much to ignore the problem any longer. She decided to seek treatment and continues in recovery, which she says will be ongoing as long as she lives. "The Betty Ford Center" in Rancho Mirage, California, was created as a result of her efforts and continues to treat thousands of individuals in need of alcohol and other drug therapy.

Types of Treatment

Varied approaches are used in the treatment of alcoholism and include not only what precipitated the originating use, but also the complex consequences of the disease. Lifestyle behavior change, stress management programs, individual counseling, spiritual renewal, hospitalization, drug therapy, support groups, and others are often used in treatment for alcoholism. Combining several of these treatment approaches is often more successful than utilizing only one.

Lifestyle Behavior Changes Lifestyle behavior changes include improved nutrition, engaging in exercise programs, developing stress management strategies, enhancement of self-worth, and recognizing a higher power. Treatment attempts to focus on making positive changes in one's life in addition to cessation of alcohol abuse.

Counseling Individual and/or group counseling assist the alcoholic in looking at issues related to the abusive behavior. Whether alcohol abuse is the result of a variety of negative situations in one's life, or the negative situations are the consequences of alcohol abuse can be determined. The counselor needs to be specifically trained in working with alcohol-dependent individuals as well as their families. Group therapy can provide an environment in which women can feel safe in discussing their alcohol-related problems and receive support from women who understand and can relate to her. Realization that others have experienced the same pain, humiliation, or shame seems to bring relief because she no longer feels she is the only one.

Treatment Centers Use of hospitals or drug treatment centers has been beneficial for some women. In this environment women can go through detoxification under medical supervision, remove themselves from the surroundings in which they've had problems with alcohol, and begin to work toward resolution of why this disease initially developed. Treatment centers usually have designed a structured routine revolving around household duties, individual and group therapy, recreation, nutritious meals, and support group meetings. All of which support reestablishment of routine, responsibility, and health. Many insurance companies provide for alcoholism treatment both on an inpatient and outpatient basis.

Women in treatment often have different needs than men. Care of small children, finances, transportation, and even distrustfulness of male professionals hinder a woman's ability to engage in treatment programs. To promote recovery for women with these needs, treatment should include child care, female counselors, transportation, reduced fees, and women-only therapies.

Chemical Treatment Chemical treatment (drug therapy) occasionally becomes necessary if a woman cannot refrain from abusing alcohol through inpatient or outpatient treatment. Antabuse is a drug that inhibits an enzyme (acetaldehyde dehydrogenase) from breaking down acetaldehyde. As a result, a toxic effect to alcohol is created; therefore, if a woman drinks alcohol and ingests Antabuse, extremely uncomfortable effects such as nausea, weakness, blurred vision, heart palpitations, and vomiting occur. These consequences are intended to impede the consumption of alcohol. Two drugs, nalmefene and naltrexone, both of which are opiate antagonist, block the brain's pleasurable response to drinking and help alcohol abusers to stop drinking compulsively. Although these drugs are still in the drug trial stage, researchers hope that in the future, drugs such as these will be most beneficial in reducing a person's desire to drink and therefore decrease the high rates of alcoholics' relapse to heavy drinking—about 80 percent.

Aftercare Aftercare, continuing care following treatment for alcohol or other drug abuse, needs to be comprehensive as well as attentive to individual needs. Provision of support groups and varied services can enable women to live drug-free lives and foster development of skills and abilities leading to self-confidence and independence. What services and support structures are most beneficial following treatment? Contact with other recovering women, recovery and personal growth literature, personal and family therapy sessions, life skills and job training, vocational training and job placement are all beneficial as women seek to move ahead to a healthy, productive lifestyle. Support and self-help groups such as twelve-step organizations, including *Alcoholics Anonymous (AA), Al-anon (AA), Adult Children of Alcoholics (ACOA), Codependency Anonymous (CODA), or Women for Sobriety,* offer emotional support and social interaction among women who can share experiences and solutions for a disease that is known best by individuals who have shared in its devastating effects. (See *FYI: "Facts about Alcoholics Anonymous."*) Involving cultural and geographic community support such as phone chains, hotlines, and recovery group gatherings can help regular contact with one another about their welfare continue. Women out of treatment programs need to have follow-up contact for as long as the woman, her counselor, and/or the case manager deem it important and necessary. (Please see resources and suggested readings at the end of the chapter.)

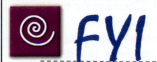

Facts About Alcoholics Anonymous[39]

- More than 87,000 groups worldwide in 134 different countries
- 35 percent of AA members are female
- Approximately one-third of the members have been sober over 5 years; one-third have been sober between 1 and 5 years
- About 50 percent of AA members are between the ages of 21 and 50
- Average member attends about three meetings per week
- Other treatment programs follow the AA model (for example, Co-dependent Anonymous and Cocaine Anonymous)

PREVENTION

Of course, the most effective way to prevent developing problems associated with alcohol abuse and the disease of alcoholism is to abstain from alcohol consumption. Because there are millions of women who drink, and many of them do develop alcohol dependency problems, it is important to look at how those problems can be avoided.

Primary prevention programs are aimed at women, especially young women, who have not begun to use alcohol, and focuses on reducing the rate of possible new alcohol users. This type of prevention program attempts to provide and promote activities that reduce the factors related to early use of alcohol. The factors include: lack of awareness in school and community of alcohol-related problems, insufficient knowledge about alcohol and other drugs, lack of understanding about negative effects of alcohol abuse, student's need for life skills training, infrequent involvement in school of parents and students, lack of awareness of positive alternatives, insufficient knowledge about regulations, and laws pertaining to alcohol use/abuse.

In consideration of each of these factors, activities can be developed to combat each one and thus reduce the possibility that young women will begin to use alcohol in their lifestyle.

Suggestions for Prevention   Suggested activities pertaining to these contributing factors include, but are not limited to some of the following:

- Raising awareness through involvement of community organizations, church groups, or parent groups by developing a media campaign using local newspaper, television, and radio; promoting a community alcohol awareness day designated by wearing certain colors or driving with headlights on; or proclamations by community officials. The more segments of community involvement, the greater the opportunity to enhance awareness in school and community of alcohol-related problems.
- Accurate, current, and age-appropriate information can affect good communication between parents, teachers, and their children/students. As part of a comprehensive approach to alcohol use prevention, purchasing materials and curricula and providing inservice programs for teachers, as well as providing opportunities for parents to become educated about alcohol use, can help to reduce the insufficient knowledge about alcohol and other drugs.

Young women often believe that alcohol use does not produce any negative consequences and therefore using this substance is okay. By developing strong anti-use policies in schools and communities and involving students in anti-use and alcohol-free campaigns and activities, young women are likely to behave accordingly and develop negative attitudes toward the use of alcohol.

Like all individuals, young women need life skills training. Activities and organizations that promote the resistance of peer influence, enhance decision-making abilities, and aid young women in coping with personal and social issues can provide a basis for choosing not to use alcohol. Developing leadership qualities, learning resistance, and developing problem-solving skills can also reduce the likelihood of alcohol use by females.

Enhancing positive family influence and reducing infrequent involvement of parents and students in school can be accomplished by promoting parenting skills through parent training programs in education systems or community organizations. More involvement and allegiance to school usually means that students often adopt behaviors and values expounded by the school and have less time for alcohol-related activities or peers who may choose to drink. Club, sport, and other student–parent organizations involve the students and provide reasons for parents to come to school events.

Giving young women opportunities to engage in many of the activities discussed in the preceding paragraph can provide healthy alternatives to alcohol use. Youth centers, community and school recreation, alcohol-free dances and parties can offer alternative activities to involvement with alcohol.

Regulations and laws can be useful in preventing abuse of alcohol and other drugs. Creating barriers to alcohol access and enforcing restrictions to curtail underage drinking and use of fake identification cards can be a deterrent to early use of alcohol. Increased supervision of youth and expanded security at places where young people congregate helps prevent the influx of alcohol by underage consumers.

The majority of these suggestions are directed toward young women, because that is exactly when alcohol abuse prevention must begin. The younger the age females initially abuse alcohol, the greater the probability they will encounter negative consequences.

Prevention can yield the greatest benefit if initiated at an early age (e.g., preschool) and continue throughout the school years and into adulthood. During this process, many of the risk factors can be ameliorated and alcohol abuse prevented.

> Yes there is pain in being severed from the red shoes. But being cut away from the addiction all at once is our only hope. It is a severing that is filled with absolute blessing. The feet will grow back, we will find our way, we will recover, we will run and jump and skip again someday. By then our handmade life will be ready. We'll slip into it and marvel that we could be so lucky to have another chance.[40]

AS WE GO TO PRESS . . .

On August 30, 1997, one of the most well-known and photographed women in the world, Diana, Princess of Wales, was killed in a high-speed car crash. Although reports that the tabloid press (known as the papparazzi) and possibly other vehicles contributed to the crash, the driver of the Princess' car was found to have a BAC at least three times higher than the legal limit. A bodyguard in the car was the only person to have been wearing a seatbelt, and was the sole survivor.

Chapter Summary

- Women and alcohol have a historical association that produced both positive and negative outcomes.
- Alcohol is the most commonly used psychoactive drug and its use has a number of health benefits; the abuse of alcohol results in serious physical, psychological, social, and economic consequences.
- Women and men respond differently to alcohol both physically and behaviorally.
- Alcohol and pregnancy do not mix; there is no safe level of alcohol ingestion for pregnant women; fetal alcohol syndrome can result from drinking alcohol during pregnancy.
- Alcohol is an addicting, depressant drug that can cause the disease of alcoholism and result in serious consequences for the addict, her family, and other important components of her life.

- There are indicators that can be utilized as a means of informal assessment to determine if someone is alcohol dependent.
- Children of Alcoholics (COAs) develop family roles that enable them to attempt to cope with the chronic distress and chaos present in an alcoholic's family. Without assistance, these roles may be taken into adulthood.
- Finding resources, intervention, seeking treatment, and changing lifestyle behaviors can all be beneficial when recovering from alcohol addiction.
- Alcohol abuse prevention is important if women are to avoid the possible devastation that can occur from alcohol abuse and addiction.

Review Questions

1. What have been some of the attitudes toward women and alcohol held by society at different times in history?
2. What are the four different types of alcohol? What does the term *proof* mean?
3. What is the process of alcohol absorption in a woman's body?
4. Why does alcohol affect women differently than men?
5. What are the criteria used to classify different levels of drinkers?
6. What are the possible consequences for the mother and her fetus and infant if she drinks alcohol during pregnancy?
7. How does the addiction process relate to alcohol dependency?
8. If alcohol is a disease, why don't we know exactly what causes it, how to successfully treat it, and how to prevent it?
9. What indications may be displayed by a woman who is either developing or has developed an addiction to alcohol?
10. What is codependency? How does it relate to alcohol abuse?
11. What characteristics may develop in children who grow up in homes where either one or both parents are alcoholic?
12. What are some approaches that can be taken to assist a woman in overcoming alcohol dependency?
13. What are some of the methods that can be used to prevent alcohol abuse in women?

Resources

Organizations and Hotlines

Adult Children of Alcoholics
P.O. Box 3216
Torrance, CA 90519
Telephone: (310) 534-1815

BACCHUS (Boost Alcohol Consciousness Concerning the Health of University Students)
P.O. Box 10430
Denver, CO 80210
Telephone: (303) 871-3068

Children of Alcoholics Foundation, Inc.
555 Madison Ave., 20th Floor
New York, NY 10022
Telephone: (800) 359-COAF

Al-ANON Family Groups, Inc.
World Service Office
P.O. Box 862, Midtown Station
New York, NY 10018
(212) 302-7240
Telephone: (800) 344-2666

Alcoholics Anonymous
P.O. Box 459, Grand Central Station
New York, NY 10163
Telephone: (212) 870-3400

Mothers Against Drunk Driving (MADD)
511 East John Carpenter Freeway
Suite 700
Irving, TX 75062
Telephone: (214) 744-6233
Telephone: (800) GET-MADD

Students Against Drunk Driving (SADD)
P.O. Box 800
Marlboro, MA 01752
Telephone: (508) 481-3568

Women for Sobriety
P.O. Box 618
Quakertown, PA 18951
Telephone: (800) 333-1606

Women's Health Network
1325 G Street NW
Washington, DC 20005
Telephone: (202) 347-1140

Secular Organization for Sobriety (SOS)
P.O. Box 5
Buffalo, NY 14215
Telephone: (716) 834-2922

Drug Alcohol Tobacco Education (DATE)
3426 Bridgeland Drive
Bridgeton, MO 63044
Telephone: (314) 739-1121

National Clearinghouse for Alcohol and Drug Information
P.O. Box 2345
Rockville, MD 20847-2345
Telephone: (800) 729-6686

National Council on Alcoholism and Drug Dependence, Inc.
12 West 21st Street
New York, NY 10010
Telephone: (212) 206-6770
Telephone: (800) NCA-CALL

Indian Health Service
Colorado River Service
Route 1, Box 12
Parker, AZ 85344
Telephone: (602) 669-2137

Institute on Black Chemical Abuse
Resource Center
2616 Nicollet Avenue, South
Minneapolis, MN 55407
Telephone: (612) 871-7878

National Asian Pacific American Families Against Substance
Abuse, Inc. (NAPAFASA)
420 E. Third Street, Suite 909
Los Angeles, CA 90013-1647
Telephone: (213) 617-8277

National Coalition of Hispanic Health Services Organization
(COSSMHO)
1501 16th Street, NW
Washington, DC 20036
Telephone: (202) 387-5000

Center for Substance Abuse Treatment
Drug Abuse Information and Treatment Referral Hotline
Telephone: (800) 662-HELP

National Alcohol Hot Line
Telephone: (800) ALCOHOL

Remove Intoxicated Drivers (RID)
Telephone: (518) 372-0034

Websites

National Clearinghouse for Alcohol and Drug Information
URL: http://nhic-nt.health.org/cgi-shl/...e=/htmlgen/
Entry.dbm&HRCode=HR0027

National Council on Alcohol and Drug Dependence
URL: http://www.ncad

National Council on Alcoholism
URL: http://www.health.org/reality/links.htm

Web of Addictions
URL: http://www.well.com/user/woa

Suggested Readings

Beattie, M. 1987. *Codependent no more: How to stop controlling others and start caring for yourself.* New York: Harper and Row, Publishers, Inc.
Discovering normal: A parenting program for adult children of alcoholics and their parents. 1992. New York: Children of Alcoholics Foundation.
Youcha, G. 1986. *Women and alcohol: A dangerous pleasure.* New York: Crown Publishers, Inc.

References

1. Blume, S. 1990. Chemical dependency in women: Important issues. *American Journal Drug Alcohol Abuse,* 16 (3&4): 297-307.
2. Ibid.
3. Pinger, R., W. Payne, D. Hahn, and E. Hahn. 1998. *Issues for today: drugs, 3rd ed.* St. Louis: Mosby.
4. Thompson, D. S. 1993. Edited by H. MacLean *Every woman's health: Complete guide to body & mind.* New York: Simon & Schuster.
5. Engs, R., and D. Hanson. 1990. Gender differences in drinking patterns & problems among college students: A review of literature. *Journal of Alcohol and Drug Education,* 35 (1): 36-47.
6. Ibid.
7. *National survey results on drug use in monitoring the future study, 1975-1992, vol. 2. College students & young adults.* 1993. In NIH Pub. no. 93-3598 Washington, DC: Government Printing Office.
8. Kinney, J., and G. Leaton. 1995. *Loosening the grip: A handbook of alcohol information,* 5th ed. St. Louis: Mosby.
9. Celis III, W. 1994. Drinking by college women raises new concern. In *New York Times,* New York, 16 February.
10. Brown, R., R. Wyn, W. G. Cumberland, Y. Hongjian, E. Abel, L. Gelberg, and L. Ng. 1991. *Women's health-related behaviors.* The Commonwealth Fund Commission on Women's Health, Los Angeles: UCLA Center for Health Policy Research.
11. UC-Berkeley School of Public Health. 1994. The alcohol/breast cancer connection. *University of California at Berkeley Wellness Letter,* 10 (6): 1-2.
12. Tivis, L., and J. Gavler. 1994. Alcohol, hormones, & health in postmenopausal women. *Alcohol Health & Research World,* 18 (3): 185-88.
13. Ray, O., and C. Ksir. 1996. *Drugs, society, & human behavior.* St. Louis: Mosby-Year Book, Inc.
14. Beckman, L. J. 1994. Treatment needs of women with alcohol problems. *Alcohol Health & Research World,* 18 (3), 206-11.
15. Alcohol and estrogen supplements may increase breast cancer risk. 1996. (URL: http://www.healthnet.ivi.com/ivi/hnews/9612.htm/alcohol.htm)
16. Tivis and Gavler, Alcohol, hormones, and health in postmenopausal women.
17. Dieting coeds more likely to drink. 1992. In *USA Today* (December), p. 11.

18. Blume, S. B. 1986. Women & alcohol: A review. *Journal of the American Medical Association,* 256 (11): 1467–70.

19. Center for Substance Abuse Treatment. 1994. *Practical approaches in a treatment of women who abuse alcohol and other drugs.* Department of Health and Human Services, Public Health Service, Rockville, Md.

20. Ibid.

21. Gilbert, M. J. 1991. Acculturation & changes in drinking patterns among Mexican-American women. *Alcohol Health and Research World,* 15 (3): 234–38.

22. Steel, C., and R. A. Josephs. 1990. Alcohol myopia. *American Psychologist,* 45, 921.

23. Klee, L., C. Schmidt, and G. Ames. 1991. Indicators of women's alcohol problems: What women themselves report. *The International Journal of the Addictions,* 26 (8): 879–95.

24. Norris, J. 1994. Alcohol & female sexuality. *Alcohol Health & Research World,* 18 (3): 197–201.

25. U.S. Department of Health & Human Services. 1990. *Alcohol and health: Seventh special report to the U.S. Congress.* Washington, D.C.: U.S. Government Printing Office, Report No. (ADM) 90–1656.

26. Kinney and Leaton, *Loosening the grip.*

27. Payne, W. A., and D. Hahn. 1998. *Understanding your health, 5th ed.* St. Louis: Mosby.

28. Department of Student Life. 1994. *Women's programs.* College Station, Tex.: Texas A&M University.

29. Alcohol and acquaintance rape: Strategies to protect yourself & others. 1996. (URL: http://www.edc.org/HHD/HEC/pubs/rapefly.htm)

30. Jennings, P. 1997. *Alcohol & pregnancy.* ABC Evening News, 23 April, Television news report.

31. Center for Substance Abuse Treatment, *Practical approaches in a treatment of women who abuse alcohol and other drugs.*

32. Asetoyer, C. 1990. Fetal alcohol syndrome chemical genocide. Copenhagen, Denmark: International Workgroup for Indigenous Affairs. Document #66, p. 87–92.

33. Little, R. E., and C. F. Sing. 1986. Association of fathers drinking and infants birth weight. *New England Journal of Medicine,* 314 (25): 1644–45.

34. Cicero, T. 1994. Effects of paternal exposure to alcohol on offspring development. *Alcohol Health & Research World,* 18 (1): 37–41.

35. Jones, V. H., and E. Hutchins. 1993. *Finding common ground: A call for collaboration, promoting state interagency efforts to reduce the impact of perinatal alcohol & other drug use on families.* Arlington, Va.: National Center for Education in Maternal and Child Health.

36. Anderson, K. N. 1994. *Mosby's medical, nursing & allied health dictionary, 4th ed.* St. Louis, Mo.: Mosby-Year Book, Inc.

37. Ray and Ksir, *Drugs, society, and human behavior.*

38. Estés, C. P. 1995. *Women who run with the wolves.* New York: Ballantine Books, p. 248.

39. Pinger et al., *Issues for today.*

40. Estés, *Women who run with the wolves,* p. 251.

Eleven

Using Other Psychoactive Drugs

◼ chapter objectives

When you complete this chapter you will be able to:

- Identify laws that have improved the quality and control of medicinal drugs.
- Explain physical and psychological dependency and the relationship to tolerance and withdrawal.
- Compare and contrast generic and brand name prescription drugs.
- Identify the types of information written on drug labels.
- Identify medicinal drugs prescribed for common disorders such as weight control, depression, anxiety, and hormone replacement therapy.
- Explain the difference between prescription and over-the-counter drugs and provide examples of both.
- Describe the consequences of illicit drug use and its impact on a woman's lifestyle, health, and pregnancy.
- Describe some of the social problems that women encounter as a result of illegal drug use.

WHERE DID ALL THESE DRUGS COME FROM?

Medicinal products have been in existence for tens of thousands of years. For most of those years very little scientific evidence was available to determine if medicines really treated what they were purported to treat. Trial and error, often at the expense of human life determined if substances cured what ailed a person. Herbal medicines made from all types of plants were used prior to the research and manufacture of synthetic drugs, whose ingredients are now regulated and controlled. During the mid-to-latter years of this century, herbal medicines have regained popularity as people search for different methods for treatment as well as improvement of well-being.

Patent medicines, drugs overseen by the U.S. Patent Office, were extremely popular in America during the nineteenth century. These medicines claimed to cure everything from cancer and paralysis to tuberculosis and uterine problems. Most products were not harmful, nor were they helpful. However some of these patented concoctions were poisonous. *Dr. Kilmer's Female Remedy,* a woman's medicine of this era, claimed to treat chronic weakness, ovarian dropsy, and suspicious growths as well as other problems.

> **patent medicines**—those medicines available to the general public without a prescription; information pertaining to the drug is usually available on the drug label.

HEALTHY PEOPLE 2000 OBJECTIVES

- Reduce drug-related death to no more than 3 per 100,000 people. 1995 progress toward goal: -70 percent
- Extend adoption of alcohol and drug policies for the work environment to at least 60 percent of worksites with 50 or more employees. 1995 progress toward goal: data unavailable

During the twentieth century, the federal government has endeavored to pass legislation to ensure the safety and quality of medicinal drugs. To promote truth in labeling and to reduce misleading advertising of patented drugs, the Pure Food and Drug Act was passed in 1906. The 1914 Harrison Narcotic Act authorized physicians to prescribe drugs that cured diseases and reduced suffering rather than prescribe the patented drugs that claimed to cure everything. Even though the 1938 Food, Drug, and Cosmetic Act increased consumer protection against drug misrepresentation, there was little difference between the labeling requirements for prescription and nonprescription drugs. The Kefauver-Harris Amendment of the Food, Drug, and Cosmetic Act became law in 1962. It prevents new drugs from being sold to the public without first providing evidence to the **Food and Drug Administration (FDA)** that the drug is safe and effective. The FDA regulates the manufacture and distribution of food, drugs, and cosmetics to protect the American public against the sale of impure or dangerous substances.

ADDICTION AND DEPENDENCY

Addiction to drugs is a compulsive and uncontrollable dependence on the substance, habit, or practice to such a degree that cessation of the drug causes severe emotional, mental, or physiological reactions.[1] Components of addiction include *tolerance, physical dependence, psychological dependence,* and *withdrawal.*

Dependency: What Is It?

Drug dependency can result from use of prescription, over-the-counter, recreational, and illegal drugs.

The pharmacological makeup of a drug often dictates the type and sometimes the degree of dependency.

Physical dependency means that body cells have become dependent on a chemical. As the body cells begin to rely on the presence of the drug in the body, the body cells will need to replenish the drug supply in order to maintain *homeostasis,* or biological balance within the body. Drug tolerance will often develop. More of the drug will be needed to maintain previously felt sensations. Once a woman has developed a physical dependence upon a drug, she will experience *withdrawal symptoms* once her body is deprived of it. Withdrawal symptoms can be extremely uncomfortable, and even fatal.

Psychological dependency is a learned process and affects the behavior of the woman who uses a dependency-creating drug. Desiring or craving the effects that a drug delivers is an indication that psychological dependency has developed. Stimulant drugs often create a psychological dependency in which the "high," the mind alteration or mood swing felt by the user, is continually sought by the user. However, these feelings are often short-lived. The user comes down from the high only to seek out the drug again to renew the feeling. Over time, the highs do not get quite as high. The lows become lower, and the user seeks the drug more often, not to reach the high, but to avoid the low. Additional information on physical and psychological dependency can be found in chapters 9 and 10.

PRESCRIPTION DRUGS

Currently, the FDA has approved more than 2,000 prescription drugs, all of which are intended to prevent, treat, or cure various types of illnesses. Prescription drugs are made of natural and/or synthetic chemicals and can only be obtained with a physician's written authorization. Prescription drugs are potent, but when used as directed, can produce positive results for treatment and healing. The FDA regulates prescription drugs for form, strength, safety, purity, effectiveness, and method of administration.

Prescription drugs have three names: the generic name, the chemical name, and the brand name. *Generic* names pertain to the kind of drug and also describe the drug, such as penicillin. Although generic drugs are identical in their chemical compounds with the same brand name drug, generic drugs may *not* be equivalent in therapeutic effect. Legally, drugs are identified by their generic names and are listed by that name in the **United States Pharmacopoeia (USP).**

Table 11.1

Generic and Brand Names of Commonly Prescribed Drugs	
BRAND NAME	**GENERIC NAME**
Zovirax	Acyclovir
Xanax	Alprazolam
Valium	Diazepam
Tylenol	Acetaminophen

The USP is responsible for conferring the official standards of identity, purity, and effectiveness for all prescription drugs. In laboratories, drugs are called by their chemical name, which usually refers to the chemicals from which the drugs have been developed. The *brand* name, under the control of the FDA, is patented by the pharmaceutical company, which develops, manufactures, and distributes the drug to pharmacies. The company that develops and tests the drug has exclusive rights to produce it for 17 years. Once the patent expires, other pharmaceutical companies are then permitted to manufacture the drug under another brand name or under its generic name. Table 11.1 provides a few examples of brand and generic names of commonly prescribed drugs.

Pharmacists can dispense generic drugs instead of brand name products with a doctor's approval in almost all states. This happens because brand name drugs can be 30–50 percent more expensive than their generic counterparts. Approximately 400 different generic drugs can presently be substituted for brand name drugs.[2] The equivalent effectiveness of generic and brand name drugs is determined by scientists who measure the time it takes the generic drug to reach the bloodstream. The rate of absorption, called **bioavailability,** is then compared to the brand name drug. If it is found that the generic version delivers the same amount of active ingredients into a patient's bloodstream with equal absorption rates, the two drugs are considered to be equivalent. The FDA ensures the equivalency of generic and brand name drugs.[3] However, even if drugs are therapeutically equivalent, they may not produce the same effects on all women.

Understanding Drug Labels

Carefully following the directions on a prescription label enables the consumer to receive the most effective results when taking a drug. A prescription label provides the patient's name and the physician's name as well as the name, address, and phone number of the pharmacy dispensing the drug. Drug-related information includes the name of the drug, the dosage form (liquid, capsule, tablet) and the strength of the drug, either in milligrams (mg) or ounces. How much, how often, and when to take the drug is indicated along with any special instructions and refill information. Essential information regarding warnings about drug-drug or food-drug interactions is also provided.

Almost half of all prescription drugs will fail to produce the desired effects because they will be used incorrectly. Patients do such things as take too much or too little of a drug, take it too often or not often enough, skip doses, take it with food or alcohol, or save and use outdated drugs. A woman needs to ask her physician and/or pharmacist critical questions and seek information that will permit her to use the medication safely and effectively. She should tell her physician about any previous allergic reactions to foods or medicines, any medication being taken on a regular basis, and any physical conditions for which she is being treated by other physicians. Certainly let her physician know if she is pregnant or breast-feeding.

Health Tips: "Questions to Ask When Taking Prescription Medicine" lists questions women should ask their physicians about prescription drug use. For practice, complete *Journal Activity:* "Questions to Ask When Purchasing Medications."

Commonly Prescribed Drugs

Two-thirds of the women who visit a doctor's office this year will have a written prescription for a drug or drugs in their hands when they leave the office. The average physician will write about 8,000 prescriptions annually.[4] What are the most frequently prescribed drugs for women? Substances that assist in weight management are among the most commonly

Food and Drug Administration (FDA)—the federal agency charged with approval and control of drug-related products in the United States.

United States Pharmacopeia (USP)—describes the properties of medicines and assures the purity of the drug.

bioavailability—rate of absorption.

➤ health tips

Questions to Ask When Taking Prescription Medicine

Asking basic questions and seeking information from your physician or pharmacist can assist you in receiving the proper medication for your health, as well as result in the most effective use of your consumer dollars.

- What is the purpose of this medicine?
- What are the possible side effects?
- What foods, beverages, or other medication should I avoid while taking this medicine?
- Exactly when and how do I take the medication?
- What should I do if I experience side effects?
- How long should I take this medication?

JOURNAL ACTIVITY

Questions to Ask When Purchasing Medications

Try this activity the next time you visit a pharmacy: ask the pharmacist the questions in *Health Tips:* "Questions to Ask When Taking Prescription Medicine." You can do this activity when obtaining prescription medicine or purchasing an OTC medication. Consider the following:

- Did the pharmacist answer your questions in language that you could understand?
- If you were unsure of the information, did you ask the pharmacist to provide additional information?
- Did the pharmacist treat you with respect and consideration?
- Did you feel comfortable with your interaction with this health professional?
- How was this activity beneficial to you regarding your own health care?

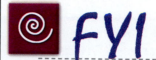

The Ideal versus Reality[5]

It is no wonder that medications to control weight are some of the most prevalent medicines used today. Consider the following:

- In the late 1960s, fashion models were 8 percent thinner than the average-sized woman; today, models are 23 percent thinner!
- Today, the average fashion model is 5'10" and weighs 110–115 pounds; the average American woman is actually 5'4" and weighs 140–145 pounds.
- If Barbie were a "real" woman, she would be 5'9" and have measurements of 36–18–33.
- One-third of American women wear size 16 or larger.
- The diet industry brings in revenue of approximately $33 billion annually.
- The estimated cost of obesity and obesity-related diseases is $70 billion annually.

think that this is the image we must have. Trying to create this image for herself, a woman may use various drugs to find this thin, ideal person she believes can be uncovered if she could just lose those extra pounds. (See the *FYI:* "The Ideal versus Reality.")

To aid in weight management and reduction, weight control substances can be obtained with a doctor's prescription or purchased as an over-the-counter product. Drugs prescribed to help weight management often help in achieving short-term weight loss. However, unless an appetite suppressant drug is combined with a behavior modification program, once the drug is stopped, a woman will probably regain any weight she has lost.

A few of the many types of prescription drugs that women can use to control their weight include:

Pondimin (**pon**-di-min); generic name: fenfluramine hydrochloride) is an immediate, time-release anorectic drug used in the short-term management of obesity (usually a few weeks). It is used as an adjunct component of a weight management program when a woman wants to restrict her caloric intake by appetite suppression. The usual dose is one 20 mg tablet three times daily before meals. This can be increased over time, but the maximum dose should not exceed 120 mg per day. Women may experience drowsiness, diarrhea, and dry mouth. More serious side effects include possible dizziness, depression,

prescribed drugs for women. Additionally, antidepressants, sedative-hypnotics, and hormone regulation substances are also among the most commonly prescribed drugs for women.

Weight Control   Media sources portray the ideal and desirable woman as one who is tall, thin, well-toned, and usually having long, blond hair. Although we cannot change our height, we can, if we choose, become blond and, in some instances, thin. This may not be everyone's "ideal," nor should we be expected to conform to the media's image. Yet we seem to

anxiety, or insomnia. Women who have glaucoma, alcoholism, or psychosis are warned not to use this substance. There also are some concerns about using this drug prior to undergoing surgery due to the negative interaction between anesthesia and fenfluramine. Tolerance and severe psychological dependency has been noted among some women who use this appetite suppressant for long periods of time.

Fastin (**fas**-tin; generically known as phentermine hydrochloride) is an appetite suppressant intended for short-term use as part of a comprehensive weight reduction plan. Fastin should not be taken for more than a few weeks because of possible side effects and decreased effectiveness as an appetite suppressant. Side effects can include constipation, dizziness, dry mouth, mood swings, loss of sex drive, and the inability to fall or stay asleep among other effects. Fastin can create psychological dependency. Abrupt discontinuance can cause extreme fatigue, depression, and/or sleeping disorders.

Another often prescribed weight control substance is *Tenuate* (**ten**-you-ate; generic name: diethylpropion hydrochloride). Similar to Fastin, it is also a short-term diet suppressant. However, it comes in two forms: immediate-release tablets and controlled-release tablets. It is essential that Tenuate be taken as prescribed because of its habit-forming and addicting qualities. Side effects such as blood pressure elevation, abdominal discomfort, mood swings, or sleep disruptions among others are possible. As with any other prescription drug, any changes or special concerns and situations should be discussed immediately with your physician.

Antidepressants

Feelings of sadness, disappointment, or helplessness, collectively known as depression, affect about 15 percent of the population at any given time. About two-thirds of individuals diagnosed with depression are women.[6] Relief from depression often comes in the form of a prescription drug such as those that follow. Physicians consider age, symptoms, general health status, and side effects when deciding which antidepressant drug to prescribe. There are a variety of antidepressant medications from which to select. Each has its own unique benefits and limitations. A detailed discussion concerning depression in women is found in chapter 5.

Zoloft (**zoe**-loft; generic name: sertraline) is prescribed for major depression including symptoms such as lack of interest in activities, disturbed sleep, reduced appetite, and feelings of worthlessness. It is thought that Zoloft alters part of the brain chemistry to balance its natural chemical messengers. Avoid Zoloft if you have taken any MAO inhibitors within the last two weeks. (See the following discussion.) Side effects may include dry mouth, constipation, dizziness, or headaches. Check with your physician if any of these or other side effects occur. You may initially lose one to two pounds and it may take a few days or weeks to see any improvement with the depression. Do not drink alcohol while using this medication.

Prozac (**pro**-zak; generic name: fluoxetine hydrochloride) is prescribed for continuing depression that can interfere with daily functioning. Prozac, a type of *selective serotonin reuptake inhibitor (SSRIs),* increases the level of serotonin, but not norepinephrine. Because SSRIs have fewer side effects than the tricyclic antidepressants, they are becoming the most frequently prescribed antidepressants in the country. There are no negative cardiovascular side effects, sedative effects, or weight gain effects associated with SSRIs. Keep in mind however, as with most medications, there are some potential unpleasant effects from using these drugs. Common side effects include diarrhea, increased or decreased appetite, nervousness, or abnormal dreams. Some evidence suggests that Prozac inhibits female orgasm. A word of caution: a woman should not take SSRIs with MAO inhibitors, which are other types of antidepressant drugs.

Monoamine oxidase inhibitors (MAOIs) increase the levels of numerous neurotransmitters in the body. These antidepressants, for example *Nardil* (**nar**-dill), are prescribed when no other antidepressant is effective and for individuals who have manic–depressive conditions. Studies indicate that MAOIs are somewhat more dangerous than other antidepressants because of the different neurotransmitters they affect. A long list of foods and other drugs cannot be taken with MAOIs. Physicians must be alerted to any and all medications being taken prior to prescribing these antidepressants.

Sedative Hypnotics

Anxiety is a feeling of unrest, excessive alertness, and hypervigilance. It may be caused by a chemical or hormonal imbalance, or emotional traumas. Anxiety can be debilitating and interfere with everyday happiness and responsibilities. Anxiety disorders, discussed more fully in chapter 6, are divided into seven categories: generalized anxiety disorder, simple phobias, agoraphobia, panic

Table 11.2

Methods of Hormone Replacement Therapy	
METHOD	**ADVANTAGES AND DISADVANTAGES**
Hormone pills	+ Processed in the liver, increases high-density lipoproteins (HDL), beneficial for the prevention of cardiovascular disease. – High doses produce negative side effects.
Injections	+ No daily intake, given once a month. – No steady hormone levels in the blood; cost and inconvenience of seeing a physician.
Patch	+ Convenient, nonpainful patch placed on buttocks or upper arm that lasts several days. – No apparent increase in HDL levels.
Creams	+ Easily applied (rubbed into skin of the abdomen, arms, or thighs); no high-dose side effects; maintain a specific dose. – Can be messy; produce too high a level of estrogen; blood estrogen levels have to be monitored.
Vaginal Creams	+ Benefits of other methods of estrogen. – Risks of other methods of estrogen.

disorders, obsessive–compulsive disorder, and post-traumatic stress disorder. In addition to treating these disorders through means of behavioral modification and therapy, medication is often prescribed in the form of sedative hypnotics.

A group of sedative hypnotics, called *benzodiazepines,* have proven to be effective and safe when used to treat anxiety disorders. These medications have fewer side effects than do barbiturates. One of the best-known benzodiazepines is *Valium* (**val**-ee-um; generic name: diazepam) which was the largest selling prescription drug in the 1970s. *Xanax* (**zan**-ax; generic name: alprazolam) is presently the drug most widely prescribed to treat anxiety disorders. Xanax is used for short-term relief of symptoms associated with anxiety or panic and, though it is most effective, it can lead to tolerance and dependency. A number of common side effects may occur following benzodiazepine use, including agitation, confusion, constipation, drowsiness, dry mouth, and fluid retention. These medications are effective for the treatment of anxiety disorders, but they must be used as directed.

Hormone Therapy Hormone therapy is the process by which a woman increases the level of estrogen in her body. Decreased estrogen levels result from either natural or surgically induced menopause. Estrogen Replacement Therapy (ERT) raises levels of estrogen in the body, but produces some unpleasant side effects. An alternative to ERT is Hormone Replacement Therapy (HRT), which provides both es-

trogen and progestin in the body. Many of the serious side effects resulting from ERT can be greatly reduced by prescribing the combination of estrogen and progestin. Hormone therapy continues to be controversial among physicians who prescribe it and women who receive it. Physicians and women find weighing the health benefits against possible health risks both confusing and stressful.

Just who is it that can benefit from hormone therapy? Physicians agree that women who either have nonfunctioning ovaries or ovaries that have been surgically removed are good candidates for hormone therapy. Additionally, early menopause, prior to age 45, and women who experience severe discomfort while going through menopause probably need hormone therapy as well. Hormones can also be beneficial for women who are at high risk for cardiovascular disease and osteoporosis.

Equally important to consider are those women who should not use this type of medical treatment. Women whose family members have had ovarian, uterine, or breast cancers may not want to have HRT. Hormone therapy should also be avoided by women who have fibroids, benign uterine tumors, blood clotting conditions, and liver or gallbladder disease. Of course, a pregnant woman should not take hormones, or most other drugs, for that matter. Table 11.2 lists the methods to receive hormone therapy.

One of the most frequently prescribed drugs for ERT is *Premarin,* (**prem**-uh-rin; generic name: conjugated estrogens). Reducing the symptoms of menopause, Premarin can also be used to reduce dry,

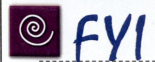

Side Effects of Premarin[7]

- Tenderness, swelling, or pain in the abdomen.
- Unusual vaginal bleeding or coughing up blood.
- Lumpy breast(s).
- Chest pains or severe headaches.
- Changes in vision or yellowing of the skin.
- Quick or shortness of breath.

health tips

Guidelines When Taking Medications

Following safe guidelines can help enhance drug effectiveness and safety:

- Take the prescribed dosage; do not take more or less than instructed.
- Follow the directions on the label; modify only as your physician specifies.
- Ask the pharmacist or physician about directions if you are unsure about using the medication properly.
- Finish the prescription even after you are feeling better; women often relapse when they fail to finish all their medication.
- Seek a second opinion if you are concerned about taking the drug.

itchy vaginal irritation, and more importantly to prevent osteoporosis. As with other medications, Premarin can have serious side effects, including an increased risk of developing uterine cancer and/or breast cancer if taken for a long time or in large doses. Additionally, Premarin may increase the risk of blood clots and if taken after menopause can promote the development of gallbladder disease. See *FYI:* "Side Effects of Premarin" for signs to watch for when using Premarin.

Estraderm (**Ess**-tra-derm; generic name: Estradiol) and *Ogen* (**oh**-jen; generic name: Estropipate) are female hormone replacement drugs that help reduce menopausal symptoms and can be prescribed for female teens who do not mature at the usual rate. Benefits as well as negative side effects closely resemble those of Premarin.

Hormone replacement drugs are most beneficial for many feminine concerns but like other drugs, they are not without consequences. A woman and her physician must weigh the benefits of hormone replacement medicines against the risks and determine the right course of action.

Using Prescription Drugs Safely

Our bodies are chemical-laden machines. When we add additional chemicals such as prescription drugs, we may be brewing a chemical mix in our bodies that could result in undesirable, uncomfortable, and in some instances, unsafe **side effects.** Side effects often result from using the drug incorrectly, such as skipping a dose, taking too much, taking it at the wrong time, taking it with beverages other than water, or taking it with or without food when directions suggest differently. However, most side effects can be reduced, or even better, eliminated.

Weight, age, gender, health status, and/or diet can affect how drugs react when used by women. *Health Tips:* "Guidelines When Taking Medications" provides guidelines to follow when taking medications.

Getting the most out of the medication you have been prescribed is as important as taking it correctly. *Assess Yourself:* "Safety Tips When Taking Medications" is a checklist to determine it you are using medicines safely.

The benefits resulting from using drugs that prevent, treat, and heal diseases correctly outweigh any risks one might encounter. Although medicines are powerful drugs, wise and careful use does eliminate most complications. (See *Health Tips:* "Caution.")

OVER-THE-COUNTER (OTC) DRUGS

Twenty-six different classes of over-the-counter (OTC) drugs containing between 250,000 and 300,000 drug products are available without prescription in markets across the country today. These include such categories as analgesics, antihistamines, stimulants, laxatives, topical analgesics, antacids, and

side effects—undesirable, uncomfortable, or unsafe reactions when using any type of drug in which the effects are unexpected.

Assess Y O U R S E L F

Safety Tips When Taking Medications

DO YOU:	YES	NO
Alert all your physicians to all medications you are currently taking?	_____	_____
Refuse to share your medications with friends and family?	_____	_____
Store medication properly and away from light, heat, and moisture?	_____	_____
Use nonmedical treatment for occasional illnesses?	_____	_____
Review with your physician any medications used on a long-term basis?	_____	_____
Dispose of any medications that are outdated or no longer used?	_____	_____

h e a l t h   t i p s

Caution: Watch for Tampering

Although prescription and over-the-counter drugs are considered to be packaged safely in the United States, manufacturers cannot make a *tamper-proof* package. It is important to know how to protect yourself from possible tampering and contaminating of medicines. You can protect yourself by doing the following:

- Inspect the outer package for tears, cuts, or punctures.
- Inspect the medicine and look for discoloration or damage.
- Look for tablets or capsules that appear to be different from others in the package.
- Never take medicine in the dark.
- Pay attention to the safety features provided by the manufacturer.
- Use time and care, and good common sense. It is your own best safety feature!

Table 11.3

FDA Categories for OTC Drug Ingredients

Category I	Ingredient is *GRAS* and *GRAE*.
Category II	Ingredient is either not *GRAS* and/or not *GRAE* and would be removed from stores within 6 months if the manufacturer did not prove its safety and effectiveness.
Category III	Insufficient data to determine the ingredients' safety and/or effectiveness. If the manufacturer cannot prove GRAS within one year, the drug becomes a Category II rather than a Category I drug.*

*(Only drugs that have been proven to be safe and effective are now placed in the OTC market.)

others. Are these drugs safe and effective? The 1962 Kefauver-Harris Act required scientific evidence to prove that OTC drugs were safe and effective. A regulatory program was developed by the FDA in 1972 in which active ingredients of OTC drugs were assigned to one of three categories: *GRAS* (Generally Recognized as Safe), *GRAE* (Generally Recognized as Effective), and *GRAHL* (Generally Recognized as Honestly Labeled). These categories with their FDA-developed acronyms are used to effectively describe the safety of the ingredients found in OTC drugs. (See Table 11.3.)

In 1992, an account by the U.S. General Accounting Office reported that the FDA is unable to determine the exact number of OTC products that are marketed each year, and that all of them may not be safe and effective. However, as more prescription drugs become OTC drugs, these OTC drugs are becoming safer and more effective. *FYI:* "How a Prescription Drug Becomes an OTC Drug" explains how this is done.

OTC Drugs Used by Women

Rising medical care costs is a major concern for those women who have little, if any, money for professional health care. Thus, self-diagnosis of illness is on the increase, and leads to more frequent purchasing of OTC prescriptions. Hundreds of thousands of OTC prescriptions are purchased each year simply

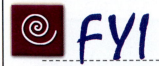

How a Prescription Drug Becomes an OTC Drug

Manufacturers who own a patent for a prescription drug must apply to the FDA for permission to reconstruct the formula for the drug. Usually, the active ingredients are made less concentrated and safer to use without a doctor's prescription. Products do retain their prescription brand name. Once approval is given by the FDA, the former prescription drug can be marketed and sold as an OTC medicine. Examples of such products include Aleve for premenstrual discomfort, Monistat and Gynelotromin which are creams to treat vaginal infection, and Ibuprofen for headaches. ☜

by consumer choice. Therefore, consumers must be informed about the advantages and the potential hazards of those medicines purchased without benefit of a physician's consultation or prescription.

To help reduce the misuse of OTC medicines, labeling and package inserts are provided with each drug and have become more reliable since the FDA assumed control over OTC medicines. Information provided on each label includes the product name, quantity of drug, active ingredients, manufacturer's or distributor's name and address, directions for use, and purpose. Drug warnings, expiration date, and possible drug interactions are also included on the packaging of the medication. By reading the information on each label, a women should not have any problem in determining the purpose of the drug, and the safe and effective way to take it.

The following discusses the major categories of OTC drugs purchased by women.

Weight Management Products

Want to make a million? Develop a diet pill that promises to remove unwanted fat without any physical exertion nor reduction in food intake and you will certainly be wealthy. Although they may be an aid to weight loss or weight control, appetite suppressants simply cannot provide a healthy approach to quick weight loss.

Diet pills, creams, liquids, and supplements are available to either suppress one's appetite, increase metabolism, and/or make a woman feel full and therefore less likely to eat large amounts of food.

Some OTC weight management products have been removed from the marketplace because they either failed to meet their claims or were shown to be dangerous. Products that "burn fat," "dissolve cellulite," and provide a "natural" way to rid one's body of unsightly fat have failed to match their advertising claims and, in some cases, have created health problems for the user.

Are there any weight management OTC products that do work? If we mean that by taking them we can lose weight, then the answer is yes. OTC drugs that contain **phenylpropanolamine (PPA)** suppress the appetite and have been declared safe by the FDA. The recommended dose for suppressing the appetite is 75 mg per day.[8] But there are some concerns about the safety of this dosage. Products such as *Acutrim* and *Dexatrim* contain PPA and come in tablet or capsule forms. Some contain vitamins and some contain less than 75 mg of PPA.

However, this is often a less healthy method because a woman may not receive the nutrients she needs if she is not eating food properly. Additionally, by changing her eating habits, any weight loss may only be temporary. She often does not include regular exercise in her weight management plan. So, although there are pills that can certainly reduce appetite and speed up metabolism, there are better methods or combinations of methods to reach a desired goal than by taking pills to lose weight.

Laxatives A laxative is a medicinal aid to help the body eliminate waste products, or "stool," from the body. OTC laxatives increase the bulk and water content of the bowel, thereby loosening it for better elimination. Laxatives are available in a number of different dosage forms: liquid, tablet, suppository, gum, power, enema, and granule. Table 11.4 lists the different types of laxatives available.

Although it is occasionally necessary to use a laxative product, frequent and continual use can lead to addiction and even the loss of muscular and neurological control of the bowels. Use of laxatives can lead to depletion of body fluids, salts, and essential nutrients. Another serious concern is that habitual

phenylpropanolamine (feen ul pro **pan** oh la mean) **(PPA)**—an OTC drug that suppresses the appetite.

Table 11.4

Types of Laxatives[9]

TYPE	ACTION	PRODUCTS
Stimulant	Agitates intestinal walls causing muscular contractions that expel fecal matter	Ex-Lax, Feen-a-Mint, Fletcher's Castoria, Modane
Lubricants	"Greases" stools, facilitating excretion	Agoral Plain, Fleet Mineral Oil Enema
Saline	Draws water into the bowel, and allows for easier passage of stools	Milk of Magnesia, Citrate of Magnesia, Epsom Salts
Stool softeners	Softens hard stools so they can absorb more liquids and pass more easily	Colace, Dialose, Regutol, Surfak
Hyperosmotics	Draws water into the bowel to allow for easier passage of stool; less risk of salt depletion than saline	OTC hyperosmotics like glycerin are only for rectal use; oral hyperosmotics require prescriptions
Carbon-dioxide-releasing agents	Produces carbon dioxide in bowels; gas pushes stool toward excretion	Ceo-Two (suppositories)
Bulk	Absorbs water into the intestine swelling the stool into an easily passed soft mass; must be taken with 8 ozs. of water	Metamucil, FiberCon, Serutan; and bran products, such as found in cereals

use of laxatives can inhibit the absorption and effectiveness of other prescriptions and OTC drugs. Depending on the type of laxative used, side effects such as belching, dizziness, fatigue, skin irritation, and irregular heartbeat may be experienced. (See *Her Story:* "Aimee.")

The FDA has taken a number of measures to help regulate OTC products such as laxatives, as well as remove products from the market that contain ingredients that cause serious side effects. Information about how the product works, how to use it properly, and the length of time needed to achieve the desired results can be found on packaging labels. Products with ingredients such as agar, guar gum, tartaric acid, ipomea, aloin, and ox bile have been removed from the marketplace until further research can prove them safe as well as effective.

Women can usually promote stool excretion regularity by making simple and healthful changes in diet and lifestyle. Increasing the intake of fiber-rich foods such as whole-grain breads, bran cereals, kidney, navy, and pinto beans, and fresh fruits and vegetables while reducing foods such as cheeses, white bread, and meat are helpful ways to replace the need for laxatives. Irregularity can also be caused by stress, depression, an underactive thyroid gland, and even colon–rectal cancer. Seeing a physician to address these concerns can produce positive results. An increased exercise routine can promote regular-

Her Story

Aimee

Aimee used a variety of laxative products to help her manage her weight. Even though she was aware of the possible consequences of habitual use of these products, Aimee relied on them to maintain the body image she felt she needed. Her roommate, Liz, began to see some negative effects upon Aimee's physical appearance and demeanor. Usually an easygoing and even passive individual, Aimee became irritable, quick-tempered, fatigued, and developed a nasty-looking skin infection. It was not until Liz found Aimee vomiting and in severe abdominal pain that Aimee was willing to seek help for her habitual use of laxatives.

- What can Liz do to help Aimee find help for her problem?
- What resources are available for women in your college or community to assist with abuse of any type of drugs?

ity as can slowing down a fast-paced lifestyle to let nature take its course. If irregularity persists, or if the use of laxatives to achieve weight management continues, then visiting a physician or psychotherapist is in order.

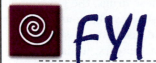

Is Melatonin a Miracle Drug?

Drug companies that promote the sale of melatonin promote it as an antiaging drug, an antioxidant, a jet-lag reducer, and as a non-habit-forming sleep aid. Is this really a miracle drug? Probably not! Melatonin has not been researched in long-term, large-scale trials that would provide support for or dispute these claims. What we do know is that melatonin induces sleep and it helps to keep the body's circadian rhythm synchronized with a 24-hour day.[10] Like all vertebrates, as human beings we make melatonin each night. Fading light alerts cells in the retina to direct the *suprachiasmic nuclei (SNC)* to signal the pineal gland, located in the brain, to produce melatonin. As a result, we soon fall asleep. Synthetic melatonin places more of this natural substance into the body. So what's the problem? Maybe nothing. However, melatonin is classified as a dietary substance and therefore it is not regulated for purity, quality, or dosage. Until this changes, anyone who takes melatonin is taking a substance that has not had to meet safety and quality regulations. ☜

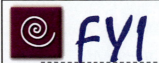

New Labeling Prototypes

The FDA has developed prototypes for easier-to-read labels for OTC drugs to provide information in a more clear and concise form. The labels use bulleted statements rather than paragraphs to highlight ingredients, uses, directions, and warnings. These prototype labels provide a standard format similar to the new food labels so that consumers can easily find information. OTC drugs that were formerly prescription drugs are all using the new labeling. Most other OTC drugs are expected to utilize this consumer-friendly labeling system. ☜

include *Extra Strength Tylenol PM* and *Sominex Pain Relief.* (See *FYI:* "Is Melatonin a Miracle Drug?" about melatonin.)

Be aware of potential side effects and warnings related to the use of sleep aids. **Contraindications** are included for individuals with asthma, glaucoma, or prostate gland enlargements. Products should not be used without a physician's advice.[11] Of course sleep aids should not be taken when driving or operating power machinery, or when any task or responsibility calls for alertness. Pregnant or lactating women need to be cautious about the use of any sleep aid. Such women, however, should not use any OTC drugs containing doxylamine. Do not use sleep aids with alcohol or other sedatives and tranquilizers. (See *FYI:* "New Labeling Prototypes" about drug labeling.) Instead of using sleep aids, try the suggestions listed in *Health Tips:* "Natural Sleep Aids."

Prescription and OTC Drug Use During Pregnancy

Rubin and colleagues[12] analyzed the drug use of over 2,700 pregnant females. Of these women, 68 percent used at least one drug during their pregnancy. The average intake of drugs was 1.2 drugs per female while pregnant. Educated, married, white women with higher than average incomes

Sleep Aids With the stress-filled lifestyles we all tend to live, getting a good night's sleep is sometimes difficult to achieve. If you do what millions of other women do, you probably visit the local pharmacy or discount store and select from a multitude of sleep aids that help promote sleep. Occasional use of some form of sleep aid is usually not harmful for temporary help. However, for sleep difficulties or insomnia lasting longer than 3 weeks, one needs to consult a physician to receive a diagnostic evaluation.

The causes of sleep difficulties can be multiple and complex. Worries about school, relationships, or finances; overconsumption of products containing caffeine; too much activity or excitement before bedtime; or poor time management skills can all lead to sleep deprivation.

Among OTC products available for insomnia, most contain one of two types of an antihistamine: diphenhydramine (found in *Compoz, Miles Nervine Caplets,* and *Nytol*) or doxylamine succinate (found in *Unisom,* and *Ultra Sleep*). In some instances, products contain analgesics, or painkillers, for insomnia caused by pain. Examples of this type of product

contraindications—conditions adversely affected by specific actions.

health tips

Natural Sleep Aids

Try these "natural" suggestions to help with sleep inducement before you go to bed.

- Engage in quiet and relaxing activities.
- Avoid any drinks containing caffeine.
- Have a bedtime routine such as warm shower, a soothing lotion, cleaning your teeth, etc.
- Listening to quiet music and/or read for a while.
- Avoid exercise too close to bedtime.
- Avoid late meals.
- Sleep in clean, comfortable bed clothes, and bedding.
- Try deep breathing and calming thoughts.

were more likely to use legal drugs, especially OTC products, while pregnant. The majority of these women gave birth to normal infants. However, women must be aware that each pregnancy is unique and the best approach is to avoid exposing the fetus to unnecessary drug substances. Therefore it is strongly recommended that women avoid all medication, both prescription and OTC, if possible during the pregnancy. Communication between pregnant women and their physicians, and strict adherence to the warnings about taking any drugs during pregnancy *must* be a priority.

ILLICIT DRUGS

Although both women and men use and abuse illicit drugs, the abuse of drugs by women can generate more health problems that may progress differently from men. In any given month, more than four million women in the United States abuse an illicit drug. In the last several years, illicit drugs were abused by more than nine million women. Almost one-half of all women between 15 and 44 years of age have used illicit drugs at least once. This includes cocaine (two million) and marijuana (six million) use, plus hundreds of thousands have sniffed inhalants. Over 70 percent of AIDS cases among women are drug-related, either because of unprotected sex with an HIV-infected male or the sharing of HIV-tainted needles.[13]

Many of today's illicit drugs were yesterday's legal drugs (such as cocaine and marijuana). Due to the potential for dependency and the devastating ef-

fects produced by using these drugs, the government declared them illegal substances. They are not now intended to be bought, sold, used, or possessed.

As child carriers and bearers, abuse of illicit drugs among women is of special concern. As women, we are responsible not only for our own personal health and well-being, but for the health and well-being of future generations. The discussion that follows explains how the abuse of drugs during pregnancy can produce devastating effects for both mother and fetus.

Drug Use and Pregnancy

Consequences to the fetus due to a woman's abuse of illegal drugs during pregnancy are of grave concern. Information about these consequences is not complete because of the ethics involved in conducting drug research on human babies. However, data from research conducted on animals have been the next best alternative. It has yielded important information about drug transmission to the fetus, the development of fetal abnormalities, effects on the fetal brain and growth patterns, and effects on fetal behavior.[14] However, with the potential for better research using ultrasound and other new techniques, a clearer and more conclusive correlation can be drawn between drug abuse by the mother, and the consequences to the fetus.

Research reveals that most drugs pass easily from the mother's blood through the placenta.[15] (See Table 11.5.) However, the time between drug intake, its transmission to the fetus, and the metabolism of the drug varies with the type used. For example, marijuana can take hours to reach the fetal bloodstream, while opiates reach the fetus quickly. Data support the contention that alcohol causes congenital abnormalities, but research on various other illicit drugs is inconclusive. Some studies with questionable research methodologies have revealed inconsistencies about fetal abnormalities and drug intake during pregnancy. Cocaine causes a decline in the delivery of oxygen and nutrients to the fetus because it is a *vasoconstrictor*. This results in an increase in blood pressure and heart rate. Marijuana increases the level of carbon monoxide in the blood, which decreases the amount of oxygen available to the fetus. Overall, drug use results in lower levels of oxygen and nutrients reaching the rapidly growing cells of the fetus. Read further to learn about the negative consequences of using various drugs.

Medical personnel should routinely ask pregnant women questions concerning the use of medications, alcohol, and other drugs. This information is important for administering proper medical care. Table 11.6 is an example of an indicator chart a physician might use to determine whether there is a need for urine and/or blood toxicology screening tests. Additional information regarding women and pregnancy can be found in chapter 17.

If the outcome of the screening tests reveal that the woman is indeed using a particular drug, then immediate medical and antidrug treatment needs to be started. Additionally, drug therapy in the form of detoxification, support groups, and individual therapy should be sought. Upon delivery, the infant should be screened for drugs in the blood and, if the screening is positive, medical treatment as well as evaluation of the home environment is needed.

Cocaine and Crack

Cocaine is derived from a plant, *Erythroxylon coca,* which grows best in the mountains of South America. Substances in its leaves produce an exhilarating effect, providing quick energy, stimulation, and a sense of well-being. Early research led physicians to believe that cocaine was a new miracle drug. It appeared in patent medicines, tonics, and even leading soda drinks. Cocaine was found to be an effective topical anesthetic during surgery and beneficial for alleviating depression. As individuals became dependent upon the products and medicines that contained this miracle drug, serious behavioral and health consequences resulted. Consequently, laws were enacted to tightly control cocaine. The Pure Food and Drugs Act in 1906 and the Harrison Act of 1914 reduced the legal availability of cocaine.

Crack is a rock-like substance that is the result of mixing cocaine with baking soda or ammonia. It is both easy to make and inexpensive to buy. Usually smoked in small pipes, it produces an almost immediate but brief high that is followed by depression and a strong longing for repeated use. Crack users quickly become dependent upon the substance often resulting in serious physical, legal, and financial consequences.

Consequences of Use The effects of cocaine upon a woman's brain depends upon the strength of the substance and the route of administration into the body. Cocaine can be inhaled by smoking, which only requires 8 seconds to the brain, absorbed by snorting, which requires 3 minutes to reach the brain, injected, which requires 14 seconds to reach the brain, or orally ingested, which requires 20 minutes to reach the brain.

Table 11.5

The Effects of Drugs on Mother and Baby[16]	
ON MOTHER	**ON BABY**
Poor nutrition	Premature birth
High blood pressure	Low birthweight
Fast heart rate	Infections
Low weight gain	Small head size
Low self-esteem	Sudden infant death syndrome (SIDS)
Preterm labor	Birth defects
Sexually transmitted diseases	Stunted growth
Early delivery	Poor motor skills
HIV/AIDS	HIV/AIDS
Depression	Learning disabilities
Physical abuse	Neurological problems

Table 11.6

Indicators of Drug Abuse[17] during Pregnancy		
INDICATOR	**YES**	**NO**
1. History of alcohol and other drug use?	_____	_____
2. Little or no prenatal care?	_____	_____
3. Mental condition such as incoherence or lethargy?	_____	_____
4. Lost custody of children?	_____	_____
5. Preterm delivery, labor, or membrane rupture?	_____	_____
6. Third trimester vaginal bleeding?	_____	_____
7. Physical indicators of alcohol and/or drug use?	_____	_____
8. Symptoms of intoxication or withdrawal?	_____	_____

Psychological and physical dependency develop with short- and long-term cocaine use. Research on both lab animals and humans reveals that the desire for the effects of cocaine are strong, and tolerance occurs with continual use. "Cocaine abstinence syndrome," are the feelings and behaviors associated with the cessation of cocaine use.[18] Individuals are likely to experience three stages of withdrawal:

Stage 1 (lasting several days) includes psychological depression, needing more sleep and food than usual, and cocaine cravings.

Stage 2 (lasting several weeks) includes boredom, anxiety, lack of motivation and little pleasure.

Stage 3 (lasting indefinitely) may include cravings produced by events, people, and places where cocaine was formerly used.

The effects of cocaine use produce immediate bodily responses: increases in heart and respiratory rates and coincidentally, an increase in blood pressure and elevated temperature. Appetite decreases and the user will feel more alert, excited, euphoric, and energized. However, due to lack of tolerance and experience and/or the high potency of cocaine, the user can also convulse, hemorrhage, or even experience heart failure.

Long-time users of cocaine will develop significant serious health consequences including: nasal inflammation, loss of appetite leading to malnourishment, coughing, heart rhythm irregularity, sleep disturbance, and even sexual dysfunction. Irritability, agitation, and paranoia can also result from continual use. Psychological consequences can be as severe as paranoid psychosis. Fortunately, with the cessation of cocaine use, time seems to repair most of the physical and psychological damage.

Effects on Pregnancy Cocaine use has increased among women in the past decade. As a result, the effects on women and the number of cocaine and crack-exposed infants has also increased. Research has found a variety of consequences that occur from cocaine and crack use during pregnancy:

- **Intrauterine growth retardation,** which is delay in the development and maturation of the fetus, appears to be an outcome of cocaine use during pregnancy.
- Sudden and severe pregnancy complications such as premature separation of the placenta from the uterus; fetal and maternal death can result.
- Premature labor and spontaneous abortion can result.

Consequences to the Fetus and Newborn The consequences of cocaine and crack use upon the fetus and the newborn can be profound. Studies have shown increased congenital anomalies, mild neurodysfunction (reduced nervous system function), cerebral (or brain) infarction, seizures, and heads with smaller circumference. Although it can be caused by other problems, *Sudden Infant Death Syndrome (SIDS)* has also been linked with cocaine abuse by pregnant women.[19]

Does the length of time a woman uses cocaine during pregnancy make a difference in the damage to the infant? Some studies indicate that the answer is yes! One study[20] compared the drug-related consequences of fetuses from mothers who used cocaine only during the first trimester with the fetuses from mothers who used cocaine throughout the pregnancy. Cocaine use throughout the pregnancy revealed a greater increase in early preterm delivery, low birthweight, and intrauterine growth retardation. However, both groups of mothers did seem to harm their offspring: The babies from both groups exhibited an impairment of orientation and motor regulation as well as temperament regulation.

Marijuana

Resurging after a decade of decline, marijuana (*Cannabis sativa*) is now more potent and troublesome than when it was widely used in the 1960s and 1970s. The current trend can be attributed to references to the substance on popular television shows, in music and movies, and merchandising or marijuana symbols. Proponents of marijuana can be found on personal internet home pages expounding upon its virtues and calling for legalization and decriminalization.

As a result of advances in plant genetics and growing methods, *Cannabis* growers have produced a more potent plant containing stronger substances, particularly with its plant's active ingredient, **tetrahydrocannabinol (THC).** Drug products from *Cannabis sativa* include marijuana, which can be smoked in joints or pipes, or ingested in teas or other foods; **hashish,** which is the dried resin from the flowering and leafy parts of the plant; and hash oil, consisting of resins and other juices often spread onto tobacco cigarettes. Depending on the part of the plant used for consumption and its preparation, the percentage of THC can vary from 1 percent in the domestic *sativa* plant to 8–14 percent or more THC found in hashish. The higher the THC, the greater the consequences are to the marijuana user.

Smoking marijuana produces peak effects within 30 minutes after inhalation. The effects usually decline after one hour. Effects from oral ingestion are usually not felt for 30 to 60 minutes and last from 3 to 5 hours.[21] Use of marijuana at moderate doses produces "feelings" of euphoria, relaxation, and peacefulness. Individuals may experience mood swings and an altered sense of time, space, and distance. There appears to be few immediate negative effects from short-term moderate marijuana use, but because of the altered sense of time, space, and distance, it is wise not to drive or use any type power tools or devices.

Consequences of Use *Cannabis* is a unique and complex plant. Containing over 400 chemicals with the most active ingredients being the cannabinoids (of which THC is the most active), marijuana can produce sedating, hallucinating, intoxicating, and/or analgesic effects. After decades of research, we know that a multitude of negative consequences can result from chronic, long-term use of marijuana. Consider the following effects that are concerns for the body systems.

- *Central Nervous System:* Reduces short-term memory, alters judgment, increases chances of developing mental illness, reduces cognitive skills, blurs and impairs vision perception, produces personality change, and alters motor coordination.
- *Respiratory System:* Can cause lung cancer, lung damage, pulmonary diseases, chronic bronchitis, and may cause trachea damage due to inhalation.
- *Cardiovascular System:* Produces tachycardia (irregular heartbeat), increases heart rate, blood pressure, concerns related to angina, diabetes, and aggravates high blood pressure in women who already have these disorders.
- *Reproductive System:* Disrupts the menstrual cycle, impairs ovulation and fertility, increases levels of testosterone in females, and may cause irreversible damage to the female ovum supply.

Effects on Pregnancy Research on marijuana and its effects on pregnancy and the fetus is lacking. However, once inhaled, THC easily crosses the pla-

centa of the mother to the fetus and causes similar levels of THC in both the mother and fetus. Studies have shown that infants born to women who smoke marijuana are likely to weigh less, and are shorter in length than infants born to nonsmoking women. Other studies revealed that babies exposed to chronic marijuana chemicals had poor nervous system responses and less response to visual stimulation. Additionally, THC is transported to nursing babies through breast milk.

Heroin and Methadone

Originally marketed as a cough suppressant, heroin is a very addictive, semisynthetic narcotic produced from chemically changed morphine, a naturally occurring opiate derived from the opium poppy plant. In its early history, heroin was thought to be safe and a substance that would aid in recovery from morphine addiction. Interestingly enough, by producing this drug from morphine, chemists made a drug that is three times more addicting than morphine.[22]

Consequences of Use *Heroin* is a fast acting narcotic which is injected directly into a vein or under the skin ("skin poppers"). Producing a dream-like state and a feeling of euphoria, users often feel they have found the panacea for all their problems and a way to temporarily escape to paradise. Like most other narcotics, heroin creates a strong physical and psychological dependency. Tolerance develops and withdrawal is usually severe and extremely uncomfortable though not life-threatening. Addiction to this chemical creates a situation in which women become so dependent on this drug that they may engage in life-threatening activities such as prostitution

intrauterine growth retardation—abnormal process in which the development and maturation of the fetus is impeded or delayed by a number of factors, including genetics, drugs, and malnutrition.

tetrahydrocannabinol (tetra hydro canuh **bin all) (THC)**—the active ingredient in the hemp plant *Cannabis sativa;* found in marijuana, hashish, and ganja.

hashish—concentrated resin from the *Cannabis* plant.

Viewpoint

Some Pros and Cons of Methadone Maintenance

Methadone Maintenance Programs (MMP) substitute one physically addicting drug, methadone, for another physical addicting drug, either heroin or morphine. But the intent of a MMP is to provide a chemical that reduces the negative physical, social, and legal impact of illegal drugs while assisting women with rehabilitation of their emotional and professional lives. There are opponents and proponents of MMPs and each side has logical arguments.

PROS

- Reduces use of illegal drug
- With counseling and support, it is a viable option for opiate treatment
- MMPs help slow the spread of HIV
- Reduces crime activity related to obtaining illegal drugs

CONS

- Methadone clinics are just drug distribution centers
- Just replaces one addiction with another
- Questions the ethics of physicians giving an addictive substance to people already having addictive disorders
- Does not prevent the addict from abusing other drugs, such as cocaine, alcohol, marijuana

What do you think about MMPs? Are you aware of any MMPs located near you? Call a local drug treatment center to learn if they have an MMP, and if not, why not!

---

or stealing, in a never-ending pursuit to calm the addiction. As a result, their health and quality of life suffers as do those, especially children, who live with and around her.

Methadone is a synthetic narcotic that can be taken orally and provides a longer duration of its effects, usually lasting from 24 to 36 hours. It was developed during World War II as a substitute for morphine. It also produces physical and psychological dependency, as well as tolerance and withdrawal symptoms. Many of the same physical problems can result from the use of methadone. However, because it is intended to be used as a legal, prescriptive replacement for heroin or morphine, the quality and the dose of the drug is controlled. (See *Viewpoint:* "Some Pros and Cons of Methadone Maintenance.")

Effects on Pregnancy   A woman who uses heroin and methadone during pregnancy can produce very serious consequences for herself and her fetus. **Toxemia,** also called blood poisoning, can occur in the blood of a pregnant woman, resulting in intrauterine growth retardation, and even premature rupture of the amniotic membrane. Heroin and methadone can adversely affect delivery because these drugs may cause preterm labor, breech birth (delivery of the baby bottom-first), and miscarriage. Of course, there also may be no effect from drug abuse during pregnancy. However, the risks are not worth the harmful effects the drug might produce.

Newborns of heroin-addicted mothers tend to have low birthweight and smaller head circumference. These babies may be born either premature or stillborn, and are more likely to die from SIDS. Infants born to methadone-addicted women may have normal birthweight, but soon may experience weight loss due to lack of sleep and hyperactivity. Drug withdrawal, lasting days or weeks, as well as irritability were experienced in varying degrees by infants born to heroin- and methadone-addicted women. As these children grow, they continue to have serious problems related to heroin and/or methadone exposure while in utero. Children, ages 2 to 4, exposed to narcotics while in utero tend to be very talkative, easily distracted, have brief attention spans, and are extremely energetic. Lower levels of learning, difficult behavior, and poor adaptation abilities were found in pre-school children who were born to women addicted to methadone and heroin.[23]

The harmful effects of drug use notwithstanding, this lifestyle often creates negative outcomes during pregnancy for mother and child. Lack of prenatal care, poor nutrition, and vitamin and mineral deficiencies can occur due to the time, energy, and money the mother must spend engaged in finding, obtaining, and using heroin. Consequences of using dirty needles include bacterial infections, sores, and hepatitis, as well as the risk of contracting HIV infection. There is also a greater likelihood of contracting other STDs such as chlamydia, herpes, or gonorrhea.

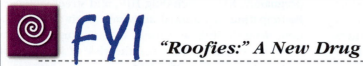

"Roofies:" A New Drug

A white pill the size of a dime has gained popularity in high schools and colleges in this country. Rohypnol (ro-**hip**-nol), called "Roofies," is colorless, odorless, and quickly dissolves in liquid. Within 10 minutes, it can produce a drunk-like effect that lasts approximately 8 hours. Effects include loss of inhibition, extreme sleepiness, relaxation, and even amnesia. An illegal drug in this country, it is prescribed as sleeping pills and used as a surgical anesthetic in other countries.

Roofies, as they are called by the students who use them, have created situations in which individuals, especially women, are unaware that the "pill" is slipped into any drink (from alcohol to Diet Coke) and produces the effects just mentioned. Costing only about $3.00, they are easily available in high schools, college dorms, frat houses, or any place individuals gather for a "good time."

One horror story after another is emerging that connects Roofies with the rape of young women. A 16-year-old girl at a high school dance was raped by three male high school students after they slipped a "Roofie" into her drink. One man was arrested after finally being identified by one of the 50 women he had raped after he had "doctored" their drinks with Rohypnol. Sadly, hundreds of such "Roofie rapes" are occurring throughout this country. Because the victim has temporary memory loss, these types of rape are hard to prosecute. Often the victim does not remember anything that happens during the time she is under its influence.

Suggestions to avoid this dangerous situation include:

- Do not accept a canned drink that is already open from anyone.
- Carefully watch your drink while in a crowded situation.
- Use a "team" approach to safety with friends when in a "party" situation by watching for suspicious behaviors.
- Avoid taking any type of drink from someone you do not know. ∽

Each of these, of course, can be passed on to the fetus in utero or during delivery.

ILLICIT DRUGS AND SOCIETAL PROBLEMS FOR WOMEN

Women, Drugs, and HIV Infection

Although men still have the greatest number of cases of AIDS, the number of women who contract HIV is increasing at a rate almost four times faster than men. Additionally, there is a chance that women will pass the virus on to their unborn children thereby doubling the tragic consequences. HIV is transmitted through direct exposure to body fluids (such as blood, semen, vaginal fluids, and mother's milk) when a woman has this virus in her body. Women can contract HIV as a result of vaginal or anal intercourse with an infected partner, injecting an illegal drug with a needle that contains HIV-infected blood, as well as other methods by which body fluids are exchanged. (Refer to chapter 18 for more information about HIV and AIDS.)

Researchers are looking at the use of psychoactive drugs that are not necessarily injected, such as al-cohol, marijuana, and cocaine, but can cause activity that increases the risk of contracting HIV. This is because women are more likely to have unsafe sex while under the influence of alcohol and other drugs. Therefore, women have an increased opportunity to contract or transmit HIV. For example, one study revealed that female crack smokers were six times more likely than nonsmokers to have had twenty or more sexual partners, fifteen times more likely to sell sexual favors, and four times more likely to have other STDs.[24] This extent of sexual activity will increase the chances of contracting HIV and other pathogens that cause sexually transmitted diseases.

The association between contracting or transmitting HIV as well as other STDs while under the influence of drugs is a serious concern. Wambach and others[25] conducted a study of 694 women and, among other concerns, examined the relationships between HIV-risk behaviors and substance use. The researchers found a significant relationship between

toxemia—presence of bacterial toxins in the blood; also called blood poisoning.

using drugs, such as alcohol, cocaine, crack, and/or heroin, and having multiple sex partners. Women who abused drugs were more likely to have partners who were also drug abusers; were unaware of their main partner's sexual history, sexual orientation, or HIV status; were more likely to be involved in prostitution; and were less likely to use condoms. The women in this study tended to believe they were more at risk for HIV only if they injected drugs. However, this study found a strong link between use of these drugs and poor decision making about the main partners and safer sex practices of these women. The research suggests that it is of primary importance to address the use of other substances as well as IV drugs when attempting to educate high-risk women about HIV infection.

Awareness, prevention, and support services are needed to help diminish the connection between women, drugs, and HIV. Refer back to chapter 10 for suggestions about drug abuse prevention strategies.

Women, Drugs, and Homelessness

Use of drugs, including alcohol, is a major risk for women and children as it relates to homelessness. Seeking, buying, and consuming illegal drugs can interfere with a woman's ability to locate employment, and purchase essential resources such as housing, food, and medical services necessary for her and her children's well-being. Although this may not be the "cause" of homelessness for many women and children, it certainly can be a contributing factor.[26]

Even though homelessness is less prevalent among women than men, it is the woman who often has the responsibility for children. Therefore, if a mother is homeless, then her children are homeless as well. Although the effects of drugs themselves have serious consequences, abusing drugs has serious effects on the personal health of homeless women and children. In an attempt to "score" or purchase various drugs, women may engage in risky sexual activity that places them at risk for unintended pregnancy, STDs, including HIV, and street violence. Participating in criminal activities, such as prostitution, drug dealing, and theft, to buy drugs, or even basic necessities, increases the risk of jail, loss of work, and loss of her children.

Children also suffer greatly because of drug abuse by their mother, sometimes even prior to birth due to her drug abuse and illnesses. Substance-abusing women, especially homeless women, often have no prenatal care, no post-birthing care, and are prone to neglect, abuse, abandonment, and placing their children in dangerous circumstances and environments.

What barriers do these women face? Many! Too few substance abuse treatment facilities to meet the special needs of addicted, homeless women, is a serious problem, especially if they have children or are pregnant. Lack of money and insurance, often lack of family support, and inability to receive outpatient treatment due to lack of a home all present almost insurmountable barriers for homeless women and children.

Solving the complex issues related to drug abuse among homeless women with children are difficult to overcome. They need treatment programs that address a woman's drug addiction, her basic survival needs, health care, and care for her children. As federal and state assistance policies are developed, each of these concerns must be considered. Funding demonstration projects that show success through the use of innovative strategies is essential.[27]

Women who suffer drug addiction have been found to have a higher physical vulnerability to drugs, especially alcohol; a higher degree of wide-ranging emotional concerns; and a briefer time between recognizing drug-related problems and seeking treatment.[28] Usually the model for drug treatment programs has been directed toward recovery for the male addict. However, treatment specific to women who abuse substances is needed.[29] For women who have substance abuse problems, treatment should include assessment and treatment of the family, and involvement of female role models.[30]   ∞

Chapter Summary

- Prescription, over-the-counter (OTC), and illicit drugs can cause physical and psychological addiction as well as tolerance and withdrawal symptoms.
- Prescription drugs are legal drugs used to treat and/or cure diseases and may be obtained in genetic or brand name forms.
- Disorders such as obesity, depression, anxiety, and hormonal imbalances can be treated with a variety of prescription drugs.
- OTC drugs are purchased without a physician's prescription and can be used to treat various common ailments.

- Reading labels, following instructions, and consulting a physician as needed, are important precautions to remember when taking OTC drugs.
- The physician's instructions should be strictly followed by pregnant women who use prescriptions and OTC drugs.
- Illicit drugs such as cocaine, marijuana, and heroin can produce devastating results for women and their unborn fetus or newborn infant.
- Social problems such as homelessness and sexually transmitted diseases often result for women who abuse illicit drugs.

Review Questions

1. What are patent medicines and for what purposes were they once used?
2. What is the process of physical and psychological addiction?
3. What is the difference between brand name and generic drugs?
4. What information is available on drug labels and what are the benefits of providing this information?
5. What are three types of weight control prescription drugs and the pharmacological function of each?
6. Why are antidepressant drugs prescribed more for women than men, and what precautions should be taken while using these drugs?
7. What are the benefits and the drawbacks of Hormone Replacement Therapy? Which ones are currently on the market?
8. How should women use medicinal drugs safely?
9. What are the pros and cons of purchasing an OTC drug? Which are purchased specifically by women?
10. What are the various types of laxative products that are currently on the market?
11. What precautions should be taken when using OTC sleep aids?
12. Which of the illicit drugs were discussed in this chapter? What are the physical responses to each of these drugs in the body? What are the physical, social, and emotional consequences of abusing these drugs? What are the possible effects use of these drugs can have on the fetus?
13. What methods could be utilized to combat societal problems that occur to women as a result of abusing illicit drugs?

Resources

Organizations and Hotlines

Cocaine Hotline
Telephone: (800)-cocaine (262-2463)

Prescription Drugs and Over-the-Counter Drugs

American Pharmaceutical Association
2215 Constitution Ave. NW
Washington, DC 20037
Telephone: (202) 628-4410

American Society of Addiction Medicine
12 West 21st St
New York, NY 10010
Telephone: (212) 848-6050

Food and Drug Administration
Office of Consumer Affairs, Public Inquiries
5600 Fishers Lane
Rockville, MD 20857
Telephone: (301) 443-1544

National Association of Retail Druggists
205 Dangerfield Rd.
Alexandria, VA 22314
Telephone: (703) 683-8200

National Library of Medicine
Public Information Office
8600 Rockville Pike
Bethesda, MD 20894
Telephone: (800) 638-8480, or
Telephone: (301) 496-6308

Pharmacists Against Drug Abuse
Welsh and McKean Rd
Spring House, PA 19477

Illicit Drugs

American Council for Drug Education
204 Monroe St., Suite 110
Rockville, MD 20850
Telephone: (301) 294-0600

Coalition on Alcohol and Drug Dependent Women and
Their Children
Washington Office of HCADD
1511 K Street, NW Suite 926
Washington, DC 20005
Telephone: (202) 737-8122

CSAP's National Resource Center for the Prevention of
Alcohol, Tobacco, Other Drug Abuse and Mental Illness in
Women
515 King Street Suite 420
Alexandria, Va 22314
Telephone: (703) 836-8761

Do It Now Foundation
PO Box 5115
Phoenix, AZ 85010
Telephone: (602) 257-0797

Drug Enforcement Administration
700 Army Navy Dr.
Arlington, VA 22202
Telephone: (202) 307-1000

Drug Information and Strategy Clearinghouse
Telephone: (800) 729-6686

Narcotic Educational Foundation of America
5055 Sunset Blvd.
Los Angeles, CA 90027
Telephone: (213) 663-5171

Narcotics Anonymous (NA)
World Service Office
PO Box 9999
Van Nuys, CA 91409
Telephone: (818) 780-3951

National Association of Perinatal Addiction Research
Education (NAPARE)
11 East Hubbard, Suite 200
Chicago, IL 60611
Telephone: (312) 541-1272
Telephone: (800) 638-BABY

National Clearinghouse for Alcohol & Drug Information
PO Box 2345
Rockville, MD 20847-2345
Telephone: (301) 468-2600
Telephone: (800) 729-6686

National Drug Information Treatment and Referral Line
Telephone: (800) 662-HELP
Telephone: (Espanol) (800) 66-AYUDA

National Institute on Drug Abuse (NIDA)
5600 Fishers Lane
Rockville, MD 20857

NIDA Cocaine Hotline
Telephone: (800) 662-HELP

Printed Information on Drugs
Telephone: (800) 729-6686

Women for Sobriety
PO Box 618
Quakertown, PA 18951
Telephone: (800) 333-1606

References

1. Anderson, K. N., ed. 1994. *Mosby's medical, nursing, and allied health dictionary, 4th ed.* St. Louis: Mosby.
2. Cornacchia, H. J., and S. Barrett. 1997. *Consumer health: A guide to intelligent decisions, 6th ed.* St. Louis: Mosby.
3. Yorke, J. 1992. FDA ensures equivalence of generic drugs. *FDA Consumer: DHHS Publication* (September), DHHS No. 93-3206.
4. Questions about your medicine? Go ahead-ask. 1991. *FDA Consumer: DHHS Publication,* DHHS No. 91-3166.
5. Kapusniak, L. 1997. Women's bodies should figure into standards. In *The Bryan-College Station Eagle* (College Station, Tex., 28 May), B3.
6. Depression. 1995. *Harvard: Women's Health Watch,* II (7): 2-3.
7. Sifton, D. W., ed. 1994. *The PDR family guide to women's health and prescription drugs.* Montale, N. J.: Medical Economics.
8. Ray, O., and C. Ksir. 1996. *Drugs, society, & human behavior, 7th ed.* St Louis: Mosby.
9. Cummings, M. 1991. Overuse hazardous: Laxatives rarely needed. *FDA Consumer: DHHS Publication* (April), DHHS Pub. No. 92-1182.
10. Melatonin. (1996, April). *Harvard Women's Health Watch,* III, (8): 6.
11. *Drug facts and comparisons.* 1995. St. Louis: Facts and Comparisons.
12. Rubin, J. P., C. Ferencz, and C. Loffredo. 1993. Use of prescription & non-prescription drugs in pregnancy. *Clinical Epidemiology,* 46 (6): 581-89.
13. National Institute of Drug Abuse. (1994, March). Women and drug abuse. CAD 45. Rockville, Md.: U.S. Dept. of Health and Human Services.
14. American Public Health Association. 1993. Effects of inutero exposure to street drugs. *American Journal of Public Health,* 83 (supplement), 8-32.
15. Ibid.
16. National Institute of Drug Abuse. 1994. Women and Drug Abuse. Pamphlet No. 94-3732, Rockville, Md.: Department of Health and Human Services.
17. Mitchell, J. L. (panel chair). 1993. Pregnant, substance-abusing women. SMA 93-1998. Rockville, Md.: Department of Health and Human Services.
18. Ray and Ksir, *Drugs, society, & human behavior.*
19. Mitchell, Pregnant, substance-abusing women.
20. Chasnoff, I. J. et al. 1989. Temporal patterns of cocaine use during pregnancy: Perinatal outcomes. *JAMA,* 261 (12): 1741-44.
21. Doweiko, H. E. 1996. *Concepts of chemical dependency, 3rd ed.* Pacific Grove, Cal.: Brooks/Cole Publishing Co.
22. Pinger, R. R., W. A. Payne, D. N. Hahn, and E. J. Hahn. 1998. *Drugs: Issues for today, 3rd ed.* St. Louis: Mosby.
23. Hayford, S. M., R. P. Epps, and M. Dahl-Regis. 1988. Behavior & development patterns in children born to heroin-addicted & methadone-addicted mothers. *Journal of the National Medical Association,* 80 (11): 1197-99.
24. Crack smokers pose high risk of contracting AIDS (particularly women). 1994. *Narcotics Demand Reduction Digest* (January): 6-7.
25. Wambach, K. G., J. B. Byers, D. F. Harrison, P. Levine, A. W. Imershein, D. M. Quadagno, and K. Maddox. Substance use among women at risk for HIV infection. *Journal of Drug Education,* 22 (2): 131-46.
26. Robertson, M. J. 1991. Homeless women with children: The role of alcohol and other drug abuse. *American Psychologist,* 46 (11): 1198-1204.
27. Weinreb, L. F., and E. L. Vassuk. 1990. Substance abuse: A growing problem among homeless families. *Family and Community Health,* 13, 55-64.
28. el-Guebaly, N. 1995. Alcohol and polysubstance abuse among women. *Canadian Journal of Psychiatry,* 40 (2): 73-79.
29. Nelson-Zlupko, L. E. Kauffman, and M. M. Dore. 1995. Gender differences in drug addiction and treatment: Implications for social work intervention with substance abusing women. *Social Work,* 40 (1): 45-54.
30. el-Guebaly, Alcohol & polysubstance abuse among women.

Twelve

Becoming a Wise Consumer

■ chapter objectives

When you complete this chapter you will be able to:
- Define consumerism and identify the various components of consumer health.
- Describe the benefits of making intelligent consumer choices.
- Identify the practices of wise health consumers.
- Identify characteristics of effectual and qualified health-care providers.
- Differentiate between quackery and effective alternative healing and treatment methods.
- Explain the influence that advertising has on the images of and attitudes toward women.
- Explain the impact of advertising on the financial, emotional, and social aspects of consumer practices.
- Evaluate beauty-enhancing products that claim to be safe and beneficial.
- Analyze the benefits and risks of beauty-enhancing procedures.
- Describe the appropriate actions necessary to become a wise and effective health consumer.

CONSUMERISM: WHAT IS IT?

Being a wise consumer takes time and energy! The lack of effective consumer skills and practices can cost you money. Which do you have more of—time or money? If you are like most people, there is precious little of both. If you develop wise consumer skills and know where to seek assistance, wouldn't you save both time and money? Yes! This chapter will help you to achieve this. (See Fig. 12.1.)

HOW WE CONSUME

Is there a "trick" to wise use of health-enhancement dollars? Perhaps the only trick is to become in-

formed about the varied, and sometimes complex, health-related costs. We are deluged with consumer information everyday from an array of sources, some of which are reliable, and some are not. Included among these are news releases, public service media campaigns, publications for women, their families, and their health-care providers, toll-free hotlines, governmental clearinghouse services, and of course, advertisements via various mediums. Consumer in-

> **consumerism**—the intelligent purchase and use of products and services that will directly impact one's health.

FIGURE 12.1 Reading package labels is an easy way to become an informed health-care consumer.

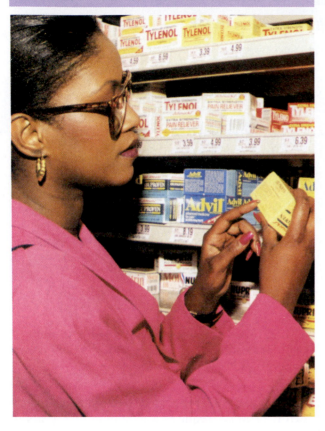

HEALTHY PEOPLE 2000 OBJECTIVES

- Increase to at least 75 percent the proportion of local television network affiliates in the top twenty television markets that have become partners with one or more community organizations addressing one of the health problems covered by the Healthy People 2000 objectives. 1995 progress toward goal: data unavailable
- Increase to at least 50 percent the proportion of primary care providers who provide their patients with the screening, counseling, and immunization services recommended by the U.S. Preventative Services Task Force. 1995 progress toward goal: data unavailable

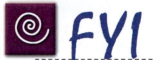

Consumer Bill of Rights[1]

1. *The right to safety:* To be protected against the marketing of goods that are hazardous to health or to life.
2. *The right to be informed:* To be protected against fraudulent, deceitful, or grossly misleading information, advertising, labeling, or other practices, and to be given the facts needed to make informed choices.
3. *The right to choose:* To be assured, whenever possible, access to a variety of products and services at competitive prices; in those industries in which government regulations are substituted, an assurance of satisfactory quality and service at fair prices.
4. *The right to be heard:* To be assured that consumer interests will receive full and sympathetic consideration in the formulation of governmental policy; and fair and expeditious treatment in its administrative tribunal.

formation from these varied sources can increase awareness and knowledge, influence attitudes and choices, and promote demands for better consumer services. But they have to be credible and proven sources of information. Otherwise the information is of little value.

Public access to both health information as well as health misinformation abounds. It seems that health misinformation is more easily obtained than sound, effective, and proven health information. Americans spend billions of dollars on unproven, worthless, and sometimes dangerous health remedies, with more money spent on "disease-curing" quackery than on research to prevent or cure these same diseases. As women, we often want to attain the body and beauty promised via weight loss gimmicks, miracle potions, or unnecessary elective surgeries. Knowledge about health products and health-care personnel, procedures, and facilities is valuable. You can protect both your money and your health by developing and using wise consumer skills. (See *FYI:* "Consumer Bill of Rights.")

CHOOSING A HEALTH-CARE PROVIDER

Selecting your health-care providers is an important consumer skill. You will be sharing some of the most intimate concerns of your life with these persons. The providers' qualifications, training, reputations,

health tips

Selecting Your Health-Care Provider

Upon entering the university, Elizabeth wants to begin a search to locate quality health-care providers of the same calibre of her family-selected health-care providers that she had for a number of years. She has two objectives: to locate two or three reputable physicians and then determine which one best meets her health-care needs. To do this, she will do the following:

To locate a provider:

- Ask local friends and relatives for their recommendations.
- Check with the local medical society for suggestions specific to providers' specialty, sex, and age.
- Call local and/or regional women's health groups or organizations for suggestions.
- Call local hospitals to ask professional personnel about specific physicians.

- Check with the state medical society or licensing board to determine whether any complaints have been registered about a particular provider.

Once located, to select a provider:

- Discuss his or her general health-care practices; is he or she a member of a group or a single provider?
- What is the office location, the hours, fees, insurance requirements, and waiting period for appointments?
- Ask about the use of local health-care facilities and other physicians.
- Is the physician an HMO member or in another health-care group?
- Request a preliminary interview to determine rapport, mutual respect, treatment approaches, and when referrals to specialists are needed.

availability, and patient-relation skills are important to know. See *Health Tips:* "Selecting Your Health-Care Provider" for suggestions about how to find the right provider for you.

Once you have visited the health-care provider, consider the following questions: Do I like this provider? Do I feel respected? Does she or he take the time to patiently answer my questions? Would my health concerns and opinions be considered as a part of a satisfactory treatment plan?

Health-Care Providers

Health-care providers are comprised of a variety of medical practitioners who have completed training in an accredited medical school and passed a medical examination. They can be divided into three groups:[2]

1. Independent practitioners who have been trained and licensed for all types of medical practices. These are medical and osteopathic physicians.
2. Independent practitioners with restricted practices such as podiatrists, dentists, psychologists, and optometrists.
3. Ancillary practitioners who practice only under the supervision of a medical practitioner. These include nurses, physical therapists, physicians' assistants, pharmacists, occupational therapists, and X-ray and laboratory technicians.

The following information gives a thumbnail sketch of health-care providers with differing education levels, skills, abilities, and responsibilities.

Physician   The process of becoming a medical doctor, or M.D., requires a minimum of 3 years of premedical college work for admission to medical school. However, 97 percent of premed students have a baccalaureate degree prior to admission.[3] Of those medical school students admitted in 1994, approximately 42 percent were women.[4] Students then spend 4 years in medical schools, which should be accredited by a joint committee representing the American Medical Association (AMA) Council on Medical Education and the Association of American Medical Colleges. Following graduation, state or national board examinations must be passed to become a licensed practitioner.

Ever-changing research outcomes, improved technology, and new medicines create the need for developing medical specialties. Becoming a specialist such as a pediatrician, neurologist, or psychiatrist requires 3 or more years of additional training. This may be followed by additional clinical hours and then becoming board certified, which means that the doctor has additional training and has passed a national examination in his or her specialty.

A doctor of osteopathy, a D.O., is legally equivalent to a medical doctor and is licensed to practice

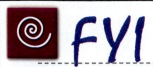

FYI   *Periodic Checkups and Screening Tests*[6]

Your doctor should ask about your:

- Family history, personal medical history, and any current medications, if any, that you take
- Dietary habits with special attention to fat, calories, fiber, iron, and calcium
- Exercise habits
- Use of any drugs including alcohol and tobacco
- Safety practices (seat belt, safety equipment)
- Sexual practices related to disease prevention
- Birth control method (if any)
- What concerns you most about your health

Screening tests for generally healthy women include:

- Blood pressure measurement: checked at least once or twice per year and during every doctor visit

- Clinical breast exam: yearly for all women over 40; every 3 years for women aged 20 to 40 years
- Mammography: yearly for women over 50; every 1 to 2 years for women aged 40 to 49 (depending on family history of breast cancer)
- Pap smear: every 1 to 3 years beginning at age of first intercourse
- Colorectal cancer: annual fecal occult blood test for age 50 and over (recommendation may change so that the test is less often)
- Cholesterol screening: check every 5 years beginning at age 18, and more frequently as age increases or risks become prevalent

---

in all states. Prior to admission to an osteopathy school, the student must have 3 years of college work related to the profession. During the 4 years of osteopathic college, the candidate will have over 5,000 hours of training, followed by a 1-year rotating internship at an approved hospital. If the D.O. decides to specialize, which about half do, a 2- to 6-year residency follows, depending on their chosen specialty.[5] Osteopathic doctors specialize in such areas as obstetrics, neurology, psychiatry, and anesthesiology. There is very little difference in the training of D.O.s and M.D.s. The difference is more in the philosophy of treatment. The American Osteopathic Association states that osteopathic medicine must closely follow the Hippocratic approach to medicine in that the body's musculoskeletal system is central to a person's well-being. Osteopathic medicine, because of its hands-on approach to diagnoses, can provide an alternative to surgery and/or drugs. The profession maintains its independence in order to provide a unique and comprehensive approach to health care.

Getting a Good Checkup. Ordering a wide range of tests and X rays, taking blood, poking, prodding, and peering often comprises the medical checkup. However, a more comprehensive look at an individual's lifestyle can often help provide better quantity and quality of life. A preventive health exam tailored to the age, risk factors, and lifestyle of the patient can promote an enhanced quality of life and is more predictive of potential disease development. So what constitutes a good periodic exam? See *FYI:* "Periodic Checkups and Screening Tests."

Physician's Assistant. A physician assistant (PA) works in the primary care medical setting under the supervision of a physician. He or she can give physical exams, prescribe drugs or therapies, and offer health counseling. Trained in community colleges, universities, or medical schools, it usually takes 2 years to complete the requirements. Because PAs do not make a salary like physicians, health-care programs often use them to help reduce the cost of health care. Physician assistants can work in private doctor's offices, hospitals, clinics, and other health-care settings.

Nurse Practitioner. A nurse practitioner can function as a primary care provider, but often performs under a physician's supervision. Training includes additional nursing education, usually at the master's level, and beyond the requirements needed to become a registered nurse (RN). Licensed by the state, registered nurses assess patient's physical and emotional needs and, assist physicians and patients in prevention and treatment practices. Nurse practitioners can be certified through the American Nurses Credentialling Center (ANCC) for work in geriatric, pediatric, and family health care, as well as in elementary and secondary school nursing. (See Fig. 12.2.)

Midwife. Midwives are usually RNs who have received additional training, and are certified to perform

FIGURE 12.2 Bev Teagle, a nurse practitioner, examines 4-year-old Antonio.

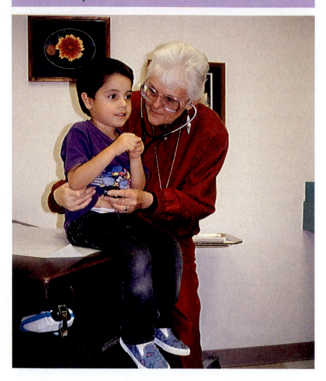

specific health-care activities. One to two years of additional training is required from an approved school of midwifery. They can also earn certified nurse-midwife certification, C.N.M., which allows them to practice in almost every state by passing an exam from the American College of Nurse-Midwives.[7] Responsibilities include caring for pregnant women, managing labor and delivery, and caring for mother and baby after childbirth. A midwife may also be a vital part of obstetrical teams in physicians' offices, clinics, and hospitals. Midwives often are certified in CPR as well as Neonatal Resuscitation. In some states, midwives are required to obtain continuing education credits to maintain current knowledge in the field.

Dr. J. M. Smith, author of *Women and Doctors*, states that he would like to see midwives assume a significant role during uncomplicated prenatal care, labor and delivery, and postpartum care.[8] He promotes the concept of midwives to serve as stand-along professionals as part of the professional staff of hospital birthing facilities and birth centers. Medical care costs would thus be limited to the institution's fee and the midwife's fee thereby helping to reduce costs. Obstetricians would only be paid if their services were needed, or if they provide professional consultation.

Mental Health Therapists. Mental health professionals are individuals who work to treat a variety of conditions related to one's mental and emotional well-being. Treatment can range from occassional outpatient counseling with single or group meetings to inpatient confinement using medication and electroshock. Seeking professional counseling and locating a competent and highly trained therapist are essential to know when concerned about your mental or emotional health.

If you have determined that you need professional assistance with a mental or emotional health problem, what type of therapist should you seek? A wide range of mental health professionals have special training to work with a variety of issues. *FYI:* "Therapists for Mental and Emotional Health" indicates what the letters following the names of therapists mean and the significance of each in helping you to select the best therapist.

Therapists should be trustworthy, nonjudgmental, empathetic, respectful, sincere, and well-trained in their area of therapy. Consider the following criteria when determining the merits of a potential therapist:

- What are the credentials of the therapist?
- Is she or he a licensed therapist?
- Will my insurance cover the costs of this therapy?
- What type of treatment does the therapist use?
- Will he or she prescribe medication?
- Do I know anyone who this therapist has treated for a similar problem? Was the treatment successful?
- Are any complaints about this therapist filed with the local medical personnel or professional licensing boards?

There are always "professionals" who will take our money and provide poor quality, and even harmful health care. In some states, it is legal to use such titles as "therapists, counselors, and sex therapists" without any specific or certified credentials. Be smart! Check for the appropriate credentials before investing time and money with a mental health professional. Locate trusted physicians, and check with family, friends, or coworkers who can recommend competent and qualified professionals to work with you.

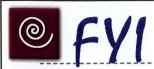 **FYI** *Therapists for Mental and Emotional Health*[9]

ACADEMIC DEGREES

Psychiatry
Doctorate in Medicine: M.D. Has completed medical training and has specialized residency in psychiatry. May also have additional training in psychoanalysis or psychodynamic training. Psychiatrists are the only therapists who can prescribe drugs.

Psychology
Doctorate in Psychology: Psy.D. Has 6 to 7 years of graduate work and training with an emphasis on practical clinical course work rather than research.

Doctorate in Philosophy: Ph.D. Has 6 to 7 years of graduate work with training in research methodology and had a psychotherapy internship. Can administer psychological testing.

Doctorate in Education: Ed.D. Training similar to that received by a Ph.D. However, this degree is issued through graduate schools of education rather than science or psychology.

Therapy
Master of Science: M.S. Has completed a 2-year program in clinical psychology after receiving a baccalaureate degree. Usually has training in psychotherapy techniques, but not psychological assessment or work.

Master of Social Work: M.S.W. Has completed a 2- to 3-year graduate program that emphasizes training psychotherapy and social work.

LICENSURES BY STATE PROFESSIONAL BOARDS*

Licensed Clinical Social Worker: L.C.S.W.
Licensed Marriage and Family Child Counselor: L.M.F.C.C.
Licensed Professional Counselor: L.P.C.
Licensed Marriage and Family Therapist: L.M.F.T.

*Note that each of these designations are licensures awarded by state professional boards. They do *not* refer to academic degrees. Licensure related to a professional specialty should be obtained. Otherwise the "professional" may not truly be qualified.

Reporting Unprofessional Treatment

Knowing what to do if you have received inadequate, unprofessional, or unethical health-care treatment is important. Taking action immediately by contacting proper authorities and providing written statements and any supporting documentation will aid you and other potential patients to avoid unnecessary, painful, incorrect, or even fatal treatment at the hands of a health-care provider. To report this concern, write a letter to the hospital or doctor involved and send a copy to any or all of the following: a referring doctor, the administrator or director of the hospital or clinic, the local medical society, the state licensing board, your insurance carrier, and any local health consumer or women's health group. A doctor-patient relationship should be one of equality and mutual respect with your doctor and you making responsible and health-enhancing decisions together.

HEALTH-CARE DELIVERY

The socioeconomic circumstances and roles of women continue to evolve and change as they relate to parenting, employment, and relationships. Today, the health-care needs of women vary significantly from the time when the "typical" female was a stay-at-home wife and mother and sheltered under her partner's health-care plan and the long-time family physician. Meeting the changing needs of women's health care is the responsibility of the health-care system, health-related institutions, and women themselves. What is needed to meet this challenge? There is a need to *improve* health-care delivery for women and to *provide* for health needs whether women live in the inner city, rural America, or the "burbs." This could be accomplished by having health-care clinics near public transport or in inner-city neighborhoods. An awareness of the differing health needs of women could be developed via better training in medical and nursing schools and by fostering an understanding attitude toward the special health needs of women.

Removal of barriers to quality health-care services is essential if women are to garner the necessary examinations, treatment, and rehabilitation that is needed. Barriers may include too little money for health care, lack of insurance, no transportation to and from health facilities, distant travel to health-care providers, job-related demands, and no sick leave or time allotted away from the job among others. (Health insurance concerns are covered later in this chapter.)

Solutions to effective health-care delivery specific to the needs of women must include experts in medical, community, and government factions. All of these factions must identify the problems related to health care for women, determine the various alternatives, the positives and negatives of each, assess the possible solutions, and then act accordingly. A health-care delivery system that addresses all women must be accessible, culturally relevant, affordable, and available.

HOME HEALTH TESTS

What Are They?

At-home methods to determine the status of one's health have come a long way from only using scales, thermometers, and taking your pulse. Over-the-counter home health test kits have expanded our access to faster results and vital information related to numerous health concerns. The purchase and use of these test kits has risen from approximately $667 million in annual sales in 1986 to over $2.2 billion today.[10] Home health tests can mean lower medical costs, better monitoring of chronic conditions, and earlier detection of health problems. Additionally, home health tests can be an easy-to-use method for providing private information in a brief amount of time. However, overreliance on these various tests (e.g., used as an indicator of diagnosis or cure) or misinterpretation of the results can be dangerous; a

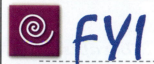

Some Common Home Health Tests[11]

The value and accuracy of home health tests varies with the individual user. The following information assumes that the user follows the directions exactly, and that the test kit has not been damaged in some way.

Pregnancy Tests:	Overall Ratings
Answer	excellent
Confirm	very good
Be Sure Plus	fair
Ovulation Tests:	
Clearplan	excellent
OvuQuick	very good
Conceive	fair
Blood-Glucose Meters	
Glucometer Elite	excellent
Accu-Chek Advantage	very good
Accu-Chek 111	good

wise consumer will not make medical decisions without consulting with a medical professional.

There are basically three types of home tests: (1) diagnostic tests (for STDs, ovulation, pregnancy, urinary tract infections), (2) continuous monitoring tests (for blood glucose, blood pressure) that are often recommended by one's physician to assist in overseeing an existing disease, and (3) screening tests (for hidden fecal blood test) to determine if a disease is present even though symptoms are not present. The best known are the pregnancy tests, whereas the biggest sellers are the blood glucose monitors and test strips used by individuals with diabetes. (See *FYI:* "Some Common Home Health Tests.") Together they account for 90 percent of home health test kits sold nationally.

It has been estimated that one in seven medical tests, even including those administered by health professionals, result in false findings. Certainly, the margin for error associated with the general consumer administering a test at home can be even greater. However, many of the use-at-home test kits, when used properly, can provide accurate and cost-effective results. Complete *Assess Yourself:* "Improving Your Chances for Accurate Test Results" to help improve the effectiveness of your test results.

Assess Y O U R S E L F

Improving Your Chances for Accurate Test Results

If you have purchased a home health testing kit, answer the following questions: This information will assist you in obtaining more accurate test results.

Question	Yes	No
1. Has the expiration date expired?	_____	_____
2. Has the kit been exposed to extreme heat or cold?	_____	_____
3. Are the directions for using the kit and chemicals clear to you?	_____	_____
4. Have you read and do you understand the special precautions, if any?	_____	_____
5. Did you follow the directions exactly as stated?	_____	_____
6. Did you time the test accurately and precisely as instructed?	_____	_____
7. Do you understand what the test kit is intended to find?	_____	_____
8. Do you know what to do when you obtain the results whether they are positive or negative?	_____	_____
9. Do you know who to contact to follow-up with the results of the test?	_____	_____
10. Do you know where to get help administrating the test if you are unsure about the directions?	_____	_____

If you answered 8 or more of the questions with a positive response, your health kit test results should be accurate. If you answered less than 8 with a positive response, you need to read directions more accurately and discuss the procedures with a medical professional.

ALTERNATIVE HEALTH CARE

Unconventional health therapies (alternative health care) such as herbal medicine, acupuncture, chiropractic care, and massage therapy are being recognized, in some areas, as having the potential for relief, treatment, and cure of certain diseases. Unconventional therapy has been defined as "commonly used interventions neither taught widely in U.S. medical schools nor generally available in U.S. hospitals."[12] One study found that one in three people use unconventional medical therapies, such as acupuncture, chiropractic care, or massage therapy and spent almost $14 billion on these therapies in 1990.[13] Further, Americans made 388 million trips to primary care physicians in 1990 and researchers calculated that 425 million visits were made to providers of alternative health-care practices. Who is most likely to use alternative therapy? The "typical" person most likely to seek alternative therapy is the non-black, college-educated individual between the ages of 25 and 49 earning more than $35,000 a year.[14]

The National Institutes of Health now has an Office for the Study of Unconventional Medical Practices, which investigates varied healing regimens. Numerous medical schools such as Georgetown University, University of Louisville, and University of Massachusetts in Worcester now offer courses and lectures on unorthodox medical therapies.[15] *Good Morning America,* a morning show on ABC television, ran a segment on alternative healing on June 25, 1995, and during the interview, two alternative healing practitioners, Joseph Pizzorno, N.D., a naturopathic doctor and Fredi Kronenberg, Ph.D., of Columbia University discussed the explosive growth of this type of health care over the last 10 years.[16]

Why has interest in alternative therapies experienced such phenomenal growth? Although we have seen amazing progress in high-tech medical practices, these procedures are often painful, expensive, and even dehumanizing. People began to seek therapies that would take healing a step beyond "treatment." Milestones in the women's movement toward alternative therapy began in the early 1960s as publication of such books as *The Feminine Mystique* by Betty Friedan, which enlightened many women and led to new heights of competence and empowerment. Near this time, such practices as yoga, meditation, and macrobiotic diets emerged as the idea of mind-body connection in illness and wellness found its practitioners and patients. *Our Bodies, Ourselves* was published in 1973, creating the desire in many women to take charge of their own well-being through increased knowledge about their own bodies and better education. A redefinition of the doctor-female patient relationship was desired in which a partnership was formed that enabled women to become part of the decision-making healing process. Books such as the 1974 *Type A Behavior and Your Heart* written by Drs. Friedman and Rosenman, *The Relaxation Response* written in 1975 by Dr. Herbert Benson, Norman Cousin's *Anatomy of an Illness in 1979,* and *Psychoneuroimmunology* written in 1981 by Robert Ader each discussed the connection between our mind, emotions, and our health leading us to believe, with effective training, we could become a partner in our own level of health. Visiting a bookstore today, you will find an uncanny array of books related to alternative health-related practices. An important next step would be for women to find the "right" type of alternative approach and the "right" practitioner, so the ability to control pain, reduce stress, and improve well-being would be ours!

Unfortunately in some instances, the results have not been what was hoped for! Women were/are too often the victims of scam artists or quacks; our money is taken, but the results are less than desirable, even worse, harmful or deadly. However, there are certainly reputable alternative practitioners, medicines, and methodologies that offer, in some instances, more favorable results than orthodox medicine. Let's take a look at a number of alternative therapies and answer the questions of what they are, how they "work," and possible risks and benefits of each.

Herbalism

Herbs could be called alternative "drugs" that promote the premise that many disorders or injuries can be treated with a plant or parts of a plant. Herbal medicine was practiced in ancient Rome, Greece, and Babylon and is still used throughout the world, especially in less-developed countries. Historically, plants such as myrrh, oil of cloves, peppermint, and caraway have been used to treat a range of disorders such as sexually transmitted diseases, inflammation, and heart disease. Patent medicines contained a variety of plants such as ginger root, castor oil, juniper bush, and alfalfa. Herbalists claimed that drinks made of herbs soothed the nerves, aloe can soothe the skin, leaves from foxglove contain digitalis, and so on.

It only takes a visit to a "health food" market to realize that herbs and products containing herbs are widely available. In fact, in the quest for a more "natural" approach to healing, Americans spend over $1.5 billion a year on herbal medicines, bulk herbs, and other herbal products.[17] Brochures, books, and pamphlets espouse the benefits of available herbal "medicines," yet researchers state that we need to be wary of some of these medicines. Concerns about herbal medicines include lack of scientific "proof" that they indeed treat and heal health problems; most reports of herbal healing abilities are based on unfounded claims from folklore and some outdated reports. Herbs can be dangerous, even deadly in fact, many herbs have been banned from sale and others must carry a warning on their labels. Herbs contain many hundreds of chemicals and their reaction in the body can be unknown, perhaps helpful, but perhaps harmful. Herbal medicines are not controlled by the FDA and certainly strengths of the herb can vary from product to product. Safe and effective medicines are available to treat conditions for which they are known to work. Purchasing and using unproven and potentially dangerous herbal medicines is not wise. It appears that it would be advantageous for Western researchers to research and determine the benefits and detrimental effects of herbs.

Acupuncture

Acupuncture has been used by more people in its 5,000-year-old history than any other form of alternative medicine. Acupuncture claims to restore balance (Qi) to promote healing and functioning through inserting needles at precise points on the body. Heat is sometimes applied to the acupuncture point to promote the healing process. The premise is that meridians, channels of energy, run like energy throughout the body. When blockage in one part of a channel occurs, it impedes the flow to others. Acupuncture claims to remove the blockage and allow the usual flow through the meridians, restoring Qi and aiding the bodily organs with imbalances. The *World Health Organization* acknowledges acupuncture for treatment of such conditions as digestive and respiratory disorders, neurological and muscular ailments, and urinary, menstrual, and reproductive problems.

Her Story

Ping

Ping found that she continued to have more and more frequent bouts of anxiety and emotional outbursts close to her menstrual period. After consulting with three physicians and trying several tranquilizers, a coworker recommended acupuncture to Ping. Ping was open to, but skeptical of the suggested treatment. However, she located a reputable acupuncturist and began a series of treatments with needles inserted at points along her back, arms, and legs. After 6 weeks of treatments, not only was she less anxious during premenstrual days, but all the time.

• Based on Ping's experience, would you be willing to try acupuncture for yourself?

health tips

Finding a Reputable Acupuncturist[19]

First, with the help of a physician, rule out conditions that cannot be helped with acupuncture: infections, cancer, and heart disease. Use the following suggestions when choosing an acupuncturist.

■ Check credentials: state licenses (25 states have training standards) and/or certification by the National Commission for the Certification of Acupuncturists (NCCA). Call NCCA at 202-232-1404 or a member physician of the American Academy of Medical Acupuncture (AAMA 1-800-521-2262).
■ Insist on disposable needles.
■ Determine treatment styles: Japanese (uses smaller needles), Chinese, Korean.
■ Determine the costs: first visits range from $40–$100; follow-up visits are $30–$70.
■ Insurance coverage: most companies do not cover; check your policy.
■ Set realistic goals: don't expect a miracle. If you are not satisfied, return to your physician for other possible options.

It appears to be especially helpful for physical difficulties related to stress and tension.

This alternative healing method has over 9,000 practicing acupuncturists in the United States with over one-third possessing medical degrees. Annually, Americans make between 9 and 12 million visits to acupuncturists.[18] National Commission for the Certification of Acupuncturists is the certifying agency in this country. Acupuncturists have submitted scientific evidence to the FDA that shows that the needles used in acupuncture do have the ability to heal. If the FDA decides to recognize the tools of acupuncture as bona fide medical instruments, then certain acupuncture treatments could be reimbursed by Medicare, Medicaid, and private insurers.

Women find relief with acupuncture for a variety of ailments; menstrual cramps, headaches, nausea, backaches, and depression. (See *Her Story:* "Ping" and *Health Tips:* "Finding a Reputable Acupuncturist.") Pain relief is the most common and well-documented use of acupuncture. With a certified acupuncturist using sterile equipment, this form of therapy has almost no side effects or risk of complication. However, it is important to remember that using acupuncture does not preclude seeing a physician and using medicinal drugs in conjunction with this type of alternative medicine.

Chiropractic Care

Reports of spinal manipulation appear in written records of ancient Chinese and Greece. Indians in early America had family members walk on and maneuver their backbones to reduce problems with their spine.

Another form of spinal manipulation, chiropractic, was founded around 1895 by Daniel David Palmer, a grocer and "magnetic healer" in Iowa.[20] After a number of battles with the AMA and other medical and political groups, chiropractic medicine became recognized as a method to treat disorders, with some degree of success, which chiropractors attribute to spinal manipulation.

There are 50,000 licensed chiropractors in this country and they comprise the third largest group of health-care practitioners, after physicians and dentists.[21] Chiropractors must complete 4,200 hours of study over a 4-year period and take both national and state board examinations to be licensed to practice. Although chiropractic is practiced in all 50 states, a chiropractor must pass the state board exam to be able to treat in a particular state. In many instances, their services are reimbursed through private as well as state and federal insurance providers. Even though chiropractors have gained some acceptance among the medical community, a 1993 member survey of the American Chiropractic Association (ACA) revealed that only 3 percent of chiropractic patients were referred for chiropractic care by medical or osteopathic doctors.[22] This is out of the 15 to 20 million Americans who visit chiropractors each year.

Chiropractic medicine is a pseudoscience based on the belief that good health depends on the proper functioning of nerve impulse transmission through the nervous system. Therefore, when nerve impulse transmission encounters any type of interference, such as an ill-aligned spine, the person develops an illness. Chiropractic medicine claims that restoring the flow of nerve impulses through proper spinal manipulation can return the person to good health.

The medical science community is concerned about the claims of chiropractors because the concept that interference of nerve impulses as a cause of disease has not been scientifically proven. Additionally, the anatomical structure of the body does not lend itself to the healing and pain relief claims made by chiropractors. However, there does seem to be evidence that chiropractic medicine can be helpful in relieving lower back pain and menstrual pain, which has a back-related component. There are also claims that manipulating and stretching muscles in the back of the head can be beneficial for migraine and tension headaches.

Concerns arise about chiropractic care when chiropractors treat disorders for which they have not had specific training such as physical therapy, "sports chiropractic," acupuncture, and sometimes nutritional and homeopathic medicine. Conventional medical practitioners worry that spinal manipulation may do more harm than good, especially if the pain has been long-lasting, or if a tumor or fracture is present. Additionally, some chiropractors keep patients returning for unnecessary treatments and X rays.

There is movement in chiropractic medicine to focus on a scientific approach to musculoskeletal problems and eliminate procedures for which chiropractors have little or no training. Should you and your physician determine that you have a condition for which chiropractic medicine may be beneficial, such as low back pain, refer to *Health Tips:* "When to See a Chiropractor" and *FYI:* "Assessing the Chiropractor."

Massage

Massage, in addition to feeling good, appears to offer healthful benefits for the promotion of healing of disease and injuries. In recent research studies, children with asthma, diabetes, and arthritis received daily massages of 15 to 20 minutes and realized a significant reduction of their symptoms related to these diseases.[25] Children receiving a nightly massage also experience less anxiety, depression, and had lower

---

health tips

When to See a Chiropractor[23]

1. See your physician to determine the reason for your condition.
2. Select a chiropractor who is referred by the National Association for Chiropractic Medicine or the Orthopractic Manipulation Society International. (See Resources at the end of this chapter.)
3. Call first to find out about the kind of treatment offered:
   - Does the chiropractor primarily treat musculoskeletal problems?
   - Will he or she cooperate with your medical doctor to reach the best treatment for you?
   - How long and how often should you expect to be in treatment?
   - What are the charges and financial expectations?
   - To which professional associations does the chiropractor belong?
   - Can the chiropractor be reimbursed by your insurance company?

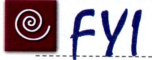

Assessing the Chiropractor[24]

Avoid the chiropractor who engages in the following practices:

- Takes repeated or full-spine X rays
- Does not attempt to professionally assess the nature of the problem
- Claims that benefits to organ systems, immune function, or even a cure will result
- Offers vitamins, or nutritional and/or homeopathic treatment
- Asks you to sign a contract for long-term care
- States that you will be kept healthy by regular checkups and manipulations
- Solicits other family members from you for treatment

---

stress hormone levels. As a result of this study, researchers believe that massage helps to counteract the body's stress response thereby reducing the ill effects stress hormones can have upon the body.[26]

Viewpoint

Holistic Medicine Practices

Some characteristics of holistic medicine practices follow. Which ones do you consider to be worthwhile and which ones lend themselves to questionable practices? Explain your position for each one.

- Uses nonscientific approaches to diagnose and treat medical problems.
- Use of lay people and other professionals in the treatment process.
- Examines the lifestyle of the individual: nutrition, exercise practices, environment, emotions, use of chemicals, social interactions, and/or spirituality.

- Encourages the woman's participation in all aspects of diagnosis and treatment.
- Views illness as a means to evaluate and change one's lifestyle.
- Emphasizes health as promotion of a healthy lifestyle rather than the absence of disease.
- Emphasizes self-care rather than treatment and dependence on medical personnel.
- Desires to reduce dependence on medicines, surgery, and treatment.
- Promotes healing through meeting the needs of mind, body, and spirit of the individual.

Many active women, such as athletes, have experienced some relief from soreness, injury, and pain as a result of using massage therapy. This approach may eliminate the use of drugs and/or surgery to realize these benefits. **Trigger-point massage** promotes the healing of muscle sprains, chronic tendinitis, and chronic muscle spasms, and **cross-fiber friction massage** assists in breaking up adhesions and stretches and realigns scar tissues with healthy muscle fiber.[27] Massages can also help to reduce fatigue and soreness in muscles by promoting muscle relaxation, increasing blood flow to muscles, and reducing inflammation and swelling.

Using massage, or any other alternative healing method, in lieu of determining the exact cause of the injury or pain through scientifically proven tests is not being a wise consumer. Also, locating a licensed massage therapist may not be an easy task. Only 15 states offer massage licenses and the requirements to receive a license varies according to the state in which it is issued. Other states allow massage certification of individuals who acquire training and pass written and practical exams; these criteria vary according to state requirements. Either ask someone who has had a positive outcome using a masseur or contact the American Massage Therapy Association, phone number (312) 761–AMTA, for the name of the nearest licensed masseur. Time of massage sessions may be anywhere from 15 to 60 minutes and range in costs from $20 to $80 or more. Be sure the masseur you choose treats you in a respectful and professional manner. If not, as with any other practi-

tioner, she or he should be reported to their professional association as well as local authorities.

Holistic Medicine

Holistic, or wholistic, medicine had its origin in ancient times and is derived from the Greek term, *holo,* which means "whole." The whole person, which includes the physical, mental, emotional, social, and spiritual dimensions, is considered in the treatment and healing process. Although certain components of holistic medicine can be beneficial, other components embraced by holistic healers lend themselves to questionable medical practices.

Of the major concerns related to holistic medicine, the potential for nonscientific medical practices and practitioners to provide useless, harmful, or even deadly care (for a large fee) is of greatest concern. Two professionals who concern themselves with the holistic healing movement believe it to be "a pabulum of common sense and nonsense offered by cranks and quacks and failed pedants who share an attachment to magic and an animosity to reason."[28] (See *Viewpoint:* "Holistic Medicine Practices.")

trigger-point massage—placing pressure on a muscle where the ligaments or tendon is attached.

cross-fiber friction massage—massaging an area where injury or surgery has occurred to break up possible adhesions and scar tissue.

There is promise of effective treatment in many holistic health-care practices but until more funding is available for research to determine scientific proof of positive results, this concept of alternative health care will continue to be just that—an alternative.

Other Types of Alternative Health Care

Consider the following brief descriptions of various other alternative health-care practices and you will see why the consumer needs information and guidelines in order to make wise choices.

Naturopathic medicine promotes the concept of the body's own natural healing ability through use of herbal medicine, nutrition, relaxation exercises, and acupuncture. *Reflexologists* use foot massage as a means to stimulate peak functioning of body systems. Massaging certain areas of the body to promote healing or pain reduction is the major premise of *craniosacral therapy*—skull, spine, and sacrum areas; *myofascial and rolfing* massage connective tissue for pain relief and promote structural integration; *myotherapists* manipulate trigger points in elbows, knuckles, and fingers to relieve pain and tension. *Yoga* attempts to integrate body, mind, and spirit with the universe through movement, relaxation, breathing techniques, and music. *Aromatherapy* is a practice for which aromatic oils are used in warm baths. They can also be massaged or breathed into the body for treatment of common disorders and influence mind and emotions. Sometimes aromas are used in a birthing environment to promote tranquility during the birthing process.

Using the best of Western medicine (orthodox health care) and the best of alternative health-care practices may be a wise approach to obtaining the best health care possible. Although surgery, medicine, and physical therapy is essential treatment to the injured or critically ill woman, however, preventing major disease, promoting well-being, and providing the opportunity for partnership in health care also has a place. Antibiotics and diagnostic tools for acute health problems combined with healing touch and needles and herbs for tension, pain, and relaxation can be effective.

Health Quackery

In the search for "hope" when no other was offered, or a "quick and painless fix" to any ailment or problem from wrinkle reduction cream to weight loss plans, U.S. citizens spend over $15 billion annually on a variety of products that purport to address these concerns.[29] When there is a health-related concern, there will often be some gimmick, potion, or practitioner available—for a price—to remedy the concern. These products promise that we can eat all we want and still lose weight, build a bigger bustline, melt away cellulite, or increase our libido. This type of alternative therapy is called **quackery**—the promotion of a medical remedy that doesn't work or hasn't been proven to work.[30]

Protecting Yourself

To protect yourself from loss of time, money, and possibly your health, use *Assess Yourself:* "Assessing Alternative Health-Care Claims and Products" to determine if the product and person is promoting quackery.

BEAUTY-ENHANCING PRODUCTS AND PROCEDURES

Products

Women, and sometimes men, elect to use products to improve the way we look and feel about ourselves. Cosmetics of all descriptions, creams, lotions, hair products, or fragrances are developed and sold, for large profits, because there is a demand for them. As purchasers of these products, knowledge and awareness is important in order to select products that meet our needs and desires.

Cosmetics Cosmetics as defined by the U.S. Food, Drug, and Cosmetic Act are "articles other than soap which are applied to the human body for cleansing, beautifying, promoting attractiveness, or altering the appearance."[31] Strangely enough, premarket approval is not required by the FDA for cosmetics. However, if a product proves to be harmful after the product is on the market, the FDA can take legal action in order to obtain the manufacturer's safety data. Cosmetics are classified into thirteen categories that include: deodorants, eye makeup, skin care, fragrances, makeup other than eye (lipsticks, for example), hair coloring preparations, shampoos and other hair products, manicure products, shaving products, baby products, bath products, mouthwashes, and sunscreens.[32] Cosmetics containing poisonous or substances that can harm consumers may not, by law, be placed on the market. With the exception of color additives and a few prohibited

Assess YOURSELF

Assessing Alternative Health-Care Claims and Products[30]

Does the practitioner or promoter exhibit these characteristics?	Yes	No
1. Promises quick, painless, drugless treatment or cure	___	___
2. Uses anecdotes or testimonials to support claim	___	___
3. Displays questionable credentials/titles	___	___
4. Uses pseudoscientific terminology	___	___
5. Claims that a single treatment can cure a wide range of illness	___	___
6. Claims persecution by organized medicine	___	___
7. Claims that many illnesses can be treated by nutrition	___	___
8. Advises use of vitamins/health foods for everyone	___	___
9. States surgery/X rays/drugs do more harm than good	___	___
10. Espouses "freedom of choice" to use unproven approaches	___	___
11. Claims to have a cure that is secret or known only in foreign countries	___	___

Any positive response should be regarded as suspicious!

---

ingredients, any ingredient or raw material may be used in the manufacture of cosmetics. See *Health Tips:* "Safety tips for Beauty-Enhancing Products" for safety tips after you purchase cosmetics.

Cosmetic manufacturers must do the following in order to market their products: work in a sanitary environment and allow no filthy, putrid, or decomposed substances in the product; test for color additives and obtain FDA approval for their use in products; list ingredients on labels in descending order of predominance; and avoid the use of prohibited ingredients such as mercury compounds, chloroform, or vinyl chloride. If a manufacturer chooses to do so, it may register its manufacturing plant, cosmetic formulas, and report adverse reactions with the FDA.

An increase in the demand for ethnic cosmetics has the manufacturers of products scrambling to meet this demand. An increase in the Latino and African American populations, as well as an increase in economic status of both groups has been credited with this new market component. The youth from these particular groups appear to have boosted ethnic cosmetic sales.[33]

Skin Care Products Our skin continually renews itself by producing new cells deep within the skin layers and sloughing off dead cells on the skin's surface. Skin layers contain water and oil, but as we age less oil is produced within the skin and also loses water faster, becomes dry, cracks, and develops fine wrinkles. When we attempt to replenish water and oil in our skin with moisturizers, we only moisturize the top layer of the skin. Because this is the skin layer that dries out, moisturizers need only to moisturize this layer. That can occur in two ways: use of an occlusive type that physically blocks moisture from leaving the skin (e.g., petroleum jelly) or with a "humectant" type that attracts moisture from the skin and air and slows down the rate of water loss.[34] Most skin care products have both types of ingredients as well as water. If a product is intended to be used for a dryer type of skin, it will have more oil; for oily skin types, the product should have more or only humectants.

Moisturizers for the body and the face work similarly, but we tend to pay more attention to our

> **quackery**—the promotion of a medical remedy that does not work or has not been proven to work.

health tips

Safety Tips for Beauty-Enhancing Products

Protect yourself by following these guidelines to use cosmetics safely:

- When not in use, keep containers closed tightly.
- Store products, especially liquids, in a cool, dry place.
- Keep products away from sunlight as ingredients may degrade.
- Never moisten dry cosmetics or applicators with saliva.
- Toss out any cosmetics that smell strange, separate into layers, or have different colors or consistencies than when purchased.
- Do not share cosmetics or applicators or use in-store samples and applicators.
- Do not use cosmetics if you have an eye or skin infection.
- Be sure to wash cosmetic sponges and brushes with warm water and soap frequently; throw them away if they degrade or lose bristles.

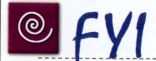

Reasons for Beauty-Enhancing Procedures[37]

- Anxiety over appearance based on a societal prejudice against aging females
- To increase feelings of worthiness, often dependent upon childhood development situations
- To maintain positive feelings about appearance
- To fulfill a personal desire to achieve the best appearance possible
- To attain an unconscious obligation to be a youthful and attractive member of society

face. Therefore, the advertiser more often promotes moisturizers for the face and the consumer will find that face moisturizers are more expensive. An excellent article in *Consumer Reports*[35] rates moisturizers according to how well they help the skin retain water.

Procedures

In attempting to obtain the image of women publicized by print and electronic media, women undergo intrusive and sometimes painful and disfiguring procedures. Breast augmentation, face-lifts, chemical peels, tummy tucks, and liposuctions have increased on the average of 24, 25, 42, 32, and 95 percent, respectively, according to a study conducted by Marcene Goodman of the Philadelphia Geriatric Center.[36] Why do women elect to go through these unpleasant and expensive procedures? (See *FYI:* "Reasons for Beauty-Enhancing Procedures.")

Cosmetic Surgery Cosmetic surgery is more prevalent than ever in our society and we are more aware of the improved technology to achieve the

image desired by the female. **Cosmetic surgeons** now advertise their practice, and provide "in-office" operating rooms and financing. What is the difference between a "cosmetic" and a "plastic" surgeon? A cosmetic surgeon specializes in procedures that enhance appearance such as face-lifts, breast reduction/augmentation, or "nose jobs." A **plastic surgeon** is trained in reconstructive surgery and performs procedures such as facial reconstruction, skin grafts, or hand surgery as well as cosmetic surgery. In selecting a cosmetic or plastic surgeon, look for the following: board certified in the area of surgical specialty; experience in the procedure you desire; recommendation from someone you trust that has used the surgeon; remains current with new procedures; communicates with you about the positives and negatives of the procedure and your motivation for having the surgical procedure; and has privileges at area hospitals.

Types of Cosmetic Procedures Many types of cosmetic procedures are available to accomplish a variety of desirable changes in one's appearance. The following list provides the common and medical procedural term and briefly explains the purpose of the procedures:

- Eyelid lift (*blepharoplasty*) corrects sagging or droopy lids above the eyes and/or bags below the eye.
- Neck/face-lift (*rhytidectomy*) lifts the lower two-thirds of the face and improves sagging skin, jowls, double chin, and aging neck.

- Forehead or brow lift is accomplished with an ear-to-ear incision and removal of extra skin to reduce forehead and frown lines and to raise sagging eyebrows.
- Liposuction uses small tubes attached to a type of vacuum to remove pounds of fatty tissue from buttocks, upper arms, stomach, hips, or face.
- Chin (*mentoplasy*) or cheek (*malar*) augmentation provides for a more pleasing face contour by adding cheekbones and a stronger more prominent chin line.
- Nose job (*rhinoplasty*) reshapes nose by changing nostrils, building or removing the bridge, recontouring the tip, or cutting or adding bone or cartilage. May be helpful for improved breathing (insurance may apply in this instance).
- Chemical peel (*phenol*) helps to remove, erase, or fade fine facial wrinkles, acne scars, or sun damage by use of certain types of acid such as phenol or trichlorocetric acid, or use of certain types of laser.
- Dermabrasion scrapes top layers of the skin to help remove fine wrinkles and marred skin so that new and smoother skin will be produced.
- Collagen or fat injections help to fill out skin tissues to reduce wrinkling or scar tissue, "plump" up lips, or smooth back of the hands.

Each of these procedures can have very positive benefits, but each can also be harmful and produce unexpected outcomes. The importance of utilizing a board-certified, experienced, and highly qualified surgeon is essential in order to avoid such side effects as infection, pooling of blood under the skin, nerve damage, numbness, scarring, or ill-positioned or hardening of implants. Side effects, such as bruising, swelling, redness, throbbing, numbness and tightness, and stiffness, can be expected, but they are presumed to be temporary.

Breast Augmentation

Breast implants appeared on the market 30 years ago and since that time approximately one million women in the United States have undergone this procedure to reshape, augment, or reconstruct the breasts.[38]

Prior to April 1995, **silicone gel-filled** and **saline implants** were basically available to any woman who could afford the procedure. However, continuing problems related to silicone gel-filled implants created a need for valid and reliable clinical research to determine the safety and long-term effects of these products. Hardening of the breast because of scar tissue shrinkage around the implant, possibility of negative effects on the immune system, risks of cancer development, and potential interference with mammogram readings all contributed to the investigation and eventual restrictions of silicone gel-filled implants.[39] At this time only females who seek breast reconstruction because of cancer, breast injury, congenital disorders, or those who are involved in clinical trials are approved to have silicone gel-filled implants. The number of women who can receive gel-filled implants for breast enlargement is limited. Research is continuing to determine safety and potential health consequences related to gel-filled implants.

Of the women who get breast implants, the vast majority do so to increase the size of their breast, called **breast augmentation.** Saline pouches, filled with a saltwater solution fills the inflatable implants and then are placed between breast tissue and the chest wall. These types of implants are presently available to anyone who can afford the procedure even though the safety of saline implants has not been proven. Concerns related to saline implants relate to deflation due to leakage or rupture that can require additional surgery to correct. Calcium deposits often develop causing difficulty in reading and interpreting mammograms. Seepage of saline solution into the body may occur creating a risk of developing an autoimmune disease.

cosmetic surgeon—a physician who specializes in beauty-enhancing surgery such as face-lifts or breast augmentation.

plastic surgeon—a physician who specializes in reconstructive surgery and also performs beauty-enhancing procedures.

silicone gel-filled implant—a pouch filled with silicone gel used to reconstruct or increase the size of the breast.

saline implant—a pouch filled with saltwater used to reconstruct or increase the size of the breast.

breast augmentation (awg men **tay** shun)—surgical method to increase the size of the breast by implanting synthetic materials into the chest wall behind the breast tissue.

Viewpoint

Should Gel-Filled Breast Implants Be Available?

The consequences of gel-filled implants are not totally known, but what has been documented is: implants should not be expected to last a lifetime; all implants leak silicone through their outer envelope; the health effects of this leakage are not truly clear; the percentage of gel-filled implant rupture is not known; there is a connection between gel-filled breast implants and cancer, immune system disorders, and interference with mammogram readings; and the formation of calcium deposits is nor clear. Because we do not have definitive answers to some of these possible health effects, should women still have the choice to have gel-filled implants placed in their breasts if they so desire? There appears to be some psychological benefits for women who elect to have their breast size enlarged. Women have reported feeling more attractive, more confident, and better about themselves. Why should women who chose to take the unknown risks related to this surgery be denied the right to make this choice? What is your opinion about this issue?

health tips

Breast Augmentation Guidelines

Remember the following guidelines in order to prevent any potential danger from breast implants:

- Have regular breast exams by a qualified physician
- Perform monthly breast self-exams
- Have screening mammograms at intervals prescribed for your age group
- Stay in contact with your regular physician as well as the cosmetic surgeon who performed the surgery

Another breast augmentation procedure is called breast augmentation mammoplasty by injection (BAMBI). In this procedure, excess fat is suctioned from the buttocks, thighs, or abdomen and injected between the breast and the chest wall. The surgeon who developed this procedure, Dr. Gerald Johnson, claims that it can permanently increase the breast by one-half a cup size.[40] However, other cosmetic surgeons claim that the injected fat either breaks down and is absorbed into the body or develops a hard calcium mass that can mask or mimic breast cancer. Dr. Johnson, although no longer performing this procedure, claims that it is a safe and effective operation.[41] Perhaps with further study, this will be a procedure used again in future breast augmentation surgeries.

What do you think about breast augmentation? Complete *Viewpoint:* "Should Gel-Filled Breast Implants Be Available?". Women who have any type of breast implants should be reminded to have regular checkups especially if experiencing a change in size, shape, or consistency or feel any discomfort. *Health Tips:* "Breast Augmentation Guidelines" provides guidelines that women should diligently follow.

The resources at the end of this chapter provide additional information about breast implants.

Although this information about different types of and precautions about cosmetic surgery is important for women to have if they choose to have any type of cosmetic surgical procedure, perhaps the more important questions are: Why are we seeing such an increase in the number of women who desire a "beauty-enhancing procedure" that carries so many risks? Why shouldn't women be able to appreciate their "natural" qualities without feeling the need to undergo risky surgery, painful recovery, and undue expense for cosmetic procedures that may or may not yield positive results? Reading the next section about advertising and the media's portrayal of women may assist us in understanding the desire to enhance our physical being, even at the potential risk of experiencing negative health consequences.

EFFECTS OF ADVERTISING

We see the beautiful, slim bodies of attractive people having an exciting and fun time in a lovely environment many times every day through the magic of television, or the turn of a page in a popular magazine. Everyone and everything appears to be just right! Whether it's wrinkle cream, beer, exercise equipment, or the latest weight control product, it's the advertisers job to persuade people to buy products and services. Too often consumers must follow the concept of **caveat emptor,** a phrase that means let the buyer beware. In other words, it is the consumer's problem to determine if the advertisement is misleading and she must make the decision to purchase at her own discretion or risk. Not fair!!

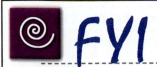

FYI *Advertising Techniques for Health-Related Products*[42]

Technique	What You Hear	What You Can Ask
bandwagon	Used by majority of hospitals/doctors, People rely on . . .	Does everyone use this, if so how do other companies stay in business?
Testimonials	By celebrities (sports, actors), by medical personnel	Do they know more than others? How much are they being paid to promote this product? Do they use the product?
Nonverbal/visuals	Music, colors, beautiful scenes & people, animation	What does this have to do with effectiveness of products?
Humor, slogans	Jokes, silly costumes, phrases, songs, comedians	Helps to sell, but what does it mean? Is a product better because its ad is funny?
Power words	Works wonders, famous, revolutionary, natural, amazing	What is the truth? What makes it amazing or revolutionary or natural?
Scientific evidence	Studies say, doctors recommend, clinical trials indicate, scientists say . . .	What test, research, or clinical trials? What doctors; what scientists?
Superior	Leading brand, more effective, stronger, no other, best	Are differences significant? Who says it's more effective?
Emotions and attitudes	Relieve tension, improve mood, feel sexier, feel better about self, feels good all over . . .	How was this determined? Where is the evidence? How do we know?

Consumers should be able to trust that the information presented by advertisements is accurate and truthful.

There have been strides toward truth in advertising and the products that are promoted. The Federal Trade Commission (FTC), established in 1914, was established to protect citizens against unfair business practices. Congress expanded the responsibilities of the FTC with the 1938 Wheeler-Lea Amendment, which was passed to protect consumers against individuals or companies engaged in false advertisements of cosmetics, foods, drugs, and devices. The Fair Packing and Labeling Act of 1966 requires the label on products involving foods, drugs, cosmetics, and medical devices to honestly inform consumers what they are buying and how it is to be used effectively.

Even with protective laws and agencies, consumers must still be aware, informed, and conscientious in regard to purchasing health-related products promoted by advertisers. Their objective is to sell a product; our objective is to purchase a product that is safe and effective for our needs. Hopefully, the following information will be beneficial in assisting you, the female consumer, in selecting products that meet your needs and do not adversely affect your pocketbook.

Types of Advertising Techniques

Strategies for promoting health-related products (as well as other types of products) range from humorous and glitzy to sophisticated and ethereal. When purchasing a product to meet your needs, keep in mind a number of questions that will aid in your decision: How does it compare to other products? What is the evidence that the product works? Can any product really do what this product claims to do? Am I buying the product or trying to purchase the image that is selling the product?

Advertisers do an outstanding job of product promotion. Some advertisements are beneficial in helping us make a decision; other products are almost camouflaged as to their real purpose due to the hype (music, lighting, gorgeous people, celebrities, good times) used to promote the product. Awareness plays a significant part of making an informed decision about consumer issues. *FYI:* "Advertising Techniques for Health-Related Products" lists the techniques used

caveat emptor (kav **vee** ott)—let the buyer beware; the opposite of *caveat vendor,* or let the seller beware.

JOURNAL ACTIVITY

Analyzing Advertisements

Select advertisements from television and women's journals and answer the following questions related to techniques presented in the previous FYI box.

1. Does the person (celebrity or otherwise) have the credentials to know about the product they are promoting?
2. Can the product, in reality, do all the things it claims it can do?
3. Where is the scientific evidence that this product can produce the results for my well-being that it claims?
4. How do I know that the clinical trials produced the outcomes that the advertisement claims occurred?
5. Does the scenery or music or imagery in this advertisement make this product a better product than another in a less-appealing advertisement? As a result of this type of advertisement, will the cost of the product become more than similar products?
6. Does the product claim to be painless, miraculous, fast and effective, FDA-approved, or guaranteed?
7. Does the product work while you sleep, cure serious disease, retard aging, reduce fat without exercise, or improve your sex life?
8. Does the product claim that it can improve your social life, make you popular, or make you more appealing to other people?
9. Does the product claim to be an effective foreign product?
10. Is the cost of this product in accord with other brands of this type?

---

by advertisers to sell their products. Which do you recognize in products you have purchased? Have any of these techniques persuaded you to purchase a cosmetic, drug, or device?

Through beautiful people, funny phrases, setting a mood, and testimonials, we are exposed to claims about products that are appealing and believable. Complete *Journal Activity:* "Analyzing Advertisements" to help you "see" beyond the image and glitz to find the real message, if there is one, about the product. Then determine if the product meets your needs.

Unrealistic Portrayals of Women

When advertisers promote products to women, it is often accompanied by the message that the product is needed in order to be thinner, more attractive, more youthful, or to improve one's lifestyle. Promoting products in this manner sends the message that women are not thin, attractive, or young enough and that our situation in life can be improved by purchasing and using a particular product. Dissatisfaction with one's physique contributes to being vulnerable to advertisements that feature thin, young women who represent the "norm" of feminine beauty. Often the heart of female-directed advertisements plays to the lack of belief in one's self-worth or attractiveness. Women of today have been programmed to believe they should be able to do and have it all—challenging careers, children and partners, and attractive,

thin, and fit bodies. Therefore, if we don't achieve this "ideal," we often feel deficient and unworthy. Thus, advertisements often portray women who use certain products as attractive and successful in all areas of their lives. Examples of these include a thin, young, fit mother riding a bike with her son; a beautiful young woman with thick, blond hair sitting on the beach promoting shampoo; a woman displaying devices that can be worn to provide a face lift effect without surgery; a gorgeous, young woman with long, thick dark hair promoting a hair conditioner; a beautiful, young Oriental woman with no wrinkles selling moisturizer; and a thin, young woman draped only in soft, see-through fabric and floating in a carefree position promoting a "soothing" line of hair products.

What about women who are of average to over-average weight, over 40 years of age, and may not have wrinkle-free complexions—are there no products for this group? Do only beautiful, thin, young, energetic women purchase products? No! Do these advertisements mean that we, of average looks and bodies, are not worthy of health-promoting and lifestyle-enhancing products? Is there some place for reality in advertising?

Advertisements also portray women as frivolous and preoccupied with self? In 1992, the Quebec's Council for the Status of Women studied women in advertisements. In the study, 3,000 prime-time television shows were reviewed over a 7-week time period. It was found that women were often depicted as frivolous, superficial, ignorant, and incapable of doing difficult tasks.[43] Magazine advertisements directed at female consumers, unfortunately, depicted women in a similar manner. A Canadian writer reported that upon reviewing women's magazines, she observed an inordinate amount of information about dressing, eating, loving, shampooing, or exercising.[44] It can be disconcerting to be the gender viewed as superficial and be perceived as having only a decorative contribution to make to society. Advertising examples of this perception include: advertisement in which four beautiful women indicate they can express their inner self by using a particular shampoo; soap that makes a woman feel like she's never felt before; a thin, lovely, young woman modeling clothes being compared to a male who has his work tools; a series of clothing advertisements depicting young women doing nothing more substantial than playing and posing; and a tobacco advertisement in which a female is going to travel to an exotic destination just to "be."

Is the mental and physical health of women negatively impacted when only thin and attractive models, implied as the cultural norm, are used in advertisements, or when women are portrayed as self-absorbed and frivolous? Advertisements that stereotype gender has been a major concern of feminist leaders. Has the image of women portrayed in the media been partially responsible for creating and maintaining limited social roles for women? In an analysis of research studies about women in advertisements from 1950s through the 1980s, Bushy and Leichty[45] found that although there were not as many advertisements showing women in home or family settings, an increased number of advertisements showed women as decorative or in "alluring" roles in the ads.

Realistic Portrayals

How about another view? A number of advertisements are beginning to portray women as decision makers and financially independent. A phone company owned and operated by women, an automobile advertisement with a woman making the purchase decision, and a mortgage company showing a woman in the role of home buyer are examples of a more enlightened and inclusive advertisement model. Another new approach finds advertisers seeking to find a neutral position; the trend is away from either-or images, but to seek an image balanced between career and

home.[46] Advertisers must place more emphasis on portraying women as capable, confident, and caring—as individuals who want factual information about products and services, not individuals preoccupied by looks and images. A more accurate and representative portrayal of women in advertisements can only be more "healthful" for women, especially for women who are searching for their physical and psychological identities.[47]

As women continue to have a major financial impact on the marketplace, we will see advertisers present a more realistic image of women—one of an intelligent, pragmatic, attentive, concerned, and financially stable individual—because it is justified.

FINANCIAL CONSIDERATIONS

Health Insurance

All aspects of health care, ranging from prevention to treatment to cure are essential to the health and well-being of all people. The continuing exponential growth of health-care costs too often leave individuals without the benefit of this vital care, especially the uninsured. Health insurance is a contract between an individual and/or a group and an insurance company, and can assist individuals to meet the

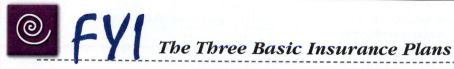

The Three Basic Insurance Plans

The type of insurance plan a woman has will determine the type of medical services, procedures, and practitioners she will be able to use. Following is a brief look at three basic types of insurance plans.

- *Private, fee-for-service plan:* The individual or employer pays a certain amount each month that ensures a woman can receive health care on a fee-for-service basis. A deductible, paid by the patient, must be met and then the insurance pays a major portion, usually 80 percent, after the deductible is met. To lower costs of insurance, **preferred providers organizations (PPO),** which are comprised of private medical practitioners, provide services at a lower rate to a particular insurance company. Use of the PPO physicians produces lower health-care fees; use of non-PPO physicians cost more.

- *Prepaid group insurance:* **Health maintenance organizations (HMOs)** are comprised of various medical personnel who provide a wide-range of

medical services (e.g., specialists, lab work, etc.) for a prepaid amount that is usually deducted from each paycheck. There is often a co-pay amount (usually minimal amount such as $5 to $10) each time an HMO service is used. The HMO is usually associated with a hospital and provides care from a limited group of medical practitioners.

- *Government-financed insurance:* For women of certain ages and socioeconomic levels, the local, state, and/or federal government provides health-care insurance under various types of plans. Briefly, two types of government insurance plans are: Medicare, which is paid from social security benefits for people 65 and older and individuals with specific health concerns, and (2) Medicaid, which provides some health-care coverage for individuals who meet certain financial criteria. These two types of coverage are discussed in greater detail in the information on the following page.

---

demands and needs of paying for their health care. What types of health insurance plans are available and how do we select one that meets our health needs and financial ability? See *FYI:* "The Three Basic Insurance Plans."

Health insurance plans will vary according to the types of services offered and price for coverage. *Basic health insurance* covers hospital, surgical, and medical expenses and individual health plans differ according to the company and the contract. *Major medical insurance* (or catastrophic coverage) assist with any major and/or long-term illness, such as heart disease or cancer, and is usually a supplement to basic health insurance. *Comprehensive major medical insurance* combines basic health and major medical insurance plans to provide for the majority of health-care needs. There is usually a deductible, ranging from between $50 to almost any amount, which must be paid by the insuree before the insurance company is required to pay anything.

Not only do too many people not have health insurance, people continue to lose the coverage they have—the number of people who lose their health insurance each month is 100,000. By early 1997, over 43,000,000 did not have any health insurance.[48]

Women and children are disproportionately represented among all uninsured individuals. Only 37 percent of employed women, compared to 56 percent of employed men, have health insurance coverage through their employment. People who work part-time, two-thirds of whom are women, are only one-third as likely as full-time workers to have health insurance.[49] Women, whose wages are only 70 percent of men's, are disproportionately represented in the job market that pays less than $20,000. At this level over 93 percent of workers are uninsured.[50]

A comprehensive health insurance plan that meets the unique needs for women, especially low-income women, should have the following components: (1) universal access—especially for women who work part-time or are seasonal, or who move in and out of the workforce; (2) affordable—especially because women have average earnings 30 percent less than men; (3) reimbursement for a range of providers—midwives, nurse practitioners, and other medical personnel who are effective, but less expensive; (4) nondiscriminatory; (5) equal rating factors—adopt a community rating and prohibit the insurance industry from using gender as a rating factor; (6) require a minimum benefits package with preventive care, reproductive care [family planning, abortion, infertility], mental health benefits, drug abuse care, long-term health care, HIV infections, and care for battered women.[51] When considering health-care insurance, assess the quality of the provisions by comparing these components to the policy components.

Medicare and Medicaid Services

Medicare, provided by the federal government Social Security Act, is a governmental health insurance program that provides health-care benefits for individuals 65 years of age or older. Disabled women under the age of 65 may also be eligible for Medicare. Medicare consists of two parts: *Part A* is the Hospital Insurance and *Part B* is Supplementary Medical Insurance. Part A helps to pay for inpatient care while in a hospital, in a skilled nursing facility, for home health care, or for hospice care. The Medicare plan is a mandatory hospital insurance financed by federal Social Security taxes, but paid for by employers paying into Social Security on their employees behalf. Part B helps to pay for physician services, outpatient care, lab tests, and other medical services and supplies. Monthly premiums paid by enrollees and from federal general revenues finance Part B Medicare.

Currently, Medicare covers approximately 36 million individuals, with about 3 million being disabled and some 200,000 experiencing end-stage renal disease.[52] To enroll for Medicare, contact any Social Security Administration found in the government section of your local phone book Yellow Pages.

Medicaid is a medical assistance program jointly financed by the state and federal governments to help provide health care for low-income women with no health care. Eligible recipients include needy and low-income women, blind, elderly, and/or disabled individuals, members of families with dependent children, and others with special circumstances. Currently, women comprise over 69 percent of all Medicaid beneficiaries between the ages of 18 and 64.[53] For 8 percent of all women, Medicaid is their only source of health insurance coverage for essential treatment and preventive services.[54] Additionally, Medicaid use is highest among women between the ages of 18–24; 11 percent of the women in this age group depend on Medicaid for their health insurance.[55] Federally mandated Medicaid services of significance to women include: inpatient and outpatient hospital, physician, midwife, and certified nurse practitioner, laboratory, X ray, nursing home and home health care, rural health clinics, family planning, and early and periodic

screening, diagnosis, and treatment for children under age 21. States have varying eligibility requirements and the services are administered out of the local community or state welfare office. Women can contact this office for assistance.

Social Security

Social Security (SS) is a protective program that provides benefits to workers and their families who have financial and health-care needs. The program began in 1935 as a way to assist retired workers, most of whom were men, and the families of deceased workers. In the 1930s only about 5 percent of women worked in jobs outside the home.[56] Today about 60 percent of all women are employed outside the home and earn credit toward their retirement. Women earn SS protection, not only for themselves and their children, but also assistance if they become disabled and cannot work, and survivor benefits if they should die. If women choose not to work outside of the home or if they enter the workforce for only a few years, they are usually covered by SS if their spouse retires, becomes disabled, or dies.

Retirement Benefits   Retirement benefits vary according to age of the retiree. A woman can be eligible for benefits by age 62, but the payments will be permanently reduced because she will be receiving payments for a longer period of time than if she had waited until age 65. A woman will be eligible for full retirement benefits if she waits until she is 65 years of age to retire. In the future, the age in which full benefits are payable will be gradually increased—by the year 2027, a woman will need to be 67 years old to receive full retirement benefits.

If you are married, you can receive retirement payments on your husband's as well as your own employment record. There are often special circumstances related to SS retirement benefits. They relate

preferred provider organization (PPO)— physicians who agree to provide their services for a reduced rate to insurance companies.

health maintenance organization (HMO)— a type of health insurance that provides a full-range of health-care services using specific physicians and specialists for a prepaid amount of money.

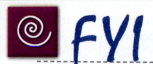

Your Social Security Benefits

Would you like to know your potential future benefits upon your retirement? That's easy to learn. Write to the Department of Health and Human Services, Social Security Administration, 300 N. Greene St., Baltimore, MD 21201–1581 and request the document entitled, "Request for Earnings and Benefit Estimate Statement," Form #SSA-7004-SM OP-7. You can complete and return the information requested and receive an estimate of your SS retirement benefits. ☜

to age, former and current marital status, and the work history of both partners.

Special situations such as never being employed, self-employment, household worker, or service in the military have some unique aspects. Information related to these and other considerations can be found in a booklet entitled, *Society Security . . . What Every Woman Should Know,* from the local or federal Social Security Office and from the toll-free number found at the end of this chapter. Social Security benefits related to remarriage, being widowed, and divorced are multifaceted and sometimes complex. The above-mentioned booklet can be helpful as well as contacting a representative from the local, state, or national Social Security Office. (See *FYI:* "Your Social Security Benefits.")

TAKING ACTION

Agencies

Food and Drug Administration (FDA) has the responsibility to regulate the following products (with examples): foods (labeling, safety), drugs (approval, advertising), cosmetics (safety, purity), biological products (blood banks, human vaccines), medical devices (registration, approval), radiological devices (microwave, X-ray equipment), and veterinary products (pet foods, vet drugs) sold in interstate commerce. States enforce regulations on products that do not cross state lines. The states are also responsible for licensing health professionals such as dentists, physicians, and pharmacists as well as inspection and regulation of restaurants and health clubs.

The FDA offers a variety of services to assist the consumer with questions or concerns related to any product under its regulatory control. Consumer affairs officers (COA) are located throughout the United States to answer questions and provide informational literature, either by print or through media. These officers (sometimes referred to as public affairs specialists) will also speak to groups on specific topics related to drugs, fraud, safety, and many other topics of interest to consumers. Your local COA can be located under the Food and Drug Administration in the federal government section of the local phone book. Consumer Inquiries Staff, located in Washington, D.C., has the responsibility of answering consumer's questions of any type. This staff has the ability to utilize the expertise of a variety of federal agencies in order to find the answer to inquiries, about 2,500 each month. Requests for information can be sent to FDA Consumer Inquiries Staff, HFE-88, Room 16–63, 5600 Fishers Lane, Rockville, MD 20857; phone # (301) 443–3170. Electronic bulletin boards are available to provide instant consumer information about drug approvals, congressional testimony, articles from the *FDA Consumer,* and a multitude of other topics.

Credit Reports

Reports of your credit history may be requested when you seek to purchase items such as an automobile, a home, or a large appliance. Credit bureaus collect and maintain great volumes of information on an individual's financial activities. If a company wants to assess your credit worthiness, it can obtain a copy of your credit report from a number of credit bureaus. Do you know what your report says about your buying and paying history? Would you like to know? You can obtain a copy of your credit report by contacting one of three national reporting systems: Equifax, Trans Union, and TRW. (Addresses are provided in *FYI:* "Credit Report Agencies.") What do you look for? Are there any inaccuracies and questionable listings of debts.

Free reports can be obtained from the credit reporting systems if you have applied for credit in the last 30 days and were denied. However, some reporting systems charge for a copy of your report.

Knowing what to do if inaccuracies appear is an important consumer skill. If you find inaccuracies, write the credit bureau and tell them which credit listing is inaccurate. The credit bureau must, by law,

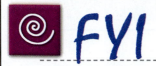

Credit Report Agencies

Equifax Information
Service Center
P.O. Box 740241
Atlanta, GA 30374-0241
(800) 685-1111

Trans Union
Consumer Relations
P.O. Box 390
Springfield, PA 19064
(800) 851-2674

TRW Consumer
Assistance Ct.
P.O. Box 2106
Allen, TX 75002
(800) 392-1122

---

re-verify the information within a reasonable amount of time (usually 30–35 days) or the credit listing must be removed from your file. Information that is inaccurate or cannot be verified must be corrected or removed from your report. If you have some negative information on your report that is accurate, you may elect to write a brief explanation (about 100 words) to the credit bureaus and explain why the negative credit incident occurred. This may be helpful in obtaining credit even though the negative report usually must stay in your file for 7 years. Bankruptcy information is kept for 10 years. If this information appeared on one credit bureau report, it may appear on others. Therefore, it is a good idea to review all three major credit reporting agencies.

Righting a Wrong

Even if we are wise consumers, there are times when we may be taken advantage of by an individual or company or we can have a faulty product. Knowing what to do and how to rectify this situation can be most helpful and save time and money. Purchase-related paperwork of a product that is intended to last for a period of time should be saved in an organized file with other product-related information. If a problem occurs, contact the business (or person) that sold you the product and describe the problem and how you would like for it to be resolved. For example, do you want the product repaired or your money back? Keep a record of calls and/or letters to and from the company and include when and with whom you spoke. If the problem has not been resolved within a reasonable amount of time, then it is time to contact the company headquarters. Look on the packaging for a toll-free 800 number or call the toll-free 800 operator at 800–555-1212 to locate the number of the company. Most local libraries have a directory of 800 numbers.

Many companies require a complaint to be in writing, therefore, knowing where to write and what to say can be valuable information. Look for the address of the product manufacturer on the packaging of the product. If it is not there, or you don't have the package, go to the reference section in your local library and search for the company address in one of the following books: *Standard & Poor's Register of Corporations, Directors and Executives; Standard Directory of Advertisers; Trade Names Directory;* or *Dun & Bradstreet Directory.* The *Thomas Register of American Manufacturers* can provide you with a list of manufacturers of thousands of products. After locating the address of the company, it is important to write a concise and reasonable, but not threatening, letter explaining what is wrong with their product and how you have attempted to resolve the problem. See Figure 12.3. Include your name, address, work or home phone numbers, and your company account number, if you have one. Provide the company with place and date of product purchase, serial or model number of the product, and include copies, not originals, of all documentation. If, after a reasonable time, usually 2 to 4 weeks, you have not received satisfaction, file a complaint, along with a copy of your letter, with the local or state consumer protection agency that pertains to the nature of your concern. Addresses and phone numbers for agencies that govern banking, hospitals, insurance, products, and utilities can usually be found in the government pages of the telephone directory. Addresses for more specific agencies and companies can be found in an excellent source, *1997 Consumer's Resource Handbook,*[57] which can be obtained free from the U.S. Department of Consumer Affairs, phone # (800) 664-4435.

FIGURE 12.3 Sample complaint letter.

Your address
Your city, state, zip code
Date

(Name of contact person if available)
(Title, if available)
(Company name)
(Consumer complaint division, if you have no contact person)
(Street address)
(City, state, zip code)

Dear (contact person):

Re: (account number, if applicable)

    On (date), I (bought, leased, rented, or had repaired) a (name of product with serial or model number or service performed) at (location, date, and other important details of the transaction).
    Unfortunately, your product (or service) has not performed well (or service was inadequate) because (state the problem). I am disappointed because (explain the problem: for example, the product does not work properly, the service was not performed correctly, I was billed the wrong amount, something was not disclosed clearly or was misrepresented, or etc.).
    To resolve the problem, I would appreciate your (state the specific action you want—money back, credit charge card, repair, exchange, etc.). Enclosed are copies (do not send originals) of my records (include receipts, guarantees, warranties, canceled checks, contracts, model and serial numbers, and any other documentation).
    I look forward to your reply and a resolution to my problem, and will wait until (set a time limit) before seeking help from a consumer protection or the Better Business Bureau. Please contact me at the above address or by phone at (home and/or numbers with area codes).

Sincerely,

(Your name)

Enclosure(s)

cc: (reference to whom you are sending a copy of this letter, if anyone)

Chapter Summary

- Effective consumer skills including having an awareness and knowledge of health products and services, making informed choices, and knowing how to obtain better consumer services.
- There are important guidelines that can be utilized when locating and selecting a health-care provider.
- A variety of health-care practitioners provide special and specific services that can be beneficial to women's health.
- Alternative health care offers options to conventional medicine, but, as a rule is not taught in U.S. medical schools. Many of these alternative practices have not been scientifically proven to be medically beneficial.
- Fraudulent health-care costs American citizens over $10 billion annually, therefore, it is essential to recognize and report acts of fraudulent behavior.
- Advertising is a major influence in the purchase of health-related products and the media uses a variety of techniques to sell these commodities.
- Women have too often been unrealistically portrayed in order to create the perception of the need to purchase certain types of products.

- Cosmetics, skin-care products, and facial and body cosmetic surgery are all products/procedures that can be expensive and risky; women can learn important guidelines for better selection of these products and procedures.
- Women have specific needs in health insurance coverage, yet are too often without important insurance coverage for themselves and their children.
- Information regarding health insurance, social security benefits, and retirement plans is needed by women in order to make health- and life-enhancing financial-related decisions.
- Medicare and Medicaid are government health insurances provided for women and children who meet specific criteria.
- Government and citizen consumer protection agencies provide avenues by which women can learn how to report problems with products/people/procedures and find assistance in correcting the problems.

Review Questions

1. What is the Consumer Bill of Rights and what is its purpose?
2. What is the difference between basic, major medical, and comprehensive major medical insurance coverage?
3. Why are women and their children disproportionately uninsured in this country?
4. What benefits are provided by Medicare and Medicaid health services?
5. What are the advantages and disadvantages of using home health tests? Which are designed specifically for women?
6. What are the processes for locating and selecting a health-care provider?
7. Why are more women turning to alternative health care? What are some of the advantages and disadvantages of alternative health care?
8. How can you protect yourself from health-care fraud?
9. What three federal laws were passed to help protect the consumer from poor-quality health products and inadequate health care?

10. What is the purpose of the various advertising techniques used by companies to sell their products?
11. What techniques do advertisers use in promoting their products? Provide an example of a product for each of these techniques.
12. Why should women be concerned about how they are portrayed in advertisements?
13. What are some safety measures that women can take when selecting and purchasing cosmetics?
14. What are some of the concerns about cosmetic surgery? Why do many women elect to have these beauty-enhancing procedures?
15. What criteria should a woman use when selecting a cosmetic surgeon?
16. What elements should be included when writing a letter of complaint about a product, a professional, an agency, or a facility?

Resources

Organizations and Hotlines

U.S. Office of Consumer Affairs
Telephone: (800) 664-4435

U.S. Consumer Product Safety Commission
Telephone: (800) 638-2772

American Society of Plastic and Reconstructive Surgeons
Telephone: (800) 635-0685

National Institutes of Health, Division of Public Information
U.S. Department of Health and Human Services
Telephone: (800) 336-4797

FDA Information and Outreach Staff
HFE-88, Room 16-63
5600 Fishers Lane
Rockville, MD 29857
Telephone: (301) 443-3170

FDA Electronic Bulletin Board (accessible free by computer modem)
Telephone: (800) 222-0185

FDA Breast Implant Information Line
Telephone: (800) 532-4440

Rural Information Center Health Service
National Agricultural Library, Room 304
10301 Baltimore Blvd.
Beltsville, MD 20705-2351
Telephone: (800) 633-7701

National Women's Law Center
1616 P. Street NW, Suite 100
Washington, DC 20036
Telephone: (202) 328-5160 *(information on insurance and health care for women)*

National Women's Health Resource Center
2440 M Street, Northwest
Washington, D.C. 20037
Telephone: (202) 293-6045 *(an educational resource and clearinghouse of women's health information; publishes a bimonthly consumer publication addressing health promotion, disease prevention, mental health, nutrition, fitness, medical research, and legislation affecting women's health)*

Websites

Better Business Bureau
http://www.bbb.org/index.html

Federal Trade Commission
http://www.ftc.gov/index.html

Alternative Medicine Homepage
http://www.pitt.edu/~cbw/altm.html

Holistic Health
http://www.hir.com/

Health Care Information Resources
http://www-hsl.mcmaster.ca/tomflem/top.html

MedAccess
http://www.medaccess.com

Suggested Readings

The American Medical Association Family Medical Guide. 1994. New York: Random House.

1997 Consumer's Resource Handbook—Obtain a free copy by writing: Handbook, Consumer Information Center, Pueblo, CO 81009 or by calling 1-800-664-4435

References

1. Consumer Advisory Council, Executive Office of the President. 1963. *First Report.* Washington, D.C.: U.S. Government Printing Office.
2. Barrett, S., W. T. Jarvis, M. Kroger, and W. M. London. 1997. *Consumer health: A guide to intelligent decisions.* Madison, WI: Brown & Benchmark.
3. Ibid.
4. Barzansky, B., H. S. Jonas, and S. I. Etzel. 1995. Education programs in U.S. medical schools, 1994-1995. *Journal of the American Medical Association,* 274, 716-22.
5. Barrett et al., *Consumer health.*
6. What is a good check-up? 1995. *Harvard Health Letter,* 20 (30): 6-8.
7. Barrett et al., *Consumer health.*
8. Smith, J. M. 1992. *Women and doctors.* New York: The Atlantic Monthly Press.
9. What therapists' degrees mean. 1996, June. *Harvard Women's Health Watch,* 111 (10): 5.
10. Farley, D. 1989. Do-it-yourself medical testing. DHHS No. 89-4206. Rockville, Md.: Department of Health & Human Services.

11. Bringing medicine home. 1996. *Consumer Reports,* 61 (10): 47–55.
12. Eisenberg, D. et al. 1993, January. Unconventional medicine in the United States. *The New England Journal of Medicine,* 328 (4): 246–52.
13. Ibid.
14. Ibid.
15. Barasch, D. S. 1994, October 4. The mainstreaming of alternative medicine. *The Good Health Magazine,* 6–9, 36, 38.
16. ABC Television. 1996, June 25. Alternative healing practices. *Good Morning America,* New York, N.Y.
17. Barrett et al., *Consumer Health.*
18. Weiss, R. 1995. Medicine's latest miracle. *Health,* 9, 70–78.
19. Ibid.
20. Chiropractors. 1994. *Consumer Reports,* 59 (6): 383–90.
21. Ibid.
22. Ibid.
23. Ibid.
24. Ibid.
25. Cohen, J. 1995, June. The therapeutic benefit of massage. *American Health,* 26.
26. Lipner, M. 1993, May/June. Different strokes. *Women's Sports and Fitness,* 31–33.
27. Witherell, M. 1995, September. Massage: De-stress in minutes. *American Health,* 70.
28. Stalker, D., and O. Glymour. 1983. Engineers, cranks, physicians, magicians. *New Journal of Medicine,* 308, 960–64.
29. Barrett et al., *Consumer Health.*
30. Cornacchia, H. J., and S. Barrett. *Consumer health: A guide to intelligent decisions.* St. Louis, Mo.: Mosby.
31. Stehlin, D. 1994, January. Cosmetic surgery: More complex than at first blush. *Current Issues in Women's Health.* FDA Consumer Special Report, 80–85.
32. Ibid.
33. Cavanaugh, T. 1995, May. Ethics expand. *Chemical Marketing Reporter,* 2 (17): SR 21–22.
34. Moisturizers. 1994. *Consumer Reports,* 59 (9): 577–81.
35. Ibid.
36. Goodman, M. 1994. Social, psychological & developmental factors in women's receptivity to cosmetic surgery. *Journal of Aging Studies,* 8 (4): 375–96.
37. Ibid.
38. Segal, M. 1994, January. Silicone breast implants: Available under tight controls. *Current Issues in Women's Health,* 76–79.
39. Ibid.
40. Margolis, D. 1993, March. Fat chance: Rearrange the unwanted mass. *American Health,* 12, 18.
41. Ibid.
42. Cornacchia and Barrett, *Consumer Health.*
43. Shier, M. 1995. On being a boy toy. *Canada and the World Backgrounder,* 60 (4): 8–10.
44. Ibid.
45. Bushy, J., and G. Leichty. 1993. Feminism & advertising in traditional and nontraditional women's magazine, 1950s–1980s. *Journalism Quarterly,* 70 (2): 247–64.
46. Kanner, B. 1995. Advertisers take aim at women at home. *New York Times,* 42.
47. Stephens, D. L., R. P. Hill, and C. Hanson. 1994. The beauty myth & female consumers: The controversial role of advertising. *The Journal of Consumer Affairs,* 28 (1): 137–50.
48. Vital statistics. 1996, March/April. *Health,* 10 (2): 23.
49. *How women fare under Clinton's health care reform.* 1994. Washington, D.C.: National Women's Law Center.
50. Ibid.
51. *Health care reform.* 1993, November. Washington, D.C.: National Women's Law Center.
52. Health Care Financing Administration. 1993. *Medicare Q&A: 85 Commonly Asked Questions.* Baltimore, Md.: U.S. Department of Health and Human Services, 1–28.
53. *Sources of health insurance and characteristics of the uninsured, analysis of the March 1993 Current Population Survey.* 1994, January. Employee Benefit Research Institute. Issue brief # 145.
54. Collins, K. et al. 1995. Assessing and improving women's health. *The American Women 1994–95, Where We Stand,* 145.
55. Ibid.
56. Social Security Administration. 1994. *Social Security . . . what every woman should know.* Baltimore, Md.: U.S. Department of Health and Human Services, 1–16.
57. *Consumer's Resource Handbook.* 1997. Washington, D.C.: U.S. Office of Consumer Affairs.

Thirteen

Preventing Abuse Against Women

■ chapter objectives

When you complete this chapter you will be able to:

- Identify the extent of violence and abuse against women in the United States.
- Classify the various types of abuse committed against women.
- Develop protective plans to avoid the possibilities of rape.
- Summarize the characteristics of women who are abused.
- Explain common elements present in all types of abuse.
- Categorize the types of consequences abused women experience.
- Develop strategies for leaving an abusive relationship.
- Utilize information and methods necessary to heal from the wounds of an abusive relationship.
- Determine methods by which violence and abuse against women can be reduced and eliminated.
- Evaluate the various sources of assistance available to abused women and their children.

THE REALITY OF VIOLENCE AGAINST WOMEN

Keisha gently pressed the cold towel against her cheek and ear. Painfully she removed the numbing cold compress and looked at her inflamed swollen face in the mirror. Why? . . . she asked herself . . . why does this happen to me? She hated it. She hated him, yet, here she was, and remained, an abused wife. As she looked once again at her physical wounds, she knew that her most profound wounds were hidden within.

In the beginning, if one were to read the Bible, women were instructed to be subservient to men, ". . . the desire shall be to thy husband, and he shall rule over thee."[1] The word "woman" is derived from the Anglo-Saxon *wifman*, which literally means "wife-man," a term implying that wifehood and woman are inseparable; that woman exists to be of service to man. The concept and treatment of women as the lesser sex is documented throughout history. For example, during the Stone Age, duties essential to survival—working the land, finding shelter, preparing food—were, for a time, shared by men and women. As metals were discovered and agriculture using heavy tools increased, man used the strength and labor of other men, reducing some men to slaves and diminishing the role of women to the position of servitude. A woman was described as the slave of a man's lust and only an instrument for the production of his children.[2] The attitude of a woman "belonging" to and serving the needs of man too often has led to men "controlling" or "disciplining" women by punishment in whatever manner was deemed necessary or appropriate. According to an old English common law doctrine, a husband could punish his wife for any behavior he considered inappropriate. This law, called the "Rule of Thumb," permitted a husband to beat his wife with a stick no larger than the circumference of his thumb.

In the early history of the United States, violence, especially domestic violence, has been met with varying degrees of concern. Scholars who have studied domestic violence believe there is a direct relationship between the degree of male dominance in a society and the extent of violence toward women.[3] Female servants in the South often fell victim to rape by their "owners"; prostitutes often are beaten by a man who "owns" them for the brief period of time for which he paid.

Historical records of U.S. court proceedings reveal that husbands tended to batter their wives less in the nineteenth century than in the late twentieth century.[4] Prior to our mobile and transient society of today, families, long-time neighbors, and friends sometimes intervened against violent husbands, and offered a buffer and a place of refuge for the abused woman and her children.

Abuse of women encompasses a wide spectrum of behaviors, from sexually derogatory remarks to rape and from battering to murder. Tragically, every 15 seconds a woman is beaten by a current or former husband or partner,[5] and every hour of every day, 57 women are raped. This equates to over 500,000 a year.[6] Over one-half of these women are raped by a family member, friend, or acquaintance.

Prevalence of violence against women varies little among all cultures, among unmarried and married couples, and among socioeconomic groups. The wife of a Fortune 500 company president may just as likely be an abused woman as might the wife or partner of a man who is a blue-collar laborer. However, women aged 19 to 29 and women in families with incomes below $10,000 are more likely than other women to be victims of violence by an intimate.[7] Abused women of all races and cultures seek refuge in safe shelters, utilize community agencies, and seek the support of the legal system.

Violence and abuse against women is a perplexing phenomenon. The perpetrator is usually someone the victim knows—and often loves—the husband, boyfriend, father, or other relative. The U.S. Department of Justice in the Redesigned Survey on Violence against Women[8] found that females over age 12 sustained almost 5 million acts of violence each year and three-fourths of all lone-offender violence was committed by someone the woman knew. Former Surgeon General Antionia Novello, at the 1991 American Medical Association National Leadership Conference, stated, "Domestic violence is a cancer that gnaws at the body and soul of the American family. It is the number one cause of injury to women. . . ."[9] An adult female today is more likely to be raped, beaten, and killed in her own home at the hands of her male partner than any place else or by anyone else in our society.[10]

Incidences, such as the following, are recounted in state and federal government reports and illustrate the extent of violence and abuse inflicted against females. A 9-year-old girl in Texas reports that she was raped by her father; a 15-year-old Connecticut girl was stabbed by her boyfriend; an Idaho woman was raped by her boss; a 46-year-old woman in New Mexico was thrown out of a moving car by her husband; a 31-year-old Baltimore woman was beaten, choked, and raped by a former friend who was helping her move; and an Arizona woman, 8 months pregnant, fled from her home after her husband beat her with a broomstick and threatened to kill her. The wide diversity of these incidences reveals that no one is immune; violence happens to women from all walks of life, old and young, rich and poor, homemakers and homeless, and it is usually inflicted by someone they know. These incidences are called **acquaintance violence,** meaning violence and abuse committed by a parent, relative, coworker, neighbor, or friend.

Women may be victimized more by individuals they know due to the fact that society and/or the legal system has not, in the past, disapproved of acquaintance violence. Abuse committed in the home, called **domestic abuse,** is often perpetrated by an individual whose belief system is grounded in extremes—it can only be right or wrong: the dinner was prepared or it was not, performance of some duty was carried out or it was not. Family violence, according to Dobash and Dobash,[11] has existed for centuries and has been an accepted, as well as a desirable part of a patriarchal family system. By virtue of observation and/or experience, children often perpetuate family traditions by engaging and/or accepting those behaviors that they have seen or experienced in their own family environment. As a result, children who are abused and/or who observe abuse ultimately learn three lifelong lessons:

1. Those who love you the most are also those who will hit you.
2. Other members of the same family have a "right" to hit you, especially if it's to teach you a lesson.
3. If all else fails, use violence.[12]

THE EXTENT OF THE PROBLEM

How much time will you devote to reading this text today? Assuming that you read for only 2 hours, imagine that during that time period more than 114 women will be sexually assaulted and approximately 1,000 will be victims of other types of violence or abuse. The U.S. Justice Department[13] revealed that almost 4.5 million of the nation's 107 million females over 12 years of age reported being victims of an attempted or actual crime, including rape, assault, or robbery. Astoundingly, three out of four women will be the victim of a violent crime sometime during their lifetime. Violent crimes against women are consistent across racial and ethnic groups: Hispanic, non-Hispanic, black, and white.

It is apparent that the numbers of women who endure some form of violence and abuse continue to increase. Data from the Redesigned Survey on Violence Against Women[14] revealed that between 1987 and 1991, 5.4 out of every 1,000 females had been a victim of intimate victimization, but in 1992–93, 9.4

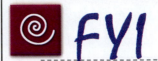

Domestic Violence

Reports of national domestic violence reveal the annual reported incidences committed by intimates.[16] These include:
- 1400 women killed by intimates (28 percent of all female homicides)
- 637 men killed by intimates (3 percent of all male homicides)
- 572,032 violent victimizations of women by intimates
- 48,983 violent victimizations of men by intimates

The consequences:[17]
- $3 to $5 billion for medical expenses related to domestic violence
- $100 million in lost wages, sick leave, absenteeism, and nonproductivity due to domestic violence

There are 1,500 shelters available for battered women in the United States, but there are 3,800 shelters available for animals. ∞

out of 1,000 women had been victimized by an intimate. Research indicates that women are 10 times more likely than men to be victimized by an intimate, and 4 women die in this country everyday as a result of domestic abuse.[15]

WHY DO WOMEN STAY?

Love for the abuser is one reason for not reporting abuse inflicted by a partner. Laura, a woman who had been abused by her husband for a number of years, cried as she said, "I love him; I don't want him arrested; I don't want to hurt him, but I don't want him to hurt me either. I don't know what to do." The partner may be the father of her children; they love him, therefore, she is reluctant to eliminate his presence from the home. Additionally, she may not have a job, job skills, or an education, which creates financial dependency for the woman and the children. Often, women who are abused remain in the abusive relationship because they have no resources and emotional support outside the relationship. Feeling trapped in the relationship, women may determine that some place to live, even if abusive, is better than no place to live, especially if children are involved.

Her Story

Pat

It wasn't easy for me to leave my spouse because, first of all, I still loved him. We had invested 24 years in our marriage, and I had never been totally on my own. Therefore, I was afraid I couldn't make it on my own financially. Until finally after several breakups, numerous arguments, and fights with some of them being near fatal on both our parts, I realized it was time for "Me" to do something different, and healthy. So I moved out for the last time. Since that time I have grown so much more spiritually and mentally. I've learned how to become an optimistic person, which means for me: things will be and are bad at times, but things won't be and aren't bad all the time. Marriage is a good example of that statement because so many years of my marriage was bad, but out of all of that, he and I have a daughter and son who we love. Through our children we were blessed with two precious and loving grandsons.

I thank God and every person that helped and encouraged me: the residential shelter, my adult children, the counseling center. Even with all of that help, it would not have worked had I not made the decision to help MYSELF, even though it took time and extreme courage. I thought I would never reach a serene point or fulfill my life goals, but I did and I have. I started college in the spring, I have a job, a car, an apartment, but most of all, I have peace of mind!! Thank you God, thank you everybody.

- What type of feelings do you have as a result of reading this story?
- What do you think was the impetus for Pat leaving the relationship?
- What do you think of Pat's explanation of being an optimistic person?

Society's view of domestic violence is often a barrier to a woman's willingness to admit that she has been abused. People may not understand why abused women do not leave the relationship, or think they may deserve the abuse, or even enjoy it. The fact is that many barriers exist that discourage this abuse from being reported. Even the legal system may create a barrier to gaining a proper perspective concerning the actual incidences of violence and abuse. Slow to respond to the needs of violated women, the legal system in some states doesn't even consider spousal violence and abuse a felony until after the second conviction of the abuser.

Once violence becomes part of a relationship, it usually escalates in severity and frequency. An innocent remark, a push, or a criticism often initiates a response that ranges from a slap, kick, or punch to permanent damage (physically and/or psychologically) or even death. The resulting consequences negatively affect the victim/survivor, her children, and perhaps the perpetrator. (See *Journal Activity:* "Do You Know Someone in an Abusive Relationship?")

TYPES OF ABUSE

Abuse against women takes many forms, each with varied and far-reaching consequences. Perhaps an awareness and understanding of the major types of violence and abuse inflicted upon women and the resultant consequences may be helpful in the prevention of abuse. Perhaps a clearer understanding of the destructive effects will motivate women to take action and resolve the abuse or dissolve the relationship, either through family counseling or by leaving. Following is a brief description of the major types of violence that women may experience during various stages in their lives.

Childhood Abuse

One of the most serious problems in our society is abuse inflicted upon children. It is often the root of abusive adult relationships. **Child abuse** is considered

---

acquaintance violence—violence and/or abuse committed by a parent, relative, coworker, neighbor, or friend.

domestic abuse—abuse committed in the home by an intimate associate, usually the spouse.

child abuse—physical or mental injury, sexual abuse or exploitation, negligent treatment, or maltreatment of a child before age 18, by a person who is responsible for the child's welfare.

JOURNAL ACTIVITY

Do You Know Someone in an Abusive Relationship?

Are you acquainted with someone who has experienced some form of abuse? Answer the following questions in the context of knowing a woman who has experienced abuse. Have you noticed any negative attitudes or behaviors this person exhibits? If so, what are they? Could these negative characteristics be due to their abusive environment? Have they shared this information with you? Do you have enough information to draw a connection between incidences of abuse, behaviors and attitudes?

---

to be maltreatment of a child before age 18 through physical or mental injury, sexual abuse or exploitation, and/or negligent treatment by the individual(s) who are responsible for the child's welfare. Childhood abuse can be categorized into four different types of abuse: physical abuse, neglect, emotional abuse, and sexual abuse.

- *Childhood physical abuse* can result in cuts, burns, contusions, frequent pain without obvious injury, bites or any other intentional pain that results in injury. Slapping, hair pulling, even tickling—especially to the point of hysteria—are also forms of childhood abuses. Physical abuse may begin as physical punishment and escalate into injurious, painful acts. Implements such as belts, switches, or paddles may be used to hit the child anywhere on the body. Frequent use of enemas or laxatives, unnecessary medical probing, and other intrusive procedures physically intrude on a child's right to privacy and respect.

- *Childhood abuse by neglect,* which is a less obvious form of physical abuse, is described as not providing a child with basic necessities (e.g., shelter, food, clothing, medical needs, or a hygienic environment). Obvious malnourishment, fatigue and listlessness, lack of personal cleanliness, or habitually dressing in torn and/or dirty clothes are noticeable signs of neglect. Less obvious types of neglect are being unattended for long periods of time, needing glasses, dental care, or other medical attention, and lack of emotional support or attention.

- *Childhood emotional abuse* is the most perplexing type of child abuse. Although there may be no physical evidence of emotional abuse, there are telltale indications that this type of abuse is occurring. Parents can inflict emotional abuse on a child by depriving her or him of an essential sense of self-worth. Emotional abuse includes continual criticizing or belittling the child, talking perpetually to the child in negative terms, threatening severe punishment or abandonment, and ignoring the child. Demanding perfection (for example, a perfect appearance or performance), excessive control by denying spontaneity and creativity, and disallowing social peer interactions are further types of emotional abuse. As a result, learning problems, behavioral extremes such as isolation or aggressiveness, expressions of depression, and apathy are often consequences of emotional abuse.

- *Childhood sexual abuse* refers to oral, anal, or vaginal intercourse, fondling, unwanted touching, and/or using instruments on a child's genitalia. Forcing a child to view adult genitalia, to watch a pornographic scene or movie, or to undress or expose himself or herself to an adult are also forms of child sexual abuse. Eighty-five percent of childhood sexual abuse is done by an individual the child knows (for example, a parent, relative, or neighbor). Harmful and serious physical and emotional consequences often are the result of childhood sexual abuse. A study conducted at Memphis State University[18] to determine the long-term effects of incestuous child abuse among college women revealed that females with a history of childhood sexual abuse by a family member experienced decreased cohesion and adaptability in the family of origin, increased perception of social isolation, and poorer social adjustment. If it is early, severe, and repeated, childhood sexual abuse may result in a permanently fragmented identity such as multiple personality disorders. This condition incorporates images of the perpetrator and possibly other individuals as well as one's self; the victim may not even be aware of the existence of the other personalities.[19]

Children who experience sexual abuse often have a poor sense of self-worth. They withdraw, isolate themselves, and may be suicidal. One common result of childhood sexual and physical abuse is **post-traumatic stress disorder (PTSD).**

PTSD develops over a period of time as a result of some traumatic event, such as war, a violent act, or abuse. Symptoms such as irritability, edginess, and insomnia among others do not arise at the time of the trauma, but occur at a late time in life. These are similar to the PTSD symptoms men experience as a result of being at war as well as other traumatic life events. As adults, women can begin to experience these symptoms, and may not understand why the symptoms are developing or the origin of the problems. Children who experience childhood sexual abuse may, as adults, develop PTSD and have involuntary memories, flashbacks, nightmares, and physical reactions when exposed to reminders of the events.

Over 2.9 million cases of child abuse were reported in 1992; 27 percent involved physical abuse, 17 percent involved sexual abuse, 45 percent involved neglect, 7 percent was emotional abuse, and 8 percent categorized as "other." More than 1,000 of these cases were fatal to the child.[20] It is a problem that has far-reaching consequences because children, both males and females, who are abused will very often grow up to be child and/or spouse abusers themselves.

Abuse and Adult Women

Females who are abused during childhood often expect to be abused or feel they deserve abuse during their adult relationships. Prevention and treatment programs often address the worthiness and respect of self as a way to overcome this misconception. Abuse inflicted on adult women often takes forms similar to child abuse as discussed below.

Physical Abuse Physical abuse, or battery, is the most overt type of domestic violence that adult women encounter. Kicking, hitting, biting, choking, pushing, hair pulling, being thrown across the room or down on the floor, and/or assaulted with some type of weapon are examples of battery. Perpetrators may target certain areas of the body for abusing, such as the breast, face, hairy areas of the body where bruises or abrasions are difficult to detect, or even the abdomen of a pregnant woman.

Abuse, especially physical abuse, tends to be cyclic in nature and typically involves three stages: increased tension building, the acute battering incident, and finally, the "honeymoon" phase, a loving, more calm, less tense period of time. The cyclic nature of this tragedy predicts that it tends to repeat itself over time. Further explanation of these phases is found in *FYI:* "The Cycle of Abuse."

Psychological Abuse Psychological abuse, unlike physical abuse, is clandestine and insidious. It is traumatic, often long-lasting, more difficult to assess, and less likely to lead to intervention and/or prosecution of the perpetrator.

Psychological abuse comes in many forms and can include some or all of the following conditions:

- *Financial disadvantages*—characterized by the perpetrator having control over household finances. The woman may not be allowed to work, and therefore she becomes entirely financially dependent on her partner. If she is working, she may have to account for all the money she earns, thus reducing her sense of any freedom or independence outside the relationship.
- *Young children at home*—includes threats to take children from their mother, abusing the children, or using the children to degrade or belittle their mother. Statements such as, "You're stupid, just like your mother," or "How can you ever amount to anything, just look at who your mother is," produce a psychological environment that hinders the development of worthiness and positive self-concept, degrading both the mother and the children.
- *Fear for herself and her children*—a woman may be frightened by her partner's looks, gestures, voice, destruction of property, or harming of children or pets. The worry that he may explode and express verbal degradation, curse, and call her or the children names can further contribute to her humiliation and fear. The home as a safe environment no longer exists.

---

post-traumatic stress disorder (PTSD)—a variety of symptoms (for example, irritability, insomnia, anxiety) that result from viewing or being involved in a traumatic event.

psychological abuse—use of children, intimidation, threats, and economic domination to control, manipulate, and cause anxiety in one's partner.

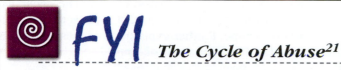

FYI The Cycle of Abuse[21]

Phase I—Tension or Buildup

This phase is characterized by increasing arguments, and minor forms of verbal or physical abuse. The perpetrator attempts to keep the woman under control, and she is aware of the consequences if she does not "obey or carry out" his demands. During this phase, the woman may be more willing to be helped by assistance from community resources or listening to a trusted friend, relative, or member of the clergy about the reality of the relationship.

Phase II—Battering Incident

In the perception of the perpetrator, situations that cause tension or anger exceed his ability to cope and result in angry and violent responses. A former batterer will know that these violent responses serve either to reduce this stress or to change "her" behavior. Intervening factors such as police involvement or injury requiring medical attention may occur during this phase.

The perpetrator and the woman may be more amenable to intervention following the battering event. She may be hurt, angry, or frightened; he may feel shame and/or guilt. Both may want the violence to cease. Arrest of the batterer and the immediate consequences are good intervention factors that may keep the violence and abuse from recurring.

Phase III—Calm or "Honeymoon" Phase

During this phase, the couple experiences feelings of reconciliation, calmness, and reminders of earlier, more loving periods in their relationship. This phase is usually shorter than the tension phase, but, it usually disappears over time as battering incidents increase in occurrence and severity. The man attempts to justify his behavior by blaming others: the victim or use of alcohol or drugs. Promises that it will never happen again are made. He usually means it, at least until the next time there is tension or disagreement.

The woman is often not amenable to assistance or counseling during this phase, especially if the battering cycle has not occurred too often. During this phase, the woman receives the most rewards (for example, loving attention, flowers, gifts) for remaining in the relationship. The perpetrator is well-behaved and caring. The woman is most receptive to this behavior and responds to his overtures for reconciliation. Both partners may minimize, forget, or distort the incident(s), which will eventually result in the cycle being repeated.

Intervention directed toward the perpetrator may be possible in this phase due to remorsefulness and the desire to please his partner. However, as this phase passes and the batterer believes his partner will remain in the relationship, he becomes less willing to be involved in any intervention process and the cycle begins again.

- *Threatening harm*—the perpetrator inflicts harm on the children or threatens to take them away. He may even elude to committing suicide. The perpetrator may also threaten to kill her, the immediate family, other relatives, or close friends. His threats are designed to create anxiety and fear in his partner and the children.
- *Ultimate control of behavior*—the perpetrator may limit his partner's activities by controlling her freedom to join organizations, limiting contact with companions, and not allowing her to go on errands or to travel. He fears the loss of control and influence over her life if she is absent too often or too long from the home environment. His extreme possessiveness or jealousy creates the need to know with whom and where his partner is at all times.
- *Isolation*—the perpetrator controls all social contacts and movements of a woman. Severe jealousy and frequent accusations serve to isolate the woman, keep her psychologically off balance, and contribute to the abusive environment.

The systematic destruction of a woman's self-esteem results from continual psychological abuse. This type of abuse is often present when physical and/or sexual violence are also present.

Sexual Assault **Sexual assault** is a term used to describe numerous forms of sexual improprieties and sexual violence toward another individual. It can result from manipulation or coercion as well as through physical force. Rape, a type of sexual assault, is sexual intercourse that is forced upon women and is considered an act of violence, aggression, power, and control rather than an act of sexual desire. Dr. Diana Scully, at Virginia Commonwealth University, interviewed 114 convicted rapists.[22] Through these interviews, she discovered that these men committed rape for numerous reasons. Some raped as a way to punish women, to "put them in their place," or to gain revenge for some deed they felt had been made against them. However, some of these rapists stated that the rape was an "afterthought" or a "bonus" following a burglary or robbery, adding the perception that "it was no big deal." Others stated that it was a form of recreation, a way to gain access to unwilling or unavailable women, or a way to express domination or control over women. However, there were no statements made that indicated any of these men committed rape because they "desired" women sexually.

The prevalence of rape is astounding. According to the 1992 report of The National Victim Center[23] entitled "Rape in America," the occurrence of forcible rape happens at the rate of:

1.3 per minute

78 per hour

1,871 per day

56,916 per month

683,000 per year

Police estimate that only 34 percent of stranger rape and 13 percent of acquaintance rape are reported. The United States is the most rape-prone contemporary society in the world. These tragic numbers reflect a dark and shameful side of human nature. Each statistic is reflective of a woman whose life is forever changed as a result of a violation inflicted on her by another human being. The amount of reported and unreported sexual assaults is staggering. But even *one* sexual assault is one too many.

A woman may be raped by a male that she knows or by a male who is a stranger to her. Each type of rape presents its own set of circumstances and consequences. **Acquaintance rape** is the sexual assault of a woman by a man whom she knows, such as a man who is in her class or lives in her residence hall. **Date rape,** a form of acquaintance rape, refers to the rape of a woman by a man who she has agreed to see socially. Some rapists prefer to know their victims because they are able to get closer to them or trap them in a vulnerable position without creating alarm. Acquaintances are also able to gain more information about the routine, friends, and living conditions of the intended victim, and perhaps believe

that a woman will be less willing to report the rape if she knows the rapist.

Date and acquaintance rape are characterized by physical attacks on the woman's breasts or genitals, sexual sadism, and forced sexual activity. Acquaintance rape occurs more frequently among college students, especially freshmen women, than any other age group. According to research conducted on a number of campuses, approximately 20 percent of college women reported being raped while on a date.[24] One study revealed that one in two college women said they had experienced some type of sexual aggression, and one in four to five reported being the victim of rape or attempted rape. Eighty-four percent of their attackers were dating partners or acquaintances at the time of the assault.

Acquaintance rape can often be prevented by being aware of certain male behaviors. A man who demonstrates a disrespectful attitude toward other individuals, especially women, may indicate that he sees women as second-class citizens. Furthermore, the potential acquaintance rapist often lacks concern for a woman's feelings, may express extreme jealousy, or attempt to be domineering. He often is highly competitive and may have a tendency to use physical violence as a means of coping with stress-filled situations. He may also speak negatively about women's rights or tell jokes that are demeaning to women. *FYI:* "Characteristics of a Rapist" summarizes characteristics to be aware of in a potential rapist.

Women should avoid individuals who exhibit the above behaviors and seek out companions who display behaviors that are conducive to developing a healthy and enjoyable relationship. *Health Tips:* "Avoiding Date Rape" offers guidelines to use to avoid being placed in a position of possible danger.

Marital rape appears to be mainly an act of violence and aggression in which sex is the method used

---

sexual assault—sexual improprieties or sexual violence directed toward another person, including rape.

acquaintance rape—sexual assault of a woman by a man she knows.

date rape—sexual assault of a woman by a man who she has agreed to see socially.

marital rape—sexual assault of a woman by her husband.

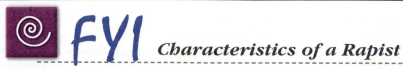

Characteristics of a Rapist

Companionship is usually welcomed, desired, and healthy. Unfortunately, not everyone is a safe companion. When deciding to associate with another person, it is important to know the traits of a person who may commit rape. Watch for the following characteristics as indicators of a potential rapist.

RAPES FOR POWER OVER WOMEN

- Needs to completely dominate and control (for example, *he* makes all decisions, gives all instructions, and makes the commands and demands)
- Covers feelings of inadequacy by acts of power
- Possessive of female friends
- Often ridicules, criticizes, and insults partners

- Wants every moment accounted for
- Checks on partner by constantly following her, calling her friends, questioning her all the time
- Believes that women should be passive and submissive

RAPES DUE TO ANGER AT WOMEN

- Expresses contempt, hostility, and hatred toward women
- Has an explosive temper
- Verbally abuses companions
- Becomes angrier or more physically aggressive when using alcohol or other drugs
- Thinks of women as sex objects
- Blames others for his anger or misfortunes

health tips

Avoiding Date Rape: Guidelines for Men and Women[25]

MEN:

- *Know your sexual desires and limits.* Communicate them clearly. Be aware of social pressures and realize it's okay not to score.
- *Being turned down when you ask for sex is not a rejection of you personally.* Women can express their desire not to participate in a single act of sex. You may think your desires are beyond control. However, your actions are certainly within your control.
- *Accept a woman's decision.* "No" means "no." Don't read other meanings into the answer. Don't continue after you are told, "No!"
- *Don't assume that just because a woman dresses in a sexy manner and flirts that she wants to have sexual intercourse.*
- *Don't assume that previous permission for sexual contact applies to the current situation.*
- *Avoid excessive use of alcohol and drugs.* Alcohol and drugs interfere with clear thinking and effective communication.

WOMEN:

- *Know your sexual desires and limits.* Believe in your right to set those limits. If you are not aware, stop and talk about it.
- *Communicate your limits clearly.* If someone starts to offend you, tell him so firmly and immediately. Polite approaches may be misunderstood or ignored. Say "no" when you mean "no."
- *Be assertive.* Often men interpret passivity as permission. Be direct and firm with someone who is sexually pressuring you.
- *Be aware that your nonverbal actions send a message.* If you dress in a sexy manner and flirt, some men assume you want to have sex. This does not make your dress or behavior wrong, but it is important to be aware of a possible misunderstanding.
- *Pay attention to what is happening around you.* Watch the nonverbal clues. Do not put yourself into a vulnerable situation.
- *Trust your intuitions.* If you feel you are being pressured into unwanted sex, you probably are.
- *Avoid excessive use of alcohol and drugs.* Alcohol and drugs interfere with clear thinking and effective communication.

to humiliate, hurt, degrade, and dominate the spouse, usually the female partner. The violence and brutality in the sexual relationship of the couple seems to escalate with time. The sexual violence is frequently accompanied by life-threatening acts or warnings.[26]

Compassion, caring, and believing a woman are important responses offered by supporters who are involved with assisting someone following an act of rape. *Health Tips:* "What to Do If You Are Raped!" provides suggestions for what to do if you find yourself or a friend to be the victim of a rape.

Alcohol and Rape. Use of alcohol can set a woman up to be the victim in a rape. Over one-half of women who have been raped and almost three-fourths of men who raped had been drinking or using drugs prior to the assault. Alcohol can cause distortion of thinking and reasoning abilities, and lessens the ability to recognize danger signals such as changes in a man's voice, his behaviors, and suggestions for being alone together. A woman may be less able to communicate her feelings about what she does and does not want to do sexually. The chances that words such as "no" or "maybe" will be

interpreted to mean "yes" is more likely if either the man and/or woman has been drinking. Sometimes women are urged to drink to increase the chances that they will be unable to resist pressure to have sex. A man may even feel that a woman who has several drinks is asking to have sex, regardless of what she says. Under the influence of alcohol, men are more likely to be more aggressive in regard to sex, and women are more likely not to recognize some of the danger signs.

Murder In this country, 4 females are killed every day because of domestic violence. This equates to approximately 1,400 annual deaths caused by an intimate partner.[27] More than half the defendants accused of murdering their spouses had been drinking alcohol at the time of the murder.[28] Each of these women are usually the victims of the one person in their lives who professed to love and honor them—their partners. Unfortunately "until death do us part" came all too soon for the female partner. Murder is frequently the ultimate end to long-term and escalating abuse; abuse that, for unknown reasons, had been tolerated over time, and was neither punished nor treated. Consider the fate of Monique in the *Her Story.*

Crisis centers across the United States report case after case of deadly outcomes of abusive relationships. For example, Christine in New Mexico was stabbed 20 times by her former husband; Louise was shot to death by her estranged husband as she picked up their children after a weekend with their father; Joycelyn's throat was slashed by a former boyfriend as she left a restaurant with a date. Although the manner in which each woman was killed differed, the underlying circumstances were quite similar: each of the woman was killed by a past or present husband or lover. Murder may be the final statement men make to their partners. A violent end to a relationship is often marked by desperate and barbarous acts on the part of the male partner.

> Men often hunt down and kill wives who have left them; women hardly ever behave similarly. Men kill wives as part of planned murder-suicides; analogous acts by women are almost unheard of. Men kill in response to revelations of wifely infidelity; women almost never respond similarly, although their mates are more often adulterous. Men often kill wives after subjecting them to lengthy periods of coercive abuse and assaults; the roles in such cases are seldom, if ever, reversed. Men perpetrate familicidal massacres, killing spouse and children together; women do not.[29]

The highest profile criminal, civil, and murder case of all time may well be that of O.J. Simpson. Simpson, a well-recognized professional athlete, TV personality, and actor was accused of murdering his former wife and her male friend. In the development of the murder case against Simpson, prosecutors uncovered a history of harassment and verbal and physical abuse of his wife. Other "well-known" men have faced similar charges. Jeffery MacDonald, a physician and Special Forces Green Beret was convicted of killing his wife and two daughters; Claus von Bulow was tried, convicted, and then won a reversed decision on appeal of murdering his wealthy wife; and John Hill, a Houston plastic surgeon was accused of murdering his wealthy, socialite wife to gain wealth and property.

Homophobia **Homophobia,** an irrational fear of homosexuality, although not a type of abuse, can result in violent acts against gay or lesbian individuals. Violence against gay individuals and gay partners has increased significantly in recent years according to a study by the National Gay and Lesbian Task Force. Incidents of victimization include verbal harassment and threats, physical assaults, and abuse by police.

In *Hate Crimes: Confronting Violence against Lesbians and Gay Men*,[30] the authors state that the link between the victimization of gay men and lesbians is due to the underlying, societal-based message that the gay lifestyle is unacceptable, and that violence is a just and rewarding punishment for homosexual behavior.

Violent actions against gay and lesbian individuals are more often delivered by males (usually "straight" males) toward either gay men or lesbians. As an example, Russell[31] surveyed 930 randomly selected homosexual women from San Francisco: 44 percent reported at least one rape or attempted rape during their lifetime, only 16 percent of the total number of rapes reported were attempted and/or completed by strangers, and only 7 percent of the women in the study reported being raped by another woman, which suggests that 93 percent of rapes against these women were carried out by males.

Sexual Harassment Although **sexual harassment** is not violent in nature, it is abusive. It represents abuse of power and position, and, furthermore, it is a criminal offense. Taking place most often in the workplace or educational setting, it can also be a different type of domestic abuse, where the abuser dominates his partner so that she feels unable to refuse sexual requests.

Types of sexual harassment include unwanted and unwarranted comments with sexual overtones or sexual innuendoes, unwanted and uninvited touching or staring, and requests for sexual favors. (See Fig. 13.1.) Jokes, comments, or personal questions with sexual overtones that are offensive to the listener are also considered sexual harassment. Sexual harassment includes working, being, or living in a hostile, offensive, or intimidating environment in which actions or talk of a sexual nature exists because of gender. Female college students may be asked to provide a sexual act in return for a favor or preferential treatment provided by a professor. Men as well as women may be victims of sexual harassment; however, more commonly women are harassed by men.

Consider the following suggestions in *Health Tips:* "Strategies for Addressing Sexual Harassment" for resolving concerns of sexual harassment. Have you ever experienced sexual harassment? Do you think these suggestions are beneficial?

INCIDENCES OF VIOLENCE AND ABUSE

Having just read about the many types of violence and abuse against women, it is easy to see that incidences of abuse appear in many forms, and range

FIGURE 13.1 Unwanted touching is a type of sexual harassment.

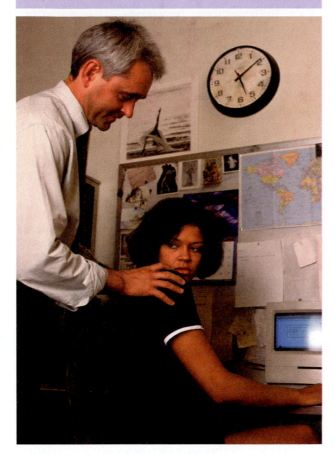

from minimal to very severe. A woman may quite easily experience several incidences, such as obscene telephone calls to being stalked, during her lifetime. No such experience should be considered inconsequential. Complete *Journal Activity:* "Incidences of Abuse" to evaluate how you would handle this situation.

health tips

Strategies for Addressing Sexual Harassment

- Do not ignore innuendoes or degrading statements, otherwise it will not stop. Clearly and firmly state your objections immediately. (Perhaps the harasser did not understand that the words or gestures were offensive.) You may need to share the incident(s) with a trusted individual in case you file charges later.
- Write down any incident(s) or written communication made by the harasser; date and file the information. Be sure to include the time, place, date, and witnesses, if any were present. Include what occurred and your response.
- Give the written information to another trusted individual as well as verbally share the incident. This person may be needed for verification if you elect to file charges either now or in the future.
- Confront the harassment by reporting it to authorities; you may be able to keep this from happening to others. If desired, talk to a professional counselor who can help you deal with any emotional distress related to the incident.
- Be truthful and accurate about the incident. Do not place the reputation of yourself and someone else in jeopardy if you are unsure about the incident. The fallout for you and the accused can have serious and embarrassing consequences.

Viewpoint

Is This Sexual Harassment?

Michelle worked in a department dominated by males. She brought to this job prior sales experience and qualities that made her effective in working with employees and customers. Her immediate supervisor developed a habit of telling his stories of sexual conquests to male employees when Michelle was near enough to hear. She politely asked him to wait until she was unable to hear the conversations before sharing the details of his sexual ventures. He refused, stating that he was not talking to her in the first place, and secondly, if she found the conversations so disturbing, to move far enough away so that she was unable to hear. If you were in Michelle's position, would you consider this a sexual harassment situation? If yes, what would you do about it? If you don't consider it sexual harassment, do you find it offensive?

homophobia (hoe moe **foe** be ya)—an irrational fear of homosexuality.

sexual harassment—unwanted attention of a sexual nature that creates embarrassment or stress; includes the use of power or position to intimidate a woman into providing sexual favors in some form to a man.

JOURNAL ACTIVITY

Incidences of Abuse

Having just read about abusive and violent acts against women, write down any incidences that you have experienced. Did you respond in any way to the perpetrator? What did you say or do? Did you share the incident with anyone? Was the incident serious enough that you needed to involve the legal system? Was there a way to handle the situation better than you did?

COMMON ELEMENTS IN ALL TYPES OF ABUSE

All forms of abuse share four common elements and are linked with concerns regarding resolution of abusive situations. These elements reflect common thought that influences public opinion and often hinders effective legal and societal resolutions, delays the victims' efforts to seek help and counseling, and/or slows the process of healing. These common elements include:

Minimization

The public often thinks that violence and abuse are rare and that official statistics accurately represent prevalence. Violence against women can be likened to an iceberg: the tip of the iceberg represents the reported amount of violence; the larger portion of the iceberg, which remains unseen, is the actual occurrence and is estimated to be two to three times greater than abuse that is reported.

Directionality

Violence occurs largely in one direction; men victimize women. Incest is generally from father or stepfather to daughter or stepdaughter; generally men make obscene phone calls to women; date rape almost always involves men assaulting women.

Trivialization

Violence against women is often viewed in a joking way: "Incest is the game the whole family can play," "If you're going to be raped, just lie back and enjoy it." Remarks and jokes tend to negate the impact and seriousness of violence against women and promote a sporting aspect to men's violence.

Blaming the Victim

This occurs not only in violence but in such crimes as car theft or house burglaries. "If you had just locked the car, this would not have happened!" Women are accused of dressing provocatively. Little girls are accused of behaving "seductively," and women are held responsible for not stopping men sooner when kissing leads to an assault. An underlying assumption is that women are careless, men are not responsible for their actions, and self-control is much more difficult for men than for women.[32]

CHARACTERISTICS OF BATTERED WOMEN

What are the traits of women who have been abused or violated? Why do they often remain in abusive relationships, either unable or unwilling to leave or seek assistance? Do these women develop these traits prior to experiencing abuse, or as a result of the abuse?

Personal Beliefs

Battered women tend to be depressed, angry, helpless, hopeless, frightened, and bewildered.[33] Mistaken personal beliefs, such as "battering is part of a loving relationship," or "if only I didn't make him mad, I wouldn't get hit," may originate in childhood and develop further in subsequent abusive relationships. These beliefs interfere with development of self-worth and prevent the victim from developing life-enhancing behaviors. Abused women often watched when their mothers or sisters were abused. They equate abuse with love and believe that this is how women are supposed to be treated by husbands, fathers, and other men. They come to believe that those who love you, abuse you.

Abused females usually hold to the traditional belief that the man is the head of the household and the female is to be subservient. Whatever her perception of marriage is before the union, his violence eventually convinces her that yielding to him, maintaining the household, and/or taking care of the relationship and the children is safer than behaviors exemplified in "liberated" marital partnerships.

Personal Feelings

Adult female victims who experience varied forms of abuse often have or will develop low self-esteem and beliefs of worthlessness. Abused women often underestimate their abilities. A woman may assess her worthiness as it relates to her success as a wife or mother. If she is involved in a stormy, abusive, and dysfunctional relationship, even if she is successful in other areas of her life, feelings of inadequacy and poor self-concept soon develop. Therefore, her perception is that her lack of abilities causes the abuse to occur. The woman often believes she is deserving of the abuse because the batterer may camouflage abusive acts under a cloak of discipline. He teaches her a lesson, just as her parents did and just as her father taught her mother during violent episodes that she may have witnessed at home.

Abused women, often blaming themselves for causing the partner's violence, are socialized to believe they are responsible for maintaining the relationship. Therefore, if the relationship is unhappy, disturbed, or abusive, she feels it is her responsibility to "repair" it or soothe whatever is bothering the abuser. She believes if only she were a better lover, wife, mother, or worker, she would not be abused. This self-blame often leads to depression if the abuse continues. However, studies indicate that as abuse increases in severity and frequency, women become less likely to blame themselves and more likely to blame their partner.

The feeling of hopelessness may be a trait of the female both before and during the abusive relationship. She may believe she cannot "do any better" than the partner she is currently with or she may be so emotionally and financially dependent on the partner that she feels afraid and/or unable to resolve the abusive situation. A woman may feel helpless in terms of her ability to move out of the relationship. She may be unaware of any type of available assistance to help her deal with the abuse. Feeling emotionally and psychologically helpless, she becomes indecisive, and unable to trust her ability to think or act outside of the relationship with her partner.

Codependency

Women often have a co-dependent relationship with the abuser. **Codependency** means developing a dependency with the abuser and the abuser's problem(s) to the point of self-neglect. Codependent women think and feel responsible for the needs of other people. These responsibilities may include their feelings, thoughts, actions, choices, wants, needs, well-being, lack of well-being, and ultimate destiny. Therefore a codependent woman who is in an abusive relationship often feels responsible for

abuse and is willing to endure it so she can be available to care for the abuser.

Perception of Partner

Her perception of the battering partner is often one of the need; that is, the batterer needs her. She may believe that she is the only person who can help him overcome his problem; therefore, she feels compassion and pity. If her partner is a chemically dependent batterer, she may believe he will stop the abuse if he stops using alcohol and/or other drugs. She may believe that if she leaves him, he may abuse alcohol and drugs to the point of illness or death. In cases of elderly or disabled female abuse, a woman may feel the partner will die or commit suicide without her. Even in relationships having a history of long-term battering, women often love the batterer and are emotionally dependent upon the relationship.

CONSEQUENCES OF ABUSE

Consequences of abuse are varied depending on the duration, type, and severity of the abuse. Over time, continual abuse will result in one or more of the following consequences.

Physical Consequences

Depending upon the type of abuse inflicted, a woman can experience a plethora of physical consequences. Cuts, burns, punctures, bites, bruises, bleeding, dislocations, and bone fractures are physical manifestations of abusive encounters. Over time, physical abuse usually escalates in both severity and frequency.

Abused women usually have a history of many visits to emergency rooms. Medical care providers are trained to screen injuries that may indicate various types of abuse. (See *FYI:* "Physical Abuse Scale.")

Physical wounds inflicted on women may eventually result in chronic, long-term disorders and disabilities. Conditions such as chronic arthritis, hypertension, gastrointestinal disorders, and/or asthma, which can develop because of stress, may be consequences of long-term physical abuse.

---

codependency—developing a dependency with the abuser and the abuser's problems to the point of self-neglect.

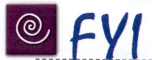

Physical Abuse Scale[34]

The acts of violence below are listed in priority of less severe to most severe. The progression of physical abuse can be used in domestic abuse evaluations to determine the level of violence at which the perpetrator is operating, and acts as a guide to determine the level of protection needed by the victim.

1. Throwing things; punching the wall
2. Pushing, shoving, grabbing, throwing things at the female
3. Slapping with an open hand
4. Kicking, biting
5. Hitting with a closed fist
6. Attempted strangulation
7. Beating up (pinned to the wall or floor, repeated kicks, punches)
8. Threatening with weapon
9. Assault with weapon

Her Story

Sue Anne

Sue Anne recounted the incestuous relationship with her father that always occurred in the mornings. After her mother left early for work, her father would come into the room as she was dressing for school. As the incest continued, it became broader in its scope, until Sue Anne had all but become her father's full-time lover. She escaped as much as possible by participating in as many school functions as possible. Sue Anne did not date until well into her college years, then married someone who was emotionally distant and withdrawn. She reported that as a married adult, it was impossible to have sexual relations with her husband in the morning and they continually argue about sexual issues. Sue Anne has difficulty with other intimate relationships even to the point of feeling uncomfortable holding her own children, believing that she will "infect" her children if she is physically too close to them.

- What are some positive steps Sue Anne could take in order to begin healing from the abuse she experienced from her father?
- How can Sue Anne establish a support system that can assist her in this issue?
- Can her husband play a role in the process of Sue Anne's healing from her early experiences?

Emotional and Psychological Consequences

Women are likely to experience negative psychological effects as a result of abusive relationships. Continual abuse will cause women to feel depressed, worthless, experience anxiety attacks, and feel they are going crazy. As a result of these feelings, women experience major emotional distress. The most devastating psychological effects appear as a result of being abused by a trusted person who was known to the victim (for example, a father, stepfather, or brothers).

As children, girls who have been sexually abused may develop feelings of anxiety, depression, anger, hostility, guilt, shame, and/or inferiority. These feelings can develop as an immediate response to the abuse or they may develop in adulthood. As adults, these women often experience nightmares, relationship distress, and sexual dysfunction. Women who were sexually abused as children may have problems relating to their own parents as well as to both men and women; these women also experience difficulty in responding to their own children in a healthy manner. The severity of emotional and psychological consequences depend on the length of time since the abuse, the length of time the abuse lasted, the

woman's age at the time of abuse, and her relationship to the perpetrator. (See *Her Story:* "Sue Anne.")

Another young woman, describing the emotional pain she experienced as a result of abuse, proclaimed her self-hatred by saying "I had an oil slick oozing goo inside me. I knew I was filled with something evil, and that evil rubbed off on everyone I came in contact with. So I didn't let anybody really get near me."[35]

A study reported in the *American Psychologist*[36] revealed that women who have been victimized will experience an immediate post victimization distress response that includes a pattern of fear and avoidance, disturbances of self-concept and self-esteem, and sexual dysfunction.

Spiritual Consequences

The very basic values of meaningful life and meaningful relationships are undermined as a result of early abuse, especially when the abuse is inflicted by individuals who are supposed to nurture and protect (for example, father, stepfather, grandfather, uncle). Females may find that core values such as trust, honesty, respect, and concern are impaired or lost as a result of abusive relationships, especially abuse inflicted by supposedly caring men. Abused women report an inability to trust and respect others, especially men. Perhaps of greater concern is the fact that these women may mistrust their *own* perceptions of other people's behaviors and motives. Abuse in the family destroys the very foundation on which healthy functioning relationships are built.

Social Consequences

Violence and abuse manifest themselves with a variety of societal consequences. For example, increased use of dwindling health-care resources causes the costs of medical care to rise, overloads medical personnel, and may lead to hasty diagnoses and sometimes too-aggressive treatments for many disorders. Emergency care is the most costly and most frequently used form of medical care following incidences of abuse. Communities experience overburdening of police, judicial, and human resources systems that lead to increases in taxes, and increases in social problems such as drug abuse, violence, and homelessness. Society as a whole suffers from abusive relationships—not just monetarily—but with the negative consequences of violence cycling into the next generation, violence of all types are continued. In general, abuse contributes to decreases in the overall quality of life.

MOVING TOWARD CHANGE

Considering the multiplicity of negative consequences resulting from violence and abuse, the question arises as to why females tolerate their abusive situations. What causes women to remain in violent and abusive relationships?

Why Women Stay in Abusive Relationships

Virginia, married 23 years to an abusive executive, remained in the relationship because she was, for many years, economically dependent upon her husband. Foregoing her education to assist him through college, she maintained the house and raised the children. Over the years, Virginia devel-

oped few job skills, had no training outside the home and no other place to live. When Virginia talked about leaving, her husband threatened her with more abuse and the possible loss of the children. Feeling trapped and fearing physical and legal retaliation, Virginia felt she had no choice but to remain in the relationship.

Situational factors such as financial dependency, lack of education, lack of job skills, and/or job inexperience are all too real for women involved in abusive relationships. Statistically, a woman with children who leaves the home has a 50 percent probability that her standard of living will drop below the poverty level. Moreover, a woman is often in greater physical danger when she attempts to leave the relationship. She fears for her safety, her children's safety, and sometimes the safety of anyone who attempts to help her.

Emotional factors such as fear of social isolation and lack of emotional and financial support from family and friends may contribute to women staying in unhealthy and abusive relationships. Abused women frequently lose touch with supportive friends and family due to the isolative nature of abuse. Cultural constraints (for example, men are the dominant sex) and religious beliefs (for example, divorce is a sin) may also keep women from leaving these relationships.

Curiously, women often are concerned about their husbands' inability to survive on their own. Women could ask themselves, "If I should die, would he be able to survive?" The answer is, of course, "Yes!" Concerns about survival if she remains in the abusive relationship and the fears associated with having independence and major life changes if she leaves creates much ambivalence about the situation. And she can live with the false hope that he will change.

LEAVING THE ABUSIVE RELATIONSHIP

Deciding to Leave

Some women stay in abusive relationships and others will leave. Abused women will typically leave an abusive environment between five to seven times before they feel safe enough and have accumulated the resources needed to leave for good. Women frequently return to perpetrators following a visit to a safe shelter or relative's home. Following her return, methods for eliminating the abuse without terminating the relationship, if both partners desire, need to be developed. However, if the abuse continues following each return, then she should seek assistance to leave the relationship permanently.

During the course of abuse, women may have involved the legal system in a number of ways. Calling the police during bouts of abuse, gaining protection for children, and obtaining restraining orders to keep the abuser at a distance are all proper and probable ways to use the legal system. As a woman prepares to leave a relationship, she may need to again use the resources of the legal system. Occasionally a safe escort out of the home is required, as well as accompaniment to secret and safe housing for her and her children. Community resources can be invaluable to a woman who has decided to remove herself and her family from an abusive environment.

Developing a Safety Plan

Once women make the decision to leave the relationship, perhaps her most critical concern is developing a safety plan and determining a means of survival. The safety plan needs to include a means of leaving, a list of people to call in case of emergency, and a suitcase containing clothing, personal items, money, social security cards, bank books, children's birth certificates and school records, and other important documents. Immediate survival needs consist of locating a safe place to live once she has left the relationship, being able to feed and clothe herself and the children, and determining a way to become financially self-sufficient. Long-term survival may include finding a job, completing some type of education, or developing necessary job skills. It may also include locating dependable and quality child care.

Answering the following questions may assist women in determining the essential elements necessary for their survival, and their children's survival. Are there family or friends where she can stay? Does she need alternative means of shelter? If so, does she know how to access the shelter? Does she need to contact the police or obtain legal aid? Does she need counseling services? What other community agencies might assist her? Let's take a close look at some possible answers to these questions.

Locating Safe Shelter

This can be as simple as calling the police and asking for help. Currently there are more than 1,200 safe shelters located throughout this country in which women can find safety, as well as advocacy, support, and other needed services. Checking the phone book under "domestic violence," "women's shelter," "shelter for battered or abused women," and "crisis hotline," can often locate the nearest safe shelter. In rural areas where safe housing may not be available, women can contact a local church, clergyman, or community center for assistance in locating temporary safe shelter.

Knowing what to expect is beneficial and may lessen the anxiety of leaving the abusive environment. Safe shelter personnel will usually transport women and their children from an emergency room, the police station, or any other designated place to the shelter and away from the abusive partner. Women and their children often arrive at the shelter with only the clothes they are wearing, and return to their home only when their partners are absent to retrieve their belongings. Women may need to utilize the shelter's resources for a time.

Women and their children are usually allowed to remain in the safe shelter for 30 days with the option of increasing the time if the situation warrants it, and providing other women are not waiting to move in. During their stay, women are usually expected to help with the routine care and maintenance of the shelter, cook meals for themselves and their children, and wash and care for personal clothing.

Planning for the future without the abusive partners is also an important task during their stay at the shelter. Depending on their individual needs, women may receive personal, group, and/or job-related counseling. Shelter personnel provide access to government assistant programs such as Women, Infant and Children (WIC), food stamps, and drug abuse counseling, if needed. Women may also receive help with obtaining Medicaid and Social Security benefits. Other important tasks may include seeking employment, locating child care, filing protective orders, and starting divorce proceedings.

Locating Other Resources

Because safe shelters are temporary and serve only as a short-term bridge, other resources beyond the abusive environment, the abuser, and the former belief system are essential to locate. Financial assistance may be temporarily obtained from Aid for Dependent Children (AFDC), American Red Cross, the Social Security Administration, or local church charities. Phone numbers and addresses for these agencies can

health tips

Locating Local Resources

Locate addresses and phone numbers for the following list of helpful resources in your town that can be used by women who are in need of assistance. Add any additional agencies or individuals who can be beneficial. Attach a city map and highlight helping agencies.

Agency	Phone #	Address
Emergency		
Crisis hotline		
Police		
Ambulance		
Safe house		
Legal Aid		
Child protective service		
Doctor		
Friend		
Other:		
Other:		

be found in local telephone directories. (See *Health Tips:* "Locating Local Resources.")

Housing can often be found through the local housing authority, Housing and Urban Development Office (HUD), and local property management offices, which often have apartments for rent at lower rates.

Addresses and information for agencies that provide child care are usually provided to women during their stay at the safe shelter. Child care arrangements, sometimes at a reduced rate, are often made between the shelter and child care providers. Additionally, churches often have day care centers that are made available to local safe shelter children on a temporary basis. Women who are making the effort to move forward following abusive relationships may elect to share child care responsibilities, caring for one another's children while each work at different times.

Job training is available through many and varied sources. Communities offer adult learning centers with computer classes, Graduate Equivalence Diploma (GED) classes, and literacy volunteers. Social Services departments offer job counseling, skill testing, and contact persons for job location through state or county employment commissions. Many temporary personnel agencies provide on-the-job training programs, which can lead to employment opportunities for women who already possess job skills. Many towns and cities have community colleges at which job training or job skill refresher courses are available for women who seek assistance. State, county, and local agencies provide emotional and financial counseling, often without monetary charge.

HEALING FROM ABUSE

Healing from violence and abuse is possible. In fact it is probable if a woman makes the choice to heal and then takes the steps, sometimes long and painful steps, to move forward and to thrive. Thriving means to flourish, bloom, to become whole, whole in one's own life, and also in friendships, family, and love relationships. Healing means moving beyond repair of the damage to body, mind, and soul. It also means being able to feel at peace, to feel genuine love, and to gain satisfaction with one's life and contribute to one's immediate and expanding environment.

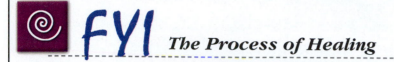

FYI   *The Process of Healing*

- Commit to heal, and begin to move toward self-change.
- Processing memories of the incidences and the accompanying feelings is often painful and depressing; remember it is transitional and will go away.
- Admit to yourself that the abuse did occur. Share this essential step with a trusted person who can help you with any feelings of shame associated with the incidences.
- Place the heavy blanket of guilt and shame on its rightful owner—the perpetrator. In no way was the abuse the fault of the victim.
- Develop realistic and appropriate feelings toward other people by getting in touch with the vulnerable child within—that child you may have lost in the process of coping with the agony that can accompany abuse.
- Listen to your instincts; listen to your own feelings, mind, and physical body. This promotes learning to trust one's self and builds a foundation from which to approach life situations.
- Recognize and feel all the losses related to an abusive relationship: loss of childhood, loss of trust, loss of idealized relationship, loss of respect, loss of joy, and so much more. This enables you to confront the pain, feel it, express it, and move forward.
- Use the freeing emotion of anger, considered the backbone of healing, and direct it to where it belongs: toward the perpetrator, and the individuals who were not protective.
- Confront the perpetrator and disclose the abuse, if possible, because this can be an empowering and freeing activity for women who choose to do it.
- Forgiving the perpetrator is highly recommended, though it is not necessary for healing. But forgiving yourself is a must.
- Spiritual renewal through religion, nature, beauty, meditation, and/or contributing to society is important to the process of resolution and moving forward.

Even though the history of the abuse cannot be erased, moving through and acting on these stages allows a woman to discover stability, develop a positive perspective, experience peace, and move forward to a satisfying and contributing life.   ⌒

One survivor said that healing and recovery are beautiful parts of life. Her healing "family" not only consisted of her present nonabusive husband, her children, and grandchildren, but also includes her fellow travelers—other survivors she has learned to love and trust. The gift she had given herself is to allow all of her healing family to express love, warmth, and kindness.

Survivors of abuse recount the stages and feelings they experienced as they progressed toward healing and moving forward with their lives. These women have come to realize that they survived the traumatic time of abuse and became adults. From this awareness, women can move forward through the necessary stages into a life of satisfying relationships and contributions.

In their book *The Courage to Heal,*[37] Bass and Davis identify fourteen stages that women experience as they progress toward healing and recovering from abuse. It should be noted that survivors may not experience every stage, and they may not go through them in any particular order. *FYI:* "The Process of Healing" is a paraphased summary of these stages.

HOW TO HELP

Helping a woman who is leaving an abusive relationship and is attempting to move forward with her life may not always be the responsibility of the legal, judicial, or social systems. Women often turn to friends and family first for support and assistance. Family, friends, and professionals who are available and knowledgeable about how to help these women can go a long way in aiding their chance to develop a healthy and contributing lifestyle.

How can friends and family help? How can you help? Consider the following suggestions developed by the National Woman Abuse Prevention Project.[38]

- Become an informed proponent for the prevention of violence and abuse against women.
- Locate all resources available in your area pertaining to abuse. These include such resources as crisis hotlines, safe shelters, support groups, social services, and legal assistance.
- Support an abused woman by listening with a sympathetic ear and by believing her. Do not blame her, underestimate the potential for continual danger, or sympathize with the abuser.

- Share all potential community resource information with her and encourage her to seek the assistance of other abuse prevention advocates.
- Provide whatever help you can: child care, financial assistance, transportation, and help with medical needs. Be especially sure to give the emotional support she needs to help her recognize her strengths and skills. (Caution: be very careful when offering and providing safety in *your* home for her. Frequently, the most danger that a battered woman frequently faces from her abuser is when she decides to leave the relationship. Keeping her with you may place you and your family in danger as well.)
- Encourage her to develop a safety plan and include a list of people she can call in an emergency (see Developing a Safety Plan, p. 284).
- Encourage her to seek professional support in addition to your support.

Time and space will be required for women to proceed through the stages of healing. As a friend or family member, express compassion for and validation of her feelings, such as feelings of fear, anger, guilt, and pain. Also, helping her through the stages of healing will produce changes in your relationship with her. Be prepared to make some changes in your attitude and behaviors toward her.

Equally important, children must be taught that the use of violence to resolve problems and exert control over others is unacceptable behavior. Children may need as much emotional support as their mother after leaving an abusive environment. Many of the same support systems that have been located for women also offer opportunities for healing and growth for children. They need both healthy role models, and structure and discipline without abuse.

MOVING FORWARD

I kept working on change ... slowly, slowly I moved ahead. My body cells replace themselves.... I can replace and remove the damage, the pain. Yes, I have more work, but I have come a long way, baby! I now have the skills and the desire to move ahead; I will use them and I will find peace.

A Survivor

Women can develop skills that enable them to heal from abusive relationships. Moreover, they can engage in activities that foster resolution of the abuse and promote progression toward a joyful and fulfilling life.

Building Resiliency

Resiliency is the ability to recover, to overcome adversity, to bend and bounce back like a willow tree in a wind storm. Resiliency can be developed as a skill and utilized to recover from the adverse effects of an abusive relationship. Finding and developing support systems outside the abusive environment can assist women in recognizing characteristics of healthy relationships. Having contact with "healthy" individuals who believe in the woman will promote belief in herself. These supportive relationships also provide conditions that enable women to feel worthwhile and valued. Susan, leaving home as a young teen following years of incest, found support and acceptance in a church group. She told of how the church group assisted her in developing a sense of purpose and value. Spirituality, too, can promote the development of resiliency because it fosters a sense of worthiness and purpose for life. As a result, women should live to discover and fulfill that purpose. Abused women report recognizing potential personal power as a way to take control of their lives and develop resiliency. Becoming self-directed, making personal decisions, taking responsibility for oneself, and/or being self-sufficient are methods by which personal power can be discovered.

Self-Caring

"Why would I care for myself when no one else cared for me? Besides I was too busy taking care of everyone else. Caring for myself made me think I was 'selfish,'" stated one survivor of domestic abuse. **Self-caring** or self-nurturing means taking care of one's own physical, emotional, and spiritual needs. Having concern for others should not be neglected but, concern for others should not be at the expense of oneself. Self-caring is often a major change in behavior for women who have been in abusive relationships. Self-care enables women to recognize the value of self and to act accordingly by making

resiliency—the ability to recover, overcome adversity, and bounce back following difficult situations.

self-caring—taking care of one's own personal physical, emotional, and spiritual needs.

Assess YOURSELF

Recognizing and Meeting Personal Needs

Identify and briefly explain some of the things a woman can do to meet the various needs that are important to moving forward with her life.

Needs	Who	How	Where
Survival			
Security			
Love/acceptance			
Self-worth			
Self-actualization			

healthy, nurturing choices. Engaging in fun and enjoyable activities is indicative of moving ahead with life and practicing the art of self-care. What would you do if you were asked to demonstrate self-care activities?

Answers to this question often reflect the stage of healing and growth that survivors are in at any given point. "Having a quiet meal or a complete night's sleep" may be indicative of initial stages of moving ahead with life. Women who, perhaps, have moved farther through the healing and growth process may provide such answers as enjoying a hot tub, working in the garden, watching movies, reading books, exercising, cooking a favorite meal, buying flowers, or sharing loving embraces. Whatever the method, engaging in self-care activities is an important move away from former negative beliefs and toward a healthier life.

Meeting Needs

Except for the most basic survival needs, such as food, shelter, and clothing, a woman's higher level needs often go unmet in an abusive relationship. Moving forward certainly means moving beyond survival needs and toward needs that promote progression and growth. Abraham Maslow, whose Hierarchy of Needs model was introduced in chapter 2, provides an excellent guide to determining human needs. The need for security, love and acceptance, self-worth, and self-actualization (the fulfillment of a woman's potential) are discussed by Maslow as nec-

essary for basic well-being and continual growth. Adhering to the suggestions found in the section titled "Leaving the Abusive Relationship," and utilizing the resource information presented here can provide the means by which these needs can be recognized and met. Now complete *Assess Yourself:* "Recognizing and Meeting Personal Needs."

PREVENTING ABUSE

Preventing abuse against women must be addressed at all levels: personal, community, state, and federal. Support and advocacy can be addressed at each level as can strategies that enable women to stop abusive episodes or, even better, prevent abusive patterns from ever occurring.

Personal Level

At the personal level consider the following suggestions that provide empowerment for women, enabling them to recognize and partner in a nonabusive and whole relationship.

- Teaching women to be intolerant of any form of abuse inflicted upon them or their children is an essential component of prevention.
- Educating girls and boys from an early age about the characteristics of healthy and long-lasting relationships. These characteristics include respect, love, shared values, trust, honesty, commitment, mutual caring, and communication.

- Improving the self-worth of women may assist them to think well enough of themselves and to accept that they do not deserve and should not tolerate any abusive behaviors. Personal self-worth leads to the desire to live in a healthy and whole family environment.
- Creating awareness of the negative consequences for women and children, both short-term and long-term, that result from involvement with an abusive partner can assist in preventing relationship abuse.

Healthy relationship awareness not only is a means of empowerment for females, but also is a way of changing patterns of socialization for the two sexes. From an early age boys must be taught that relationships are a partnership in which both participants share in all areas of decision making, responsibilities, and promotion of the relationship's success.

In thinking back on boys and young men in your life, can you remember characteristics that created an uneasy or skeptical feeling in you about them? Do you remember any of the following traits or behaviors that have been identified as characteristics of potential abusers: very little tolerance for others who have different ideas, opinions, or beliefs; low self-esteem; feelings of inadequacy as a man; quick to anger; rigid and controlling behaviors or demands; overuse of alcohol and use of other drugs; blames others for anything that doesn't work out; criticizes others; or was from a family in which there was abusive treatment of the mother and/or children.

Community Level

A community effort to prevent violence and abuse against women is essential because abuse is a social problem, and not a private or secret problem. Following are community actions that have been initiated in some areas to address this as a major social concern.

- Coordination of agencies and programs that can serve to reach families in the community has been accomplished in some areas of the country. The legal, medical, social, and educational agencies have developed formal, and in some instances, informal linkages to educate and provide services to families.
- Parenting classes, relationship-building skills, and stress management seminars are a few of the components that communities offer that can promote healthy family relationships, family

preservation, and support for families in need of these services. When the health and well-being of individuals and families are destroyed by family violence, the quality of community life deteriorates.
- Programs for men, especially abusive men, are being developed in which they learn to take responsibility for their actions, develop better partnering skills, and find support for change and growth among other participants.
- Extended-day programs for children and youth have been developed, either at school sites or at community centers. Providing recreational and educational activities and sometimes personal and social guidance, these centers offer a safe, fun, and caring environment for youth from all types of families.
- Increasing community awareness, speaking out about individual and victims' rights, and holding men accountable for their abusive actions is critical, not only in preventing, but in stopping violence and abuse against women.

State and Federal Levels

State and federal legislation, legislators, agencies, and other governing entities are making inroads into accepting the fact that women *are* abused and that not only the perpetrators, but the systems that allow this to go unchallenged must be stopped. State and federal governments are continuing to enact legislation to prevent violence and abuse against women as well as prosecute individuals who dare to commit this crime against another human being, especially human beings whom they profess to love.

- Laws to protect the rights of women against violence and abuse are being passed at the state and federal government levels.
- Reporting any injury that medical personnel, during the time of treatment, perceive to be the result of violence or abuse is required by many states. A physician who fails to report suspected abusive wounds of any type (for example, cuts, burns, bruises, or bullet wounds) is subject to fines or even a possible jail sentence.
- Passage of the most comprehensive and expensive crime bill in the U.S. history occurred in 1994, providing $13.5 billion for law enforcement, $9.9 billion for prisons, and $6.9 billion for crime prevention.[39] As a part of this crime bill, the Violence Against Women Act is a

landmark mandate that will strengthen law enforcement strategies, and promote safeguards for victims of domestic and sexual assault. This law has provisions related to safe streets, safe homes for women, civil rights and equal justice for women in the court system, stalker reduction rights, and protection for battered immigrant women and children. The Department of Justice will be coordinating efforts with other federal agencies as well as state, local, and tribal law enforcement agencies.

It is clear that violence and abuse against women are raging crimes in this country. Varied and complex negative consequences result—not only for women, but for our children, who are possibly future victims or perpetrators. To rectify and to prevent this, actions at all levels—from the individual to the federal government—must continue to be enacted. Until violence and abuse is absolutely condemned by everyone, abuse will continue and women will remain trapped in a potentially lethal cycle of violence.

Autobiography in Five Short Chapters

I.
I walk down the street.
There is a deep hole in the sidewalk.
I fall in
I am lost . . . I am helpless
It isn't my fault
It takes forever to find a way out.

II.
I walk down the same street.
There is a deep hole in the sidewalk.
I pretend I don't see it.
I fall in again.
I can't believe I am in the same place
but, it isn't my fault.
It still takes a long time to get out.

III.
I walk down the same street
There is a deep hole in the sidewalk.
I see it is there.
I still fall in . . . it's a habit
my eyes are open.
I know where I am.
It is my fault.
I get out immediately.

IV.
I walk down the same street.
There is a deep hole in the sidewalk.
I walk around it.

V.
I walk down another street.

by Portia Nelson

Chapter Summary

- Abuse against women has been documented throughout history.
- Domestic abuse, sexual assault, child abuse, and other forms of abuse against women abound in epidemic numbers in this country and produce serious physical, mental, emotional, and social consequences for men, women, and their children.
- Financial concerns, self-blame, emotional issues, codependency, and perception of her partner are reasons women often remain in abusive relationships.
- Fear for their children's lives and safety as well as their own is sometimes the impetus for leaving an abusive relationship.

- Having a plan that includes safe facilities, a support system, and accessibility to a variety of resources are important assets when leaving an abusive relationship.
- As women heal from abusive relationship(s), they generally experience the healing process in a number of stages.
- Family and friends can aid women in moving forward with their lives. Survivors can develop skills that assist their efforts to improve the quality of life for themselves as well as their children.
- Developing a wide-spread and comprehensive approach to violence and abuse prevention must be a personal priority as well as a priority at the community, state, and federal government levels.

Review Questions

1. Historically, why have women been considered the lesser or weaker sex?
2. Why is it that women often believe they deserve the abuse they receive in a relationship?
3. How and why is the perpetrator socialized into a belief system?
4. Why are women reluctant to report domestic abuse?
5. What barriers in society reduce the likelihood that domestic abuse will be reported to law enforcement authorities?
6. What is meant by psychological abuse and what are a number of their resulting consequences?
7. What are the behaviors of a potential rapist and how can rape be avoided?

8. What are some methods that can help resolve issues related to sexual harassment?
9. What characteristics are associated with women who are abused? How do they develop?
10. What are some of the physical, psychological, spiritual, and social consequences when experiencing abuse?
11. What are the types of resources available to enable a woman to leave an abusive relationship?
12. What are the indicators of healing that show that women are moving ahead with their lives after abuse?

Resources

Hotlines and Organizations

National Domestic Violence Hotline
Telephone: (800) 799–SAFE
Toll-free hotline, 24-hours providing information, referrals and support for abused women.

National Coalition Against Domestic Violence
119 Constitution Ave. NE
Washington, D.C. 20002
Telephone: (202) 544–7358
or
National Coalition Against Domestic Violence
Box 18749
Denver, CO 80218
Telephone: (303) 839–1852

Co-dependents Anonymous (CODA),
P.O. Box 33577
Phoenix, AZ 85067–3577
Telephone: (602) 277–7991
Organization for women and men from dysfunctional families who want assistance in developing healthy relationships.

Women Against Rape
P.O. Box 02084
Columbus, OH 43202
Telephone: (614) 221–447 (crisis #)
Telephone: (614) 291–9751 (business #)

Local Rape Hotline
(check local yellow pages)

National Center for Lesbian Rights
1663 Mission St., 5th Floor
San Francisco, CA 94103
Telephone: (415) 621-0674

Child Help National Child Abuse Hotline
Telephone: (800) 422-4453
Telephone: (705) 526-5647 (Canada)
A 24-hour hotline to report child abuse, for counseling and referrals for children and adults.

National Childwatch
4065 Page Avenue
P.O. Box 1368
Jackson, MI 49204
Telephone: (800) 222-1464

National Committee for Prevention of Child Abuse
Telephone: (800) 55NCPCA

National Center for Injury Prevention and Control
Centers for Disease Control and Prevention
4770 Buford Hwy., NE MS: F-36
Atlanta, GA 30341-3724
Telephone: (404) 488-4690

National Clearinghouse for the Defense of Battered Women
125 S. 9th Street
Suite 302
Philadelphia, PA 19107

Parents Anonymous
Telephone: (800) 421-0353
Telephone: (800) 352-0386
For abusive parents.

Survivors of Incest Anonymous
P.O. Box 21817
Baltimore, MD 21222
Telephone: (410) 282-3400
A twelve-step, self-help program.

Voices in Action
Telephone: (312) 327-1500
Offers meetings and publications for individuals who have been sexually abused.

Audiotapes

Don't Touch Me That Way, Again by Susan Johnston (Note: Call Texas Council on Family Violence for specifics)

Videotapes

Scenes from a Shelter: Talking about Domestic Violence by Susan Fine (Note: Call Texas Council on Family Violence for specifics)

Websites

Femina
http://www.femina.com/femina/health
Search engine for health issues including disease prevention, reproductive health, assault prevention; start here and move to many other sites.

Rape
http://www.ocs.mg.edu.au/~Korman/feminism/rape
Includes information, organizations, and resources as well as rape issues.

Sexual Assault
http://www.cs.utk.edu/-bartley/saInfoPage.html
Issues concerning rape, sexual and domestic abuse with links to additional sites.

WWWomen
http://www.wwwomen.com/
Search engine for topics related to women's health, sexual orientation, ethnic and feminine issues.

The Commonwealth Fund
http:www.cmwf.org
Provides information about various publications from this organization dedicated to helping Americans live healthy and productive lives.

Suggested Readings
Newsletters

Above and Beyond, Box 2672, Ann Arbor, MI 48106-2672
A quarterly newsletter concerned with the issues of all types of abuse.

Healing paths, Box 599, Coos Bay, OR 97420-0114
Bimonthly journal costing about $18.00 per year.

The Survivor Network Newsletter, Box 80058, Albuquerque, NM 87198.
Quarterly newsletter written by survivors of abuse.

Books

Bass, E., and Davis, L. 1992. *The courage to heal.* New York: Harper & Row.
Commission on Women's Health from The Commonwealth Fund. *Violence against women in the United States: A comprehensive background paper.* New York: Columbia University, College of Physicians and Surgeons.
Comstock, Gary David. 1991. *Violence against lesbians and gay men.* New York: Columbia University Press.
Crowell, N.A. and A. W. Burgess, ed. 1996. *Understanding violence against women,* Washington DC: National Academy Press

References

1. Genesis 3:16, *The Holy Bible*. 1962. New York: World Publishing Co., pp. 3-4.

2. Bullough, V. L. 1973. *The subordinate sex: A history of attitudes toward women.* Chicago: University of Illinois Press.

3. Dobash, R. E. and R. P. Dobash. 1977. Wives: The "appropriate" victim of marital violence. *Victimology, 11,* 427.

4. Peterson, D. 1992. Wifebeating: An American tradition. *Journal of Interdisciplinary History, 23,* 97-118.

5. Hearing before the Subcommittee of Crime and Criminal Justice of the Committee on the Judiciary House of Representatives, 1992. *One Hundred Second Congress: Second Session,* Washington, D.C.

6. Bachman, R. and L. E. Saltzman. 1995. Washington, D.C.: U.S. Department of Justice, *Violence against women: Estimates from the redesigned survey.* Report # NJC-154348.

7. Ibid.

8. Ibid.

9. U.S. Surgeon General. 1992. In American Medical Society National Leadership Conference. *Journal of the American Medical Association, 267,* 3132.

10. Gelles, R. J., and M. A. Straus. 1988. *Intimate violence: The definitive study of the causes and consequences of abuse in the American family.* New York: Simon and Schuster.

11. Dobash and Dobash, Wives: The "appropriate" victim of marital violence.

12. Straus, M., R. J. Gelles, and S. K. Seinmetz. 1980. *Behind closed doors: Violence in the American family.* Garden City, N.Y.: Anchor.

13. Bachman and Saltzman, *Violence against women.*

14. Ibid.

15. U.S. Department of Justice, 1994. *Violence against women: A national crime victimization survey report.* Washington, D.C. 1994.

16. Bachman and Saltzman, *Violence against women.*

17. National Clearinghouse for the Defense of Battered Women, Philadelphia, 1994. *General facts about domestic abuse.*

18. Harter, S., P. C. Alexander, and R. A. Neimeyer. 1988. Long-term effects of incestuous child abuse in college women: Social adjustment, social cognition, and family characteristics. *Journal of Consulting and Clinical Psychology, 56* (1): 5-8.

19. Child abuse—Part II. 1993, June. *The Harvard Mental Health Letter, 9* (12):1-4.

20. National Committee for Prevention of Child Abuse, 1993. *Report on child abuse.* Washington D.C.

21. Family Violence Prevention Programs. 1992. *Domestic violence: A guide for health care providers.* Section 111-27-29, Denver, Co.: Department of Health and Colorado Domestic Violence Coalition.

22. Scully, D. 1992, January. Who's to blame for sexual violence? *USA Today Magazine,* pp. 35-37.

23. *Rape in America—A report to the nation.* 1992. Arlington, Va.: National Victim Center.

24. Payne, W. and D. Hahn. 1998. *Understanding your health,* 5th ed. St. Louis: McGraw-Hill.

25. Ibid.

26. Walker, L. 1984. Battered women, psychology and public policy. *American Psychologist, 29* (10): 1178.

27. Federal Bureau of Investigation. 1992. *Uniform crime reporting handbook.* U.S. Government Printing Office.

28. Office of Justice Programs. 1994. *Violence between intimates.* Washington, D.C.: U.S. Department of Justice, NJC-149259.

29. Excerpted from Wilson, M. D., and M. Daly. 1992, November. Who kills whom in spouse killings? On the exceptional sex ratio of spousal homicides in the United States. *Criminology, 30.*

30. Herek, G. B., and K. T. Berrill, ed. 1992. *Hate crimes: Confronting violence against lesbians and gay men.* Newbury Park, Ca.: Safe.

31. Russell, D. E. H. 1984. *Sexual exploitation.* Beverly Hills, Ca.: Sage.

32. Leidig, M. 1992. The continuum of violence against women: Psychological and physical consequences, *Journal of American College Health,* 40:149-55.

33. Schumacher, L. 1985. How to help victims of domestic violence. *Personality Journal,* 64: 102-5.

34. Straus et al.; *Behind closed doors: Violence in the American family.*

35. Bass, E., and L. Davis. 1992. *The courage to heal: A guide for women survivors of child sexual abuse.* New York: Harper & Row, p. 181.

36. Walker, Battered women, psychology and public policy.

37. Bass and Davis, *The courage to heal.*

38. U.S. Department of Justice. 1993. *Helping the battered woman: A guide for family and friends.* Washington, D.C.: U.S. Department of Justice, National Women Abuse Prevention Project, Project #20573-0538.

39. Payne and Hahn, *Understanding your health.*

Part Four

SEXUAL AND RELATIONAL WELLNESS

CHAPTER FOURTEEN
Building Healthy Relationships

CHAPTER FIFTEEN
Examining Gynecological Issues

CHAPTER SIXTEEN
Selecting Birth Control Methods

CHAPTER SEVENTEEN
Planning for Pregnancy and Parenting

Fourteen

Building Healthy Relationships

■ chapter objectives

When you complete this chapter you will be able to:
- Distinguish between instrumental and expressive traits.
- Explain the stages of dating.
- Provide examples of different types of love based on Sternberg's triangular theory of love.
- Compare and contrast various types of relationships.
- Describe relationship success and distress.
- Explain how to resolve relationship conflicts.

GENDER-ROLE ATTRIBUTES AND SOCIOLOGICAL FACTORS

This chapter discusses current findings and beliefs about the individual and relationship characteristics that contribute to a viable, dynamic relationship. It discusses how relationships are formed, how to tell if it's love or addiction, and what it takes to keep a relationship healthy and stable.

Gender-Role Attributes

Psychological factors such as masculinity and femininity have a profound influence on the development of relationships. Early studies of gender-role attitudes used a unidimensional, bipolar concept of masculinity and femininity. Traits designated for

males or females were dichotomous and precluded each other. Masculinity was viewed as an absence of femininity; femininity was viewed as an absence of masculinity. This view was based on the belief that males and females differed in instinctive and emotional behavior, for instance, those factors that shaped personality. The female was characterized as sympathetic, nurturing, timid, prone to jealousy and suspicion, submissive, and nonaggressive. The male was described as aggressive, dominating, prone to leadership, less religious, and strong.

Later, researchers suggested that masculinity and femininity were separate principles that coexisted to some degree in all individuals, irrespective of gender. They used a multidimensional model that was independent of gender. Individuals who scored high in attributes defined as masculine and low in feminine were classified as **masculine.** Individuals who scored high in feminine attributes and low in masculine attributes were classified as **feminine.** Those who possessed a high number of masculine and feminine traits were labeled **androgynous.** Androgynous individuals were believed to possess the traits that allowed them to function more equally in a relationship and fared better psychologically.

A study of gender-role attitudes and dating behaviors in college students found differences in self-disclosure, power, and cohabitation among traditional and androgynous individuals. Traditional masculine males tended toward less self-disclosure and exerted more power in the dating relationship. Traditional masculine males and feminine females were also less likely to choose to be sexually active or cohabitate. In a follow-up of these couples, traditional feminine women were more likely than androgynous women to marry their college sweetheart and to remain married.[1] However, this study ignored one apparent paradox of gender attributes: traditionally masculine males and feminine females have far from optimal relationships. In fact, another study suggested that marital happiness appeared to be related to high feminine traits in both males and females.[2]

More recently, the terms "instrumental" or "agentic" have been used to define masculine traits and "expressive" or "communal" to define feminine traits. These terms remove gender stereotyping and de-emphasize gender differences. Instrumental or agentic traits include assertiveness, independence, and competence, whereas expressive traits include compassionate, affectionate, and interpersonal concern. An androgynous person exhibits a balance of instrumental and expressive traits, and can appropriately display the necessary traits for the circumstances.

Sociological Factors

Sociological factors also impact the development of relationships. Socialization can contribute to the respective differences in attitudes and behaviors between males and females in interpersonal interactions. Some scholars suggest that women are more relational, whereas men are more autonomous. Women are socialized to be more dependent or interdependent, thus more likely to define themselves in the context of relationships. Men, on the other hand, define themselves as more independent, thus focusing on individual rights, self-centeredness, and self-interest.

Females and males tend to be socialized differently according to the values and beliefs of their cul-

> ### JOURNAL ACTIVITY
>
> #### *Attractive and Unattractive Qualities*
>
> Create a list of ten qualities you find most attractive and least attractive in another person. Look at the qualities that you listed as most attractive in another person. Now, answer the following questions: To what degree do you possess these qualities? Would you like to develop these qualities more fully in yourself? Look at the qualities that you find least attractive in another person. To what degree do you possess these qualities? Do you try hard to avoid these qualities in yourself? Have you accepted your potential to possess these qualities? Do you accept these qualities as part of every human being's potential? Why or why not? Oftentimes, the qualities that we react to most strongly in another human being are related to issues that we need to address within ourselves.

ture. Individualistic societies focus on "the subordination of the goals of the collectives to individual goals." Men in these societies tend to pursue their self-interests and give the immediate family primary importance. Collective societies, on the other hand, emphasize interdependence and the goals of the collective over an individual's goals.[3]

The United States, as a society, is viewed as more individualist than collective. Some researchers have proposed that belonging to an individualistic society profoundly effects love and intimacy. They postulate that romantic love is more important to committed relationships in individualistic societies and that psychological intimacy (an important component in committed relationships) is difficult to develop.[4] Here, men tend to embrace the cultural and psychological aspects of an individualistic society, whereas most women tend to embrace the messages of a collective society. Men find it easier to integrate societal messages and expectations for their role in relationships because these messages and expectations are congruent with an individualistic society. Women, on the other hand, grow up with the messages of interdependence (collective values) and can experience dissonance when trying to live by the rules of an individualistic society. This dissonance may lead to confusion if a woman seeks congruity between personal and societal values. Now complete *Journal Activity:* "Attractive and Unattractive Qualities."

FORMING RELATIONSHIPS

Healthy relationships evolve, they do not happen spontaneously! Young adolescents, as they begin to date, are learning how to connect and interact with someone else. The way adolescents interact is greatly influenced by the role models (parents, caregivers, media) observed during childhood and more accurately, the adolescent's perceptions of how these role models interacted with each other. Most adults have never received training in appropriate methods and techniques for building, maintaining, and nurturing a relationship. This lack of skill development limits their ability to serve as role models of healthy interactions that their children can emulate. As a result, adolescents are faced with the difficult task of figuring out how to build healthy relationships without the benefit of previous modeling. This section addresses the stages of dating, the skills needed for healthy interaction between two people, and the characteristics of healthy and troubled relationships.

Stages of Dating

The stages of dating include attraction, ritual, appreciation, intimacy, and possibly, commitment.[5] These stages take time to evolve and if women move too quickly through them, they may find themselves repeating destructive relationship patterns over and over.

Attraction The first stage of dating is attraction, sometimes called "chemistry." Physical attraction draws us to another person. You see him standing there, on the other side of the room. You think he's attractive. You see her at a bookstore and want to begin a conversation. She looks incredible. You make eye contact. Why did he catch your eye? Why did you want to talk to her? The physical appearance that appeals to one person may or may not appeal to another. Physical attraction doesn't suggest that this person will have the attributes or personality that you like, but it is a first step. Physically attractive people often benefit from their good looks. Studies suggest that they are perceived as being more intelligent, more socially skilled, happier, more successful, and better adjusted than less attractive persons.[6,7] This perception occurs through the conscious or unconscious meaning we attach to the attraction; it isn't reality. It takes time to develop a complete picture of a person, and true reality can only occur with mutual self-disclosure and an unbiased observation of another person's behaviors.

Ritual Rituals are the practices that help us create familiarity. These are the mannerisms, experiences, and behaviors that occur to deepen the bond between two people. Rituals are the shared experiences that lead to calling something "special" or "our favorite." It may be our song, our place to go for a walk, our special nicknames, or anything that makes us think fondly about the other person. Rituals create meaning; meaning comes from doing; and doing takes time!

Information Sharing Information sharing is the stage of getting to know each other better. It begins with impersonal dialog that allows you to get to know each other: likes and dislikes, hobbies, career aspirations, worldview and politics, and other external issues. At this stage, you are attuned to how the other person communicates and interacts with you and others, what she or he says about others (either positively or negatively), and what draws you to this person. If you feel a sense of immediacy or desire to hurry through this stage, stop and evaluate why you are feeling this need. Are you feeling a need to be rescued, to rescue, to attach before he leaves or gets bored? Why aren't you willing to continue moving slowly? The information-sharing stage is only the beginning level of emotional intimacy. Eventually, you may choose to disclose more personal information about yourself, such as information about your background, your family, and your inner thoughts and feelings. This disclosure will occur at a reasonably slow pace. Physical contact, such as kissing, hand holding, and other such behaviors, may also begin at this time. If you move too quickly with physical contact, you may mistakenly think that the physical intimacy is synonymous with emotional intimacy. You may overlook characteristics and behaviors that otherwise could alert you to possible future problems (so-called red flags).

---

masculinity—possessing a high number of attributes defined as masculine and a low number of attributes defined as feminine.

femininity—possessing a high number of attributes defined as feminine and a low number of attributes defined as masculine.

androgyny—possessing a high number of attributes defined as masculine and a high number of attributes defined as feminine.

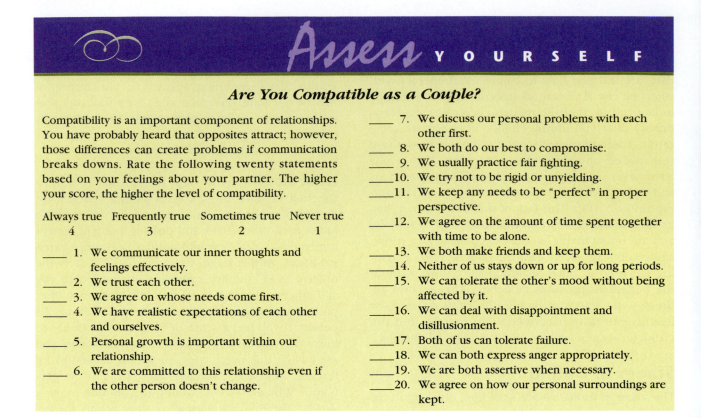

Assess YOURSELF

Are You Compatible as a Couple?

Compatibility is an important component of relationships. You have probably heard that opposites attract; however, those differences can create problems if communication breaks downs. Rate the following twenty statements based on your feelings about your partner. The higher your score, the higher the level of compatibility.

Always true	Frequently true	Sometimes true	Never true
4	3	2	1

____ 1. We communicate our inner thoughts and feelings effectively.

____ 2. We trust each other.

____ 3. We agree on whose needs come first.

____ 4. We have realistic expectations of each other and ourselves.

____ 5. Personal growth is important within our relationship.

____ 6. We are committed to this relationship even if the other person doesn't change.

____ 7. We discuss our personal problems with each other first.

____ 8. We both do our best to compromise.

____ 9. We usually practice fair fighting.

____10. We try not to be rigid or unyielding.

____11. We keep any needs to be "perfect" in proper perspective.

____12. We agree on the amount of time spent together with time to be alone.

____13. We both make friends and keep them.

____14. Neither of us stays down or up for long periods.

____15. We can tolerate the other's mood without being affected by it.

____16. We can deal with disappointment and disillusionment.

____17. Both of us can tolerate failure.

____18. We can both express anger appropriately.

____19. We are both assertive when necessary.

____20. We agree on how our personal surroundings are kept.

Activities   Activities play an important role in the dating process and keep the process moving slowly. These activities occur concurrently with the information-sharing stage and now is the time to figure out if your interests are similar to the other person's interests. Do you like the same events, movies, or restaurants? Do you equally choose activities or are you always doing the activities she or he planned for you? You should feel comfortable stating whether you prefer to do what he wants or if you prefer to do something else. You should feel comfortable saying that you want to go out with friends or have made plans to do something without him. If conflicts arise, you and your partner have an opportunity to practice compromise and negotiation. If either person begins to sacrifice interests on a regular basis and goes along with the other's suggestions, inequity soon begins to infiltrate the relationship. Complete *Assess Yourself:* "Are You Compatible as a Couple?" to help you reflect on whether you have balance between alone time, time with him, and time with other friends. Spending time alone and with other friends will help you move slowly. Throughout this dating

process, you can decide whether to move forward toward a greater level of intimacy and more exclusivity, to keep the relationship at a more superficial level, to terminate the relationship, or to compromise on an acceptable level of interaction.

Emotional Intimacy   As two people spend more time together, their level of **intimacy** continues to grow. Emotional intimacy is the feeling of knowing and being known. A key component of intimacy is good communication. It is knowing who you are and being willing to reveal yourself to someone else. It involves openly sharing important information about yourself while keeping your boundaries intact. Intimacy requires the same from your partner. Your partner must be willing to reveal herself and you must be willing to listen effectively. It is knowing where you begin and end and where she begins and ends. Emotional intimacy occurs when you disclose information in an open, honest, and authentic manner.[8]

Sometimes, as you become more intimate with a partner, you may encounter barriers that keep you from experiencing a meaningful intimate relationship. Such barriers may occur from being traumatized as a child, feeling fragmented, or having poor role models. Some children experience trauma (physical, emotional, or spiritual) as they are growing and, in response, develop a psychological wall to protect themselves. This wall was useful for them as children, but as adults, it prevents them from being vulnerable and open with others. As they gain an understanding of their barriers, they begin to work toward overcoming the walls so emotional intimacy can be attained.

As you share the parts of yourself that make you feel vulnerable, the psychological wounds you experienced as a child can begin to heal. Embracing those parts of yourself that you prefer to hide or disown and being truthful with a partner can provide a deeper level of emotional maturity. In an open, honest relationship, you can freely share those aspects while still accepting responsibility for your actions. Even small lies (whether through omission or commission) impact a relationship. Truth and honesty permit you to openly experience your vulnerability, admit your mistakes, acknowledge your fears, express anger and sadness, and ask for what you need. These inner thoughts and feelings are easier to share if your partner demonstrates empathy (compassion), praise, and encouragement, and if you moved slowly through the initial stages of dating. Strong communication skills is a major asset to intimacy and a healthy relationship.

Commitment   Commitment represents feelings of attachment and the desire to be in a more intimate relationship with the other person. People commit to a relationship for a variety of reasons, some more healthy than others. Three factors found to increase the potential of a person to remain committed to a relationship include a partner's satisfaction with the relationship, a partner's perceived lack of alternatives to the current partner, and the investment of important or numerous resources in the relationship.[9] Ultimately, staying or leaving depends on the willingness of the partners to commit to the relationship.

THEORIES OF LOVE

Love is something that everyone seeks, yet when someone is asked how they know when they're in love or what to expect from love, the answers are varied. How do researchers describe love and its various forms? What ingredients do they feel are necessary for a couple to maintain a long-term love relationship?

Sternberg's Triangular Theory

Sternberg's triangular theory of love focuses on three components: commitment, intimacy, and passion. These components explain nine different combinations of love, but not why love occurs. One side of the triangle focuses on the emotional aspect of love (intimacy); the second side focuses on the motivational aspect of love (passion); and, the third side focuses on the cognitive side of love (commitment). The combination of these three aspects explain different types of love and changes in the components are illustrated by changes to the size and shape of the triangles.

Liking occurs when only the emotional side of love (intimacy) is present. Two friends who trust each other, share similar values and beliefs, and communicate well form an intimate bond. They know the vulnerabilities and strengths of each other and form a close friendship. *Empty love* occurs when commitment alone is present. For example, when Julie states emphatically, "You know, I really don't like Ted anymore but I took a marriage vow. I said 'in sickness and in health, for better or for worse, until death do us part' and that's what I intend to honor. When I want to talk about intimate matters, I talk to my best friend. Besides, the children need a father and I can't find a job now." Julie's religious beliefs, the values instilled during childhood, and limited financial earning potential keep her from leaving to seek a more fulfilling relationship. She may not like Ted as a person, but she married him and intends to stay with him. *Infatuation* occurs when passion is the sole dimension in the relationship. This concept can be summarized as "a crush." Kenitra isn't worried about Andre's values, beliefs, background, job, or anything else; she doesn't care. Andre is awesome, she's never seen anyone more attractive, and she thinks about him all the time. *Romantic love* involves the dimensions of intimacy and passion. Two people who like and are physically attracted to each other but do not have a commitment form a romantic liaison. In one study, when men and women were asked, "What constitutes a romantic act?" both sexes cited "taking walks together" most often. The

intimacy—the feeling of knowing and being known.

women's list included taking walks together, sending or receiving flowers, kissing, candle-lit dinners, cuddling, declaring "I love you," love letters, slow dancing, hugging, and giving surprise gifts. The list for men looked similar and included taking walks together, kissing, candle-lit dinners, cuddling, hugging, flowers, holding hands, making love, love letters, and sitting by the fireplace.[10]

When passion and commitment result in a committed relationship without taking time to get to know each other, *fatuous love* results. Jill met Jackie at a softball game. It was the first game between their teams and the two players were immediately attracted to each other. After the game, they shook hands and agreed to meet later at the bar. They ended the night at Jill's place and the sex was great. The next week, Jill asked Jackie to move into her apartment. They were "in love" and ready to commit to a lifetime together. Six months later, each of them was shaking their heads, wondering how they could have possibly been attracted to each other. They ran out of things to talk about and had very little in common! *Companionate love* involves intimacy and commitment without passion. In some long-term relationships, the physical attraction may die but the intimacy and commitment provide the ingredients for a long-term friendship. The partners are best friends. When all three components are present in the relationship, *consummate love* or complete love occurs. This love is what partners strive to create and to maintain. It requires nurturing, physical attraction, vulnerability, and a commitment to growing together. When all three components are absent in the relationship, Sternberg calls this *nonlove*. These are just casual interactions that occur without any form of relationship evolving.

Lovestyles

I love him, but I'm not in love with him. I like him, but I'm not sure I love him. What do we mean by such words? John Alan Lee, in "The Colors of Love," identifies six different lovestyles.[11] He identifies three primary lovestyles (*eros, storge,* and *ludus*) and three secondary lovestyles (*mania, pragma,* and *agape*). **Erotic** love occurs when lovers get involved quickly, and base their attraction on physical attributes and sexual passion. This love is based on "chemistry" and "love at first sight." Eros is a major ingredient in relationship success.

Ludic love is an uncommitted alliance with more than one partner. The partners may be very different from one another, because love is based on game playing rather than romance. A partner is "kept guessing" and distancing occurs when dependency develops. Ludus tend to be negatively related to satisfaction with relationships.

Pragmatic love draws two people together for practical reasons such as financial security or parental potential. It is "pragmatic," and fills certain specifications such as similar background, good job, or good parent. It is often present in long-term relationships.

Manic love is often portrayed in the "heart throb" of Hollywood, the perfect match. The emotional highs and lows remind one of a roller coaster ride, and possessiveness, dependency, and jealousy abound. Mania lead to total focus on and fear of losing one's partner.

Altruistic love places the needs of the partner above one's own needs. It is selfless and nondemanding, and one chooses self-sacrifice rather than hurting a partner. This love is sometimes referred to as **agape,** a more spiritual relationship.

Storgic love is more like friendship, without the passion. It provides a secure, trusting relationship that evolves from a deep, abiding friendship and leads to long-term relationships.

TRAITS OF A SUCCESSFUL RELATIONSHIP

What attributes or characteristics are needed to create a healthy relationship in which both partners indicate happiness? Researchers have identified a number of attributes that contribute to a happy, successful relationship. Researcher Judith Wallerstein's study of fifty happily married couples indicated that nine psychological tasks had to occur for marital satisfaction to be achieved.[12] The nine tasks couples had to achieve include:

1. Separating emotionally from the families of origin and creating a new family. The lines of connection to the original families had to be redefined.
2. Maintaining autonomy and balancing it with togetherness. Mutual identification and shared intimacy are essential for overall satisfaction.
3. Establishing a vital sexual relationship that remains free from the distractions of work and family obligations. Setting aside quality time for each other is important.

4. Recognizing the changes that occur with parenthood and keeping communication open while time demands and responsibilities shift. Privacy is important and should be protected.
5. Confronting crises (they will happen in every relationship) and facing adversity together.
6. Determining safe ways to express differences, conflict, and anger, and seeking resolution when differences occur.
7. Creating humor that keeps the little things in perspective and maintains the dynamic stimulation to avoid boredom and isolation.
8. Nurturing and comforting each other, allowing dependency and vulnerability to feel safe.
9. Remembering the early romantic, idealized images of love for the partner while facing the reality of shifts in the relationship.

These tasks are important in any committed relationship regardless of whether the couple is married, cohabiting, heterosexual, homosexual, or bisexual. Happiness within the relationship requires both partners to keep the relationship a high priority. Now complete *Journal Activity:* "Attributes That Contribute to Relationship Success."

TYPES OF RELATIONSHIPS

Marriage and Committed Relationships

For most women, getting married, followed by having a baby, are the expected norm as they reach adulthood. In fact, 60 percent of Americans are married. David Olson and his colleagues have studied the marital relationships of over eight thousand couples and found seven basic types of marriage. They established profiles based on ten scales including personality issues, communication, conflict resolution, financial management, leisure activities, sexual relationship, children and parenting, family and friends, egalitarian roles, and religious orientation. These ten issues are most frequently cited as areas of conflict for couples. Seven distinguishable marriage typologies were derived from these scales: devitalized, financially focused, conflicted, traditional, balanced, harmonious, and vitalized marriages. Devitalized marriages (40 percent) were characterized by dissatisfaction in all areas. These couples were extremely unhappy and both had considered divorce at some point in the relationship. Partners tended to be

JOURNAL ACTIVITY

Attributes That Contribute to Relationship Success

Many components are important for creating and maintaining a successful relationship. Write one or two feeling statements regarding the importance and meaning of each attribute.

ability to nurture	acceptance	authenticity
commitment	competence	confidence
devotion	empathy (compassion)	generosity
honesty	ability to apologize	openness
sacrifice	remember own needs	respect
responsibility	sacrifice	self-disclosure
support	touch	trust

What other attributes are necessary for relationship success? Can any of the above attributes be removed from the list?

younger, married a shorter period of time, and less financially secure. They stayed together because of limited alternatives and often came from families with divorced parents. In contrast, vitalized marriages (9 percent) were characterized by satisfaction with all dimensions of the relationship and reciprocal liking. Partners had well-integrated personalities and agreed on most external issues. They tended to be in their first marriage, were older, Protestant, and came from intact families. Couples in financially focused marriages (11 percent) were unhappy in their

erotic—a relationship built on passion and sexual desire.

ludic—love based on game playing and maintaining distance in a relationship.

pragmatic—a relationship built on practical needs between partners.

manic—consumed or obsessed with thoughts about a lover and a strong need for love and affection.

agape—selfless and unconditional love between partners.

storgic—a relationship built on security and friendship.

communication but stayed together for money and financial rewards. Careers were more important than the relationship and financial management was their only relationship strength. Couples in conflicted marriages (14 percent) had unresolved conflicts between them but gained satisfaction from outside sources such as leisure, children, or friends. Couples in the traditional marriage (10 percent) were moderately satisfied with their relatively stable relationship. These couples tended to be older, married longer, white, and Protestant. Their major sources of distress were sexual and communication conflicts. Couples in balanced marriages (8 percent) were moderately satisfied with their relationship, particularly in areas of communication and problem solving. Their source of distress was financial stability, whereas agreement occurred in areas such as leisure and childrearing. Couples in harmonious marriages (8 percent) were extremely satisfied with each other, including sexual and affectional dimensions. They tended to be self-centered and preferred to have no children. In all seven types, women were less satisfied than men in the relationships and were more likely to have considered divorce.[13,14] Although generalizing to all types of relationships (heterosexual or homosexual) has some inherent reliability and validity problems, you might discuss the implications of this research for all types of committed relationships.

Predicting Marital Success Olson and his colleagues also have consolidated the above typologies and attempted to predict marital success in premarital couples. Couples categorized as vitalized had a high degree of overall relationship satisfaction. They preferred egalitarian roles, viewed religion as important, resolved conflicts appropriately, and liked each other. Harmonious couples had a moderate level of relationship satisfaction. They liked their partner's personality and habits, enjoyed family and friends, and resolved conflicts appropriately. They did not view religion as important and had somewhat unrealistic expectations of relationships. Their strengths were in the areas of interpersonal communication and sexual relationships. Traditional couples had a moderate level of relationship dissatisfaction. They were realistic about the relationship, were least likely to have cohabitated before marriage, and placed a higher value on religion. Their strengths were in the area of children, family, and developing well-defined plans. Conflicted relationships reported

dissatisfaction with the relationship. They disliked their partner's personality and habits, had problems with the sexual relationship and relating to family and friends. Results of their longitudinal study showed that conflicted couples were more likely to cancel wedding plans or divorce if they got married, traditional couples were least likely to divorce or separate, and vitalized couples demonstrated more marital satisfaction after three years.[15]

Peer Marriages Pepper Schwartz, coauthor of *American Couples,* coined the phrase, **peer marriages,** to describe egalitarian partnerships between two people. She found that true companionship came in the form of equity and quality with both partners sharing talents, resources, and decision-making skills. In these couples, both partners had equal say in major decisions, equal sharing of money decisions and discretionary funds, and supported and valued each other's work. Peer couples enjoyed their mutual friendship, greater emotional intimacy, and exhibited a stronger commitment and interdependence. The major difficulties faced by peer couples were the lack of role models, the lack of support by others, and keeping passion alive. Near peers emulated these couples but differed in several key areas: when arguing, the male usually dominated; in childrearing, the male did not participate equally; and in money matters, the male still assumed a provider role.[16]

Cohabitation

Cohabitation can take a variety of forms. It can be a precursor to marriage, a stage during courtship, or an alternative to marriage. More couples are cohabitating today than at any other time in history. According to the U.S. Census Bureau, fewer than 500,000 people were living together in 1970 compared to more than 3.7 million people in 1995. Not only are the numbers increasing, but the patterns of cohabitation have changed. In the past, a woman cohabitated in anticipation of marriage but she often experienced disappointment. Cohabitation was anything but a sure way to get a commitment of marriage. The primary reason women gave for cohabitating was that they wanted to get married; the major reason given by men was that they wanted a sexual partner. In reality, fewer than 25 percent of women and 20 percent of men married their live-in lover. Today, more than 50 percent of all first marriages are preceded by cohabitation and the likelihood of plans to marry in-

FYI *Racial and Ethnic Differences in Cohabitation*

A study of cohabitation patterns among whites, African American, and Hispanic women found differences that persisted independent of employment status, education, and income. Researchers found that the majority of cohabitating white women who became pregnant got married before the birth of their child. Twenty-eight percent of white women conceived their first child before marriage and only 13 percent remained unmarried before the birth of that child.

In contrast to white women, young African American women were more likely to cohabitate and most did not marry their partners. The majority of births to single African American women occurred outside of legal marriage. Seventy-four percent of cohabitating African American women conceived their first child before marriage and only a small percentage (6 percent) got married be-fore the birth of that child. These women were more likely to rely on the extended family, not the male partner, for assistance.

Among Puerto Ricans, traditional consensual unions are commonly accepted for low-income couples who do not have the resources to legally marry. These unions are an alternative to marriage and women often become pregnant and have children within them. Forty-seven percent of Puerto Rican women conceived their first child before marriage and few of them (11 percent) get married before the birth of the first child. In fact, many couples view cohabitation as a form of marriage, and continue to reside together after the birth of the child. Significantly more cohabitating Puerto Rican women were likely to get pregnant than white or African American women. ∞

creases with higher incomes.[17] However, a word of caution to those considering cohabitation: marriages in which one spouse had cohabitated previously were 50 percent more likely to end in divorce. For most couples, cohabitation is a short-term arrangement. Fifty percent of cohabitating couples break up or marry within two years and 90 percent marry or break up within five years.[18]

Researchers suggest that cohabitators share some behaviors similar to married couples, although other patterns are similar to singles. The commonalities they share with married couples include a shared residence, monogamy, and more than 10 percent conceive a child while cohabitating. Nearly three-quarters of these couples have plans to get married and their relationships are qualitatively similar to married relationships.[19] The behaviors they share in common with singles include less commitment to marriage, more acceptance of divorce, more egalitarian roles, a similar economic status, valuing independence in the relationship, and being more likely to have an outside relationship.

A determining factor in the quality and stability of cohabitation seems to be the intention to marry or the presence of a child. Children require an investment by both partners, not just one individual.[20] (See *FYI:* "Racial and Ethnic Differences in Cohabitation.")

Interracial Couples

Interracial marriages still create feelings of prejudice and discrimination despite the repeal of laws prohibiting them nearly thirty years ago. Although most interracial marriages experience some discrimination, our society tends to exhibit more animosity toward unions between African Americans and whites than Asian Americans and whites and Hispanics and whites. Yet, despite the taboo, statistics indicate that the number of interracial marriages and unions have been steadily increasing since the 1970s, including among African Americans and whites.[21] The number of African Americans involved in interracial marriages jumped from 2.6 percent in 1970, to 6.6 percent in 1980, to 10.6 percent in 1990, and to 12.1 percent in 1993. The number of African American women marrying white men has also risen sharply, from .7 percent in 1970 to 3.9 percent in 1993.[22] In

peer marriage—egalitarian partnership between two people.

cohabitation—two people living together; an alternative to marriage.

fact, the interracial marriage rate is increasing faster for African American women than African American men. A factor that may contribute to this trend is the lack of available African American men in the middle and upper middle class with nearly one-third of African American men in their twenties living in prison, on parole, or on probation.

Some researchers suggest that changing socioeconomic demographics have contributed to the increase in interracial marriages. Marriages are more likely to occur because partners share common values, goals, interests, and beliefs, factors related to socioeconomic status as much as race. As the middle class had become more racially diverse, socioeconomic status now rivals race as a major determinant of marital suitability.

Most interracial dating occurs among college students, but most interracial marriages involve women who are older, previously divorced, and working in a diverse environment.[23] However, current trends suggest that changes are occurring in the demographics of interracial marriages. More white women who marry African American men are now in their first marriages, are younger, and most intend to have children.[24] The degree of discrimination, prejudice, and animosity these couples (and their children) will face depends, to some extent, on their socioeconomic status, the diversity within their community, and their educational status. Their relationship, particularly African American and white, faces demands not experienced by other couples, including other intermarriage groups. These demands create opportunities for extraordinary growth and maturity within the couple, as well as potential downfalls than can contribute to a higher than normal divorce rate. Couples who find themselves in interracial relationships need support and encouragement, not only from each other, but from friends and family. (See *Her Story:* "Michelle.")

Lesbian Couples

Lesbian couples have a unique opportunity to experience the best and also the most challenging aspects of what it means to be "female" in a relationship. Previously, we discussed the psychological and sociological factors that impact individual roles in relationships. As women, lesbians have grown up with the same societal influences as their heterosexual counterparts. A major difference between the two groups is that lesbians must be more consciously aware of the influences they will accept or reject. For instance, lesbians usually accept the values of a collective society, thus both partners are relationship-focused. This focus on community encourages equality and equity, regardless of whether they are in a committed, long-term relationship or an intimate friendship. By the same token, lesbians often reject the influence of income on power as exemplified in a patriarchal society. "Lesbians do not use income to establish dominance in their relationship. They use it to avoid having one woman dependent on the other."[25]

Lesbians, by virtue of being same-sex couples, encounter additional challenges in their relationships. One potential hazard is maintaining personal boundaries, which easily can become blurred when both partners focus on emotional intimacy and exclude personal autonomy. Maintaining balance between autonomy and intimacy is an important consideration. Another potential difficulty for lesbian couples is the lack of adequate role models for "peer relationships." Within the lesbian community, long-term relationships are often "closeted," particularly among older lesbians who grew up during more discriminatory times. Many lesbian couples form committed relationships, but do not receive the same benefits as married couples, for example, health insurance, help in finding a job for one partner when the other is relocated, tax benefits, and family support.

In the past, lesbian couples didn't have the option of raising children, unless one or both partners had children from a previous heterosexual relationship. Today, the number of lesbian couples choosing to have children is rising steadily, and their options extend to include adoption, artificial insemination, or other arrangements. Children provide the same parental bond for lesbian couples found in heterosexual couples, but may create some additional parenting issues. Difficulty can arise when others, particularly those opposed to lesbian lifestyles, question the ability or right of lesbians to raise children. They suggest that children raised in a same-sex household may differ from other children emotionally or the children may be raised to be lesbians or gay. A study comparing men and women raised by heterosexual single mothers and lesbian mothers found that young adults exhibited similar behavioral patterns regardless of the sexual orientation of the parent. Almost all (including twenty-three of twenty-five lesbian-raised adults) described themselves as heterosexual, and indicated a desire for marriage and children.[26]

Her Story

Michelle

Michelle, a 24-year-old senior, met Tony at a nightclub. She found him physically attractive, but more importantly, she enjoyed talking with him. When she discussed her work, he showed genuine interest. When he asked her out on a date, she wondered what her parents would think. They never told Michelle that she could not date a black man. But she could recall a time when she was 9 or 10 years old and her father commented negatively about an interracial couple at a restaurant. However, she decided to go ahead with the date.

Michelle told her mother about Tony immediately, but waited nearly six months before telling her dad. Her mother was pretty open-minded about it, but her father could not accept it. She had always been "Daddy's little girl," had followed the path that made him happy, and now, she just couldn't understand his feelings. Maybe with some time, he would accept it. Why didn't he trust her to make the right decisions for herself?

Michelle noticed other changes. Her job at the fitness club required contact with the public. The businessmen who came into the club really liked her, until she started dating Tony. White men and black women caused her the most difficulty. White men gave her the least respect, treating her completely different than before, almost as if she were invisible. Black women mumbled a lot of comments under their breath, but she could hear what they were saying. At first, she felt hurt by all the looks, comments, and treatment. Eventually she got used to it, but she also noticed that it didn't happen when Tony was with her . . . only when she was alone. She wondered why?

They had been dating for 2 ½ years when Michelle became pregnant. It wasn't planned, but they were excited about having a baby. Michelle would be graduating soon, and Tony had an excellent job as a business consultant. Her mother handled the news pretty well; she didn't like the idea that they weren't married. Her dad, however, went through the roof . . . he said he hadn't accepted the relationship so he most certainly wasn't going to accept this! He didn't even want her in the house anymore; he didn't want to see her. Michelle was devastated; how could he treat his own daughter this way? Would her baby ever know her grandfather? What should she tell her little girl as she grew up and wanted to know about her grandparents?

For now, Michelle plans to move in with Tony's family until she graduates and the baby is born. Tony spends a great deal of time away from home with his current job, so they decided such an arrangement would be best. Tony's family lives in a very diverse neighborhood so she feels comfortable. And, her friends from work and school have been wonderful.

Tony and Michelle know they will have a number of obstacles along the way. They plan to get married eventually, but they want it to be for the right reasons. Michelle continues to acknowledge her father with cards for special events, and even if he doesn't respond, she wants him to know that she loves him.

- What would your parents say about an interracial relationship?
- Would they accept an interracial grandchild?

Single Lifestyle and Parenthood

One trend in the Western world is the increasing number of women who are choosing to remain single. Better education, more career opportunities, and birth control have reduced the pressure on young women to get married. These women enjoy their current lifestyle and many plan to keep it that way. Some women also choose to remain single after divorce or widowhood.

Another trend is the growing number of single-parent households. In the United States, approximately 10 percent of all households were single parent in 1950 compared to 25 percent in 1990. Seventy percent of nonmarital births are to women age 20 years or older, with 22 percent being white births and 66 percent African American. More than 20 percent of live births in the United States are out of wedlock.[27]

TROUBLED RELATIONSHIPS

When a relationship gets into trouble, a variety of patterns can ensue that exacerbate existing problems and prevent resolution. As conflict and distress increase, the familiar pattern occurs more quickly and each partner becomes more entrenched in their role of perpetuating the pattern. Couples will continue to cycle through these patterns until the relationship ends or help is sought.

Love Addiction

The idea that love might be connected to "addiction" seems contradictory, however, loving relationships built on emotional and physical intimacy differ significantly from "addictive," incomplete relationships built on faulty thinking and feeling. This pattern has been described as love/avoidance addition.[28] It occurs when one partner, the **love addict,** feels the need to be rescued and the other partner, the **avoidance addict,** attempts to avoid involvement with the partner. The primary fear of the love addict is abandonment; the primary fear of the avoidance addict is intimacy. The secondary fear of each is reversed, thus both have the same two fears: abandonment and intimacy. Unless both partners make a concerted effort to break these cycles (usually through making conscious decisions to understand and change behaviors that contribute to these patterns), the relationship will deteriorate further until one partner leaves.[29]

Terminating a Relationship

According to the U.S. Census Bureau (1992), 52 percent of all first marriages end in divorce, and more than 60 percent of second marriages fail. The rate of divorce among all couples in the United States was 4.6 per 1,000 in 1994 with rates stabilizing for younger couples, whereas the rate of divorce has increased 50 percent for couples between ages 40 and 65 and 35 percent for couples age 65 and older.[30] The states in the United States with the lowest divorce rates include Massachusetts (2.4 per 1,000) and Connecticut (2.8 per 1,000) and the state with the highest rate is Nevada (9.0 per 1,000).[31] One suggested reason for such differences is that laws vary from state to state regarding dissolution of marriage. For example, Massachusetts law has traditionally required a very long waiting period between the filing for divorce and the entry of a divorce decree. In contrast, Nevada has historically been a state recognized for quick and easy divorce, requiring very short waiting periods and limited length of residency.

It is well known that the emotional and financial effects of divorce are generally greater for women than for men. The group who suffers and fares most poorly are older women, especially when they are ending a long-term relationship, or have limited work experience, or have relied on the husband as the wage earner. Less information is available about the financial and emotional effects of breakups on cohabitating women or lesbians. However, the consequences are certainly as devastating. These women may experience more difficulty in gaining emotional support than divorcing women because their relationships are less acceptable or recognized by the general population. And, in these situations, women have limited, if any, legal recourse. A breakup of a relationship (lesbian, cohabitating, or divorcing) can cause a number of disruptive consequences in women's lives, including depression, lower self-esteem, anxiety, feelings of betrayal or abandonment, as well as changes in childrearing, career decisions, finances, and housing.

Many women, with time, will choose to remarry or become involved in another relationship. Remarriages have been found to be more fragile and break up at a greater rate than first marriages. Census Bureau data shows that more than 62 percent of remarriages of women under age 40 end in divorce and when children are involved, the rate is even higher.

A major problem for a blended family is that expectations of the adults and the children are often unrealistic. When these expectations are broken (regardless of the reason), partners may experience conflict. The partner with children may find herself caught between the needs of her current partner and her children from the previous marriage or relationship. The parent-child relationship was established before this relationship and she may feel compelled to reassure her children that they will not be abandoned again. Meanwhile, her new partner may feel slighted. He may feel like he has to compete with the children for her attention. Realistically, it takes time and patience to blend a family and unless all parties set reasonable expectations, trouble will ensue. Conflict can also ensue if unresolved differences or unfinished business exists with an ex-partner. This tension can definitely impact and affect the new relationship.

Potential Sources of Conflict

Partners can have individual-related problems that may come between them in the relationship. Some of these problems include self-absorption, excessive ambition, feelings of inferiority or superiority, criticism, contempt, or defensiveness. A self-absorbed partner always puts his own needs ahead of his partner's needs. He is unable or unwilling to meet his partner's needs if they interfere with his own. A partner with excessive ambition will make getting ahead in the material world a higher priority than the relationship. Most women prefer intimacy and relationship, not goals connected to ambition. Whether a partner has feelings of inferiority or superiority, she is masking the underlying malady, low self-esteem. The behaviors and interaction with a partner will manifest differently, but the root cause is the same. A partner with feelings of inferiority will defer to her partner because she believes he has more rights, is more knowledgeable, or is more deserving. A partner with feelings of superiority will believe she has more rights, knows more, and "is more" than her partner. A critical partner attacks his partner for who she is rather than her behaviors. This type of attack can certainly be construed as emotional abuse of a partner and creates few opportunities for changing the pattern. A partner who feels contempt for his partner can intentionally hurt her with words or actions. A partner exhibiting defensiveness may deny responsibility or make excuses for his actions. If she complains, his complaint will be louder, stronger, worse, one better. He may "dig in" on his position and not see any alternatives. The distancer will put up a wall and shut the other person out with silence. This position inhibits emotional intimacy and keeps the other person "guessing."

A number of warning signs may signal a troubled relationship including an increase in physical symptoms by a partner, an increase in alcohol or drug consumption, silence or emotional withdrawal by a partner, more frequent arguments, more fantasies of separation, or more divergent lives. These signs may manifest in actual behaviors such as a partner's affair, lying or other deceit, inattentiveness, lack of sexual interest, outside influences, and illegal activity. Several of these behaviors and issues are described below.

External Affair All affairs are not alike! Some involve accidental infidelity; others involve romantic infidelity; and, others may be a form of philandering. Some result because expectations were not met; others are viewed as a payback or punishment; whereas others involve emotional intimacy and closeness. The four words, "I'm having an affair," can be a wakeup call or a death knell to relationships. These words and the act itself certainly signal problems in a relationship. Affairs exacerbate the problems that currently exist, and the person isn't necessarily running to something as much as running away from something. The reason most cited as to why a woman has an affair is, "I wanted more warmth and intimacy."

Women often view an external affair by a partner as the ultimate betrayal. It is construed as decep-

tive and violates the commitment between primary partners. Yet, some women are known to seek an extramarital affair. In one study of dating, cohabiting, and married women, the researchers found that the length of a relationship and number of previous partners were positively related to the potential for a secondary sex partner. Women who had four or more sex partners before the current relationship were nearly ten times more likely to have another sex partner. Married women with multiple previous partners were twenty times more likely than their counterparts with no previous partners to have a secondary sex partner. And, as the length of the relationship increased, the potential for a secondary sex partner also increased. They found that cohabiting women were less committed than married women to monogamy.[32]

Nonmonogamy within the relationship, whether heterosexual or lesbian, increases the likelihood of a breakup.[33] Although an affair has the potential to destroy a relationship, it doesn't have to end. The end of an affair can be the new beginning to an existing relationship. The outcome depends on the willingness of both individuals to work through broken expectations.

Money Few people openly discuss their finances or even think about their attitudes toward money before getting seriously involved in a relationship, yet numerous studies show that money is the most discussed issue in heterosexual relationships. Money issues are often a major consideration because the amount of money earned determines power within the relationship. And, power equates with freedom to make important decisions. Blumstein and Schwartz found that the amount of money a person earned, in comparison to her partner, was the major factor in determining relative power in heterosexual, but not lesbian, relationships. They suggested, "Since women in this society are not accustomed to judging their own worth by how much money they make,

love addict—an unhealthy pattern of becoming involved with a partner to mask fear of abandonment.

avoidance addict—an unhealthy pattern of maintaining emotional distance from a partner to mask fear of intimacy.

Viewpoint

Spending Differences Can Impact Relationships

Money conflicts within relationships are common, particularly if expectations differ when it comes to the management and control of money. Money harmony is difficult to maintain, and requires flexibility and communication. Olivia Mellan, author of *Money Harmony: Resolving Money Conflicts in Your Life and Relationships,* calls money harmony "a balanced state in which both partners feel free to spend, save, or invest money in ways that support their deeper desires, values, and sense of themselves."[35] Money harmony can occur only if partners are willing to discuss and explore their beliefs and behaviors related to money. Mellan identified seven common money personality types: spenders, hoarders, avoiders, amassers, money monks, and worriers. Spenders use the slogans "shop till you drop" or "power shopping." This person enjoys spending and has a hard time saving money. Hoarders are the misers, the stingy money savers who put money away for a rainy day. The miser has a strict budget and will not part with her money unless absolutely necessary. Managing money is a difficult, over-whelming task for avoiders. This person waits until the last minute to pay her bills, and often is late with her payments. She is overwhelmed by the concept of budgeting and saving, thus seldom does. Amassers base their self-worth on net worth. An amasser will accumulate money to feel good about herself, and workaholism is common. Money monks view the love of money as the "root of all evil," therefore they tend to give money to socially worthwhile projects or religious endeavors. They seldom accumulate money so as to avoid the temptation of valuing it too highly. Worriers, on the other hand, see money as a scarcity and are extremely cautious. They review the budget and expenditures over and over, looking for corners to cut or making sure to account for every dime. Bingers use money to fill an emotional need, and the "rush" that comes from spending money dissipates with the empty feelings that follow the binge.

Which pattern of money management most describes your behavior? Which pattern does your partner practice?

we feel that lesbians do not fall into judging their partners by such a standard." Lesbians had grown to reject the male-provider philosophy and preferred to equally share financial responsibility. For heterosexuals, power and money differed according to the male-provider philosophy. Married women who accepted the male-provider philosophy had less power in the relationship, regardless of income level between the spouses. In cohabiting couples, money equated with power but these women were more likely to believe that equal contributions were important.[34] (See *Viewpoint:* "Spending Differences Can Impact Relationships.")

The key to resolving money issues in a relationship is understanding your own habits and communicating with your partner regarding the management of money and power within the relationship. A couple must set joint priorities and appreciate the differences that exist in philosophy and patterns of handling money.

Sex   Sexual feelings, desires, and activities are present throughout the life cycle and profoundly shaped by culture. Differences between male and female attitudes toward sex begin early and can be seen from the first sexual encounter. When females are asked about their first sexual encounter, they usually choose to be sexual with someone they like. When males are asked about their first sexual encounter, curiosity is usually the driving force.

Physical intimacy tends to be viewed differently by men and women. Most men view sex as a way to be emotionally intimate, whereas most women want emotional intimacy before they can be sexual. Blumstein and Schwartz found considerable differences among men and women in their sexual patterns. The majority of married couples were having sex at least once a week. Lesbians, on the other hand, were far less sexual than married, cohabiting, or gay male couples, even when compared at each stage of relationship development. But, lesbians were much more active in the amount of physical contact (cuddling, touching, hugging) between partners when compared to other couples. Genital sex was less important to lesbians even though physical intimacy, without sex, was usually an end unto itself.[36]

Keeping physical intimacy alive can be difficult for partners, particularly when schedules get busy, distractions increase, and familiarity and friendship cause the physical and sexual intimacy to wane.

Childrearing and Household Labor Gender is the major criterion used by married couples for the distribution of household tasks and childrearing. Married women do the majority of household tasks and childrearing, estimated at two to three times that of married men. Even in married couples who appear to divide household labor more equally, men do not assume more responsibility but women, in effect, choose to do less. This condition of inequity exists irrespective of education, income, and presence of children. The assigning of tasks based on gender may be efficient but it often relegates women to subordinate roles in the relationship, leading to depression and a sense of powerlessness. Married women who feel relegated to this role and powerless to change it are more likely to experience psychological distress. This sense of inequality can lead to marital distress and in a larger sense, gender inequalities with the relationship (unpaid household labor and child care) may produce gender inequalities outside the relationship.[37] Researchers have found that lesbian couples are more careful to divide household labor equally (maybe because few women enjoy doing these tasks) than married or gay couples.[38,39] This equal sharing of responsibility for menial tasks and sense of personal power in choosing to share the tasks acts as a protective factor in preventing emotional distress.

Inattentiveness Once you enter a committed relationship, you may face a variety of challenges to keeping the attraction alive. One danger you may face in a relationship is getting too busy or too tired to exercise the skills necessary to keep the relationship healthy and functional. These skills include effective communication, such as good listening skills, conflict resolution, and the ability to work toward mutual compromise.

Couples tend to slip into inattentiveness unknowingly, being too busy with taking the kids to soccer, meeting deadlines, or juggling added responsibilities. These demands are conditional real demands on the relationship but if they continue to build, problems can begin. At some time the couple needs to prioritize these demands or the relationship may terminate. Ideally, we need to nurture the relationship on a daily basis the same way we need to nurture ourselves. However, at minimum, specific time must be set aside at least once a week to focus on nurturing the relationship, time to have dinner and talk, enjoy a movie, or engage in mutually enjoyable activities. The key to success is to manage time, rather than letting time manage the partners.

Resolving Conflicts—Fighting Fair

Some experts suggest that how couples fight or handle fundamental disagreements is a major predictor of whether the relationship will last. Robert Levenson and John Gottman have studied numerous couples and monitored physiological responses to determine the impact of the disagreements. They believe that successful couples find a way to put a conflict behind them, whereas troubled couples will leave the argument unresolved, thus eroding the bond that holds them together. They found that couples who had the same fighting style were most successful. The three fighting styles they saw were validators, volatile reactors, and conflict avoiders. Validators would discuss their differences, attempting to understand the other's viewpoint, and strive to reach a compromise. Volatile reactors shouted at each other and attempted to outmaneuver their partner to a position of submission. Conflict avoiders, the least successful of the three types, did everything possible to avoid conflict. When disagreements occurred, they just agreed to disagree, not looking for compromise or a change in stance of the other partner.

In "The Dance of Anger," Harriet Lerner discusses some ineffective techniques women may use to handle anger.[40] These techniques (silent submission, ineffective fighting and blaming, and emotional distancing) can be used by women to keep a relationship harmonious, but often at the expense of authenticity. These patterns may happen during times of stress or overload, and may change depending on the individual with whom you are arguing. The patterns of expressing anger are classified as pursuers, distancers, underfunctioners, and overfunctioners. Pursuers value talking through an issue and want a partner to do the same. They seek closeness when disagreements occur and feel hurt when the other person seeks distance. Distancers want to be left alone, emotionally and physically, when disagreements occur. They attempt to figure things out away from the pressure of the moment. They will address the issue again when they are ready. Underfunctioners appear weak and submissive, fragile, or irresponsible. They fall apart under stress and become disorganized or nonfunctional. They have difficulty appearing competent to those close to them. Overfunctioners are the "fixers" who give advice and move in quickly to resolve a dispute.

Couples can learn to negotiate for their needs in a fair manner. (See *Health Tips:* "Fighting Fair.") The first step in fair fighting requires that both partners agree to engage in the discussion. The partner who is angry should ask her partner if he or she is willing to engage in a fight for change. When they are willing to engage in the discussion, the partner with the complaint should state it clearly and ask for what she needs or wants. When the other person has heard and restated the complaint, she has several options: she can agree to the request, she can ask for clarification, she can offer an alternative, or she can agree to disagree (say no). Successful negotiation occurs

health tips

Fighting Fair

Successful negotiation requires that both partners must:
- Clearly state the problem or complaint
- Agree to discuss the problem or complaint
- Commit to: +Change the pattern
        +Find an acceptable compromise
        +Disagree

when both parties have heard each other and have committed to change the pattern, found an acceptable compromise, or have reached an agreement to disagree.[41] Difficulties arise in all relationships; the difference between successful and unsuccessful resolution is the willingness of both partners to openly share their concerns and negotiate for change.

Chapter Summary

- Statistics suggest that relationships are more difficult to maintain in today's society. Over one-half of all first marriages end in divorce.
- Relationships have undergone a number of changes as gender roles and attitudes have converged.
- Sternberg's triangular theory of love suggests that relationships can be envisioned as the sides of a triangle. The sides include commitment, intimacy, and passion.
- Healthy relationships are characterized by attributes such as trust, respect, honesty, and authenticity.

- Unhealthy relationships are characterized by traits such as self-absorption, jealousy, feelings of inferiority or superiority, and distancing.
- Marriage, cohabitation, same-sex unions, and remarriages are different types of relationships.
- People spend money according to different personality profiles.
- Resolving conflicts by fair fighting is important to the happiness of partners in a relationship.

Review Questions

1. What gender role attributes seem best suited to relationships?
2. What are the differences between individualistic and collective societies?
3. What are the key components of each stage of dating?
4. What is the difference between physical and emotional intimacy?
5. What is consummate love based on Sternberg's theory?
6. What are the lovestyles described by John Alan Lee?

7. What are the differences between vitalized and devitalized marriages?
8. What is a peer marriage?
9. What characteristics do cohabitators share with married couples? with singles?
10. What are some challenges to lesbian couples?
11. What characteristics are exhibited by love addicts? by avoidance addicts?
12. What are the major issues in troubled relationships?

Resources

Organizations and Hotlines

American Association for Marriage and Family Therapy. Telephone: (800) 374-2638

Suggested Readings

Friedan, B. 1986. *Human sex and human politics.* New York: Summit.

Journal of Social Issues. 1993. Vol. 49.

Lerner, H. G. 1989. *The dance of anger: A woman's guide to changing the patterns of intimate relationships.* San Francisco: HarperCollins Publishers.

MacKinnon, C. 1987. *Feminism unmodified: Discourse on life and love.* Cambridge, MA: Harvard University Press.

Mellody, P., A. W. Miller, and J. K. Miller, 1992. *Facing love addiction: Giving yourself the power to change the way you love.* San Francisco: HarperCollins Publishers.

Rich, A. 1977. *The meaning of our love for women or what we constantly need to expand.* New York: Out and Out.

References

1. Peplau, L. A., C. T. Hill, and Z. Rubin. 1993. Sex role attitudes in dating and marriage: A 15-year follow-up of the Boston couples study. *Journal of Social Issues,* 49 (3): 31–52.

2. Antill, J. K. 1983. Sex role complementarily versus similarity in married couples. *Journal of Personality and Social Psychology,* 45: 145–55.

3. Hui, C. H., and H. C. Triandis. 1986. Individualism-collectivism: A study of cross-cultural researchers. *Journal of Cross-Cultural Psychology,* 17: 225–48.

4. Dion, K. K., and K .L. Dion. 1993. Individualistic and collectivistic perspectives of gender and the cultural context of love and intimacy. *Journal of Social Issues,* 49 (3): 53–69.

5. Presented by Michel Ann Fultz, Louisville Center for Adult Children, Louisville, Kentucky, 1996.

6. Adams, G. R. 1982. The physical attractiveness stereotype. In A. G. Miller, ed., *In the eye of the beholder: Contemporary issues in stereotyping.* New York: Praeger Publishers.

7. Berscheid, E. 1985. Interpersonal attraction. In G. Lindzey, and E. Aronson, ed., *Handbook of social psychology.* New York: Random House.

8. Lerner, H. G. 1990. *The dance of intimacy: A woman's guide to courageous acts of change in key relationships.* New York: Harper & Row Publishers, Inc.

9. Sacher, J. A., and M. A. Fine, 1996. Predicting relationship status and satisfaction after six months among dating couples. *Journal of Marriage and the Family,* 58: 21–32.

10. Livermore, B. 1993. The lessons of love. *Psychology Today:* 30–39.

11. Lee, J. A. 1976. *The colors of love.* New York: Prentice Hall.

12. Wallerstein, J. S., and S. Blakeslee. 1995. *The good marriage: How and why love lasts.* Houghton Mifflin.

13. Lavee, Y., and D. H. Olson. 1993. Seven types of marriage: Empirical typology based on ENRICH. *Journal of Marital and Family Therapy,* 19: 325–40.

14. Olson, D. H., D. Fournier, and J. Druckman. 1986. *PREPARE/ENRICH Counselor Manual,* 2nd ed. Minneapolis, MN: PREPARE/ENRICH, Inc.

15. Fowers, B. J., K. H. Montel, and D. H. Olson. 1996. Predicting marital success for premarital couple types based on PREPARE. *Journal of Marital and Family Therapy,* 22: 103–19.

16. Schwartz, P. 1994. Modernizing marriage. *Psychology Today,* 27: 54–59.

17. Bumpass, L. L., J. A. Sweet, and A. J. Cherlin, 1991. The role of cohabitation in declining rates of marriage. *Journal of Marriage and the Family,* 53: 913–27.

18. Ibid.

19. Brown, S. L., and A. Booth. 1996. Cohabitation versus marriage: A comparison of relationship quality. *Journal of Marriage and the Family,* 58: 668–78.

20. Wu, Z. 1996. Childbearing in cohabitational relationships. *Journal of Marriage and the Family,* 58: 281–92.

21. Solsberry, P. W. July, 1994. Interracial couples in the United States of America: Implications for mental health counseling. *Journal of Mental Health Counseling,* 16 (3): 304–17.

22. Besherov, D. J., and T. S. Sullivan. July/August 1996. One flesh: America is experiencing an unprecedented increase in black-white intermarriage. *The New Democrat,* 8 (4): 19–21.

23. Solsberry, Interracial couples in the United States of America.

24. Besherov and Sullivan, One flesh. *The New Democrat.*

25. Blumstein, P., and P. Schwartz. 1983. *American couples: Money, work, sex.* New York: William Morrow and Company, Inc.

26. Tacker, F., and S. Golombok. 1995. Adults raised as children in lesbian families. *American Journal of Orthopsychiatry,* 65: 203–15.

27. DeParle, J. 1994. Census report sees incomes in decline and more poverty. New York Times, p. A16.

28. Mellody, P., A. W. Miller, and J. K. Miller. 1992. *Facing love addiction: Giving yourself the power to change the way you love.* San Francisco: HarperCollins Publishers.

29. Mellody, P., A. W. Miller, and J. K. Miller. 1992. *Facing love addiction: Giving yourself the power to change the way you love.* San Francisco: HarperCollins Publishers.

30. Weingarten, H. R. 1988. The impact of late life divorce: A conceptual and empirical study. *Journal of Divorce,* 12 (1): 21–39.

31. National Center for Health Statistics, Centers for Disease Control and Prevention. October, 1995. *Monthly Vital Statistics,* 43 (13).

32. Forste, R., and K. Tanfer. 1996. Sexual exclusivity among dating, cohabitating, and married women. *Journal of Marriage and the Family,* 58: 33–47.

33. Blumstein and Schwartz, *American couples.*

34. Ibid.

35. Mellan, O. 1994. *Money harmony: Resolving money conflicts in your life and your relationships.* New York: Walker and Company.

36. Blumstein and Schwartz, *American couples.*

37. Major, B. 1993. Gender, entitlement, and the distribution of family labor. *Journal of Social Issues,* 49: 141–59.

38. Blumstein and Schwartz, *American couples.*

39. Kurdek, L. A. 1993. The allocation of household labor in gay, lesbian, and heterosexual married couples. *Journal of Social Issues,* 49: 127–39.

40. Lerner, H. G. 1989. *The dance of anger: A woman's guide to changing the patterns of intimate relationships.* San Francisco: HarperCollins.

41. PAIRS International, Inc. *PAIRS for love—for life: Resolving anger nondestructively.* FL: Pembroke Pines. Info@pairs.org

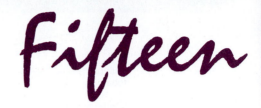

Examining Gynecological Issues

■ chapter objectives

When you complete this chapter you will be able to:
- Describe the female reproductive anatomy.
- Demonstrate the proper breast self-examination technique.
- Describe the phases of the menstrual cycle.
- Recognize the signs and symptoms of toxic shock syndrome.
- Contrast the stages of the female sexual response cycle.
- Explain the advantages and disadvantages of hormone replacement therapy.

FEMALE REPRODUCTIVE ANATOMY

This chapter covers the female reproductive system and the changes you can expect to experience from menarche to menopause. This information is important in raising your level of awareness and understanding about your physical body.

The female reproductive anatomy consists of the external genitals, the internal genitals, and the breasts. The section that follows gives you information about how the female reproductive system works.

External Genitalia

The external genitalia, or **vulva,** refers to those parts that are outwardly visible. The vulva includes the mons pubis, labia majora, labia minora, clitoris, ure-thral opening, vaginal opening, and perineum. Individual differences in size, coloration, and shape of the external genitalia are common. (See Fig. 15.1.)

Mons Pubis The mons pubis is a triangular, mounding area of fatty tissue that covers the pubic bone. It protects the pubic symphysis (the place where the pubic bones join), particularly during intercourse. During adolescence, pubic hair begins to appear on the mons pubis as a result of increased sex hormones. This hair, varying in coarseness, curliness, amount, and thickness, covers the mons and may extend to the navel.

> **vulva**—sometimes referred to as the pudendum; the outer genitals of the female.

FIGURE 15.1 (*A*), Female reproductive structures, side view. (*B*), External view of female genitalia.

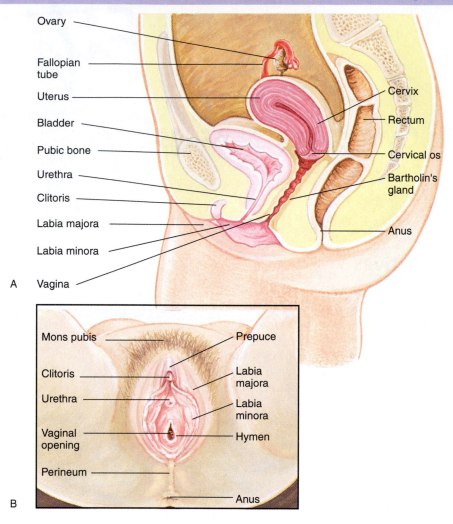

Labels (A): Ovary, Fallopian tube, Uterus, Bladder, Pubic bone, Urethra, Clitoris, Labia majora, Labia minora, Vagina, Cervix, Rectum, Cervical os, Bartholin's gland, Anus

Labels (B): Mons pubis, Clitoris, Urethra, Vaginal opening, Perineum, Prepuce, Labia majora, Labia minora, Hymen, Anus

Labia Majora The **labia majora,** sometimes referred to as the "outer lips," have darker pigmentation. The labia majora protect the vaginal and urethral openings and are covered with hair and sebaceous (oil) glands. The inner surfaces tend to be smooth, moist, and hairless. After childbirth, the labia majora may separate and no longer fully cover the vaginal area. The labia majora become more flaccid as a woman gets older.

Labia Minora The **labia minora,** sometimes referred to as the "inner lips," consist of erectile, connective tissue that darkens and swells during sexual arousal. The labia minora, located inside the labia ma-jora, are more sensitive and responsive to touch than the labia majora. The labia minora tighten to hold the penis in place during intercourse.

Clitoris The **clitoris** is a highly sensitive organ composed of nerves, blood vessels, and erectile tissue. It can be found under the prepuce, clitoral foreskin, by separating the folds of the labia majora. The clitoris consists of a shaft and a glans that becomes engorged with blood during sexual stimulation. It is the key to sexual pleasure for most women, and consequently, some misogynist cultures practice female genital mutilation. (See *Her Story:* "Samyra.")

HEALTHY PEOPLE 2000 OBJECTIVES

- Increase to at least 95 percent the proportion of women aged 18 and older who have ever received a Pap test, and to at least 85 percent those who received a Pap test within the preceding 1 to 3 years. 1995 progress toward goal achieved: 98 percent
- Ensure that Pap tests meet quality standards by monitoring and certifying all cytology laboratories. 1995 progress toward goal achieved: data unavailable
- Reduce the incidence of pelvic inflammatory disease, as measured by a reduction in hospitalizations for pelvic inflammatory disease to no more than 250 per 100,000 women aged 15 to 44. Revised goal: and a reduction in the number of initial visits to physicians for PID to no more than 290,000. 1995 progress toward goal achieved: 189 percent

Her Story

Samyra

Samyra, a 17-year-old fled from her home to escape a ritual mutilation that had been inflicted on the women of her tribe for centuries. After being forced by her relatives to go through a marriage ceremony to a man more than twice her age, Samyra was told that she would have to be "circumcised." She would be held down and her legs spread, while an elder woman of her tribe cut away her clitoris and the labia minora, scraping them to the bone. Her lower extremities would then be bound tightly for 40 days during which her wounds would heal, after which time her new husband would be permitted to have sex with her.[1] The purpose of this practice of female genital mutilation, FGM, was to diminish the pleasure a woman experiences while having sex, thus supposedly decreasing the likelihood of her being sexually promiscuous.

- What other reasons are given for genital mutilation?
- What steps can be taken to encourage countries to change this practice?

Urethral Opening The urethral opening is located directly below the clitoris. It is the opening through which you urinate.

Vaginal Opening The vaginal opening may be covered by a thin sheath called the **hymen.** Hymens vary in size, shape, and thickness, and usually have an opening in the center through which menstrual blood flows. A common myth is that an intact hymen indicates virginity and it breaks during a young woman's first experience with sexual intercourse. Using the presence of an intact hymen for determining virginity is erroneous. The hymen can be perforated by many different events, such as the first menstrual blood, the use of a tampon, strenuous exercise, or some mishap. Some women are born without hymens, and some women retain intact hymens despite several experiences of sexual intercourse.

Perineum The **perineum** is the part of the muscle and tissue located between the vaginal opening and the anal canal. It holds up and surrounds the lower parts of the urinary and digestive tracts. The perineum contains an abundance of nerve endings that make it sensitive to touch. A common practice in Western medicine is to perform an **episiotomy,**

an incision of the perineum, for widening the vaginal opening for purposes of birth. Some women's advocates and health-care personnel challenge the need for this practice, suggesting that the incision actually contributes to further tearing.

labia majora—two folds of skin, one on each side of the vaginal opening.

labia minora—two folds of skin between the labia majora, from the clitoris to the vaginal opening.

clitoris—pea-shaped projection made up of nerves, blood vessels, and erectile tissue.

hymen—fold of mucous membrane, skin, and fibrous tissue covering the vaginal opening.

perineum (per **inee** em)—part of body between inner thighs.

episiotomy (ee **pease** ee **ott** uh me)—surgical procedure to lengthen the vaginal opening during childbirth.

Internal Genitalia

The internal genitalia consist of the vagina, cervix, uterus, fallopian (uterine) tubes, and the ovaries. (See Fig. 15.1.)

Vagina The **vagina** connects the cervix to the outer body and lies between the bladder and rectum. The vaginal canal serves three important functions. First, the menstrual flow and uterine secretions pass through the vagina to the vaginal opening. Second, the vagina serves as the birth canal during labor and can expand during childbirth to several inches in width. Third, the vagina is lubricated by two Bartholin's glands, to receive the penis during sexual intercourse.

A common myth is that the size of a penis contributes to sexual satisfaction. In reality, the vagina expands to accommodate the size of any penis. Another myth is that a penis may become trapped within the vagina. In fact, unlike animals with a bone in the penis, a male's penis becomes flaccid after ejaculation and cannot be trapped in the vagina.

Cervix The **cervix** is the portion of the uterus that protrudes into the vaginal cavity. The cervical opening to the vagina is small, thus preventing tampons and other objects from entering the uterus. During childbirth, the cervix dilates to accommodate the passage of the fetus. The dilation of the cervix is an early sign that labor has begun.

Uterus The **uterus** is often described as being pear-shaped and about the size of a clenched fist. The powerful muscles of the uterus expand to accommodate a growing fetus and contract strongly to begin the birth process and push the fetus through the birth canal. The **endometrium,** the complex, inner lining of cells, consists of blood-enriched tissue that sloughs off each month during the menstrual flow if fertilization does not occur.

Fallopian Tubes The fallopian tubes, or oviducts, serve as a pathway for the ovum (egg) to the uterus and as the site of fertilization, typically in the upper third of a fallopian tube. The sperm travels through the vagina, cervix, and uterus to fertilize the egg in the fallopian tube. The fertilized egg takes approximately 6 to 10 days to travel through the fallopian tube to implant in the uterine lining.

Ovaries The **ovaries** are the female gonads (sex glands) that develop and expel an ovum each month. A woman is born with approximately 400,000 immature eggs called follicles. Very few of these follicles reach full maturity; about 400 to 500 are developed and released for reproducing during your lifetime. The follicles in the ovaries produce the female sex hormones, progesterone and estrogen, which are important in preparing the uterus for the implantation of a fertilized egg.

Breasts

The breasts function as organs of sexual arousal, contain the mammary glands that nourish a newborn baby, and consist of connective tissue that serves as support. Each breast contains 15 to 25 clusters called lobes, which have smaller sections called lobules. Lobes and lobules are connected by ducts opening into the nipple. The ducts join together to form ampulla, the collecting sacs located just behind the nipple. The nipples, composed of erectile tissue, become temporarily erect with cold temperature, sexual stimulation, or lactation. The pigmented portion around the nipple of each breast is called the areola, which usually darkens during pregnancy and in women who have had children. The core of the nipple is the opening of the 15 to 25 ducts and contains sebaceous glands that keep the nipple lubricated during breast-feeding. Figure 15.2 shows the structures of the breast. The supporting structure of the breasts is connective tissue, composed mainly of collagen, a material that also makes up bone and tendons.

Breast size is determined primarily by heredity and depends on the existing amount of fat and glandular tissue. Breasts may exhibit cyclical changes, including increased swelling and tenderness just before menstruation.

Benign Breast Changes Benign breast changes are sometimes referred to as fibrocystic disease, a catchall phrase for any signs or symptoms not related to breast cancer. Women can have cyclic periods of pain, tenderness, and swelling in the breast tissue, particularly during the 1 to 2 weeks before menstruation. These symptoms can occur concurrently with lumps or masses of overgrown breast tissue. Benign (noncancerous) breast changes are most common in the upper-outer quadrant of the breasts,

FIGURE 15.2 Structures of the breast.

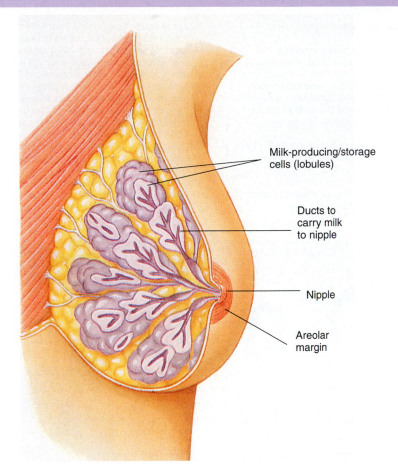

Milk-producing/storage
cells (lobules)

Ducts to
carry milk
to nipple

Nipple

Areolar
margin

followed by the lower-outer quadrant of the breasts. Many women, nearly 70 percent, experience benign breast changes, that is, breast lumps, pain, tenderness, or nipple discharge during the menstrual cycle. Remember, 85 to 90 percent of lumps are benign. Only your health-care provider can determine whether the mass is benign or malignant.

Breast Self-Examination Women can take a proactive approach to detect possible breast cancer in its early stages by examining their breasts monthly. Figure 15.3 shows the breast self-examination (BSE) technique recommended by the American College of Obstetricians and Gynecologists. Monthly breast self-examination is important, not only as a supplement to

vagina—part of female genitals that form a canal from the vaginal opening to the cervix.

cervix—part of the uterus that protrudes into the vaginal opening.

uterus—pear-shaped female organ of reproduction in which the ovum implants and develops.

endometrium (en doe **me** tree um)—mucous membrane lining the uterus.

ovaries— reproductive organs found on each side of the lower abdomen beside the uterus.

FIGURE 15.3 Breast self-examination.

The following explains how to do a breast self-examination.

1. *In the shower:* Examine your breasts during a bath or shower; hands glide more easily over wet skin. With your fingers flat, move gently over every part of each breast. Use your right hand to examine the left breast, your left hand to examine the right breast. Check for any lump, hard knot, or thickening. This self-examination should be done monthly, preferably a day or two after the end of your menstrual period.
2. *Before a mirror:* Inspect your breasts, with arms at your sides. Next, raise your arms high overhead. Look for any changes in contour of each breast, swelling, dimpling of skin, and changes in the nipple. Then rest your palms on your hips and press down firmly to flex your chest muscles. The left and right breasts will not match exactly—few women's breasts do.

3. *Lying down:* To examine your right breast, put a pillow or folded towel under your right shoulder. Place your right hand behind your head—this distributes breast tissue more evenly on the chest. With your left hand, fingers flat, press gently in small circular motions around an imaginary clock face. Begin at the outermost top of your right breast for 12 o'clock, then move to 1 o'clock, and so on around the circle back to 12 o'clock. A ridge of firm tissue in the lower curve of each breast is normal. Then move in an inch toward the nipple; keep circling to examine every part of your breast, including the nipples. This requires at least three more circles. Now slowly repeat the procedure on your left breast, with a pillow under your left shoulder and your left hand behind your head. Notice how your breast structure feels. Finally, squeeze the nipple of each breast gently between your thumb and index finger. Any discharge, clear or bloody, should be reported to your doctor immediately.

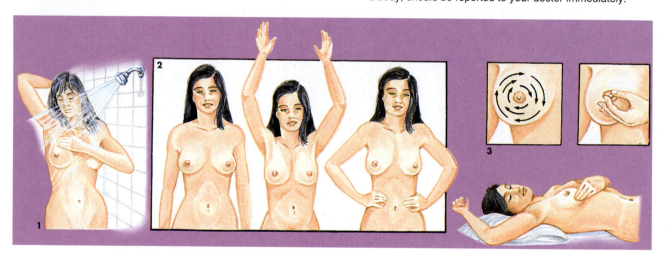

clinical breast examination and mammography, but for raising your level of awareness regarding changes that could be abnormal. Breast self-examination should be conducted on a regular basis so you become familiar with the shape and feel of your breasts. If a change occurs (lumps, dimpling changes, skin irregularities, or nipple discharge), you will recognize it immediately and should contact your health-care provider! Now complete *Journal Activity:* "Daily Breast Self-Examination."

The best time for you to conduct BSE is about a week after menstruation, because breasts are less tender at this time. Women who are postmenopausal may choose the first day of each month or a special date, such as your birthday or anniversary date of every month.

MENSTRUATION

Menarche

Menarche is a central focus of body politics. It draws attention to the female body and signifies movement from girlhood to womanhood. "Menarche is a physiological happening, framed by the biomedical metaphors of current scientific knowledge, yet also a gendered sexualized happening, a transition to womanhood as objectified other."[2]

Menarche sets the stage for how a young woman perceives her sexuality. Most young girls anticipate their first menstrual cycle (**menarche**) with a range of emotions from fear, disgust, and embarrassment to joy and excitement. Indeed, researchers have suggested that a young woman's attitude toward menstruation is influenced and shaped by how the media, popular culture, and others portray it.[3]

The preadolescent's body begins to change around age 10 or 11. She may experience an increase in body hair, the beginning of breast development, and her hips begin to get larger. She also may experience a growth spurt of several inches at this time. Over the past century, a decrease of about 3 to 4 months in age of onset of menstruation has occurred every decade. Currently, the average age is 12.8 and this age appears to have stabilized. The onset of menstruation is affected by a number of factors including genetic factors, socioeconomic conditions, nutritional status, and in some cases, exercise regimens. Record your personal recollections of your menarche in *Journal Activity:* "Your Recollection of Menarche."

The menstrual cycle consists of four phases: the follicular phase during which the egg matures in the ovaries, the ovulatory phase during which the mature egg is released by the ovary, the luteal phase during which the empty follicle becomes the corpus luteum and the endometrium prepares for a fertilized egg, and the menstrual phase when the endometrium is sloughed off due to the unfertilized egg. The amount of bleeding varies from woman to woman, and the expulsion of blood clots (pooled blood in the vagina) is common. The blood can vary in color from bright red to dark brown, usually lasts from 3 to 5 days and usually occurs every 25 to 32 days. (See Fig. 15.4.) Some women experience little discomfort, whereas others have fluid retention, cramping, mood swings, weight gain, breast tenderness, diarrhea, and constipation.

Sex Hormones Although a number of hormones are involved in the menstrual cycle, we primarily think of four sex hormones: follicle stimulating hormone (FSH) and luteinizing hormone (LH), which are produced by the pituitary gland, and estrogen and progesterone, which are produced by the follicles in the ovaries. The follicles produce estrogen throughout the entire menstrual cycle. Estrogen stimulates the endometrium to grow a thick layer of tissue each month for preparation of a fertilized egg. Progesterone, produced during the second half of the menstrual cycle, contributes to further thickening of the endometrium and if the egg is not fertilized, the levels of both hormones decline. This drop in estrogen and progesterone levels signals the endometrium to be shed during the menstrual period. FSH rises in response to low levels of estrogen and decreases as the follicle produces estrogen. However, high levels of estrogen during ovulation cause a temporary surge in FSH. Luteinizing hormone (LH) is present as the mature egg leaves the follicle and causes a structural change that becomes the corpus luteum. The sharp rise in LH during the menstrual cycle signals ovulation and the presence of LH is important for maturation and release of the follicle. The corpus luteum produces progesterone until it reaches a certain level that signals the pituitary gland to stop producing luteinizing hormone.

menarche—the onset of menstruation.

FIGURE 15.4 The menstrual cycle: As an egg matures in the ovary, the lining of the uterus prepares to receive a fertilized egg. The egg is released during ovulation (approximately day 14). If not fertilized, the lining is shed during the menstrual period.

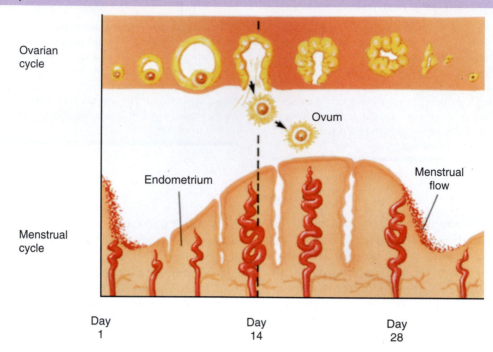

Ovarian cycle

Ovum

Endometrium

Menstrual flow

Menstrual cycle

Day 1   Day 14   Day 28

Dysmenorrhea

Dysmenorrhea is the medical term that describes painful menstrual cramps, the most cited reason for missing school or lost workdays for young women. Although most women occasionally experience menstrual cramps, 5 to 10 percent of women will experience painful, incapacitating cramps for several hours to a couple of days. Primary **dysmenorrhea,** painful menses without evidence of a physical abnormality, is believed to be a normal body response to uterine contractions resulting from enhanced production of prostaglandins. Prostaglandins cause the forceful, frequent uterine contractions associated with the pain of menses. A number of other symptoms may occur including nausea, vomiting, gastrointestinal disturbances, and fainting. Some women can alleviate painful cramps with OTC medications such as ibuprofen (Advil, Nuprin, and Motrin IB), with drugs designed specifically for menstrual symptoms (Midol, Pamprin), or with prescription nonsteroidal antiinflammatory drugs such as Naproxyn or Indocin. Other measures a young woman can take include exercising, cutting down on salt to reduce fluid retention, or resting if fatigued. Secondary dysmenorrhea

is usually due to anatomic abnormalities such as a congenital abnormality of the uterus, presence of fibroids or endometrial polyps, an IUD, pelvic inflammatory disease, or endometriosis.

Endometriosis Endometriosis is a common cause of dysmenorrhea, dyspareunia (painful intercourse), and infertility in women. **Endometriosis** occurs when the lining of the endometrium fragments and lodges in other parts of the body. It most commonly lodges in the pelvic cavity, on the uterosacral ligaments, on the ovaries, fallopian tubes, and supporting broad ligaments. The fragments build up tissue each month and then break down and bleed, causing inflammation, scarring, and adhesions. Treatment of endometriosis includes hormonal therapy, laparoscopic surgery, and major surgical management, depending upon the needs of the woman.[4] Treatment may alleviate the symptoms, but removal of endometrial tissue does not mean a woman is cured. Chronic endometriosis can be frustrating and disabling for women. The etiology of endometriosis remains unknown so scientists are continuing to explore the causes and experiment with drugs to reduce the symptoms.

Her Story

Shelly

Shelly, a 5'9", 110 pound, Division I volleyball player, remembers the first time she dropped weight. It was the summer after her sophomore year and a new coach had been hired. She reported for the first practice and hadn't even attempted her first set to a teammate when he yelled, "Shelly, you're slow. What took you so long? Have you always weighed this much? I don't want a setter who can't move!"

Shelly remembers how embarrassed she felt! No one had ever said anything about her weight before and she was faster than anyone else on the team when it came to sprints. She had even lifted weights all summer, was feeling strong, and was looking forward to the season. Doubt began to creep into her thinking. Maybe she was too fat! Maybe he was right!

Shelly had only known success until now. She had been a standout setter during high school, was heavily recruited by top universities, and had easily transitioned to college volleyball because she and the coach clicked. They understood each other! She couldn't believe it when her coach accepted another position.

Then the university hired a high-profile coach, and she decided to stay. Shelly not only excelled in sports, she was a top-notch student. She had a 4.0 G.P.A. in political science and planned to attend law school. If this coach wanted her to drop weight, she would! If he thought she'd be a better setter at a lower weight, she'd do whatever it took to excel. She dropped 15 pounds in a month, going from 125 to 110 pounds. She stayed after practice and ran sprints. She dropped to 1000 calories a day and didn't eat meat anymore. She thought the laxatives were helping too! She still felt fat and slow, and had not menstruated in six months.

The coach noticed that Shelly seemed fatigued during practice. Her performance seemed to be slipping, she was moving more slowly to the ball. He thought Jamie, an incoming freshman, might earn the starting position.

- What are the warning signs that indicate Shelly was suffering from the Female Athlete Triad?
- What would you say to her if you were her friend?

Amenorrhea

It is not unusual for women to miss some periods during their lifetime because menstruation is tied to emotional, biological, and environmental conditions. Primary **amenorrhea** indicates a significant physical disorder characterized by delayed puberty, the failure to menstruate by age 16 or lack of menses by age 14 along with the absence of secondary characteristics such as breast and increased body hair development. Secondary amenorrhea is failure to menstruate for more than six months after prior establishment of menstruation. Some missed periods are quite normal, such as after childbirth or after discontinuing birth control pills. The most common cause of amenorrhea in premenopausal women is pregnancy or the onset of menopause.

Female Athlete Triad The prevalence of amenorrhea by young female athletes, particularly dancers, gymnasts, and long-distance runners, has received considerable media attention. The Female Athlete Triad is identified as disordered eating, amenorrhea, and osteoporosis.

The combination of restrictive eating, excessive training, extreme stress, and low body fat percentage all predispose a female athlete to amenorrhea. A young, elite athlete who participates in sports for which appearance or low body fat are advantageous is at greatest risk. (See *Her Story:* "Shelly.") The endocrine profile of this athlete may show an estrogen deficit similar to menopausal women. This profile has implications for infertility, premature osteoporosis, disordered eating, and poor psychological well-being.[5] Some studies suggest that up to 60 percent of

---

dysmenorrhea—pain associated with menstruation.

endometriosis—chronic growth of endometrial tissue outside the uterus; can be painful and debilitating.

amenorrhea (a men or **ee** ah)—absence of a monthly menstrual flow.

→ **h e a l t h   t i p s**

Toxic Shock Syndrome

The following are warning signs and symptoms of toxic shock syndrome. If you experience these symptoms, remove the tampon and contact your physician *immediately*.

■ Sudden fever over 102 degrees Fahrenheit
■ Vomiting
■ Diarrhea
■ Dizziness
■ Fainting or near fainting
■ A rash that looks like a sunburn

young female athletes have episodes of amenorrhea compared to 2 to 5 percent of the general female population.[6]

Toxic Shock Syndrome

Toxic shock syndrome (TSS) is a rare and sometimes fatal disease that usually affects menstruating, young women who use highly absorbent tampons. The best protection against TSS is using sanitary napkins. If you choose to use tampons, you can protect yourself by changing tampons frequently (every 4 to 6 hours), avoiding super absorbent tampons, and alternating tampons with sanitary napkins.

Knowing the signs and symptoms of TSS can save your life. If you experience the symptoms found in *Health Tips:* "Toxic Shock Syndrome," immediately remove the tampon and contact a health-care provider.

PELVIC EXAMINATION AND PAP TEST

Pelvic Examination

Regular screening with a pelvic examination and Pap test is important for any sexually active woman. A pelvic examination should be conducted annually for 3 consecutive years for all women who are or have been sexually active or are over age 18. If the results are negative, less frequent examinations can be conducted at your discretion in consultation with your health-care provider. Women with a history of abnormal Pap smears or who have been treated for cervical abnormalities should be screened every 2 to 4 months for 1 to 2 years and then annually. Women who have had hysterectomies for treatment of a malignant lesion should be screened annually to ensure that a tumor has not recurred. Women at high risk for cervical cancer due to HPV or HIV infections, cigarette smoking, or sexual activity with multiple partners should be screened annually.[7]

The pelvic examination includes a visual screening to ensure that the reproductive organs look normal in size, shape, and location, a Pap test to screen for cervical cancer, and a bimanual check of the ovaries, fallopian tubes, and uterus. The health-care provider visually checks the vaginal area for signs of herpes, tumors, or genital warts. She then gently inserts a speculum into the vagina to view and check the internal organs for normalcy. It is helpful if you can remain relaxed during the examination. Many women feel embarrassed or get uptight about the pelvic examination, but relaxing the stomach and vaginal muscles makes the pelvic examination easier. A Pap test and then a bimanual examination follow the visual examination. The bimanual examination requires the health-care provider to place two gloved fingers (with lubricating jelly) into the vagina to feel for abnormalities in the ovaries and uterus, followed by a rectal examination. She checks for tumors, tenderness to the area, and the location of the organs.

Pap Test

The Pap test is a standard part of any pelvic examination. The best time to have a Pap test is 10 to 14 days after the first day of the last menstrual period. Avoid using douches or lubricants for 48 hours before the examination. The Pap test is conducted by taking a sample of cells from the cervical area called the squamocolumnar epithelium. This area is the site where 90 percent of all cervical cancers begin. The speculum separates the vaginal walls and exposes the cervical opening. A flat stick called a spatula is used to scrape some cells from the part of the cervix that protrudes into the vagina, and then the cells are smeared onto a slide. Another sample is also taken from the endocervical canal, wiped onto another slide, and then the speculum is removed.[8] Both slides with samples are sent to a lab for analysis. (See *FYI:* "Laboratory Errors.") Sometimes, a woman will spot blood after a pelvic examination; this is normal and does not require treatment unless the area remains tender.

Until recently, health-care providers relied on the Pap test to reveal any cellular abnormalities such

Laboratory Errors

In 1987, the *Wall Street Journal* broke a story about Pap test mills and exposed the practice by some laboratories of reading and recording high numbers of Pap results. They also reported that some cytotechnologists were reading as many as 35,000 slides a year, despite recommendations by the American Society of Cytotechnology that no technologist read more than 12,000 slides a year. The Clinical Laboratories Improvement Act, enforced by the Department of Health and Human Services, is designed to provide quality control of laboratories. Unfortunately, some labs push their workers to read more tests, more quickly than recommended.[9]

The best method of ensuring that your sample is read in a quality lab is to take control of your Pap test. Choose a health-care provider who is experienced in taking the Pap test because correctly taken samples reduces the chance of false negatives. Ask her if she has a choice about where the lab work is done, if it is done locally, and if your insurance company allows her to choose the lab. Schedule regular Pap tests because cervical cancer is slow growing and your risk is reduced by having Pap tests done more frequently. ∞

as HPV infection. Health-care providers now use the ViraPap® test as an adjunct to the Pap test to detect HPV. Test accuracy of the ViraPap® for genital HPV is almost 95 percent. If the test results are positive, a woman has an increased risk of developing precancerous lesions. Further tests will most likely be conducted to determine if cervical cancer is present.

The primary purpose for having a Pap test is to detect precancerous or cancerous lesions. Cervical cancer develops slowly and is nearly 100 percent curable if detected when localized. A minute or two of discomfort (whether emotionally or physically) is well worth the benefit of early detection. A woman's failure to undergo an annual examination is more common than a failure by the physician to obtain an accurate smear or the cytotechnologist to misread a slide. The most important preventive measure is to comply with the American Cancer Society and National Cancer Institute guidelines for annual pelvic examinations.

PREMENSTRUAL SYNDROME

Premenstrual syndrome (PMS) is a politically charged issue. Some women question whether this is another medicalization of a woman's normal cyclical pattern. The disorder was officially recognized in the medical literature in 1931, was labeled PMS in 1953, and gained notoriety in the 1980s when several women committed violent acts attributed to the PMS syndrome. Medically, PMS is recognized as a disorder with an array of physical and psychological symptoms associated with the luteal phase or the second half of menstruation. It has no known etiology despite a plethora of studies. See *Viewpoint:* "PMS."

The best approach to dealing with PMS symptoms is to alleviate them through noninvasive strategies such as relaxation techniques, biofeedback, nutritional changes, and exercise. Suggested nutritional changes include vitamin and mineral supplements, reducing salt intake, eliminating caffeine and refined sugar, and increasing foods that are high in fiber and complex carbohydrates. Medications can help alleviate most premenstrual abdominal cramping, headaches, nausea, vomiting, and diarrhea. A health-care provider can work closely with a woman experiencing PMS to alleviate discomforting symptoms. In rare instances, severe emotional symptoms may require antidepressant or antianxiety medication.

Most symptoms of PMS taper off with menstruation although some women continue to experience symptoms throughout the period. Changes in symptoms of PMS can be attributed to factors such as aging, childbearing, and menopause. Now complete *Assess Yourself:* "Physical and Emotional Symptoms and PMS" to determine which symptoms you experience.

Some researchers believe that the cyclical trigger for biochemical events contributing to PMS are due to normal ovarian function, not imbalances in hormones, prostaglandin, vitamins, or minerals. Suppressing the

toxic shock syndrome (TSS)—severe and sudden infectious disease, most commonly found in menstruating women using high absorbing tampons.

premenstrual syndrome (PMS)—nervous tension, irritability, etc., that occur a few days before menstruation.

PMS: Mental Illness or Normal Behavior?

A recent decision by the American Psychiatric Association to define premenstrual dysphoric disorder (PMDD) has sparked controversy. The APA has defined PMDD as bouts of marked premenstrual depressed mood, anxiety, sadness, or anger that occur one week before menses and impair a woman socially or occupationally. The definition is currently located in the appendix of the Diagnostic and Statistical Manual of Mental Disorders (DSM-IV), meaning further research will be conducted.

Feminists voiced concern that normal behavior (anger, sadness) may be labeled inappropriately or ex-

plained away as "that time of month." They believe that a condition that exists normally for most women should not be labeled as "clinically pathological." Young girls may use PMS as an excuse for mood swings, rather than deal with their core issues. On the other hand, approximately 3 to 5 percent of women experience emotional or physical symptoms that feel debilitating. Further debate and research regarding PMS may help answer some of these questions. What do you think about PMS? Does it exist? Is it a clinically pathological disorder? What criteria would you use to define it?[10]

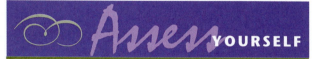

Physical and Emotional Symptoms and PMS

Over 150 symptoms have been associated with PMS, a disorder that women can experience 1 to 2 weeks before menstruation. Listed below are some common symptoms associated with PMS. Keep a daily diary of the changes in your physical and emotional state for 2 to 3 months. Record any of the following symptoms you experience before menstruation:

acne, anxiety, depression, dizziness, fatigue, eating disorders, headaches, irritability, panic, swelling, rashes, nausea, weight gain, hives, breast swelling, irregular heartbeats, joint pain, mood swings, muscle aches, paranoia, gastrointestinal symptoms, water retention, food cravings, moodiness, insomnia, withdrawal, sadness, crying, impatience, overreactivity, self-criticism, extreme sensitivity, distractibility, indecision, suicide ideation, and violence.

- Did you experience any other symptoms during your menstrual cycle?
- Do you practice any nutritional or health behaviors to alleviate these symptoms?
- What other suggestions might you try?

symptoms. Psychotropic drugs, particularly serotonin uptake inhibitors, have provided encouraging results.[11]

Nearly half of women with PMS have symptoms unrelated to a cycle dependent pattern. Health-care providers diagnose PMS by eliminating other coexisting medical disorders and charting symptoms through several consecutive menstrual cycles. Symptoms that consistently occur during the second half of the menstrual cycle may be caused by PMS and these symptoms can increase with age before tapering off after menopause.

A 1993 preliminary research study of 100 women who had been treated at a PMS clinic determined that only 44 percent actually met the criteria for PMS. Thirteen percent of the women actually met the criteria for a psychiatric disorder and half of them had been diagnosed with PMS. The authors suggested that standardization of the diagnostic criteria needed to occur.[12] If you feel as though PMS is causing emotional or physical trauma in your life, you must work closely with your health-care provider to find the best course of treatment.

HUMAN SEXUAL RESPONSE CYCLE

The human sexual response cycle was first described by Havelock Ellis and later elaborated on by Alfred Kinsey and colleagues.[13,14] It is the research of William Masters and Virginia Johnson that remains the most cited when it comes to discussion of the human sexual response cycle. With the ex-

ovulatory function of the ovaries, either through prescription drugs or surgery, may effect change in symptoms. Other researchers point to a deficiency in serotonin as a contributing factor to psychological

ception of Kinsey's study, little, if any, empirical research has been conducted regarding the physiological response of women during orgasm. Masters and Johnson reported their controversial findings in their book, *Human Sexual Responses*.[15] Several key findings from their report are that unlike men, women experience a variety of differing orgasmic responses, they could experience multiple orgasms, and that physiologically, organs are the same regardless of whether initiated by penile penetration or masturbation.

They determined that the human sexual response cycle include four predictable phases: excitement, plateau, orgasm, and resolution. The sexual response cycle follows a pattern through the four stages with individual variability in duration and intensity. Figure 15.5 shows the human sexual response cycle experienced by women.

Orgasms

Can a woman fake an orgasm? We need look no further than the restaurant scene from *When Harry Met Sally* to realize that indeed, it is possible for a woman to fake an orgasm. Unlike men, for which ejaculation is the visible sign of an orgasm, signs may be undetectable in women and uterine contractions may be minimal.

Why does a woman fake an orgasm? Women give a variety of different responses to this question. Some women fake an orgasm because they want their partner to believe that the experience was mutually satisfying. They believe the partner's ego is tied to performance and they want to give the impression that everything was great. Some women fake an orgasm because they don't believe they have a right to take an active role in getting their sexual needs met. Others don't have adequate information to know that stimulation of the clitoris is important for their sexual satisfaction. In heterosexual relationships, some women may hold the socially stereotypic image of the male as actor (dominant), and the female as receiver (submissive). They may fake an orgasm because they really don't want to be sexual and they just want to get it over. They may have been taught that having sex is their duty, and that keeping him happy is important at all costs. Do you remember your responses to the androgyny scale? If you scored high on feminine and low on masculine, you may still be holding stereotypic beliefs. What other reasons might women give for faking an orgasm?

Some reasons for faking orgasms are more bothersome than others, especially if the partner's desires are viewed as more important than your own desires. Sexual behavior entails mutual respect and desire, and has nothing to do with sexual needs. If sex were a necessary physiological need, society would be more accepting of masturbation and less tolerant of celibacy.

Can all women experience orgasm? It is impossible to say that all women can experience orgasm, but it is true that more women would experience orgasms (including multiple orgasms) if her partner knew how to provide adequate stimulation. Inhibited female orgasm is the term used to describe the persistent delay or absence of orgasm. Researchers have proposed a variety of reasons why women may not experience orgasms. The inability to have an orgasm is rarely related to a physical cause, unless alcohol or medications are involved.

Most anorgasmic experiences have psychological and sociological roots or can be caused by a lack of proper technique. Some women may not feel comfortable expressing their needs and desires, and expect their partners to know what to do to satisfy them. Feeling comfortable enough to communicate openly with your partner during sexual interactions is extremely important. Most women need continuous clitoral stimulation to experience an orgasm, otherwise they stay in the plateau phase without adequate sexual tension to create an orgasm. Some women experience guilt, shame, or feelings of being "bad" as a result of strict religious upbringing. They also may have experienced socialization in stereotypical beliefs about the feminine role, such as submissive, pleasing, and passive. These sociological and psychological experiences can be a source of inhibited female orgasm. Most women can experience orgasm with adequate stimulation, whether through masturbation, mutual masturbation, or intercourse.

Aging and Sexual Response

The aging process brings physiological changes in the human sexual response cycle. Physiologically, the excitement phase takes longer because it takes more time to lubricate the vaginal area. The orgasmic phase is shorter in duration and contractions may be less intense. And, the resolution phase has also been found to be longer.[16]

Psychologically, sexual desire continues throughout the lifespan. Studies suggest that sexual activity

FIGURE 15.5   Female sexual response cycle.

Excitement   Vaginal lubrication begins within 10 to 15 seconds of stimulation. Labia majora and minora darken. Clitoris engorges with blood, and increases in size and length. Uterus and cervix pull away from the vagina. Breasts swell and nipples become erect. Sexual tension heightens. Sex flush (darkening of the skin) may occur.

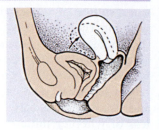

Plateau   Vagina continues to expand and outer third fills with blood. Uterus elevates into abdomen. Tenting (distending of inner two-thirds of vagina) takes place. Cervix elevates. Clitoris retracts under clitoral hood. Secretion occurs from Bartholin's glands. Breasts continue to enlarge and areola engorge with blood. Sex flush may continue and spread.

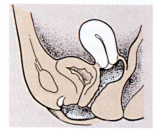

Orgasm   Rhythmic contractions (3–15) of uterine walls, first 3–6 are most intense. Involuntary muscle spasms. Clitoris remains retracted under clitoral hood. Vasocongestion and myotonia (muscle tension) release. Respiration and heart rate increase frequency. Blood pressure increases.

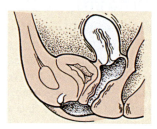

Resolution   Vasocongestion and myotonia dissipate rapidly. Vaginal color returns shortly. Uterus returns to unaroused state. Labia majora and minora return to normal size and shape. Swelling of breasts disappears.

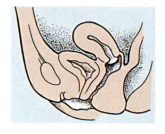

of older men is greater than older women, usually because opportunities remain higher for older men. Opportunities for sexual encounters appear to be increasing for women as retirement communities bring retirees in closer physical proximity. Physiological changes during the aging process will cause men and women to need longer periods of stimulation during sexual interaction, but enjoyment of sexual activity throughout the lifespan is certainly possible.

MENOPAUSE

Menopause is one of the hottest women's health topics as the baby boomer generation comes of age. An unprecedented number of American women, about 1.25 million annually, are experiencing menopause. This generation of women has grown up believing that informed decisions are based on adequate information. They want answers to questions that previously have not been asked. They want to know what to expect physiologically and psychologically as they go through this next life transition. This generation has removed the shroud of secrecy around a number of health topics, from breast cancer to menopause.

Menopause, physiologically speaking, is the time when ovulation and menstruation cease but, more commonly, is referred to as the period from perimenopause to postmenopause. Menopause can also be viewed positively as the life stage when women have more time to be creative and autonomous, to evaluate prior life choices, and to plan for future choices.

Perimenopause

Perimenopause is the period of time, often 3 to 7 years before menopause, during which the menstrual cycles become irregular and hot flashes may occur. One of the earliest signs of perimenopause is irregular bleeding. A woman may skip one or two periods, she may experience lighter or heavier menstrual flow, or the length of her period may be shorter or longer than usual. **Hot flashes** often accompany irregular bleeding. Some women refer to them as "power surges," a sudden burst of intense heat. Hot flashes are a feeling of warmth with corresponding flushing, profuse sweating, and even tremors or shaking in some women. Hot flashes alter skin and core temperature, and precede increases in LH and FSH. One recognized benefit of hormone replacement therapy or birth control pills is the elimination of hot flashes by regulating hormone levels. Women may prefer to explore more natural strategies such as nutritional products (soy products and *dong quai*) and exercise.

Hormone Replacement Therapy

Hormone replacement therapy (HRT) is quickly becoming another political, as well as medical, issue. Today, a woman has to assess whether HRT is appropriate based on her genetic background, medical history, and political beliefs. Women who look for research to give them a definitive answer will be disappointed. The data is incomplete and often statistically flawed, especially for the questions she may want to have answered. Does she need HRT to prevent premature heart disease or osteoporosis? Does progestin in combination with estrogen produce the same protection against heart disease and osteoporosis as estrogen alone? Can she accept the increased risks of endometrial and breast cancer caused by HRT? Does she view menopause as an estrogen-deficient disease or a natural process? She may ask, "If menopause is a natural occurrence, why would a normally healthy woman subject herself to a lifetime of medication?" Answers to these questions are not easy to find. Also, menopause is more than physiological changes. This marks a life transition and very few studies have looked at the social and psychological changes that occur during this mid-life developmental period. Most studies, whether biomedical or psychological, discuss only the negative aspects of menopause.[17]

A 1993 Gallup poll found that only 15 percent of postmenopausal women were on HRT, although a *U.S. News and World Report* stated that the number of American women between ages 45 to 64 on HRT increased nearly 30 percent between 1990 and 1993, from 5.8 million to 7.4 million women.[18] According to Wyeth-Agerst Lab, the five-year increment of number of prescriptions written for estrogen supplements increased from 12 million in 1980, 17 million in 1985, 30 million in 1990, and 48 million in 1993.

The debate about whether to use HRT accelerated after the results of the Nurses Health Study were published. Researchers found that women on *estrogen replacement therapy (ERT)* reduced their risk of heart disease by nearly 50 percent. Estrogen enhanced the cholesterol profile in women by lowering total cholesterol, elevating HDL cholesterol, and lowering LDL cholesterol. Estrogen appeared to relax the coronary arteries, thus reducing the likelihood of spasm (variant angina) and high blood pressure. When taken for at least 7 years, estrogen appeared to reduce the risk of fractures due to osteoporosis. And, estrogen maintained the vitality of the skin, hair, and nails.[18] These results led many women and their physicians to view HRT as a wonder drug. (See Table 15.1.)

---

menopause—the end of ovulation and menstruation.

perimenopause—decline in monthly hormonal cycles before menopause.

hot flashes—short periods of extreme warmth experienced by some women around the time of menopause.

On the other hand, some researchers cautioned that HRT alone may not have been responsible for lowering the risk of heart disease. They suggested that the women who chose HRT were healthier overall. These women appeared to be more affluent, better educated, and more physically active.[20] Thus, the results were skewed.

Others view the medicalization of menopause as disempowering to women. They don't want menopause to be treated like an estrogen-deficiency disease. They want it to be recognized as a natural process of aging. They suggest that medical experts, pharmaceutical companies, and the media should be closely scrutinized for the real motives behind their endorsement of HRT—profit. They suggest that women review the findings of studies supporting HRT and look at alternatives to HRT for reducing heart disease and osteoporosis.[21,22]

Studies with implications for understanding menopause include the Massachusetts Women's Health Study and the Healthy Women Study. In 1993, NIH launched the Women's Health Initiative, an 8- to 15-year study to determine the effectiveness of HRT. Until the results of these randomized studies are provided, the overall cost–benefit of HRT remains unanswered.

In January 1993, Wyeth-Agerst Labs began the Heart and Estrogen/Progestin Replacement Study (HERS) to determine the effects of hormone replacement therapy on women who already had heart disease. This randomized study should answer some questions about the benefits and risks of HRT. However, because the focus is secondary prevention (these women already have heart disease), the question of HRT as primary prevention won't be answered by this study. The increased risk of breast cancer or endometrial cancer associated with HRT or the side effect of progesterone also will not be answered.

The drawbacks of HRT include increased risks of endometrial and breast cancer. Today most HRT includes the use of progestin to reduce the risk of endometrial cancer, although a recent study suggests that the combination of estrogen and progestin appears to increase the risk of breast cancer. Progestin also causes bloating, depression, and irritability, symptoms similar to PMS. The impact of this combination therapy, adding progestin to estrogen, on heart disease is unknown. (See Table 15.2.)

Most health-care providers agree on one point. Each woman should be carefully assessed for individual risks and benefits. Many women can benefit from HRT, but others have risk factors that contraindicate its use. Natural methods would be more appropriate for many women to try before deciding to use HRT.

Table 15.1

Common Side Effects of Hormone Replacement Therapy

ESTROGENS	PROGESTINS
Breast tenderness	Symptoms similar to PMS
Breast enlargement	Headaches or migraines
Bloating	Depression
Water retention	Irritability and moodiness
Symptoms similar to PMS	Abdominal bloating
Nausea	Cramping

Table 15.2

Benefits and Risks of Hormone Replacement Therapy

BENEFITS	RISKS
Reduces heart disease	Increases risk of endometrial cancer (unopposed estrogen)
Reduces colon cancer	Increases risk of breast cancer and breast-related complications
Reduces bone loss (osteoporosis)	Increases symptoms similar to PMS (bloating, irritability, fluid retention, etc.)
Increases skin vitality	
Relaxes blood vessels so pumping is eased	Can trigger vaginal bleeding
Lowers total cholesterol	Possible weight gain
Raises high-density lipoprotein	Aggravate or cause migraine headaches
Lowers fibrinogen levels	Increases risk of gallstones
Prevents artery clogging by low-density lipoproteins	Possible reactivation of endometriosis if history exists
Reduces memory lapses and improves mental capacity	Views menopause as an estrogen-deficiency disease
Relieves symptoms of hot flashes, night sweats, etc.	Cost and inconvenience of taking medication for a lifetime
Increases vaginal lubrication	
Improves sense of well-being	

Several natural methods can be used to alleviate the symptoms of menopause. Preventive measures include exercise, proper diet, stopping smoking, and routine checkups. Complementary therapy may include a change in diet or using dietary supplements. Natural sources of estrogen and progesterone include soybean products like tofu and yams. Food sources such as milk and green leafy vegetables can be used to increase calcium, vitamin D, and vitamin E. Supplements can be taken if the diet does not adequately provide these vitamins and minerals. Herbs such as *dong quai* may help reduce hot flashes. Reducing salt intake will help prevent water retention. Some exposure to the sun (for vitamin D) and weight-bearing exercise will help increase or maintain bone density. Meditation can help reduce anxiety or insomnia. Some over-the-counter products will increase vaginal lubrication. Being a nonsmoker is extremely important in reducing the risk of heart disease, osteoporosis, and other symptoms of menopause.

The decision to choose HRT or natural methods to deal with menopause requires a knowledge of your physical and emotional risk factors and protective factors, the political aspects of HRT, your values and beliefs, and the research results that continue to accrue. The decision is ultimately yours! ∞

Chapter Summary

- The vulva refers to the external genitalia, those parts that are outwardly visible.
- Female genital mutilation is still practiced in many countries.
- The hymen is a thin sheath that covers the vaginal opening.
- The perineum is the muscle tissue found between the vaginal opening and the anal canal. An episiotomy is a surgical incision that widens the vaginal opening during childbirth.
- The vaginal opening serves as the opening for menstrual flow, the birth canal during labor, and receives the penis during intercourse.
- The endometrium is the inner lining of cells of the uterus that is sloughed off each month during the menstrual flow if fertilization does not occur.
- The ovaries produce and expel eggs each month and also the female sex hormones, progesterone and estrogen.
- Breasts can exhibit cyclic changes including benign lumps or masses of overgrown breast tissue.
- The average age of menarche, the onset of the first menstrual cycle, is 12.8 years.
- The sex hormones involved in menstruation include follicle-stimulating hormone, luteinizing hormone, estrogen, and progesterone.
- Primary dysmenorrhea is painful menses without evidence of a physical abnormality.
- Secondary dysmenorrhea is usually due to anatomic abnormalities.
- Primary amenorrhea indicates a significant medical disorder.
- The etiology of endometriosis is unknown.
- Primary amenorrhea indicates a significnat medical disorder.
- The causes of secondary amenorrhea reamin unknown.
- Toxic shock syndrome occurs when a woman uses high absorbing tampons.
- A Pap test is the best method of detecting cervical cancer.
- PMS has physical and emotional symptoms that are associated with the luteal phase of menstruation.
- The human sexual response cycle includes four phases: excitement, plateau, orgasm, and resolution.
- Menopause is the time when ovulation and menstruation cease.
- The decision to use HRT is based on medical needs, genetic factors, and political beliefs.

Review Questions

1. What are the anatomic parts of the vulva?
2. What are the anatomic parts of the internal genitalia?
3. How are the four sex hormones involved in the menstrual cycle?
4. What constitutes the components of the Female Athlete Triad?
5. Describe the differences between primary and secondary dysmenorrhea.
6. Describe the differences between primary and secondary amenorrhea.
7. What would you expect to occur during a pelvic examination?
8. How can you ensure that your Pap test is read by a qualified lab technician?
9. What are some emotional and physical symptoms of PMS?
10. What are the changes that occur during the four phases of the human sexual response cycle?
11. What are the drawbacks and benefits of HRT?

Resources

Organizations and Hotlines

National Women's Health Network
514 10th St. NW
Washington, DC 20004
Telephone: (202) 628-7814

National Women's Health Resource Center
2440 M St. NW, No. 325
Washington, DC 20037
Telephone: (202) 293-6045

Endometriosis Association
8585 N. 76th Place
Milwaukee, WI 53223
Telephone: (800) 992-3636

Websites

Planned Parenthood's Women's Health Letter
www.ppfa.org

Obstetrics and Gynecology (University of Pittsburgh)
www.falk.med.pitt.edu

North American Menopause Society
www.menopause.org

Obstetrics and Gynecology (Southern Illinois University)
www.siumed.edu

Suggested Readings

Brown, E. H., and L. P. Walker. 1996. *Menopause and estrogen: Natural alternatives to hormone replacement therapy.* North Atlantic Books.

Gold, J. H., and S. K. Severion. 1994. *Premenstrual dysphorias: Myths and realities.* American Psychiatric Press.

Grahn, J. 1993. *Blood, bread, and roses: How menstruation created the world.* Beacon Press.

Gravelle, K., and J. Gravelle. 1996. *The period book: Everything you don't want to ask (but need to know).* Walker & Company.

Greer, G. 1991. *The change: Women, aging and menopause.* New York: Ballantine Books.

Lee, J., and J. Sasser-Coen. 1996. *Blood stories: Menarche and the politics of the female body in contemporary U.S. society.* Routledge.

Love, S. 1997. *Dr. Susan Love's hormone book: Making informed choices about menopause.* New York: Random House.

Rapkin, A. J., and D. Tonnessen. 1993. *A woman doctor's guide to PMS: Essential facts and up-to-the-minute information on premenstrual syndrome.* Hyperion Press.

Stoppard, M. 1996. *The breast book: The essential guide to breast care & breast health for women of all ages.* New York: DK Publishing, Inc.

References

1. Fleeing mutilation, fighting for asylum. January-February, 1996. *Ms. Magazine:* 12-16.
2. Lee, J. 1994. Menarche and the (hetero) sexualization of the female body. *Gender & Society,* 8 (3): 343-62.
3. Chrisler, J. C., I. K. Johnston et al. 1994. Menstrual joy: The construct and its consequences. *Psychology of Women Quarterly,* 18 (3): 375-87.
4. Lichten, E. M. Medical treatment of endometriosis and pelvic pain. www.usdoctor.com/endo.htm
5. Nattiv, A., R. Agostini, B. Drinkwater et al. 1994. The female athlete triad. *Clinical Sports Medicine,* 13: 405-18.
6. Nattiv, A., and L. Lynch. 1994. The female athlete triad: Managing an acute risk to long-term health. *The Physician and Sportsmedicine,* 22 (1): 61-68.
7. Cervical dysplasia. July, 1995. *Harvard Women's Health Watch,* Boston, MA.
8. Ibid.
9. Hale, E. Reprinted from September, 1989. The controversial Pap test: It could save your life. Department of Health and Human Services, Public Health Service, Food and Drug Administration, Office of Public Affairs, Rockville, MD. Reprinted from FDA Consumer Magazine.
10. Wartik, N. Is it an illness? *American Health,* April, 1995, p. 67.
11. O'Brien, P. 1993. Helping women with premenstrual syndrome. *British Medical Journal,* 307: 1471-75.
12. Plouffe, L., K. Stewart et al. 1993. Diagnostic and treatment results from a southeastern academic center-based premenstrual syndrome clinic: the first year. *American Journal of Obstetrics and Gynecology,* 169: 295-307.
13. Ellis, H. 1904. *Man and woman: A study of human secondary sex characteristics.* New York: Scribner.

14. Kinsey, A. C., W. B. Pomeroy, C. E. Martin, and P. H. Gebhard. 1953. *Sexual behavior in the human female.* Philadelphia: Saunders Company.

15. Masters, W. H., and V. E. Johnson. 1970. *Human sexual response.* Boston: Little, Brown, and Company.

16. Ibid.

17. Rostosky, S. S., and C. B. Travis. 1996. Menopause research and the dominance of the biomedical model 1984-1994. *Psychology of Women Quarterly, 20:* 285-312.

18. Rubin, R. 1994. Estrogen anxiety: Enter menopause and pop hormone pills? Not so fast, says researchers. *U.S. News & World Report, 116:* 60-62.

19. Rinzler, C. A. 1993. *Estrogen and breast cancer: A warning to women.* New York: Macmillan.

20. Ibid.

21. Klein R. and L. J. Dumble. (1994). Disempowering midlife women: The science and politics of hormone replacement therapy (HRT). *Women's Studies International Forum* 17(4): 327-343.

22. Rostosky and Travis, Menopause research and the dominance of the biomedical model.

Sixteen

Selecting Birth Control Methods

■ chapter objectives

When you complete this chapter you will be able to:
- Prepare your own reproductive life plan.
- Identify factors that affect the menstrual cycle.
- Describe the benefits and risks of the available contraceptive choices.
- Properly explain the procedures for using a condom.
- Differentiate between Right to Life and Pro Choice positions.

ACCESS TO FAMILY PLANNING

Family planning is not just a "family" issue. It has health, social, and political implications. In many developing countries, a family still averages four or five children, whereas in the United States and other developed countries, families average less than one child. As we move into the twenty-first century, a major focus and initiative for world health continues to be population control. Women in developing countries have few family planning options available because the government determines and prescribes acceptable birth control methods. The leading causes of death for these women continue to be complications associated with pregnancy, childbirth, and abortion. Governments throughout the world can reduce population overcrowding by making a wider variety of birth control methods accessible and affordable, rather than limiting the selection. See *Viewpoint:* "Contrast in Approaches to Family Plan-

ning." Women need access to a variety of options for controlling their own reproductive health, regardless of their ability to pay.

In the United States, we also see efforts to dictate reproductive health choices for women. Power lies in the hands of government officials, rather than the women who would be served by these methods. Many women select a birth control method based on their ability to pay, and perceive other considerations as a luxury they cannot afford. Human sexuality viewed as a family matter rather than as a political or social issue creates woeful underfunding for availability of birth control methods and family planning clinics. Sexuality viewed as a family matter rather than as a health issue causes ignorance about healthy sexual functioning and family planning options. See *FYI:* "Teens and Contraceptive Use." This chapter addresses components of reproductive health related to family planning and contraceptive choices.

HEALTHY PEOPLE 2000 OBJECTIVES

- Reduce pregnancies among girls aged 17 and younger to no more than 50 per 1000 adolescents. 1995 progress toward goal achieved: -20 percent
- Reduce to no more than 30 percent the proportion of all pregnancies that are unintended. 1995 progress toward goal achieved: unavailable
- Reduce the proportion of adolescents who have engaged in sexual intercourse to no more than 15 percent by age 15 and no more than 40 percent by age 17. 1995 progress toward goal achieved: females aged 15: -150 percent, males age 15: -85 percent, females age 17: -160 percent, males age 17: -20 percent
- Increase to at least 40 percent the proportion of ever sexually active adolescents aged 17 and younger who have abstained from sexual activity for the previous 3 months. 1995 progress toward goal achieved: females (10 percent) and males (0 percent)

- Increase to at least 90 percent the proportion of sexually active, unmarried people aged 15–24 who use contraception, especially combined method contraception that both effectively prevents pregnancy and provides barrier protection against disease. 1995 progress toward goal achieved: females aged 15–19 (40 percent) and males aged 15–19 (50 percent)
- Increase the effectiveness with which family planning methods are used, as measured by a decrease to no more than 7 percent in the proportion of couples experiencing pregnancy despite use of a contraceptive method. 1995 progress toward goal achieved: unavailable
- (Added in 1995) Increase to at least 95 percent the proportion of all females aged 15–44 at risk of unintended pregnancy who use contraception

Viewpoint

Contrast in Approaches to Family Planning

In February 1995, China's government announced that the population had reached 1.2 billion, 5 years before expected. It determined to redouble its efforts to slow the growth by toughening its stance toward family planning. The government was determined to reduce infant births.

India's approach was to create a more educated society. "The birth rate began to decline, thanks to higher incomes, more education, better health and a government family-planning programme. It dropped from 45 per thousand in 1941 to 29 per thousand in 1991." The fertility rate was lowest in the states with higher education and social services.[1] India's approach of increasing income, increasing education, and providing family planning services appears to have greater effect than China's tough stance. What other factors might be occurring in these countries? What efforts can be undertaken to improve family planning in countries with high fertility rates?

SELECTING BIRTH CONTROL METHODS

A landmark decision by the U.S. Supreme Court in June 1967 created the present environment of contraceptive acceptance in the United States. *Griswold v. Connecticut* held that the state law prohibiting married couples from using birth control was unconstitutional. This decision afforded married couples the right of privacy in making choices regarding the use of birth control by placing the issue beyond state intervention. **Birth control** methods are all the strategies used to keep from having a baby and include contraceptive methods, IUDs, emergency contraception, and abortion. Another term often used synonymously with birth control is contraceptive choice. Contraceptive choices are defined more accurately as those methods that prevent fertilization of

birth control—umbrella term for all the strategies to prevent pregnancy; oftentimes used synonymously with contraception.

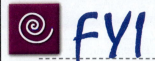

Teens and Contraceptive Use

The Alan Guttmacher Institute (AGI) published a report in 1994 called *Sex and America's Teenagers.* The following information was drawn from one component of the study, for example, the use of contraceptives by teenagers:

- A sexually active teenage female who doesn't use contraception has a 90 percent chance of pregnancy within 1 year.
- Two-thirds of teenagers use some form of contraception the first time they have sex, usually a condom.
- Teenage women's contraceptive use the first time they have sex increased from 48 percent to 65 percent during the 1980s, which correlated with the increased use of condoms by males.
- One-fourth of the 1.7 million teens who use the pill also use condoms.
- Single teens who use contraception are less likely to become pregnant than are single women in their early twenties who use contraceptives.
- Eighty-five percent of teen pregnancies are unplanned, accounting for about one-fourth of all accidental pregnancies annually. ∞

the ovum such as hormonal methods, barrier methods, and sterilization. However, throughout this chapter, these words are used interchangeably.

Contraceptive Choices

This section discusses a variety of available **contraceptive** methods for family planning, the health benefits and drawbacks, the relative failure rates, and the cost estimate of each method. Failure rates are determined as "method failure," which means the method itself fails when used as prescribed, and "user failure," which means the user makes a mistake. Contraceptive methods can be classified according to the method of protection, such as fertitility awareness methods, barrier methods, and hormonal methods.

Abstinence

Many teenagers and young adults decide to delay sexual intercourse for a variety of reasons. Abstinence is the only sure method of birth control to prevent an

unintended pregnancy or unwanted STDs. Abstinence from sexual intercourse does not necessarily equate with being nonsexual. Teenagers can be sexually intimate without risking pregnancy or STDs. A group of Iowa high school students came up with a list of "101 Ways to Make Love Without Doin' It." Some ways provided in the brochure include: "Hold hands; Relax in a whirlpool; Kiss; Give or get a hug; Hold one another close."[2] The message was clear: intimacy and love do not have to be associated with sexual intercourse.

Healthy People 2000 states: "The proportion of young people who choose abstinence has increased. In 1988 an estimated 23.6 percent of every sexually active female, aged 15–17, abstained from sexual intercourse. In 1991, 25 percent abstained from sexual intercourse. Among adolescent males, the percent increased from 33 percent in 1988 to 36 percent in 1991."[3] Unfortunately, despite these encouraging statistics, "only limited success has been realized by concerted attempts to reduce pregnancy rates among adolescents, to convince teenagers to delay sexual activity, and to reduce repeat pregnancies among this age group."[4]

Fertility Awareness Methods

Fertility awareness methods of contraception include the *calendar method, basal body temperature method,* and the *symptothermal method,* a combination of basal body temperature tracking and mucosal sampling. Withdrawal, referred to as coitus interruptus, is common and will be discussed, but cannot be considered a birth control method. Natural family planning methods or fertility awareness methods help women understand their menstrual cycle better, but require high motivation and cooperation by both partners. These methods have high method and user failure rates, are not suggested for couples who could not tolerate a pregnancy, and offer no protection against STDs. (See Fig. 16.1.)

Calendar Method The **calendar method** (or rhythm) is a form of contraception that relies on abstinence during the period of time a woman is ovulating. It is the least user effective method of contraception and should be supplemented with another option if pregnancy cannot be tolerated. The average menstrual cycle is 21 to 35 days long and **ovulation** can occur anytime between days 11 to 21 depending on cycle length. Ovulation occurs near the mid-point of a menstrual cycle, or put another way, approxi-

FIGURE 16.1 Fertility awareness, also known as natural family planning, can combine each method to identify when a woman is fertile. However, it must be remembered that the cycles for most women are not consistently 28-day cycles.

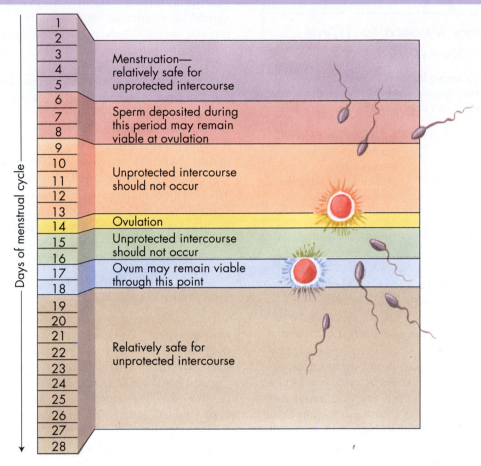

mately 14 days after ovulation, menses begins. The calendar method would be very effective if a woman knew the exact day of ovulation; however, pregnancy has been known to occur with isolated intercourse on virtually every day of the menstrual cycle. To use the calendar method, a woman determines the length of time between menstrual cycles, including the shortest and longest times between cycles. To be safe, a couple should refrain from intercourse during the entire time that ovulation is possible, including 3 to 5 days after ovulation. The egg can be fertilized anytime between the release by the ovary and its exit from the fallopian tube.

The calendar method has a 30 percent failure rate, meaning that 3 in 10 women will become pregnant within a year when using this method alone. The primary advantage of this method is its acceptance by most religious organizations. The pri-

mary disadvantage is the unpredictability of a woman's menstrual cycle, particularly during stress or illness. (See *FYI:* "Factors Known to Affect the Menstrual Cycle.")

contraceptive—variety of methods to prevent pregnancy.

calendar method—natural family planning. method that does not require a drug or device to avoid pregnancy.

ovulation—the releasing of an egg from the ovary, usually occurring 14 days before the start of menstruation.

Factors Known to Affect the Menstrual Cycle

Ovulation is often unpredictable because the menstrual cycle can fluctuate. Numerous factors have been found to affect the menstrual cycle. Some of these factors are listed below.

alcohol	holidays
stress	illness
travel	medication
changing work schedules	gynecological problems
excessive exercise	perimenopausal status

What other factors have impacted the length of your menstrual cycle? ∽

Basal Body Temperature Method The **basal body temperature** method is designed to determine when a woman is ovulating. A woman's basal body temperature drops slightly 1 to 2 days before ovulation and then rises sharply by approximately one-half to 1 degree during ovulation and remains elevated until the menstrual cycle begins. The basal body temperature should be measured each morning before rising from bed for reliability. One problem with basal body temperature, as with the calendar method, is that sexual activity should not occur 3 to 4 days before ovulation because the sperm can remain viable in the genital tract for several days. Sexual activity also should be stopped for 3 to 4 days after the temperature elevates. Intercourse before ovulation carries a greater risk than intercourse during the post-ovulatory infertile phase, which is somewhat easier to determine. The sperm can remain viable for nearly 72 hours so predicting the time of ovulation is extremely important with this method.

Symptothermal Method The **symptothermal method** is a combination of basal body temperature and cervical mucus monitoring. In addition to monitoring basal body temperature, a woman can detect changes in consistency of the cervical mucus at ovulation when it becomes more watery. Sexual intercourse should be avoided until the mucus thickens or dries. Monitoring both basal body temperature and mucus consistency are better methods than the

calendar method for determining ovulation. This method still has a failure rate of nearly 20 percent, thus 1 in 5 women will become pregnant during the year using this method of birth control. Intercourse should be avoided or other methods considered during the months before a woman becomes familiar with her menstrual cycle.

Withdrawal Withdrawal, **coitus interruptus,** is not a contraceptive method; it is a method that leads to many unintended pregnancies. Some young teenage women believe that pregnancy cannot occur if the penis is withdrawn from the vagina before ejaculation. In reality, the pre-ejaculate carries sperm that may be released into the vagina before withdrawal. This method requires an inordinate amount of self-control by both partners, and has an extremely high failure rate. If a woman wants to prevent an unwanted pregnancy or protect herself from STDs, this is one method to avoid!

Barrier Methods

Barrier methods include spermicides, condoms, diaphragms, and cervical caps. Spermicides and condoms are inexpensive and available without a health-care provider's prescription. Diaphragms and cervical caps require a prescription and are more difficult to use. Barrier methods have become increasingly popular because of the protection they provide against HIV and other STDs. However, their use as contraception for young women remains questionable because of high failure rates. Many health-care providers recommend using a combination of the condom and oral contraceptives to protect against unintended pregnancy and unwanted STDs.

Spermicides Vaginal **spermicides,** a chemical method of contraceptive use, come in a variety of forms: creams, gels, suppositories, and foams. (See Fig. 16.2.) Spermicides prevent contraception by killing sperm before they reach the uterus. They serve as a lubricant and can be used alone or with another barrier method, such as condoms, diaphragms, or cervical caps. Spermicides must be reapplied before each ejaculation to prevent loss of effectiveness. Douching should be avoided, or if practiced, should be delayed for 8 to 10 hours after intercourse because sperm can be forced into the uterine cavity. Contrary to the messages seen in advertisements, douching does not enhance feminine hygiene or provide health benefits.

FIGURE 16.2 Vaginal spermicides are placed deep into the vagina no longer than 30 minutes before intercourse.

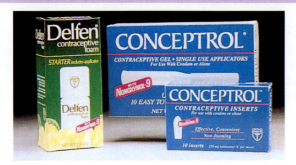

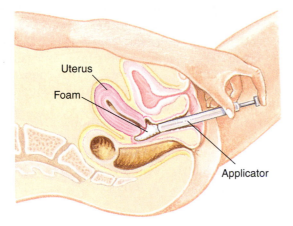

Uterus

Foam

Applicator

Spermicides, particularly those containing nonoxynol-9, have proven to be somewhat effective in preventing gonorrhea, herpes simplex 2 virus, chlamydia, and HIV infection.[5] In addition, they are inexpensive, readily available, and highly effective when used with a condom. The drawbacks include loss of spontaneity because the spermicide must be reapplied before each ejaculation and of allergic reactions such as rash or itching. The complaint of loss of spontaneity can be overcome by using spermicides as part of foreplay.

Condom, Male The latex condom has increased in use, primarily because it helps to protect against HIV and other STDs such as herpes simplex 2 virus, chlamydia, and cytomegalovirus. They also reduce transmission of gonorrhea, hepatitis B virus, and Trichomonas vaginalis.[6] The **condom** is a thin sheath and should contain the lubricant, nonoxynol-9. (See Fig. 16.3.) The condom is 86 to 90 percent effective when used alone, and 98 percent effective when used with a spermicide. (See *Health Tips:* "How to Use a Condom.")

FIGURE 16.3 Condoms.

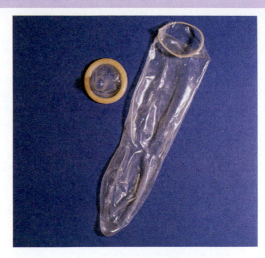

Drawbacks to using a condom include reduced spontaneity and possible allergic reactions. Using condoms as part of foreplay can help reduce a lack of spontaneity. The complaint of an allergic reaction can be addressed by a procedure called double bagging. If the male exhibits an allergy, he can roll a sheep-skin condom onto the penis, followed by a latex condom to offer protection against HIV and other STDs. If the female exhibits an allergic reaction, the procedure can be reversed with the latex condom applied first, followed by the sheep-skin condom. Sheep-skin condoms, made from lamb intestines, are not recommended for preventing AIDS and other STDs because of their porousness. The new polyurethane condoms could also be tried to avoid an allergic response.

basal body temperature method—natural family planning method that requires taking temperature in the morning, orally or rectally, after 8 hours of sleep and before doing anything else.

symptothermal method—uses ovulation and basal body temperature methods of family planning.

coitus interruptus—an unreliable birth control method; the penis is withdrawn from the vagina prior to ejaculation.

spermicide—chemical substance that kills sperm.

condom—latex sheath designed to cover the erect penis and hold semen upon ejaculation.

How to Use a Condom

1. Roll the condom down on the penis as soon as it is erect. Do this as soon as possible as part of foreplay.
2. Your partner should leave one-half inch of space at the tip of the condom. If the condom has a reservoir tip, this is easy to remember. This extra space is for the ejaculate (see Fig. 16.4).
3. If using another lubricant, choose something like K-Y jelly, which is water based. Do not use an oil-based lubricant, which can break down the latex.
4. After ejaculation, hold the condom at the rim and withdraw the penis. Be careful so semen does not leak out of the condom.
5. Remove the condom, wrap it in tissue, and dispose of it safely in a waste container. Do not flush the condom in the toilet.

FIGURE 16.4 Pinch the end of the condom to leave one-half inch of space at the tip.

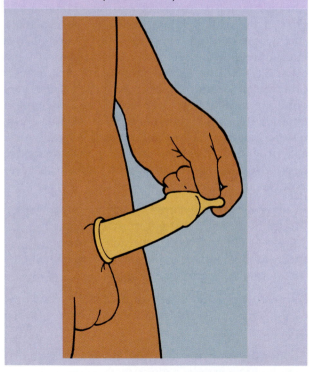

The condom must be applied before intercourse, and a new condom should be used before each act of intercourse. Condoms should be stored in a cool place to prevent deterioration, and Vaseline and other petroleum products that contribute to break-down of the latex should be avoided. Proper application of the condom is essential for maximizing its user effectiveness. The male condom should not be used concurrently with the female condom.

Condom, Female The **female condom,** Reality®, was approved with restricted labeling for use by the FDA in 1993. Reality® is marketed by Wisconsin Pharmacol Company and is a one-size-fits-all barrier method. It is the first barrier contraceptive for women and offers protection against HIV and other STDs. The restrictive labeling suggests that this method is not as effective in protecting against HIV and other STDs as the male latex condom. Some women advocates suggest that the female condom has been subjected to much greater scrutiny and testing than the male condom. They suggest that its more limited effectiveness results from user failure, not product failure. Laboratory tests demonstrate that the HIV virus and other STD viruses cannot permeate the polyurethane material.

Reality® consists of a pre-lubricated, soft, polyurethane pouch with two flexible rings, one inserted into the vagina to cover the cervix and the other ring partially covers the labia. It is approximately $6\frac{1}{2}$ inches in length (see Fig. 16.5).

FIGURE 16.5 The female condom.

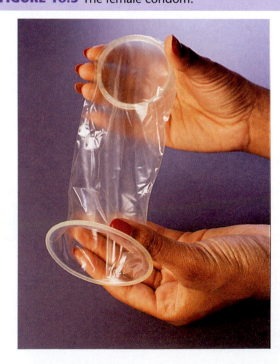

Polyurethane is strong, soft, and transfers heat so it warms to body temperature soon after insertion. The advantage of Reality® is that it does not require fitting and its use is controlled by the woman. The major disadvantage of Reality® seems to be its lack of aesthetic appeal. However, increased advertising of its availability has increased sales.

The condom costs $2–3 and should be discarded after one use. The failure rate is approximately 26 percent, primarily due to user error. Again, women advocates suggest that the high failure rate is exaggerated and the FDA is biased toward male condom use. The actual rip and tear rate may actually be considerably lower than latex. The expected rate of pregnancy among women not using any contraceptive method is 85 percent.

Diaphragm

Diaphragm The **diaphragm** is an oval, dome-shaped device with a flexible spring at the outer edge (see Fig. 16.6). A spermicide is applied into the dome and a small amount is spread around the rim with your finger. Then the diaphragm is inserted with the back rim below and behind the cervix and held in place by the back of the pubic bone (see Fig. 16.7). The diaphragm is not felt by either partner when fitted properly. The diaphragm should be left in place for 6–8 hours after intercourse, and then removed.

The diaphragm lowers the probability of contracting several STDs, including chlamydia and HPV. It appears to lower the risk of cervical cancer, tubal infertility, and PID but increases the risk for urinary tract, bladder, and yeast infections.[7] The failure rate ranges from 3 to 16 percent. The diaphragm must be initially fitted by a health-care provider and costs approximately $75–180 per year. Refitting may be necessary after weight change, childbirth, or pelvic surgery.

Cervical Cap The **cervical cap** is designed to fit tightly over the cervix, and should be filled with spermicide before intercourse (see Fig. 16.8). Like the diaphragm, it must be fitted by a health-care provider; however, it can remain in place for 48 hours without spermicidal reapplication. Method effectiveness ranges from 87 to 98 percent, with higher failure rates among young women. The advantages of the cervical cap include its smaller size and lower cost when compared to the diaphragm, and it can be left in place up to 48 hours with no need for additional spermicide. It also provides some protec-

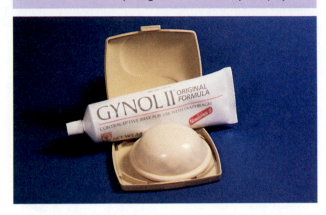

FIGURE 16.6 Diaphragm and contraceptive jelly.

tion against STDs. The disadvantage to many young women is that the smaller size makes it more difficult to ensure that the cervical cap is covering the cervix properly. The cervical cap costs approximately $15 to $150.

Hormonal Methods

Oral contraceptives, *Norplant,* and *Depo-Provera* constitute the hormonal methods available in the United States. Hormonal methods provide *no* protection against HIV and other STDs.

Oral Contraceptives Oral contraceptives are the second most popular form of birth control in the United States with 25 percent of women choosing this method. Most women who take oral contraceptives receive a combination of synthetic estrogen and a derivative of progesterone. When first introduced in 1960, the pill contained 150 mg of ethinyloestradiol and 10 mg norethisterone. Modern pills contain

---

female condom—thin, polyurethane pouch with two flexible rings: one covers the cervix and the other partially covers the vagina.

diaphragm—oval, dome-shaped device that covers the lower end of the uterus to prevent sperm from entering cervical canal.

cervical cap—small rubber cup fitted over narrow lower end of the uterus to prevent sperm from entering cervical canal.

FIGURE 16.7 (*A*), Spermicidal cream or jelly is placed into the diaphragm. (*B*), The diaphragm is folded lengthwise and inserted into the vagina. (*C*), The diaphragm is then placed against the cervix so that the cup portion with the spermicide is facing the cervix. The outline of the cervix should be felt through the central part of the diaphragm.

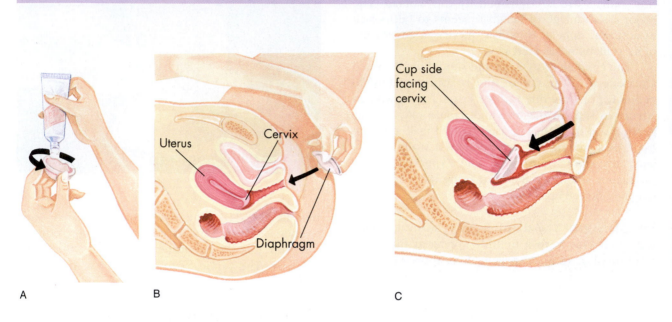

A   B   C

FIGURE 16.8 After the spermicidal cream or jelly is placed in the cervical cap, the cap is inserted into the vagina and placed against the cervix.

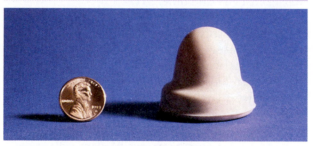

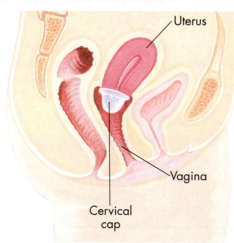

less than 35 mg of ethinyloestradiol and less than 1.5 (if any) norethisterone. A progestin-only pill is available on the market for women for whom estrogen has been contraindicated.[8] Oral contraceptives come in 21- or 28-day packages. With the 21-day pack, you take one pill each day at the same time for 21 days. You will start your period during the 7 days that you are not taking the pill and you begin taking the pills again after 7 days. The 28-day pack is designed for you to take one pill at the same time every day. The last seven pills do not contain hormones and you will have your period during that time. The pill is 94 to 97 percent effective in preventing pregnancy when used properly. However, consult the back-up methods in *Health Tips:* "Back-up Methods of Contraception" if you use oral contraceptives.

Research suggests that oral contraceptives provide several benefits including protection against ovarian and endometrial cancer, lowered risk for ectopic pregnancies and PID, reduced menstrual flow, and decreases in iron deficiency anemia.[9]

Oral contraceptives have several drawbacks. Estrogen use is associated with a number of side effects including nausea, breast soreness, and fluid retention. Progestin-only pills are associated with increased irregular menstrual cycles and they must be taken at the same time each day. Research results remain mixed regarding the effect of oral contracep-

Back-up Methods of Contraception

You should use a back-up method of contraception, such as a condom or spermicide when:

- Your period begins on a day other than Sunday just before you begin taking a Sunday-start pill. Use a back-up method for the first 7 days that you take the pill.
- You have vomiting or diarrhea. Your body may not absorb the pill. Use a back-up method for the rest of your cycle.
- You forget to take two or more pills. Call your health-care provider and ask what you should do.

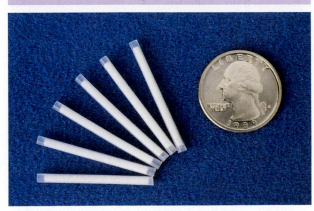

FIGURE 16.9 The Norplant subdermal implant.

tives on breast cancer, cardiovascular disease, and liver cancer. Although estrogen does increase the level of HDL (the good cholesterol) in women, progestin appears to increase the level of LDL (the bad cholesterol). Most importantly, women at risk for cardiovascular disease, particularly smokers over age 35, those with diabetes mellitus, or hypertension should be advised of the high risk of oral contraceptives containing estrogen.

Norplant Norplant (levonorgestrel) is a progestin-only implant that is inserted under the skin of the upper arm. The implant consists of six flexible, matchstick-like capsules filled with levonorgestrel that dissipate slowly over a 5-year time frame (see Fig. 16.9). The implant procedure is performed under local anesthesia in the health-care provider's office. Norplant prevents pregnancy in several ways, by suppressing ovulation, decreasing the thickness of the endometrial lining, making penetration of sperm difficult by reducing the amount and thickening cervical mucus, and decreasing the likelihood of fertilization. It has an extremely low failure rate, particularly in the first several years. The failure rate does increase for women who weigh more than 150 pounds, particularly during the latter years of use. The advantages of Norplant include its low failure rate, 5-year effectiveness, lack of estrogen side effects, high reversibility (nearly 80 percent of women who discontinue use were pregnant within 1 year), and ease of use for women with compliance difficulty.[10]

The major side effects of Norplant are irregular menstrual cycle changes including heavier bleeding, spotting between periods, infrequent bleeding, or amenorrhea. Other reported possible side effects include headache, nausea, dizziness, acne, hair loss, increase in facial or body hair, and breast tenderness. The major drawbacks are the initial high cost of Norplant, varying from $500 to $750, and the difficulty some women experience in having the implants removed. Norplant is effective for 5 years, but must be removed at that time. Many physicians have discontinued implanting Norplant because tissue scarring at the site of the implant can make the capsules very difficult to remove. Another concern regarding this contraceptive is that current research has not determined the impact of extended use. Controversy continues about the relationship between the risk of cancer and injectables.[11,12]

Shortly after Norplant's approval by the FDA, controversy regarding the coercion of lower income women to use Norplant began to surface. Several court cases pointed to the apparent coercion. A California woman agreed to use Norplant at a sentencing when her lawyer was not present, and her failure to comply resulted in her being sent to jail. A Texas woman agreed to use Norplant as part of her sentence. She experienced complications and later underwent a tubal ligation. Other court cases have followed, raising the issue of whether coercion is an undue influence on women.[13]

Norplant—trademark name for contraceptive method utilizing six capsules under the skin in a woman's upper arm.

Depo-Provera Depo-Provera is the most widely used progestin injection. It is injected into the gluteal or deltoid muscle of a woman once every 3 months. Depo-Provera contains medroxyprogesterone acetate, a chemical similar to the natural hormone progesterone that is produced by the ovaries during the last half of the menstrual cycle. It prevents the egg from ripening, thus suppressing ovulation so the egg cannot be fertilized by the sperm. It also causes changes in the endometrium so that implantation cannot occur. Depo-Provera lasts approximately 4 months and was approved for contraceptive use by the FDA in 1992. It is similar to Norplant in that it has high effectiveness (99.7 percent) and reversibility. Nearly 50 percent of women who stop using Depo-Provera to get pregnant are expected to become pregnant within 10 months after their last injection, 66 percent of women are expected to become pregnant within a year, and 93 percent are expected to become pregnant within 18 months after their last injection. Side effects may include amenorrhea, weight gain, headache, nervousness, dizziness, stomach cramps, and decreased sex drive.[14]

Contraindications for Hormonal Methods

A woman considering any hormonal method should be asked whether she is pregnant, if she has active liver disease, heart problems, breast cancer, diabetes, hypertension, migraine headaches, epilepsy, or a history of blood clotting. Research regarding the effect of hormonal methods on these conditions remains mixed and a woman may choose another method. A woman should be asked about her sexual history, including whether she or her partner have other sexual partners. Although hormonal methods are highly effective in preventing pregnancy, they provide no protection against HIV and other STDs.

Other Birth Control Methods

Other birth control methods also deserve consideration. These methods include emergency contraception, intrauterine devices, and sterilization. Emergency contraception is gaining public awareness as a "morning after" method. Even though intrauterine devices have lost favor in the United States, they remain one of the most common forms of birth control in other countries. And, sterilization is the leading form of birth control in the United States.

Emergency Contraception If you experience an episode of unprotected intercourse or method failure (e.g., condom breakage), you can seek help within the first 12–24 hours to reduce the risk of an unwanted pregnancy. In fact, the method may work up to 72 hours after unprotected intercourse. In numerous countries (including Great Britain, Denmark, Sweden, Germany, and others), emergency contraceptive pills are packaged in appropriate dosages and with instructions for clinicians and patients.

Emergency contraception has not received FDA approval in the United States; however, the contraceptives used in emergency contraception are legal and have been approved for ordinary contraception. Numerous physicians, particularly on college campuses, have been prescribing this contraceptive method for years. Emergency contraception reduces the risk of pregnancy by approximately 75 percent and involves the administration of high doses of oral contraceptive, which causes changes in the endometrium. The egg, if fertilized, cannot implant in the endometrium and the tissue will be sloughed off as part of a menstrual cycle. This emergency contraceptive method has also been called the "morning after pill."

In February 1997, the FDA published a Federal Register notice asking manufacturers to submit supplemental new drug applications for emergency oral contraception. The FDA is attempting to increase the information available to young women and the health-care provider by making a statement as part of the product's official labeling. Several recent news articles have reported that a few pharmacists have refused to fill prescriptions for women who were using the oral contraceptives as emergency contraception. These pharmacists believe this procedure is a form of abortion.

Other less-used techniques for emergency contraception include administration of "mini-pills" within 48 hours or the insertion of a copper-T IUD up to 7 days after unprotected sex. These methods interrupt the process of an egg becoming fertilized and implanting in the uterus. An Emergency Contraceptive Hotline (1–800–584–9911) provides information about emergency contraception and refers you to a health-care provider in your area.

Intrauterine Devices Only two **intrauterine devices** (IUDs) are currently available in the United States, the copper-T and Progestasert (see Fig. 16.10). IUDs have decreased in popularity since the lawsuit involving the removal of the Dalkon shield from the

FIGURE 16.10 *(A)* Progestasert IUD. *(B)* Copper T380A (ParaGard) IUD.

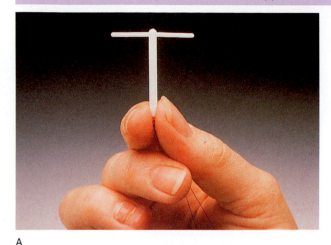

A

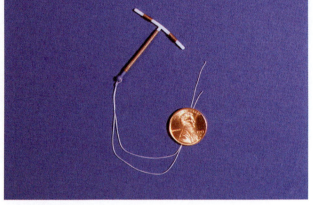

B

United States market was filed in 1974. Less than 1 percent of contraceptive users in the United States choose this method of protection. However, IUDs are the most popular form of temporary birth control worldwide with nearly 85 million women using them. Some IUDs can remain in place for 4 years, whereas others must be replaced yearly.[15]

The IUD is usually inserted into the uterus during menstruation by a health-care provider. A string leading from the uterus, through the cervix, and out into the vaginal area should be checked regularly after your menstrual cycle. The IUD appears to prevent pregnancy in a number of ways. It reduces the number of sperm cells that reach the fallopian tubes, it decreases the viability of sperm cells, and it prevents the implantation of a fertilized egg within the uterus. Common side effects include increased menstrual flow and cramping, and common drawbacks are increased risk of sterility, ectopic pregnancies, uterine perforation, PID, and spontaneous expulsion. IUDs are contraindicated in women who are currently pregnant, have had previous ectopic pregnancies, or have experienced endometriosis, an abnormal pap test, unusual vaginal bleeding, a current infection, uterine abnormalities, or PID.

An IUD with time-releasing Levonorgestrel, (a progesterone also found in Norplant) is being tested and is waiting to become available. A silastic capsule containing Levonorgestrel has been added to an IUD that releases 20 mg daily for up to 6 years. It reduces the risk of ectopic pregnancy, and decreases the amount of menstrual flow.[16]

Sterilization Sterilization methods, *tubal ligation* and *vasectomy,* are the most common form of contraceptive used by women over age 30 and men (see Fig. 16.11). Sterilization is the choice of one-third of women who want to prevent an unintended pregnancy; 25 percent have a tubal ligation and 11 percent of their partners have a vasectomy.[17] These methods have low method and user failure rates and low reversibility so they should be considered only when voluntarily choosing to have no more children. Women with multiple partners or who have a partner with multiple partners still need to consider using a condom for protection against STDs and HIV.

Tubal Ligation **Tubal ligation** can be performed on an outpatient basis or it can require hospitalization, depending on the type of procedure. It is the most prevalent form of birth control used in the United

Depo-Provera—trademark name for contraceptive method utilizing progestin injection into the gluteal or deltoid muscle once every three months.

intrauterine device—birth control device made of plastic or other material; inserted into the uterus to prevent pregnancy.

tubal ligation—sterilization process in women in which the fallopian tubes are blocked to prevent pregnancy.

FIGURE 16.11 (*A*) Vasectomy. (*B*) Tubal ligation.

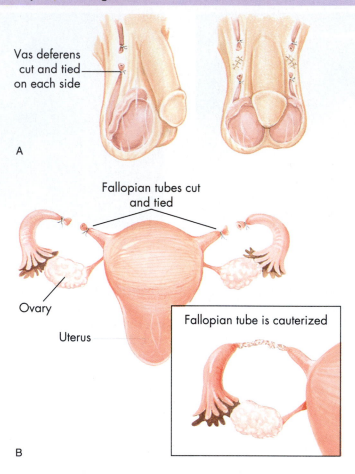

Vas deferens
cut and tied
on each side

A

Fallopian tubes cut
and tied

Ovary

Uterus

Fallopian tube is cauterized

B

States. The surgery involves closing the fallopian tubes, either by cautery, tying, cutting, or clamping; thus preventing the egg from becoming fertilized. Laparoscopy, sometimes referred to as "band-aid" surgery, is completed through a small incision near the navel. A laparoscope is inserted into a small incision allowing the health-care provider to locate the fallopian tube. Then, another incision is made through which the fallopian tubes are closed or an instrument is inserted through the laparoscope. Tubal ligation is most often performed immediately after childbirth. The one incision is made into the abdomen through which both fallopian tubes can be tied. Tubal ligation is a permanent procedure for a women who is certain she does not want to have any more children.

A review of the Nurses Health Study showed that women who underwent tubal ligation had a one-fourth lower risk of ovarian cancer.[18] Women experiencing unusual symptoms (bleeding from the vagina, fever, or discharge, bleeding or redness at the surgi-

cal site) should contact their health-care provider immediately.

Vasectomy **Vasectomy** is the third most popular form of contraception available with nearly 500,000 men choosing this method each year. The traditional vasectomy is an office procedure, including one or two incisions by the surgeon to access each vas deferens. Each vas is then cauterized, tied, or sutured to prevent sperm from being ejaculated. A technique called the no-scalpel vasectomy (NSV) procedure was developed in China in 1974 and introduced in the United States in 1985. With NSV, the surgeon makes a small puncture to access each vas deferens after both vas deferens have been anesthetized. Each vas can be cauterized, lasered, sutured, or hemoclipped for occlusion. NSV, when compared to conventional vasectomy, reduces the psychological barrier for many men, the surgical time from 20–30 minutes to 5–11 minutes, and the risk for infection, bleeding, and pain.[19]

Table 16.1

Comparison of User Effectiveness and Cost

METHOD	USER EFFECTIVENESS (PERCENTAGE)	COST
Fertility awareness		
Calendar	70–80	Charts are free
Basal body temperature	85–90	Temperature kit $5–10
Symptothermal	85–98	Temperature kit $5–10
Barrier		
Spermicides	80–85	$8–10 kit with 20–40 applications
		Refills $2–5
Male condom	85–88	Free at clinics to
(with spermicide)	90–95	$6–10/dozen
Female condom	75–80	$1.50–4.00
(with spermicide)	85–90	
Diaphragm/cervical cap	82	$70–80
(with spermicide)	85–90	
Hormonal methods		
Oral contraceptives	94–97	$1.50/month in
		clinics to $30/month
Norplant	96–99	$450–600 to implant
Depo-Provera	98–99	$60–90 every 3 months
Other methods		
Intrauterine device	97–98	$350–400
Tubal ligation	99.9	$1000–2500
Vasectomy	99.9	$250–600

Sources: Birth Control: Your Choices. Texas Department of Health, Bureau of Maternal and Child Health.

Planned Parenthood Federation of America: www.ppfa.org

Alan Guttmacher Institute: www.agi-usa.org

Couples should use another form of contraceptive control until all sperm have been cleared from the ampullar storage area, which takes several weeks. A semen sample should be taken to determine that the sperm count has reached zero.

The advantages of vasectomy, whether conventional or NSV, include its greater safety and cost effectiveness compared to tubal ligation, its low failure rate, and better rates of reversibility than tubal ligation. A common myth about vasectomy is that males will lose their masculinity. Research has found no relationship between vasectomy and loss of masculinity. Furthermore, no relationship has been shown between vasectomy and prostate cancer, testicular cancer, and atherosclerosis, although studies are still being conducted.

SELECTING A BIRTH CONTROL METHOD

Choosing an appropriate birth control method requires planning and informed decision making. The first consideration is whether to involve your partner in the decision. He can assist with the choice of the appropriate contraceptive, go with you for scheduled physical examinations if a prescription is required, and share the cost for the contraceptive (see Table 16.1). Is he willing to participate in the decision and management of birth control? Will the cost be shared? The next consideration is acceptability. The method you select should be congruent with your personal values and beliefs (e.g., religious) about the likelihood of pregnancy or STDs. If you believe that premarital sex is not acceptable, your only choice is abstinence. If you are in a monogamous relationship and your partner is STD-free, you might choose hormonal methods. If you have not had a previous ectopic pregnancy, you might want to consider a method other than an IUD. The next consideration is availability of the method you

vasectomy—sterilization process in men in which the vas deferens are blocked to prevent the ejaculation of sperm.

select. If a prescription is required, you must have access to a health-care provider who can prescribe the method. If you are a minor, you may need to secure parental consent. Is the product easily accessible or is a prescription necessary? Fourth, you need to consider the cost of the method. You must weigh the cost of the method against the cost of an unintended pregnancy or unwanted STD. Can you afford this method of protection (both monetarily and in terms of method and user effectiveness)? Check the user effectiveness rate, rather than the method effectiveness rate. If you choose to use the pill, you must remember to take it at the same time every day. If you forget, you will need to use another method during the month. Are you knowledgeable about the method and will you use it dependably? Can you afford (financially and emotionally) to become pregnant? Another factor to consider is health risk. A method you may want to select may be contraindicated for medical reasons. For example, women smokers over age 40 or women who are breast-feeding should choose a method other than the pill. If you have a family history of breast cancer, you may want to consider a nonhormonal method. If you had a previous pregnancy, the IUD may not be appropriate. If a partner has an STD, you may want to choose an appropriate method to reduce your risk of contracting it. Are you in a monogamous relationship or do you need to protect yourself from HIV and other STDs? Is the method you want to use contraindicated? Now complete *Journal Activity:* "Making an Informed Decision."

Birth control and STD prevention are not just a woman's issue. Decisions regarding family planning and STD protection are a joint effort with both partners sharing responsibility. If you feel you are solely responsible for contraceptive choices, you may want to reevaluate the relationship. We strongly encourage you to protect your body from unwanted diseases and unintended pregnancies. We encourage you to discuss birth control considerations with your partner. Your partner should be willing to take an active and supportive role in family planning. (See *FYI:* "Male Contraception.") Remember, family planning is a joint venture.

ABORTION

The Centers for Disease Control (CDC) and Prevention reports that the abortion rate has continued to decline during the past 4 years. In 1994, 1.2 million

> ### JOURNAL ACTIVITY
> #### *Making an Informed Decision*
> The major factors to consider when choosing an appropriate contraceptive method (including abstinence) include whether or not to involve your partner, acceptability, accessibility, cost (money and effectiveness), and health risks. Choose a birth control method that is right for you at this time. Write about each major factor and how it affects your decision. Are there other factors you may need to consider?

abortions were performed compared to 1.3 million during the previous year. The CDC estimated that 321 abortions per 1,000 live births occurred in 1994 compared to 312 abortions per 1,000 live births in 1976, which was the lowest recorded rate since the CDC began tracking abortion rates in 1972, a year before *Roe* v. *Wade.*[20] Right to Life members suggest that this decline is due to better education efforts, whereas Pro-Choice advocates suggest that the decline is due to increased harassment and difficulty in finding clinics willing to conduct abortions. They suggest that women's right to choose is being hampered by lack of access because physicians and facility personnel are fearful for their safety. A 1995 Planned Parenthood fact sheet states that lack of access to abortion is a problem for low-income women and teenagers. It states:

- Eighty-four percent of all U.S. counties have no abortion provider, 94 percent of nonmetropolitan counties and one-third of metropolitan areas are underserved. Thirty percent of women of reproductive age live in counties with no abortion provider. The number of abortion providers has declined 18 percent since 1982.
- With very limited exceptions, the federal "Hyde Amendment" has prohibited the use of federal funds for abortions for poor women. Approximately 20 percent of the women who are denied publicly funded abortions go on to bear unwanted children at considerable emotional and physical cost.

Low-income women and teenagers often face fewer options than other women. (See *FYI:* "Teenagers and Abortions." Only fifteen states currently fund abortions for low-income women.

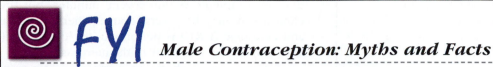

Male Contraception: Myths and Facts

When it comes to male contraception, many sayings get repeated because they *sound* good; most people haven't thought too hard about them. Here are some common "soundbites" and some new ways of thinking about them:

Myth	Fact
"Men aren't interested in contraception or in taking responsibility."	Men are already using their only two options, vasectomy (which makes up 10–12 percent of the world's contraceptive use) and condoms. A safe new reversible, nonsurgical method used separately from the sex act could attract 41–75 percent of men, according to one WHO study.
"It's easier to stop one egg than millions of sperm."	Only hormonally; *physically,* it's easier to stop millions of sperm than one egg! The sperm all travel through the vas deferens, a small, easily accessed tube where they can be incapacitated or blocked. Much simpler than hormones!
"Why develop these methods when they don't prevent the spread of AIDS/HIV?"	Why develop Norplant?
"Women won't trust men to use these methods."	Unlike the "pill" concept, most nonhormonal methods are easy for a female partner to verify. She can go to the doctor with the man when he gets a shot, for example, or help him with the method herself. Also, see below.
"Men would never use this method because . . ." • It's too permanent • It's not permanent enough • It requires dedication • It requires a shot • It's not perfect for younger men • It's not perfect for older men • Etc. (Fill in the blank)	No one method is right for everybody. A "contraceptive supermarket" (a variety of choices) best suits everybody's needs.
"Why develop these methods when we're not sure they'll be completely safe and effective?"	If we never try, we'll never know.

"Hawaii, Maryland, New York, North Carolina, Washington (in addition to the District of Columbia) provide funding voluntarily under Medicaid for low-income women. Alaska, California, Connecticut, Idaho, Massachusetts, Minnesota, New Jersey, Vermont, and West Virginia, as a result of litigation, fund 'medically necessary' abortions for low-income women. Challenges to funding restrictions based on rights guaranteed under state constitutions, are pending in Florida, Illinois, and Texas."[21]

Defining Abortion

Abortion is described as the spontaneous or deliberate termination of a pregnancy. There are a number of different types of abortion including therapeutic, spontaneous, and voluntary. Spontaneous abortions (miscarriages) occur for a variety of reasons. These abortions can result from a chronic infection (i.e., PID or endometriosis), hormonal imbalances, fetal abnormalities, or problems with the uterus. Some women experience habitual abortions. Habitual abortions are defined as the abrupt end of three pregnancies in a row before the twentieth week.

Therapeutic abortions are procedures conducted to terminate a pregnancy that threatens the life of the mother or fetus. An infected abortion is conducted when an immature pregnancy shows signs of infection to the fetus. Fever is present and the uterus must be emptied. A septic abortion occurs when the womb is infected and the life of the mother is threatened. This abortion may be spontaneous or induced by the health-care provider. A threatened abortion is a condition with symptoms of bleeding of the uterus

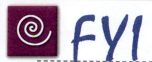

Teenagers and Abortions

The 1994 report by the Alan Guttmacher Institute addressed the issue of abortion and teenagers. The following findings were reported:

- Nearly 4 in 10 teen pregnancies (excluding miscarriages) end in abortion. Teens had about 308,000 abortions in 1992.
- Since 1980, abortion rates among sexually experienced teenagers have declined steadily because fewer teens are becoming pregnant, and in recent years, fewer pregnant teens have chosen to have an abortion.
- The reasons most often given by teens for choosing an abortion are concern about how having a baby would change their lives, feeling that they are not mature enough to have a child, and having financial problems.
- Sixty-one percent of minors who have abortions do so with at least one parent's knowledge; 45 percent of parents are told by their daughter. The great majority of parents support their daughter's decision to have an abortion. ∞

and cramping before the twentieth week. A woman with this condition requires rest and observation.

A voluntary (elective) abortion is the ending of a pregnancy by choice. Twenty-five states currently have mandatory parental involvement laws in effect for a minor seeking an abortion. These states include Alabama, Arizona, Delaware, Georgia, Indiana, Kansas, Kentucky, Louisiana, Maryland, Massachusetts, Minnesota, Mississippi, Missouri, Nebraska, North Carolina, North Dakota, Ohio, Pennsylvania, Rhode Island, South Carolina, Utah, West Virginia, Wisconsin, and Wyoming.[22] Women who undergo abortions are more likely to be young, white, and unmarried; most had no previous live births and were undergoing their first abortion. Only five deaths of women were associated with legal induced abortions in 1990.[23] The procedures most used in the United States include surgical techniques, vacuum aspiration or D&C, and more recently, a drug combination therapy.

Surgical Procedure

Vacuum aspiration, also called suction curettage, is the most common method of first trimester abortion. The cervix is dilated, and a small plastic tube is inserted into the uterus to gently suction out the contents. The procedure is completed within several minutes, but the clinical stay may be several hours. When a dilation and curettage (D&C) is performed, the cervix is dilated and the endometrium of the uterus is scraped.

First trimester abortions performed in a safe, sterile environment by a qualified health-care provider carry less risk than a full-term pregnancy. Appointments are usually required and some clinics require proof of pregnancy such as a physician's letter or lab results.

Drug Therapy

Two drug therapies deserve explanation. The first method is a combination therapy, using two drugs approved for other medical purposes but effective in inducing abortion. The second method is RU-486, a drug still lacking FDA approval.

The discovery of a two-drug combination to induce abortion offers women another choice. The two legally prescribed drugs are methotrexate, a widely used cancer drug, and misoprostol, an ulcer medication. The combination of these drugs works effectively to induce abortions although they have not been prescribed for that purpose.

RU-486 (mifepristone) was first developed in 1982 by Roussel UCLAF, a French pharmaceutical company, and has been used throughout France, England, China, and Sweden to induce abortions. RU-486 belongs to a class of steroid drugs known as antiprogestins. It is not a "magic pill" that makes abortion easier. In actuality, women who choose RU-486 as a method for inducing abortion are more involved in the process than those who choose a surgical procedure. Surgical abortions often take less than a half hour and occur in a sterile environment. The procedure is performed under local anesthesia, and the embryo is not seen by the woman. With the RU-486 procedure, the woman initiates the process herself by consciously taking the pill, available only at abortion clinics.

RU-486 works by blocking the action of progesterone, the hormone that bonds the fertilized egg to the uterus (implantation). Two days after taking RU-486, a woman returns to the clinic and takes a prostaglandin tablet, which causes the muscles to contract and expel the embryo. Unlike the surgical procedure in which the woman does not physically experience the process, RU-486 initiates a process in which the woman actually experiences the feelings and sensations of aborting the embryo. Some women experience no pain, others experience pain and bleeding similar to a menstrual cycle, whereas others

Her Story

La Shonda

I met Greg at a campus meeting for graduate students in business administration. Greg was incredible! He was witty, gentle, and a competitive bodybuilder. I had waited my whole life to meet someone like him! We began dating regularly; he used condoms for STD protection until we received confirmation of HIV-negative tests. He wasn't immediately worried about contraceptive protection; he was still facing the effects of steroid-related infertility. I decided to take the pill anyhow because graduate school would take another year and getting pregnant was out of the question. So I scheduled an appointment with the campus health-care provider.

We had a great relationship, and we were happily living together for a year when I *accidentally* got pregnant. I took the pills regularly (except for a few missed days) and Greg was supposedly infertile anyhow. We agonized over what to do. Should we get married? We weren't emotionally and financially ready to have a family. Should I quit school? Should he quit school? The discussions went on and on, including the possibility of an abortion. I wanted to get married and have the baby. Greg wasn't ready for the responsibility and wanted me to have an abortion. He was angry about the whole situation! I thought he might leave me if I decided to continue the pregnancy. I couldn't raise a child by myself, I just wasn't ready to quit school, give up a career, and possibly lose Greg. So, with his insistence and support, I called the Medical Center and scheduled an abortion.

The abortion changed our relationship! We had residual feelings about the events leading up to the abortion, and the abortion itself. I was grieving a loss and at the same time resented Greg's sense of relief. I was angry that he had been unwilling to commit to marriage. I grew more distant! He wanted out! We suffered from the experience, quit communicating, and soon the relationship failed.

- What would you have done?
- What other issues have you heard from women about whether to continue or abort an unintended pregnancy?

experience enough pain to require a mild pain killer. Some women prefer this method because it can be done several weeks earlier than a surgical abortion.

RU-486 has been in use for over a decade in Europe, but has not received FDA approval in the United States. Abortion opponents continue to pressure pharmaceutical companies by threatening to boycott the one that produces the drug.

The Grief and Acceptance Process

Studies of women who choose abortion have found that the majority experience relief after the abortion, and the immediate feelings of guilt, loss, and/or depression are usually transient.[24] The circumstances leading to the decision to abort a pregnancy may include fear or threat of losing one's partner, financial hardship, missed educational opportunities or career advancement, loss of a job, detectable fetal defects, responsibility to other children, lack of social support, rape or incest, maternal age, and others.[25] A woman's feelings and emotions often are shaped by the political, religious, and social climate she experiences. Thus, support for the woman's right to choose may facilitate better recovery. (See *Her Story:* "La Shonda.")

Like most major life events, a woman needs to handle the event in her own way. A woman should reach a stage of accepting the loss (regardless of the reasons), rather than live in secrecy and guilt. If grief exists, the resolution of the process may be facilitated by sharing one's feelings with accepting friends, family members, health-care providers, mental health professionals, or clergy. Guilt, depression, or other emotional trauma can linger if grief remains unresolved.

Political Debate

The question isn't whether abortion is a political issue, rather the question is just how did it become such a major issue? Look at politicians, political appointees, and Supreme Court justices who can be

vacuum aspiration—suction method by which the fetus and placenta are removed up to 14th week.

RU-486—drug therapy used to induce abortion.

Viewpoint

Legal vs. Illegal Abortion: A Worldview

In 1993, nearly 30 to 40 million legal abortions were reported worldwide. Approximately one-third of the reported cases occurred in the former Soviet Union and Eastern Europe in which one-tenth of the world population resides.

In these countries, abortion has been legal since well before modern contraceptive methods. However, countries with strong ties to the Roman Catholic Church distanced themselves from legal abortions, and clandestine operations flourished in this repressed environment. In Romania, where hundreds of women die each year from illegal abortions, the ban on abortion and contraception continues. In Eastern Europe, abortion rates range from 1.5 to 4.0 per woman and the profile of a woman seeking an abortion includes married with children, over age 25.[27]

Can we expect to reduce the requests for abortion without offering some contraceptive alternative? At the 1994 World Population Conference, the Roman Catholic Church continued its stance against any form of contraception other than natural family planning. How does this stance affect famine, poverty, and overpopulation? What solutions would you suggest?

elected, appointed, or denied based solely on their view of this issue. Their personal beliefs about abortion cause more political consternation than their public stance on fiscal responsibility, health care, environmental control, and other national and international issues. Look at the political platforms adopted by the political parties over the past several elections! Why is abortion such a "hot" issue? Is the issue the rights of the fetus versus the rights of the mother? Is the underlying issue "controlling" women? Is the underlying issue lack of access to contraceptives? What do you think? (See *Viewpoint:* "Legal vs. Illegal Abortion.")

A variety of political maneuvers have occurred since the *Roe* v. *Wade* decision in 1973. In 1981, the Hyde Amendment eliminated federal funding (Medicaid) for all abortions except those in which the life of the mother was endangered if the pregnancy should be carried to term. This measure made it more difficult for low-income women to seek assistance for an abortion, even in cases of rape and incest. As a result of public outcry, Congress did amend the law in 1993 to include funding for women in cases of rape and incest.[26]

In 1996, President Clinton vetoed an amendment, passed by Congress, to prevent late term abortions. Then again, in 1997, Congress reintroduced and debated a similar amendment to prevent late term abortions in an attempt to further restrict a woman's right to choose. The amendment was passed by the Congress and congress*men* suggested that the debate would now shift to the issue of when life begins and protection of the unborn. They also insinuated that members who voted against the amendment would surely lose their bids for reelection. The discussion about the events leading to a late term abortion and the medical consequences for women in this situation are far different than the discussion of induced abortions for ending an unintended pregnancy. Yet, shouldn't the discussion focus on how to prevent unintended pregnancies rather than how to prevent abortions?

Right to Life and Pro-Choice

Is it Right to Life, Pro-Life, or Anti-Choice? Is it Pro-Choice, Pro-Abortion or Anti-Life? Even the titles we use to describe the stances toward abortion give some indication of a person's views. What do we know about the individuals who describe themselves as Right to Life or Pro-Choice advocates? Researchers have found that Right to Life advocates tend to have a more unified attitude structure than Pro-Choice advocates. Because attitude structures are more unified, Right to Life advocates tend to be more monolithic in their beliefs. This position can best be summarized as people advocating for the rights of the fetus and as people who believe that life begins at conception. Right to Life advocates are more dogmatic and conservative religiously, politically, and socially. They view abortion as a moral issue and often will vote for political candidates on the basis of this single issue.[28,29]

Pro-Choice advocates tend to have less unified attitude structures, thus they are more open-minded to interpreting and organizing reality. The Pro-Choice position maintains that women should have control over their own bodies, including reproductive rights. The reasons that Pro-Choice advocates give for choosing this stance are varied. They advocate for individual rights. Some may take a stance that the fetus is not a viable life, others may have strong feelings about a woman's right to choose, and others may consider the circumstances of the pregnancy.[30]

Right to Life advocates sometimes appear to be more effective politically, but this is due to their single issue politics. This appearance should not suggest that Pro-Choice advocates are less committed to their values and beliefs. Rather, Pro-Choice advocates have a variety of issues on which to focus whereas Right to Life advocates are monolithic and unidimensional.

Another question we might ask is how children are being influenced by this "moralistic" (right versus wrong) debate? Look at Right to Life and Pro-Choice rallies at which children often stand next to sign-carrying parents. At Right to Life rallies, young children carry signs with graphic pictures of aborted, discarded fetuses. These children are led to believe that the women who have abortions are murderers and baby killers. At Pro-Choice rallies, children tote signs saying, KEEP CHOICE LEGAL. They are led to believe that individual rights and freedoms will be sacrificed if abortion isn't legal and that all Right to Life advocates are violent.

At what age did you form your opinion about abortion? How did you reach this decision? Do you think it might change? Now complete *Assess Yourself:* "Attitudes Toward Induced Abortion" to determine your attitudes toward abortion.

Human Dimension

Reproductive rights can be debated from moral, political, health, and social dimensions. The political arena tends to make Right to Life versus Pro-Choice views to seem dichotomous and bipolar opposites (much like ultraliberal and ultraconservative). Sometimes we forget that many men and women find themselves somewhere other than on either extreme end of a continuum. We also forget that abortions are about women (younger and older) making difficult choices. This is the human dimension of pregnant girls and women making difficult decisions.

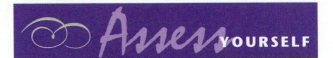

Attitudes Toward Induced Abortion

For each statement about induced abortion indicate your feelings based on the values in the following scale:

Strongly Agree	6
Moderately Agree	5
Slightly Agree	4
Slightly Disagree	3
Moderately Disagree	2
Strongly Disagree	1

_____ 1. Abortion is a moral issue.
_____ 2. The rights of a fetus should be protected because the unborn child can't protect herself.
_____ 3. A woman who has an abortion is selfish and self-centered.
_____ 4. Societies with high moral standards should prohibit abortions.
_____ 5. Life begins at conception.
_____ 6. If two people have unprotected sex, they should be willing to live with the consequences of their action.
_____ 7. Abortions are not an alternative when contraception has failed.
_____ 8. All abortions should be banned.
_____ 9. Parental consent should be required for all young girls under age 18 who seek an abortion.
_____ 10. Every young woman seeking an abortion should be required to watch a video about the procedure before making a final decision.

Total your score. Higher scores indicate a more Right to Life attitude and lower scores indicate a more Pro-Choice attitude.

How long will this issue continue to polarize persons, communities, and countries? What will it take to focus the debate on other dimensions of reproductive rights and to forge a middle ground? The recent bombings of family planning clinics in Tulsa and Atlanta indicate that Right to Life supporters have distanced themselves from the violence associated with extreme polarization. Dialog is the only strategy we can use to tolerate differences and decrease the number of unintended pregnancies and unwanted STDs. ∞

Chapter Summary

- Family planning is a health, social, and political issue.
- Fertility awareness methods include the calendar method, basal body temperature method, and symptothermal method.
- Withdrawal, coitus interruptus, is not a birth control method.
- Barrier methods include spermicides, condoms, diaphragms, and cervical caps.
- Hormonal methods include oral contraceptives, Norplant, and Depo-Provera.
- Emergency contraception can help women within the first 12–24 hours after unprotected intercourse or method failure.
- Intrauterine devices are the most popular worldwide forms of temporary birth control.
- Sterilization methods include tubal ligation and vasectomy.
- Sterilization methods are the most common form of contraceptions used by women over age 30.
- Choosing a birth control method should be a joint decision. However, a woman must take precautions to protect against unintended pregnancies and unwanted STDs.
- Categories of abortion include spontaneous, therapeutic, and voluntary.
- The abortion rate has declined over the past several years, to 1.2 million abortions in 1994.
- Twenty-five states have mandatory parental involvement laws in effect for a minor seeking an abortion.
- Surgical procedures include vacuum aspiration and dilation and curettage.
- Drug therapy for inducing abortions includes a combination of two drugs usually prescribed for other purposes.
- RU-486 has been used for years in Europe and other countries but has not received FDA approval in the United States.
- Women choose voluntary abortions for a number of reasons.

Review Questions

1. Describe the techniques for the fertility awareness methods.
2. What are the benefits and drawbacks among the fertility awareness methods? barrier methods? hormonal methods?
3. What factors affect the length of a menstrual cycle?
4. What is the leading method of birth control? Why?
5. What is the difference between method failure and user failure?
6. Discuss the procedures for applying a condom.
7. What is emergency contraception?
8. What are some of the causes of spontaneous abortions?
9. What reasons might a woman give for choosing a voluntary abortion?
10. Discuss the surgical procedures and drug therapy options available to women seeking an abortion.
11. What are the arguments offered by Pro-Choice and Right to Life regarding abortion?

Resources

Organizations and Hotlines

Alan Guttmacher Institute
1120 Connecticut Ave, NW
Suite 460
Washington, D.C. 20036

Planned Parenthood Federation of America, Inc.
810 Seventh Avenue
New York, NY 10019

Centers for Disease Control and Prevention
Atlanta, GA.

Websites

Planned Parenthood Federation of America, Inc.
www.ppfa.org

Alan Guttmacher Institute
www.agi-usa.org

National Abortion and Reproductive Rights Action League
www.naral.org

Pro-Life in Canada
home.istar.ca

National Right to Life Committee
www.nrlc.org

California Link to Pro-Choice Websites
www.choice.org

Suggested Readings

Ginsburg, F. D., and R. Rapp (eds). 1995. *Conceiving the new world order: The global politics of reproduction.* Berkeley, CA: University of California Press.

Hatcher, R. A., J. Trussell, and F. Stewart. 1994. *Contraceptive technology.* New York, NY: Irvington Publishers.

Matteson, P. 1995. *Advocating for self: Women's decisions concerning contraception.* Binghamton, NY: Haworth Press.

Petchesky, R. P. 1990. *Abortion and women's choice: The state, sexuality, and reproductive freedom.* Boston, MA: Northeastern University Press.

References

1. India's long multiplication. *The Economist, 334* (February 19, 1995): 34.
2. 101 ways to make love without doin' it. 1991. Santa Cruz, Calif.: ETR Associates. (pamphlet)
3. Public Health Service. 1996. *Healthy People 2000: Midcourse review and 1995 revisions.* U.S. Department of Health and Human Services.
4. Ibid.
5. DaVanzo, J., A. M. Parnell, and W. H. Foege. 1991. Health consequences of contraceptive use and reproductive patterns: Summary of a report from the U.S. National Research Council. *JAMA, 265:* 2692-96.
6. Ibid.
7. Ibid.
8. Szarewski, A., and J. Guillebaud. 1991. Contraception: Current state of the art. *British Medical Journal, 302:* 1224-26.
9. DaVanzo, Parnell, and Foege, Health consequences of contraceptive use and reproductive patterns.
10. Heath, C. B. 1993. Helping patients choose appropriate contraception. *American Family Physician, 48:* 1115-26.
11. McCauley, A. P., and J. S. Geller. 1992. Decisions for Norplant programs. *Population Reports, 20:* 1-31.
12. DaVanzo, Parnell, and Foege, Health consequences of contraceptive use and reproductive patterns.
13. Norplant contraceptive implant. 1993. Planned Parenthood Fact Sheet, Planned Parenthood Federation of America, Inc.
14. Depo-Provera contraceptive injection. November 1992. Upjohn Pharmaceutical Company.
15. Planned Parenthood. September 1989. Facts about birth control. Planned Parenthood Federation of America, Inc.
16. Szarewski and Guillebaud. Contraception.
17. Planned Parenthood. 1995. Planned Parenthood Fact Sheet: Thirty years at a glance. Planned Parenthood Federation of America, Inc.
18. Hankinson, S. E., D. J. Hunter, G. A. Colditz, and others. 1993. Tubal ligation, hysterectomy, and risk of ovarian cancer: a prospective study. *JAMA, 270:* 2813-18.
19. Goldstein, M. 1994. No-scalpel vasectomy: a kinder, gentler approach. *Patient Care, 28:* 55-67.
20. Stets, J. E., and R. K. Leik. 1993. Attitudes about abortion and varying attitude structures. *Social Science Research, 22:* 265-82.
21. Luker, K. 1984. *Abortion and the politics of motherhood.* Berkeley, Calif.: University of California Press.
22. Stets and Leik, Attitudes about abortion and varying attitude structures.
23. Centers for Disease Control and Prevention. www.cdc.gov
24. Planned Parenthood, Thirty years at a glance.
25. *State Reproductive Health Monitor,* June 1996.
26. Centers for Disease Control and Prevention. Abortion surveillance—United States, 1992. *MMWR Surveillance Summary, 45,* SS-3 (May 17, 1996).
27. Stotland, N. L. 1992. The myth of the abortion trauma syndrome. *JAMA, 268:* 2078-79.
28. Ibid.
29. Perotti, D., and C. Blayo. 1994. The long march from abortion to contraception. *World Health, 47:* 18-19.
30. Planned Parenthood, Thirty years at a glance.

Seventeen

Planning for Pregnancy and Parenting

■ chapter objectives

When you complete this chapter you will be able to:
- Describe the major fetal development stages during each trimester.
- Describe how to plan for a pregnancy.
- Explain the benefits and risks of special prenatal tests.
- Differentiate between true and false labor.
- Compare and contrast birthing options.
- Describe the reasons for female and male infertility.
- Explain appropriate and inappropriate parenting styles.

PREGNANCY TODAY

In an ideal world, all pregnancies would be planned and all children would be wanted. In reality, nearly 45 percent of all pregnancies are unplanned and every year nearly 1 million U.S. teenagers become pregnant, twice the rate of England and Canada and nine times that of Japan and the Netherlands. The birthrate for U.S. teenagers aged 15–17 has begun to decline in recent years, but it was still 37.6 per 1,000 in 1994, a mere decrease of 3 percent since 1990. Thirty percent of all live births in the United States were to unwed mothers (69 percent of African American births, 39 percent of Hispanic births, 23 percent of white births, and 15 percent of Asian births).[1] These young women, especially those under age 18, are more likely to have problems with pregnancy and low birthweight babies. On the oppo-

site end of the spectrum, a growing number of women have postponed pregnancy until later in their career when risks for complications also increase and infertility is more common. This chapter addresses issues of reproductive health, including pregnancy, childbirth, birthing options, breast-feeding, infertility, fetal health, and parenting.

Pre-Pregnancy Planning

Pre-pregnancy planning encompasses non-drug use, nutritional planning, exercise, a time lapse of one menstrual cycle between contraceptive use and conception, immunizations, and folic acid supplements. These lifestyle changes should begin as soon as a woman is contemplating pregnancy, that is before conception and before stopping birth control. If a woman smokes cigarettes, she should quit before

HEALTHY PEOPLE 2000 OBJECTIVES

- Reduce the infant mortality rate to no more than 7 per 1,000 live births. 1995 progress toward goal achieved: 60 percent
- Reduce the fetal death rate (20 or more weeks of gestation) to no more than 5 per 1,000 live births plus fetal deaths. 1995 progress toward goal achieved: 10 percent
- Reduce the maternal mortality rate to no more than 3.3 per 100,000 live births. 1995 progress toward goal achieved: -40 percent
- Reduce the cesarean delivery rate to no more than 15 per 100 deliveries. 1995 progress toward goal achieved: 20 percent
- Increase to at least 75 percent the proportion of mothers who breast-feed their babies in the early postpartum period and to at least 50 percent the proportion who continue breast-feeding until their babies are 5 to 6 months old. 1995 progress toward goal achieved: 10 percent
- Increase abstinence from tobacco use by pregnant women to at least 90 percent and increase abstinence from alcohol, cocaine, and marijuana by pregnant women to at least 20 percent. 1995 progress toward goal achieved: 20 percent
- Increase to at least 90 percent the proportion of all pregnant women who receive prenatal care in the first trimester of pregnancy. 1995 progress toward goal achieved: 15 percent
- Increase to at least 90 percent the proportion of babies aged 18 months and younger who receive recommended primary care services at the appropriate intervals. 1995 progress toward goal achieved: data unavailable
- Reduce the prevalence of infertility to no more than 6.5 percent. 1995 progress toward goal achieved: data unavailable
- Increase to at least 90 percent the proportion of family planning counselors who offer accurate information about all options, including prenatal care and delivery, infant care, foster care, or adoption and pregnancy termination to their unmarried patients with unintended pregnancies. 1995 progress toward goal achieved: data unavailable

getting pregnant because smoking during pregnancy increases the risks of lower birthweight, a premature birth, or having a newborn with increased respiratory problems. If a woman drinks alcoholic beverages, she should stop drinking before getting pregnant because alcoholic beverages can cause infertility and birth defects, and no amount is safe. One woman may drink heavily and be fortunate to have a "normal" child, whereas another woman may drink lightly and give birth to a child with fetal alcohol syndrome. Any drugs, including over-the-counter drugs, should not be taken without the consent of a health-care provider. Proper nutrition and exercise includes eating appropriately from the food pyramid, avoiding megadoses of vitamins and minerals, and working out in moderation. Folic acid is a nutritional supplement that provides protection against neural tube defects (defects of the brain and/or spinal cord) to the fetus. The U.S. Public Health Service recommends 0.4 milligrams of folic acid (the amount found in vitamin supplements) beginning one month before conception and through the first trimester. If a woman is contemplating pregnancy, it is important to discuss pre-pregnancy planning with her health-care provider.

Conception

Ovulation, the release of the egg from the ovary into the fallopian tube, typically occurs 12 to 14 days before the onset of menstruation. Just before ovulation, the cervix produces a clear, watery mucus that facilitates the transport of sperm into the reproductive tract. The corpus luteum, the remaining structure after ovulation, secretes progesterone, which is the hormone needed to prepare the uterus for implantation. When conception occurs, the corpus luteum continues to produce progesterone. **Conception** occurs when the sperm and ovum unite to form a **zygote** and typically takes place in the outer third of the fallopian tube (see Fig. 17.1). The fertilized egg then takes several days to travel to the uterus in the

conception—the beginning of pregnancy; when the sperm enters the egg.

zygote (zie goat)—the developing egg from the time it is fertilized until implantation in the uterus.

FIGURE 17.1 After its release from the follicle, the ovum begins its week-long journey down the fallopian tube. Fertilization generally occurs in the outermost third of the tube. Now fertilized, the ovum progresses toward the uterus, where it embeds itself in the endometrium. A pregnancy is established.

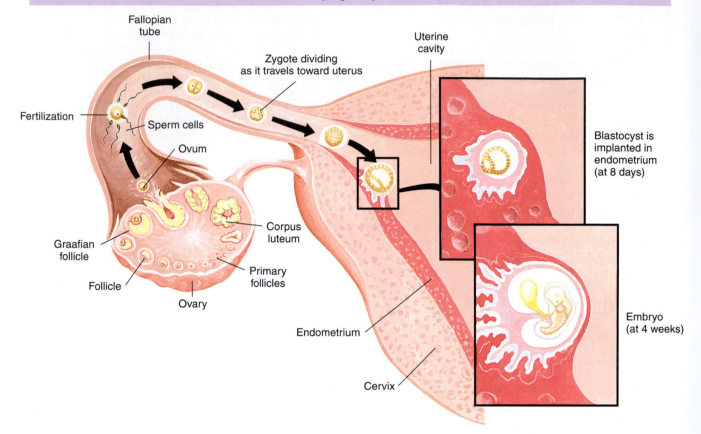

form of a **blastocyst** (early embryonic cells before a cell layer has formed), which implants into the endometrium to become an **embryo.** In most circumstances, one sperm and one ovum unite to form one zygote. However, if two (or more) eggs are released during ovulation and fertilized during conception, multiple births can occur. *Fraternal* twins come from different fertilized eggs and will be no more genetically similar than siblings from different births. *Identical* twins develop from the division of a single fertilized egg and share the same genetic material.

Early Signs of Pregnancy

A woman usually becomes pregnant before she recognizes the signs of pregnancy because fertilization occurs approximately 2 weeks before menstruation. The major organs of the fetus develop before the eighth week of pregnancy while the embryo is devel-

oping. The importance of practicing positive health behaviors before conception and during the early pregnancy to prevent birth defects and low birthweight cannot be emphasized strongly enough. The early signs of pregnancy consist of one or more of the following signs: a missed period; a light period or spotting; tender, swollen breasts; fatigue; upset stomach or vomiting; feeling bloated; or needing to urinate often.[2]

Home Pregnancy Tests

A missed period is usually the first sign of pregnancy. When this happens, you may decide to buy a home pregnancy test to determine whether you are truly pregnant. Most home pregnancy tests are urine tests that measure human chorionic gonadotropin (HCG). Some tests require urine to be combined with chemicals whereas others require placement of urine on a treated surface. Small traces of HCG can be detected as quickly as 6 days after conception. False negatives are much more common than false positives. False negatives often occur when the test if taken too early in the pregnancy, when HCG levels are undetectable. A positive test is usually accurate, however some contaminants can create false positives.

A variety of products such as e.p.t., First Response, Clearblue Easy, Advance 1-Step Pregnancy Test, and Fact Plus Pregnancy can be purchased without a prescription. Some home tests (First Response and e.p.t.) contain monoclonal antibodies that bond to HCG. Others (Clearblue Easy) give quick results by a testing method called rapid assay delivery system. These tests claim 99 percent accuracy in laboratory tests.[3] The cost for a home pregnancy test varies from $8–14 for one test kit, and $12–18 for 2-test kits. Test results can be obtained within 2 to 20 minutes depending upon the product.

The following guidelines are suggested for proper use of a pregnancy test. First, the test kit instructions should be read thoroughly and the directions should be followed precisely. Second, the urine (preferably the first urine in the morning) sample should be collected in a clean, dry container. The test should be conducted in a well-lighted area with a cold water faucet and a watch or timer that measures time in seconds nearby. Last, the color of the test should be compared with the color chart on the package when the timing period has ended. These results should be recorded (time and date) so you can discuss them with your health-care provider.[4]

Fetal Development

The development of the fetus begins at conception. During the next 9 months, a sequence of changes occurs to the fetus and the mother. Table 17.1 shows the stages of development during each trimester with descriptions of the changes for both.

Ectopic Pregnancy

One in 60 pregnancies result in implantation of the embryo in the fallopian tubes or other extra-uterine site such as the ovaries, abdominal cavity, or cervix. Ninety to 95 percent of ectopic pregnancies are tubal pregnancies, primarily in the ampulla. The women at greatest risk include those with a prior history of ectopic pregnancy, a previous pelvic infection or surgery to the fallopian tubes, endometriosis,

uterine fibroids, and the use of an intrauterine device. An **ectopic pregnancy** presents a potential risk to a mother and can cause infertility and maternal mortality. The symptoms vary and may mimic those of various other pathologies such as appendicitis, salpingitis, or spontaneous abortion. The symptoms may include menstrual irregularities such as spotting or missed periods, unilateral pelvic pain, elevated temperature, internal bleeding before rupture, and external bleeding if rupture occurs. The degree of risk to a mother depends upon the stage of diagnosis and the presenting symptoms.

PRENATAL CARE AND DELIVERY

Prenatal care is extremely important to the health and well-being of mother and child. Young teenage women who unexpectedly get pregnant are at greatest risk for complications, especially if they live in a low-income environment. They can usually receive services through local health department clinics or community health centers. These clinics offer low-price or free services, depending on income.

Pregnant women over age 35 were once labelled "high risk." Now, these pregnancies are becoming more commonplace as women who delayed pregnancy to pursue careers are beginning to plan for a family. These women have the advantage of being emotionally prepared for a pregnancy. The disadvantage is an increased risk due to chronic diseases. A review of several studies of pregnant women over age 35 found no relationship between pregnancy outcome and maternal age after exclusion of coexisting maternal disease. The risk of preterm delivery in women in their thirties and forties was comparable to that of women in their twenties.[5]

---

blastocyst—a cluster of embryonic cells; the stage between the zygote and embryo.

embryo—the developing egg from the time of implantation (about 2 weeks after conception) in the uterus until the seventh or eighth week of pregnancy.

ectopic pregnancy—implantation of the embryo in the fallopian tube, ovary, abdominal cavity, or cervix.

Table 17.1

Growth and Changes During Pregnancy

	WOMAN	FETUS
0–14 Weeks (First Trimester)	• Your period stops or is light. • You may have nausea and vomiting. This usually goes away by the end of this time. • Your breasts become larger. They may be tender. • Your nipples may stick out more. • You may have to urinate more often.	• The heart begins to beat. • Bones have appeared—the head, arms, fingers, legs, and toes are formed. • The major organ and nervous systems are formed. • The placenta forms. • Hair is starting to grow. • 20 buds for future teeth have appeared. • By the end of this time, the fetus is 4 inches long and weighs just over 1 ounce.
14–28 Weeks (Second Trimester)	• Your abdomen begins to swell—your uterus will be near your ribs by the end of this time. • The skin on your abdomen and breasts stretches. You may see stretch marks. • At about 16–20 weeks, you may start to feel the fetus move. • You may get a dark line from the navel down the middle of the abdomen or brown, uneven marks on the face. You may get a brown ring around your areolas.	• The fetus grows quickly from now until birth. • The organs are developing further. • Eyebrows and fingernails form. • The skin is wrinkled and covered with fine hair. • The fetus moves, kicks, sleeps and wakes, swallows, can hear, and can pass urine. • By the end of this time, the fetus is 11–14 inches long and weighs about 2–2 ½ pounds.
28–40 Weeks (Third Trimester)	• The movements of the fetus are stronger. • You may have abdominal pains. These may be false or true labor pains. • You may feel short of breath as the uterus pushes against the diaphragm (a flat, strong muscle that aids in breathing). You will be able to breathe better when the baby drops. • When the baby drops, you may need to urinate more often. • Yellow, watery fluid (colostrum) may leak from the nipples. • Your navel may stick out. • Your cervix may begin to thin out and open slightly.	• The fetus kicks and stretches, but as it gets bigger it has less room to move. • Fine body hair disappears. • Bones harden, but bones of the head are soft and flexible for delivery. • The fetus usually settles into a good position for birth. • At 40 weeks, the fetus will be full term. It is about 20 inches long and weighs 6–9 pounds.

Primary Care Services

A primary care team may include an obstetrician-gynecologist, certified nurse-midwife, and a child-birth educator. The initial visit may occur before conception and entails a discussion of maternal nutritional needs; exercise and weight management; current drug use including tobacco, alcohol, OTC drugs, prescription drugs such as those for diabetes or hypertension control, illegal drugs such as marijuana or crack cocaine, and other drugs; immunizations; and genetic counseling. The first prenatal visit will include a history (if not taken previously); a physical examination to determine height, weight, and blood pressure; an examination of the reproductive organs including changes to the cervix and the size of the uterus; an estimation of the due date; blood, urine, and Pap tests; and a plan for future visits and tests. Typically, visits occur monthly during the first 28 weeks, every 2 weeks during weeks 28 to 36, and weekly thereafter.[6]

Each subsequent visit will consist of a check of weight; blood pressure; fetal heartbeat, growth, and position; and a urine test for protein and sugar. In addition to routine tests, a health-care provider may suggest special tests for birth defects or stress to the fetus. These tests include ultrasound, chorionic villus sampling (CVS), maternal serum screening, amniocentesis, a nonstress test, a contraction stress test, and a biophysical profile. Table 17.2 describes these tests, what they check for, who should have them, and when they should be given.

Table 17.2

Special Pregnancy Tests

TEST	WHAT IT IS	WHAT IT LOOKS FOR	WHO SHOULD HAVE IT	WHEN
Ultrasound	Test that creates an image of the fetus from sound waves by either moving an instrument across the abdomen or placing a small device in the vagina	Information about the fetus, such as age; rate of growth; placement of the placenta; fetal position, movement, and heart rate; number of fetuses; some, but not all, fetal problems	Women whose doctors want to tell how old the fetus is, confirm a condition, or check a suspected problem	Depends on the reason for performing ultrasound
Maternal serum screening	A blood test that tests for substances from the pregnancy that are also in the woman's blood	Signs of birth defects such as open neural tube defects (NTDs) or Down syndrome	Every woman should be offered maternal serum screening	15–18 weeks
Chorionic villus sampling (CVS)	A sample of the chorionic villi is taken from the placenta, either through a needle passed through the abdomen and uterus or through a thin tube passed through the vagina and cervix	Certain conditions, such as Down syndrome; other tests may be run depending on a woman's risk factors	If available, test will be offered to women who already have a child with certain birth defects, who have a family history of birth defects, who will be 35 or older on their due date, or if they and their partner are at risk for certain genetic diseases	10–12 weeks
Amniocentesis	A sample of amniotic fluid (the liquid around the fetus inside the uterus) is drawn through a thin needle that is inserted through the abdomen into the uterus. Ultrasound is used to guide the needle	Certain conditions, such as Down syndrome and NTDs; other tests may be run on amniotic fluid depending on a woman's risk factors. May be used late in pregnancy to see if baby's lungs are likely to work if birth occurs soon	Test may be offered to women who already have a child with certain birth defects, who have a family history of birth defects, who will be 35 or older on their due date, or if they and their partner are at risk for certain genetic diseases	14–18 weeks
Nonstress test	Test that measures the fetal heart rate as the fetus moves. An instrument is attached to the woman's abdomen (an electronic fetal monitor). Fetal movements are felt by the woman or noted by the doctor or nurse	Whether enough oxygen is getting to the fetus	Women with diabetes or high blood pressure; who smoke or use drugs; who have twins; or who have decreased fetal movements. Sometimes recommended in other circumstances	As doctor recommends, usually in the last 10 weeks of pregnancy
Contraction stress test	Test that measures how the fetal heart rate reacts to a uterine contraction. An electronic fetal monitor is used	Whether the fetus is under stress	Women with diabetes or high blood pressure; who smoke or use drugs; who have twins; or who have decreased fetal movements. Sometimes recommended in other circumstances	As doctor recommends, usually in the last 10 weeks of pregnancy
Biophysical profile	Combination of the nonstress test and ultrasound	Checks the fetus's "breathing" movements, muscle action, movement, amount of amniotic fluid, and the result of the nonstress test	Women with diabetes or high blood pressure; who smoke or use drugs; who have twins; or who have decreased fetal movements. Sometimes recommended in other circumstances	If nonstress test results are not normal. Some doctors use this test instead of the nonstress test

Weekly prenatal checkups are recommended after week 36. A woman will know that pre-term labor has begun when contractions:

- Are regular and evenly spaced apart (e.g., every 10 minutes)
- Happen more than five times an hour
- Last for 30 to 70 seconds
- Get worse as you move around[7]

Labor and Delivery

Throughout the pregnancy, a woman will experience irregular contractions that increase in frequency and intensity as the pregnancy progresses. These preliminary contractions, known as **Braxton Hicks contractions,** prepare the uterus for childbirth. Near the end of pregnancy, these contractions are difficult to distinguish from true labor. (See Table 17.3.) A woman will know that it is time to go to the hospital, call the nurse-midwife, or prepare for home birth when contractions are 5 minutes or less apart, her "water breaks" (the amniotic sac ruptures), and the pain remains constant and more intense. True labor occurs in three stages. (See Fig. 17.2.) Although the length and experience may vary among women, it also varies for a woman from the birth of her first child to ensuing births. The average length of time in labor for a first birth is approximately 13 hours and subsequent births average around 8 hours. Stage 1 begins with regular, uterine contractions at 15- to 20-minute intervals and throughout the first stage, the contractions become longer and stronger. The signs of stage 1 include "show," a slight flow of bloody mucus, and effacement (flattens out and gets longer) and dilation (opening) of the cervix. Stage 2 signs include a fully dilated cervix of approximately 10 centimeters, and strong contractions that facilitate the movement of the baby through the birth canal. (See Fig. 17.3.) This stage can last several hours and ends with expulsion of the baby. The baby is cleared of any mucus from the mouth and nose, and the umbilical cord is clamped. Stage 3 occurs after the baby is born. Uterine contractions continue until the placenta is delivered. This stage usually lasts between 3 to 20 minutes.[8] If an episiotomy was performed, the health-care provider will stitch up the incision after the placenta has been delivered.

The health-care provider will immediately evaluate the physical condition of the infant at 1 minute and 5 minutes. She will assess heart rate, respiratory effort, muscle tone, reflexes, and color with a score

Table 17.3

True and False Labor Contractions: How Do You Know?	
TRUE LABOR	**FALSE LABOR**
Regular intervals	Irregular intervals
Dilation of cervix	No dilation of cervix
Shortened intervals	Intervals remain longer
Increase in intensity	No increase in intensity
Back and abdominal discomfort	Minimal abdominal discomfort

of 0 to 2 for each sign. This is the infant's *Apgar score,* which averages 7 or higher for healthy infants.

Birthing Options

You have a wide variety of birthing options available today that are more empowering than the passive, clinical procedures typical of the past 30 years. More women today are choosing natural birth options whether with home birthing, birth centers, or hospitals. Childbirth classes provide you and your partner with an opportunity to find ways to be more actively involved in the birth process. These classes provide information to empower a couple, including suggestions on the available birthing options, breathing techniques, relaxation strategies, exercise, and methods to transition through labor. Natural birth is a process that includes an active mother as the participant in the birth experience. A misunderstanding about natural birth is that medication and assistance by medical personnel are avoided regardless of circumstances. Sometimes, when labor is difficult or complications arise, additional support may be needed. If normal labor becomes high risk, a couple should be flexible and may need to amend their choices.

Midwifery   **Midwives** assist pregnant women who are expecting low-risk pregnancies with prenatal care, childbirth, and infant care. A review of fifteen studies by the American Nurses Association

Braxton Hicks contraction—irregular tightening of the uterus during pregnancy, sometimes called false labor.

midwife—assists women in childbirth.

FIGURE 17.2 The three stages of childbirth.

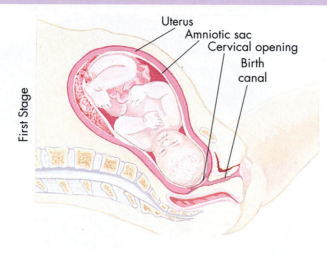

First Stage

Uterus
Amniotic sac
Cervical opening
Birth canal

Uterine contractions thin the cervix and enlarge the cervical opening

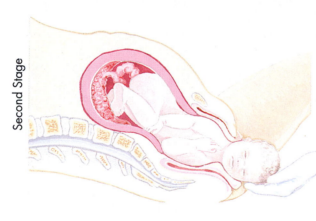

Second Stage

Uterine contractions are aided by mother's voluntary contractions of abdominal muscles

Fetus moves through dilated cervical opening and birth canal

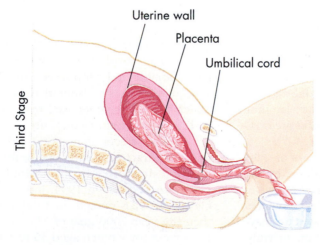

Third Stage

Uterine wall
Placenta
Umbilical cord

Placenta detaches from uterine wall and is delivered though the vagina

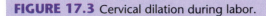

FIGURE 17.3 Cervical dilation during labor.

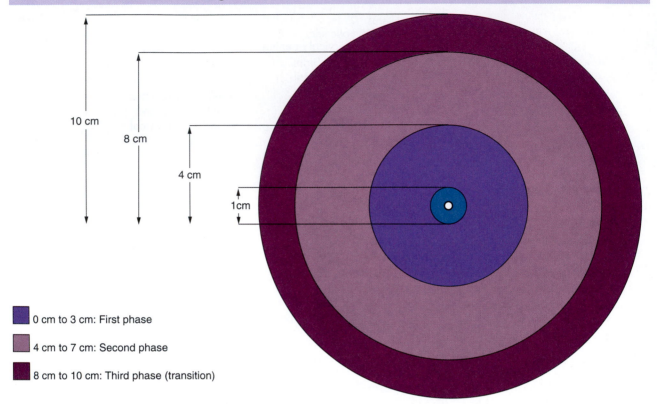

10 cm

8 cm

4 cm

1cm

■ 0 cm to 3 cm: First phase

■ 4 cm to 7 cm: Second phase

■ 8 cm to 10 cm: Third phase (transition)

found that women choosing Certified Nurse-Midwife (CNM) assisted births compared to physician-assisted births had fewer premature deliveries, fewer induced labors, shorter hospital stays, and less physical trauma to the mother. Carrying the fetus to full term has the added benefit of reducing the likelihood of low birthweight, a major factor in infant mortality. Infants born to mothers attended by a CNM tend to score similarly on the Apgar scale of vital signs at 1 and 5 minutes after birth.[9]

Nearly 10,500 practicing midwives are located in the United States and 6,000 of them are lay midwives. Approximately 4,500 nurse-midwives are certified and registered in the United States. CNMs are registered nurses with two additional years of training from a midwifery program accredited by the American College of Nurse-Midwives. Lay midwives have no formal midwifery education.[10] The number of lay midwives has steadily decreased as states have restricted or prohibited their practice. Concurrently, the number of certified nurse-midwives has continued to grow. A recent movement to certify lay midwives may once again increase the number of options available to pregnant women.

Hospital Deliveries Hospitals are changing their approach to birthing methods as women demand increased alternatives. In 1992, physician-attended births in hospitals declined to 94.2 percent while midwife-attended deliveries in hospitals increased to 4.4 percent of all births. This change has been gradually occurring since 1975.[11] Some hospitals have added all-in-one labor, delivery, and recovery rooms. Hospital staff have been trained to be more flexible and supportive. Another option available to women is collaborative management, during which a CNM is supervised by a physician and the mother knows both medical providers.

Some aspects of hospital deliveries continue to be unattractive. Nearly one in four (21.2 percent) hospital deliveries in the United States were by **cesarean section** in 1994, indicating a gradual decline from 22.8 percent in 1989, but still far higher than the year 2000 goal of 15 percent. The highest rates were for women aged 35 to 39 delivering their first child or women over age 40 delivering their first or second child.[12] Fetal monitoring and ultrasound devices appear to have contributed to the ever-increasing number of cesarean section deliveries. Continuous fetal monitoring was initially reserved for high-risk cases such as breach delivery, diabetes, and prematurity. Now, nearly three-quarters of all women are monitored, and studies suggest that fetal monitoring of low-risk women doubles their likelihood of having a cesarean delivery. Electronic fetal monitoring was the most prevalent obstetric procedure in 1994 and the rates of use are continuing to rise. A MMWR Weekly Report in 1995 also shows a changing trend in length of hospital stay. The average length of stay in the hospital for women who gave birth vaginally has decreased from 3.9 days in 1970 to 2.1 days in 1995. The average length of stay in the hospital for women who had Cesarean section stayed an average of 7.8 days in 1970 and 4.0 days in 1995. The researchers also found that women released earlier suffered more complications than women who stayed in the hospital longer.[13]

The reanalysis of another surgical procedure, episiotomies, is currently being debated. An episiotomy, an incision of the perineum (between the vagina and rectum), is designed to widen the birth canal and prevent severe tears during childbirth. Nearly 90 percent of first-time mothers have been subjected to this surgical procedure. Evidence suggests that this procedure actually may cause further tearing, rather than reduce tearing. A comparison between natural births and hospital births suggests that less trauma to the mother occurs with natural births.

Hospitals and medical procedures certainly have advantages for some women. Women who are at risk for having a high-risk pregnancy need the attention of a health-care provider. Even women at low risk for having a high-risk pregnancy may find they need medical attention because nearly 40 percent of high-risk pregnancies occur in low-risk women.

Birth Centers Nearly 135 licensed birth centers exist in the United States with the majority in Florida, Pennsylvania, Texas, and New York. Birth centers emphasize a close collaboration between OB-GYNs, nurses, and nurse-midwives. Birth centers provide couples with an alternative, professional environment to hospitals. Some are free-standing, whereas others are connected to a hospital. They are often arranged comfortably and provide the feelings of a quiet, home-like atmosphere in which births can occur with minimal intervention. Family members and friends are invited to participate fully in the birthing process. This participation further separates birth centers from hospitals. Some medical equipment is available for emergencies; however, certified birth centers collaborate closely with local hospitals and have a consulting physician who handles complications. If complications arise, the woman is transferred to the hospital because birth centers do not perform cesarean sections or seldom provide drugs for pain relief. Birth centers have been endorsed by the American College of Obstetricians and Gynecologists, and birth centers can be located through the National Association of Childbearing Centers.[14]

Birthing Positions

Homebirth Australia studied 4,523 planned home births in which women were free to assume a comfortable position. In hospital births, nearly 80 percent of women gave birth in recumbent positions. However, the Australian study found that given the freedom to move around, the most frequent position chosen by first-time mothers was a squatting position (36 percent), whereas experienced mothers chose hands and knees (28 percent). Other nonrecumbent positions include kneeling, standing, sitting, and the use of a birth chair. Birth chairs range from those designed with technical features to facilitate the birth to a simple stool with a high, slanted back for support and a hole in the seat. The upright position allows gravity to help in shortening the period from labor to delivery. The rate of episiotomies was considerably lower for home births than hospital births, and the amount of tearing was very low with less than 1 percent experiencing third-degree tears.[15]

BREAST-FEEDING

Breast-feeding has prevented nearly 6 million infant deaths each year worldwide and has the potential to prevent an additional 1 to 2 million child deaths each year. The percentage of women in the United States who are breast-feeding has been increasing, particularly among racial and ethnic minorities. The advantages of breast milk over formula are well known and include its inexpensiveness, its better nutritional quality, its ability to act as a birth control measure to

> **cesarean section**—surgical procedure in which the abdomen and uterus are cut open for the birth of the child.

limit fertility, and its role in reducing ovarian and pre-menopausal breast cancer.[16]

Breast milk is unique and because of its qualities, more women should be encouraged to breast-feed their infants. Breast milk has been described as "dynamic," ever changing in content to meet the needs of a growing infant. It consists of fat, protein, carbohydrates, minerals, and vitamins, in varying degrees. Lactose, the predominant sugar in milk, cannot be found in any other natural state. **Colostrum,** the initial milk produced by the mother, has numerous infection fighting agents and is tailored to the needs of the infant. One author wrote, "The colostrum present in mothers delivering premature infants contains a much higher concentration of protein, anti-infection fighting components, and infection fighting cells than colostrum of full term infants. Also, the more premature the infant, the higher the concentrations of these components."[17]

Breast-feeding has beneficial health results for the mother as well as the infant. Maternal benefits when breast-feeding begins immediately include reducing the risk of hemorrhage by helping the uterus contract, reducing the risk of breast and ovarian cancer, reducing the risk of osteoporosis, and assisting in family planning. The Lactational Amenorrhea Method (LAM), a family planning method, uses three measures to determine a woman's fertility: the return of a menstrual period, the pattern of breast-feeding, and the length of time since birth. The chance of getting pregnant is less than 2 percent if menstruation has not begun, breast-feeding is regular and on demand, and the infant is less than 6 months old.[18]

Breast-feeding is awkward for some mothers and babies to learn. It is a specific learned skill and given adequate assistance, both mother and infant will be successful unless unusual circumstances exist. The Baby-Friendly Hospital Initiative was introduced in 1989 as a joint project by the World Health Organization and UNICEF. Nearly 170 countries with 4,282 hospitals have participated in the program since its inception. *FYI:* "Ten Steps to Successful Breast-Feeding" presents the criteria for successful breast-feeding, which a facility must satisfy to qualify as a baby-friendly hospital.

In 1998, Minnesota became the first state to pass a law encouraging businesses and industry to provide a private room (not a toilet stall) in the work environment for nursing mothers to express breastmilk for their infants. The Senator who introduced the bill

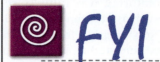

Ten Steps to Successful Breast-Feeding

Every facility providing maternity services and care for newborn infants should:

1. Have a written breast-feeding policy that is routinely communicated to all health-care staff.
2. Train all health-care staff in skills necessary to implement this policy.
3. Inform all pregnant women about the benefits and management of breast-feeding.
4. Help mothers initiate breast-feeding within a half-hour of birth.
5. Show mothers how to breast-feed and how to maintain lactation even if they should be separated from their infants.
6. Give newborn infants no food or drink other than breast-milk, unless medically indicated.
7. Practice rooming-in: allow mothers and infants to remain together 24 hours a day.
8. Encourage breast-feeding on demand.
9. Give no artificial teats or pacifiers (also called dummies or soothers) to breast-feeding infants.
10. Foster the establishment of breast-feeding support groups and refer mothers to them on discharge from the hospital or clinic.

stated that breastfed infants are healthier, and keeping infants healthy translates into less absenteeism by working mothers. Hopefully, other states will follow suit and assist working mothers to practice healthy childbearing behaviors.

MATERNAL AND INFANT MORTALITY

Maternal mortality is the best indicator of the status of women, particularly their health status. Maternal mortality is defined as the "death of a woman while pregnant or within 42 days of termination of pregnancy . . . but not from accidental or incidental causes."[19] New estimates of maternal mortality rates worldwide average 430 per 100,000; 27 per 100,000 in developed countries compared to 480 in 100,000 in developing countries and with rates as high as 1 in

10 in some parts of Africa. Maternal deaths are classified as direct or indirect obstetric deaths due to complications of the pregnancy. Direct obstetric deaths account for 80 percent of all maternal deaths and result from complications such as incorrect treatment, labor, pregnancy, or omissions. The most common complication is hemorrhage, usually during the postpartum phase. Indirect obstetric deaths account for 20 percent of all maternal deaths and result from previous existing diseases or diseases caused by the physiological complications of pregnancy.[20] In the United States, the maternal mortality rate is higher among African American women compared to white women. In 1990, the maternal mortality rate was 5.7 per 100,000 live births for white women and 18.6 per 100,000 live births for African American women. African American women were three times more likely to die from complications of pregnancy, childbirth, and puerperium than white women.[21]

The World Health Organization has determined that three interventions are essential to meet the goal of cutting maternal deaths by half:

- Reducing the number of high-risk and unwanted pregnancies
- Reducing the number of obstetric complications
- Reducing deaths among women who develop complications[22]

The best mechanism for preventing maternal deaths is continuing to improve the status of women. This improvement includes access to education, health care, and proper nutrition. The long-term goal of bettering the status of women can be supplemented by the short-term goals of providing universal access to family planning and skilled health care.

Infant mortality, like maternal mortality, is an important indicator of a country's health status. Infant mortality is defined as the "deaths of infants under 1 year; neonatal mortality is deaths of infants under 28 days; and postneonatal mortality is deaths of infants aged 28 days up to 1 year." The United States ranks twenty-fourth in infant mortality compared to other developed countries and the disparity between African American and white infant deaths has remained constant since 1987. Neonatal mortality accounts for 70 percent of all infant mortality and the overall U.S. infant mortality rate is 8.5 per 1,000 live births. The primary cause for neonatal and infant mortality is low and very low birthweight due predominately to an increase of preterm births.[23]

INFERTILITY

A growing number of couples are having difficulty with conceiving. Some couples have delayed childbirth decisions until their late thirties to early forties, a time when women are less fertile. Others face the challenge of infertility at a younger age. Regardless of the age of the couple, advances in assisted reproductive technology have allowed couples who previously were childless to experience the joy of childbirth. The initial step for the health-care provider is to determine the cause of the infertility. **Primary infertility** is recognized as the inability of a woman to become pregnant within 1 year of having unprotected sexual intercourse. **Secondary infertility** is her inability to carry the pregnancy to full term. In 10 to 15 percent of the cases, no cause for infertility can be established. Overall, women and men account equally for cases of primary infertility.

The most common reasons for primary infertility in women are failure to ovulate or having a damaged uterus or fallopian tubes. In men, low sperm count or abnormal sperm development cause primary infertility. The risk of infertility increases as women age. Women aged 35 have a 50 percent pregnancy rate after 1 year of unprotected sexual intercourse. Women aged 40 to 44 have a 1-year pregnancy rate of 27 percent.[24] *FYI:* "Reasons for Infertility" presents some of the recognized reasons for infertility in women and men. Also, see *Health Tips* for information on where to go for help.

Fertility clinics have proliferated over the past decade with approximately 300 clinics operating in

---

colostrum (kol **os** trum)—the initial breast milk produced by the mother.

maternal mortality—death of a mother while pregnant or within 42 days of termination of the pregnancy.

infant mortality—statistic rate of infant death during the first year of birth expressed as the number per 1,000 live births.

primary infertility—inability to conceive after a year of unprotected sexual intercourse.

secondary infertility—inability to carry a pregnancy full term.

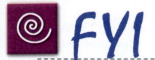

FYI

Reasons for Infertility

Failure to Ovulate

- Hormonal imbalance
- Obesity and/or weight gain
- Prolonged stress
- Ovarian tumor or cyst
- Abbreviated menstrual cycle
- Weight loss including eating disorders
- Alcohol, tobacco, or other drug abuse, including caffeine

Damaged Fallopian Tubes or Uterus

- PID or other STD infection
- Birth defect
- Previous removal of ectopic pregnancy
- Endometriosis or uterine fibroids
- Irregularly shaped or tipped uterus

Low Sperm Count

- ATOD abuse, including steroids and marijuana
- Prolonged stress
- Previous STD infection
- Exposure to toxic substances in the workplace

health tips

RESOLVE, Inc.

RESOLVE, Inc., established in 1974, is a national, non-profit organization of over 20,000 fertility-impaired persons. It offers assistance, medical referral, emotional support, and education to many people. RESOLVE provides immediate, compassionate, and informed help to people who are experiencing the infertility crisis and provides visibility of the issues through advocacy and public education. To contact RESOLVE, Inc., see the Resources section at the end of this chapter.

JOURNAL ACTIVITY

Medical and Ethical Issues

Assisted reproductive technologies raise a number of social, medical, and ethical issues. The Roman Catholic Church clearly opposes all assisted reproduction. This stance causes dismay for many infertile couples who are practicing Catholics. Their dilemma is whether to adhere to the church's position or seek medical help to have their child. The social and ethical issues are weighed against medical advances. What are your feelings about the dilemma some women face? How would you handle this dilemma? What would you suggest to a friend who may be infertile?

the United States. These clinics have functioned with limited oversight and take in nearly $2 billion a year. The average success rate of most clinics is between 18 to 20 percent, but some clinics have rates as high as 30 percent. Keep in mind that some clinics with low rates may still be as good as others; these clinics may accept more difficult cases. Fertility clinics provide a number of procedures and methods of assisted reproduction including fertility drugs, surgery, artificial insemination, surrogacy, in vitro fertilization, and a variety of newer high-tech techniques.

Fertility Drugs

Fertility drugs such as Pergonal (HMG), Metrodin, Humegon, and Clomid (clomiphene citrate) can be given to induce ovulation. These hormones function in different ways with the intent of stimulating a woman's ovaries to produce extra eggs. A woman may also receive the drug Lopron to suppress natural hormonal increases. When the eggs ripen, an injection of human chorionic gonadotropin (hCG) is ad-

ministered to facilitate the release of eggs. The eggs are then retrieved and a method is chosen for transferring the embryo, such as IVF, GIFT, or ZIFT.[25] Several questions have arisen about the use of fertility drugs. Do these hormones increase the woman's risk of ovarian cancer? What are the long-term risks from these procedures or drugs? What should be done with the remaining embryos? How should the risks associated with multiple births be handled? Now complete *Journal Activity:* "Medical and Ethical Issues."

Artificial Insemination

Artificial insemination involves the use of sperm from a donor or partner to fertilize an egg. Sperm are collected and placed in the woman's vagina or uterus through a catheter. During the 1970s, a self insemination movement arose among single women and lesbians. This effort moved the medical community to be less se-

Her Story

Toni and Kelly

Toni and Kelly, a lesbian couple, chose artificial insemination as their route to having children. They have been together in a committed relationship for 8 years. When Toni decided she wanted to have a baby, she was 35 years old. Kelly thought it was a great idea and they immediately started asking friends about their options. Soon, they found a health-care provider who was willing to work with them and who informed them about a fertility clinic in California that would mail-order sperm to them. They contacted the clinic and received an information packet with the description and background information on a variety of sperm donors who were identified only by a code number. After careful consideration, they chose donor number 872 from the cryobank. After working with their health-care provider to determine the best time to inseminate the sperm, Toni placed a call to the clinic, and the sperm, frozen in liquid nitrogen, was delivered to their front door by UPS when the time was most optimal. Kelly and Toni carefully followed the directions, thawed out the sperm, and Kelly inseminated Toni with the sperm using a small plastic syringe. Toni got pregnant on the second try and gave birth to a beautiful girl, Jana. When Jana was 2 years old, Toni and Kelly decided to

have a second child. They were disappointed to learn that 872 was no longer an active donor because they wanted Jana to have a full biological sibling and they were pleased with Jana's disposition. They decided to try another donor, but Toni didn't get pregnant. When they contacted the clinic a second time, they discovered that 872 had begun donating sperm again. They were thrilled! Toni got pregnant on the first try and nine months later, Kindra was born. Jana and Kindra are surrounded by loving parents, grandparents, and friends. The donor, 872, has provided a waiver to the clinic, giving permission to the girls to learn the identity of their father when they are 18 years old.

Although the birth of these children occurred in a loving family, Toni and Kelly knew that their children may face profuse challenges as they grow up. Not all people are going to share their joy and happiness. Not all people are going to understand their desire to be a family.

- What do you think?
- What are the obstacles facing Jana and Kindra?
- What is the strength of this family unit?
- How did you react when you read this story?

lective about the recipients of donated sperm. However, the fear of AIDS has increased the need to be more cautious with this procedure. The lack of regulations regarding who can donate sperm and the number of times sperm can be donated has led to some self-regulation. The case of a physician in Virginia who was believed to impregnate dozens of women with his sperm indicates a flaw with voluntary regulatory procedures.[26]

A controversy regarding artificial insemination is whether HIV-negative women should be allowed to be inseminated by their HIV-positive partner. Some HIV-negative women have wanted to be inseminated after HIV has been washed from the sperm of their partners. The CDC has recommended against sperm washing, a technique that removes HIV from sperm, because the procedure cannot reliably eliminate HIV from semen. U.S. couples wanting children despite the HIV-positive status of the male have sought support in other countries. In one study, a method known as the Percoil configuration method, con-

ducted by researchers in Milan, Italy, appeared to reduce the amount of HIV in semen by 99 percent. Other studies suggest that the woman's risk can be reduced by 30 to 40 percent.[27]

Another controversy exists regarding whether single women, particularly lesbians, should be permitted access to assisted conception. More and more lesbians and single women are deciding to have children. Some factions would like to deny these women the opportunity to use sperm banks. Is it right to deny some women access to artificial insemination? If so, who should be denied access? (See *Her Story:* "Toni and Kelly.")

artificial insemination—placing semen in the vagina or uterus by mechanical means rather than intercourse.

Surrogacy

Surrogacy has been practiced throughout history. The major question asked by many is how can a woman carry a pregnancy to full term and then walk away from the baby? And, if the motivating factor is money, how does this differ from selling babies? In surrogacy, a woman, other than the partner, agrees to become pregnant and carry the fetus to full term. Usually the surrogate woman's own egg is fertilized by the sperm of the male from the couple seeking a baby. If IVF is attempted the woman's fertilized egg may be placed in the surrogate woman's uterus. This child is the biological offspring of the couple.

Since 1977, nearly 4,500 children were born to surrogate women in the United States. Few of these cases have resulted in legal battles; however, some situations have led to national attention. By 1992, many states had banned or restricted the practice of commercial surrogacy and five states had criminalized surrogacy. Most states have restricted the amount of payment the surrogate mother can receive for medical expenses and have eliminated the expenses of a broker. The cost of surrogacy can range from $15,000 to $40,000 and cover lawyer fees, medical costs, a possible surrogate fee, and miscellaneous expenses. Legal issues can arise if the surrogate woman tries to gain custody of the baby. Should the child be denied access to his or her biological mother? Who has the parental rights to raise this child? Can a surrogate woman change her mind? Now see *Viewpoint:* "Surrogate Grandmothers."

In Vitro Fertilization

Louise Brown, the world's first "test tube" baby, was born in July 1978. Since 1977, **in vitro fertilization (IVF)** has been practiced extensively. The IVF process begins with a 2-week regimen of daily drug injections to prepare the ovaries for producing a number of mature eggs. The mature eggs are extracted from the ovaries and placed in a petri dish with the partner's sperm. The embryos are incubated for 3 days and then implanted into the woman's uterus. IVF boasts a success rate of approximately 17 percent, as high as 19 percent for women under age 35 and as low as 6 percent for women over age 40.[28] *FYI:* "Clinic-Specific Report" provides an example of the information available from the American Society for Reproductive Medicine and Society for Assisted Reproductive Medicine regarding assisted reproduction. How important would this information be for couples dealing with infertility?

Newer high-tech techniques, including **GIFT** (gamete intrafallopian transfer), **ZIFT** (zygote intrafallopian transfer), and **ICSI** (intracytoplasmic sperm in-

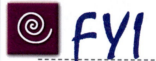

Clinic-Specific Report

Clinics throughout the United States and Canada are encouraged to provide data regarding their success rates and outcomes of all pregnancies. Reports have a 2-year delay in processing but they are available to couples through the American Society for Reproductive Medicine. These reports include information based on the type of procedure and its success. Information may include:

- Number of clinical pregnancies that occurred
- Number of egg retrievals performed
- Number of embryo transfers performed
- Live baby delivery rates
- Number of multiple births
- Number of ectopic pregnancies
- Number of miscarriages or stillbirths

Information is provided on a regional basis and a fee is assessed. This information can be accessed through the Internet. See the Resources section at the end of this chapter. ☞

Surrogate Grandmothers

A grandmother in England gave birth to her own grandchild. Her daughter was born without a uterus and she wanted her daughter and son-in-law to have their own child.

A grandmother in South Dakota gave birth to her own grandchild. Her daughter, a librarian, was unable to have children so she carried the fertilized embryos for her daughter and gave birth to twins.

Should surrogacy remain legal? When should the children be told about this event?

Viewpoint

Aging and Assisted Reproduction

As menopausal or postmenopausal women choose to become impregnated, the demand for donor eggs will continue to increase. Research suggests that when donor eggs from younger women are used, older women increase their likelihood of conceiving and the risk of congenital defects decreases.[30]

On November 7, 1996, a 63-year-old California woman gave birth to a healthy baby girl. She is believed to be the oldest woman in the world to give birth to a healthy child. Her husband is 60 years old. She entered the USC Fertility Center 3 years ago with medical records showing an age of 50. She was inseminated with donor eggs and her husband's sperm. Only after she had been pregnant for 13 weeks did she confess to lying about her age. Dr. Mark Sauer, the infertility specialist who pio-

neered the use of donor eggs in older women, believes it is becoming more common for older women seeking donor eggs to lie about their age. His concern is the quality-of-life issues for the child.[31] Some ethicists believe this woman had a right to have a child. They view arbitrary age cutoffs for women as discriminatory. Other ethicists believe that just because technology can create this opportunity, it isn't necessarily right to give limited donor eggs to older women when young, healthy women are seeking fertility assistance. Unlike sperm donors, the person assuming most of the risk with donor eggs is the donor. What do you think? Should there be age cutoffs? Are there quality-of-life issues for the child? Is there a double-standard between older women and older men?

jection), require surgery and are more expensive than single IVF. However, many clinics quickly incorporate these procedures because couples often are willing to give large sums of money for the remote chance of conceiving a baby. The cost of these procedures can vary from $8,000 to $15,000 depending upon the location and the type of procedure.

Donor Eggs and Egg Retrieval

Immature oocyte collection, a method similar to IVF, has received considerable attention recently because it reduces or eliminates the need for fertility drugs. This method, first used successfully in Australia, removes the immature eggs from the follicles, matures the egg outside the ovary, fertilizes the egg with sperm, and places the fertilized egg in the uterus. A number of social and ethical questions have arisen with the issue of donor eggs. (See *Viewpoint:* "Aging and Assisted Reproduction.") The immature oocyte collection procedure raises issues such as whether retrieval and storage of eggs from aborted fetuses, accident victims, or women undergoing a hysterectomy should occur. A female has 300,000 to 400,000 eggs at birth, with approximately 400 mature eggs released during her lifetime. These mature eggs are the ones sought by fertility specialists. Immature eggs, often four to seven viable eggs with each monthly cycle, can be removed from the follicle.[29]

Multiple Births

Multiple births have increased 33 percent since 1980, many because of the increased use of assisted reproduction. Multiple births are a major issue for

surrogacy—a woman, other than the partner, agrees to become pregnant and carry the fetus to full term.

in vitro fertilization (IVF)—multiple eggs are removed from the ovary, fertilized with sperm within glass and the resulting embryos are inserted into the woman's uterus.

GIFT (gamete intrafallopian transfer)—multiple eggs are removed from the ovary, mixed with sperm, and surgically inserted into the woman's fallopian tubes.

ZIFT (zygote intrafallopian transfer)—multiple eggs are removed from the ovary, fertilized with sperm in a petri dish, and surgically inserted into the woman's fallopian tubes.

ICSI (intracytoplasmic sperm injection)—a type of IVF in which a single sperm is injected into the center of an egg; can be used with sperm that are less mobile and weaker.

fertility clinics. Over 50 percent of births through IVF are multiple births, creating higher medical expenses and greater risk of maternal or infant mortality. Multiple births are common because several embryos are transferred to the woman's uterus. The transfer of a number of embryos increases the likelihood of pregnancy during that cycle and it also increases the likelihood of multiple births.

ADOPTION

Adoption is an alternative to assisted reproduction. Adoption issues have changed because the rights of adoptees are now viewed as being equal to the rights of birth parents and adoptive parents. Couples who are making a decision on whether to adopt a child have a variety of issues to consider. First, they need to decide on the age, race, and health status of the child they want to adopt. Do they expect to raise a normal, healthy child from infancy? Does the child's background matter? Should they consider intercountry adoption or adopting a special needs child, a minority child, or an older child? Once they decide on the kind of child they desire, they need to find an appropriate agency to meet their needs. Agencies can vary from public agencies such as county social services to private adoption by a lawyer, physician, or church. Services can vary from matching children and adoptive parents to educational and support services throughout the parenting years.

Adoptions can be closed or open. **Closed** (confidential) **adoption** means that contact between birth parents and adoptive parents is nonexistent. **Open adoption** means that contact occurs between birth parents and adoptive parents. This contact can vary from occasional letters to regular contact with the child. Open adoption eliminates the need for children to fantasize about their birth parents; they get actual knowledge of their ancestry. However, open adoption also brings the inherent risk of birth parents interfering or intruding on the life of the adopted family. Bonding can become difficult if competition arises for the child's attention.

Such attachment and identity issues in adopted children may not develop during the early years, especially if the child is adopted as an infant. Rather, these issues may develop during the adolescent years, when many young adults feel that they have a need to know their birth parents. This process can be difficult; the anticipation and expectation of being

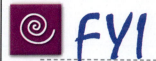

National Adoption Registry, Inc.

The National Adoption Registry is a private registry that accepts registrations from adoptees, birth parents, and other interested individuals. Vital statistics of the adoptee are entered into the data base and matched with existing information in the file. A fee is assessed for registration. (See the Resources Section at the end of this chapter.) ∞

accepted by their birth parents are usually mixed with the fear of experiencing further rejection. The Internet has become a ready source for exchange of information between adopted children seeking birth parents and birth parents seeking information about the child they gave up for adoption years ago. (See *FYI:* "National Adoption Registry, Inc.")

Foster Care

Many children, over 100,000 in all, were once thought unadoptable. These children, labeled "special needs," live in foster care and await adoption. Special needs children include school-age or older children, children who have suffered emotional or physical abuse or neglect, children with physical or mental handicaps, siblings who desire to be kept together, children with racial or ethnic differences, or children born with HIV or other medical problems. The criteria for parents seeking to adopt special needs children are often more relaxed compared to adoption of infants. Foster parents, parents with large families, single parents, and others will find reduced fees and sometimes reimbursement for adopting these children.[32]

PARENTING

A critical and essential aspect of child development is the parenting process during the formative years. Each child is born with inherent characteristics, called temperament, that make him or her unique. The parent's responsibility is to get to know the child, his or her likes and dislikes, activity level, personality, skills and abilities, and then to guide the

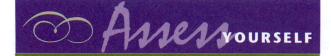

How Do You Rate Your Competence to Be a Parent?

Rate each of the items below by indicating how competent you feel about your abilities according to the following scale:

a—Very competent
b—Fairly competent
c—Somewhat competent
d—Not very competent
e—Not at all competent

How do you feel about your competence and ability to:

_____ 1. Care for a child when he or she is sick or upset?
_____ 2. Help a child solve problems?
_____ 3. Provide adequate time for a child?
_____ 4. Be a good parent?
_____ 5. Provide emotional support for a child?
_____ 6. Maintain a close relationship with a child?
_____ 7. Provide a good role model for a child?
_____ 8. Discipline a child?
_____ 9. Give advice to a child?
_____10. Meet the needs of a child?
_____11. Establish and enforce rules for a child's behavior?
_____12. Obtain needed resources for a child?

Using a rating of a=5, b=4, c=3, d=2, e=1, total your score. Which competencies are you most comfortable doing? What skills would you need to improve some of the other competencies?

vary widely among biological parents, foster parents, institution parents, adopted parents, single parents, stepparents, and others. The caregiver's perceived role may differ based on culture, ethnicity, and other background variables. Researchers have studied parental roles and determined that certain attitudes and practices are more conducive to effective parenting irrespective of family patterns or background variables. Table 17.4 shows how parental love and control can contribute to the self-esteem, emotional stability, and social adjustment of children.

Acceptance involves recognizing the uniqueness of each child and appreciating the similarities and differences that exist among children. It suggests that each child is valuable, has a right to his or her point of view, and should be encouraged to develop the strengths he or she possesses. The parent allows the child to evolve and enjoys the process of discovering the essence of the child. A child raised in this environment is treated as an individual, not a possession. A rejecting parent criticizes the child for not adhering to a set of standards, often unrealistic in nature. A child lives under constant scrutiny and falls short in most situations.

A restrictive parent sets appropriate limits and establishes clear boundaries. Consequences for inappropriate behavior are determined in advance, so the child is not surprised when the consequences are implemented. Individuality is encouraged and good communication skills are practiced. The roles and responsibilities of the parent and child are clearly defined and separate. Appropriate restrictiveness implies flexibility, and open communication between the parent and child. The permissive parent has a difficult time setting limits, and boundaries are diffuse. Here, the child is uncertain of the consequences of his or her actions, which often change from circumstance and time. The roles and responsibilities of parent and child are diffuse and confuse the child. Diverse viewpoints are strongly discouraged so the

child to know himself or herself. Parenting is not imposing our will and interests on the child, nor imposing our likes and dislikes, our beliefs, values, and desires upon him or her. As a parent, you may have aspirations for your child to become a musician, but he or she may not have musical talent. If they try to please you, they may try to succeed in music and forego developing his or her own talents. If they rebel, they will be labelled as difficult and uncooperative. Now rate your competence as a parent by completing *Assess Yourself:* "How Do You Rate Your Competence to Be a Parent?"

Parenting is facilitating the growth of children and teaching through modeling. Caregiver patterns

closed adoption—confidential and no contact between birth and adoptive parents.

open adoption—contact between birth and adoptive parents occurs as the child is being raised; contact can be occasional to regular depending upon the agreement.

Table 17.4

Parental Love and Control

Love: Acceptance vs. Rejection

The Accepting Parent:	*The Rejecting Parent:*
Is satisfied with child	Is critical of child
Seeks out and enjoys child	Does not seek out or enjoy child
Provides much positive reinforcement	Provides little positive reinforcement
Is sensitive to child's needs and viewpoints	Is insensitive to child's needs and viewpoints

Control: Restrictiveness vs. Permissiveness

The Restrictive Parent:	*The Permissive Parent:*
States rules clearly and provides consequences for violations	Does not state rules clearly or provide consequences for violations
Firmly or consistently enforces rules	Does not firmly or consistently enforce rules
Rarely gives in to coercive demands	Is likely to give in to coercive demands

Table 17.5

Productive and Destructive Parenting Patterns

A productive parenting pattern	*A destructive parenting pattern*
High parental acceptance	Low acceptance
Moderate to high restrictiveness	Unyielding restrictiveness
Insistence on mature behavior	No insistence on mature behavior
High responsiveness	Inconsistent responsiveness
High positive involvement	Primarily negative involvement

child loses his or her individuality and becomes easily influenced by family, friends, or outside factors. The child may not know his or her own values and beliefs, but rather takes on the values and beliefs of his or her caregivers and others.

These parenting patterns impact the child's emotional and social development. Parenting that includes acceptance and moderate restrictiveness appear to have a positive impact on the child's development. Another dimension of parenting patterns that impact the child includes the parent's behavior toward the child. Table 17.5 distinguishes the characteristics of productive and destructive parenting patterns.

The productive parenting pattern is associated with independence, competence in social and academic arenas, assertiveness, social responsibility, and self-esteem. The destructive parenting pattern appears to create withdrawal, lack of spontaneity, and either passivity or aggression.

Parents assume various roles during the child's growth and development. Their ability to function in these roles is influenced by several factors including the ability to distinguish between appropriate and inappropriate parenting behaviors; understanding of appropriate child behaviors; cultural and religious values; and marital, work, and household characteristics. Now complete *Journal Activity:* "Roles and Responsibilities for Appropriate Caregiving," which provides an overview of the parental roles and responsibilities assumed by primary caregivers.

Parenting can be challenging and rewarding. Parenting skills aren't an innate talent you are born with, instead, they are skills you can learn. If you are considering parenting, you need to gather knowledge, develop positive attitudes, and practice the necessary skills needed for effective parenting. A parent can learn to control his or her actions and behaviors, thus modeling the patterns that help the child learn to be a productive, contributing member of society. A parent who is experiencing problems in childrearing may need and should accept help from others. Childrearing is more than a parental issue, it is a community issue. Support and assistance can come from other parents, pastoral or therapeutic counseling, or agencies that deal with parental assistance. We all have an investment in the children of today; they become the parents of tomorrow! ∞

Roles and Responsibilities for Appropriate Caregiving

Review the roles and responsibilities for appropriate caregiving. Are there other roles and responsibilities that caregivers should assume? Can you describe situations in which your caregivers showed guidance by providing these roles and responsibilities?

Role Models

Children imitate the behaviors of parents. They are influenced by the modeling they observe. Positive modeling of appropriate language, social responsibility, expression of feelings, and decision making can help the child mature. Children tend to pay as much attention to what we do as what we say.

Educators and Information Resources

Children listen to the verbal communication of their caregivers. Parents can influence the child's intellectual, social, and emotional well-being through responsible, clear verbal communication. Communication skills that provide open discussion are more effective than closed statements or stoppers such as "Why can't you _____" or "You're such a _____."

Family Policymakers and Rule Setters

Rules can protect and limit freedom. Rules provide consistency and boundaries for acceptable behavior. As children mature, they need an opportunity to have input into the rule making, and to recognize the relationship between rules and consequences. Threats and physical punishment seldom work. Statements like "If you don't _____, I'll _____." immediately set up a conflict between children and parents. Communication that begins with "When" or "As soon as" will be more effective.[33]

Originators of and Participants in Enjoyable Family Activities

Children need interaction with caregivers that provides fun. Spontaneity, humor, and play are important for everyone. Children also need opportunities to be involved in family governance, household responsibilities, and money management. These activities provide essential situations for learning skills to become productive family members.

Consultants

Children need parents to be listeners and providers of insight regarding solutions to problems that may arise throughout their lifetimes. Parents can provide suggestions, offer assistance in the decision-making process, and support their children as they face a multitude of situations while growing and maturing.

Monitors and Supervisors

Children need to learn the rights and responsibilities of freedom. House rules are important, with rewards and consequences kept reasonable and well defined. Negotiation occurs as the child gets older, and the supervision and monitoring plan can be reviewed and revised. Disciplining with dignity and respect will help children learn skills of negotiation.

Collaborators

Parents need to network with others in the community and collaborate on creating an environment conducive to the well-being of all children. They can share suggestions for handling problems that arise in the parenting process, and build support for effective parenting practices.

Identifiers and Confronters

All parents face the difficult task of how to confront their child when inappropriate behavior has occurred. Parents must identify the behavior (not ignore it) and confront the child in an appropriate manner. Denying or postponing confrontation is not beneficial.

Interveners

Sometimes, early intervention is necessary if a pattern or behavior is destructive. When the parent's efforts at intervention are unsuccessful, professional assistance may be necessary and parents must be willing to follow through on consequences. Seeking professional help is now more acceptable than in the past; however, admitting to problems can be difficult.

Managers of Their Own Feelings

Parents need to express their feelings in appropriate ways, including anger, hurt, sadness, and happiness. They can stand firm and/or be forgiving and compassionate, depending upon the situation and the circumstances.

Chapter Summary

- Nearly 40 percent of all pregnancies are unplanned.
- The birthrate for teenagers declined by 3 percent since 1990.
- Lifestyle changes should begin before pregnancy. These changes include exercise, nutritional planning and necessary supplements, nondrug use without first consulting a health-care provider, a time lapse if using oral contraceptives, and appropriate immunizations.
- Early signs of pregnancy include a missed period, a light period or spotting, tender or swollen breasts, fatigue, nausea and vomiting, and frequent urination.
- One in sixty pregnancies result in ectopic pregnancies.
- Home pregnancy tests are reliable when used properly. You must follow directions carefully when attempting to determine if you are pregnant. These tests are sensitive to the presence of human HCG in the urine.
- A sequence of changes occurs to the fetus and the mother during the 40-week gestational period.
- The maternal mortality rate is higher among African American women compared to white women.
- Prenatal checkups are recommended monthly through the first 28 weeks, biweekly during weeks 28 to 36, and weekly thereafter.
- A variety of birthing options are available including hospital, birth center, or home births.
- Certified nurse-midwives and lay midwives provide primary care to women expecting low-risk pregnancies.
- Nearly one in four deliveries in the United States was by cesarean section in 1994.
- Breast-feeding is beneficial to both mother and infant.

- Breast-feeding saves 6 million infants each year.
- Primary infertility is recognized as the inability of a woman to conceive within 1 year of having unprotected sexual intercourse.
- Secondary infertility is the woman's inability to carry the pregnancy to full term.
- Women and men account equally for cases of primary infertility.
- Artificial insemination involves the use of sperm from a donor or partner to fertilize an egg.
- Surrogacy has been banned or restricted in many states.
- In vitro fertilization involves the implantation of a fertilized egg into a woman's uterus.
- Multiple births are more likely to occur with assisted reproduction.
- Closed adoption is confidential and eliminates contact between birth and adoptive parents.
- Open adoption means the possibility of contact between birth and adoptive parents.
- Foster care occurs most often with special needs children.
- Parental love and control contribute to self-esteem and social adjustment of children.
- Productive parenting patterns include high parental acceptance, moderate restrictiveness, high responsiveness, and other aspects.
- Destructive parenting patterns include low acceptance, inconsistent responsiveness, and high negative involvement in child interaction.
- Primary caregivers have a variety of roles and responsibilities in childrearing.

Resources

Organizations and Hotlines

National Association of Childbearing Centers
3123 Gottschall Rd.
Perkiomenville, PA 18074
Telephone: (215) 234-8068
To locate a birthing center

American College of Nurse-Midwives
818 Connecticut Ave, NW Suite 900
Washington, DC 20006
Telephone: (202) 728-9860
Directory of certified nurse-midwives

American Society for Reproductive Medicine (ASRM)
1209 Montgomery Highway
Birmingham, AL 35216-2809
Up-to-date report of fertility clinics in your region

Stars of David International, Inc.
3175 Commercial Ave, Ste. 00
Northbrook, IL 60062
Telephone: (708) 205-1200
Services for Jewish and part-Jewish adoptive families

National Adoption Information Clearinghouse
11426 Rockville Pike
Rockville, MD 20852
Telephone: (301) 231-6512
Copies of state and federal laws related to adoption

Websites

American Society for Reproductive Medicine
www.asrm.com
A listing of resources and clinic success rates for fertility clinics

Resources for Adoptive Parents
Internet Adoption Photolisting
www.adoption.com
A listing of agencies, facilitators, attorneys, and exchanges
for adoption services and information

InterNational Council on Infertility Information
Dissemination
(INCIID)
P.O. Box 6836
Arlington, Va. 22206
www.inciid.org

National Adoption Registry, Inc.
Telephone: (800) 875-4347
www.searchint.com/adopt.htm

RESOLVE, Inc.
1310 Broadway
Sommerville, MA 02144-1731
Helpline (617) 623-1156
www.resolve.org
Services for fertility problems and adoption information

National Parent Information Network (NPIN)
www.npin.edu
A resource for parents provided by ERIC clearinghouses

Dinkmeyer, D., and G. D. McKay. STEP: Systematic
Training for Effective Parenting.
Telephone: (800) 328-2560
STEP, STEP/teen, Early Childhood STEP, Next STEP
www.agsnet.com

Suggested Readings

American College of Nurse-Midwives, and Sandra Jacobs.
1993. *Having your baby with a nurse-midwife:
Everything you need to know to make an informed
decision. New York: Hyperion Press.*

Blank, Robert H. 1992. *Regulating reproduction.*
Columbia University Press.

Gilman, L. 1992. *The adoption resource book.* New York:
HarperCollins Publishing.

McCutcheon, S., and E. Ingraham. 1996. *Natural
childbirth the Bradley way.* New York, NY: Plume
Publishing.

Toussaint, P.A., and D. Brown. 1997. *Mama's little baby:
The black woman's guide to pregnancy, childbirth
and baby's first year.* New York, NY: NAL/Dutton
Publishing, Dutton Publishing.

References

1. Lancashire, J. January/February, 1995. National Center for Health Statistics data line. *Public Health Reports,* 110: 105-6.
2. You and your baby: Prenatal care, labor and delivery, and postpartum care. April 1994. Washington, D.C.: American College of Obstetricians and Gynecologists.
3. Iannucci, L. November 1990. The perplexities of pregnancy. *FDA Consumer Magazine,* DHHS Publication No. (FDA) 91-1170.
4. Pregnancy test kits for home use. 1994. *USP DI- Volume II. Advice for the patient: Drug information in lay language.* 14th ed., pp. 1148-49.
5. Catanzarite, V., M. Deutchman, C. A. Johnson, and J. E. Scherger. 1995. Pregnancy after 35: What's the real risk? *Patient Care,* 29: 41-50.
6. American College of Obstetricians and Gynecologists. 1994. *You and your baby: Prenatal care, labor and delivery, and postpartum care.* Washington, D.C.: ACOG Patient Education.
7. March of Dimes. 1994. *How your baby grows: A monthly diary of your baby's development.* Wilkes-Barre, Pa.: Birth Defects Foundation.
8. Ibid.
9. Lucas, V. A. 1993. Birth: Nursing's role in today's choices. *RN,* 56: 38-44.
10. Ibid.
11. Lancashire, National Center for Health Statistics data line.
12. Ibid.
13. Trends in length of stay for hospital deliveries—United States, 1970-1992. May, 1995. *Morbidity and Mortality Weekly Report,* pp. 335-37.
14. Jacobs, S. 1993. *What birth centers are, what they are not.* Washington, D.C.: American College of Nurse-Midwives.
15. Homebirth Australia Newsletter, no. 36, February 1994.
16. A warm chain for breastfeeding (editorial). 1994. *Lancet,* 344: 1239-41.
17. Pellman, H. 1994. The advantages of breastfeeding. *Pediatrics for Parents*: 4-5.
18. What is LAM? www.ihr.org/LAM.html
19. AbouZahr, C., T. Wardlaw, C. Staton, and K. Hill. 1996. Maternal mortality. *World Health Statistical Quarterly,* 49 (2): 77-87.
20. Ibid.
21. Lancashire, National Center for Health Statistics data line.
22. AbouZahr, Wardlaw, Staton, and Hill. Maternal mortality.

23. Public Health Service. 1996. Healthy People 2000: Midcourse review and 1995 revisions. U.S. Department of Health and Human Services.

24. Catanzarite, V., M. Deutchman, C. A. Johnson, and J. E. Scherger. 1995. Pregnancy after 35: What's the real risk? *Patient Care,* 29: 41–50.

25. Assisted reproduction. April, 1995. *Harvard Women's Health Watch II* (8): 4–5.

26. Phillips, S. C. 1994. Reproductive ethics: Is it ethical to tamper with the reproductive process? *CQ Researcher,* 4: 291–306.

27. Sperm washing study encouraging but U.S. researchers leery of risks. April, 1993. *AIDS Alert,* 8: 53–56.

28. Brownlee, S. December, 1995. The baby chase: Millions of couples have fertility problems, and many try high-tech remedies. But who minds the pricey clinics they turn to? *U.S. News & World Report,* 117: 84–90.

29. Phillips, Reproductive ethics.

30. Sauer, M. V., R. J. Paulson, and R. A. Lobo. 1992. Reversing the natural decline in human fertility: An extended clinical trial of oocyte donation to women of advanced reproductive age. *JAMA,* 268: 1275–80.

31. Hellmich, H. April 24, 1997. Oldest new mom is 63: California birth renews debate on age and motherhood. *USA Today,* D, 1: 2.

32. Gillman, L. 1997. Before you adopt. Adoptive Families of America, Children Youth and Family Consortium Electronic Clearinghouse. Email: cyfced@maroon.tc.umn.edu Phone: 612-626-1212.

33. Samalin, N., and D. B. Hogarty. 1995. "You're such a slob!" . . . and other things you should never say to kids. *Parents Magazine,* 70: 37–40.

COMMUNICABLE AND CHRONIC CONDITIONS

CHAPTER EIGHTEEN
Preventing Aids and Other Sexually Transmitted Diseases

CHAPTER NINETEEN
Managing Cardiovascular Health and Other Chronic Conditions

CHAPTER TWENTY
Reducing Your Risk of Cancer

Part Five

Eighteen

Preventing AIDS and Other Sexually Transmitted Diseases

■ chapter objectives

When you complete this chapter you will be able to:

• Describe the consequences of untreated STDs in women.
• Compare and contrast the incidence and prevalence of various STDs.
• Identify the signs and symptoms of the common STDs.
• Describe the three most common types of vaginitis.
• Differentiate among the various forms of contraception that reduce the risk of transmitting STDs and AIDS.
• Describe safer and riskier sexual behaviors.
• Explain various ways to prevent the spread of STDs and AIDS among women and children.
• Identify the highest risk groups for various STDs and AIDS.

THE PRIMARY BURDEN OF STDS

Sexually transmitted diseases (STDs) can be physically and emotionally devastating for women, so information about the prevention, signs, symptoms, and treatment of these diseases is imperative. Ignorance is not bliss, because what you don't know *can* hurt you. The physical risks of STDs are potentially serious and long-term complications such as pelvic inflammatory disease (PID), impaired fertility, and ectopic pregnancies, whereas the emotional risks can manifest as feelings ranging from shame to fear of social scrutiny. Sexually transmitted infections can lead to chronic pain, cervical cancer, and chronic liver disease.

Women and children suffer the primary burden of STDs and they have a right to know what might

happen if STDs go undiagnosed. Pelvic inflammatory disease is one of the insidious outcomes of some STDs. STDs are responsible for over 2.5 million cases of pelvic inflammatory disease (PID) each year, 275,000 hospitalizations, 150,000 cases of infertility, and 45,000 ectopic pregnancies. The estimated cost of sexually transmitted diseases exceeds $3.5 billion annually, and PID and PID-associated infertility and ectopic pregnancies exceed $2.6 billion.[1]

Until the 1980s, only five venereal diseases (STDs) were regularly monitored. Today, nearly fifty different STD-related organisms and syndromes are recognized, and the complexity and scope of these STDs has changed dramatically.[2] The list includes the traditional sexually transmitted diseases, previously called venereal diseases such as syphilis and gonorrhea, as well as chlamydia, genital herpes,

HEALTHY PEOPLE 2000 OBJECTIVES

- Reduce chlamydia trachomatis infections, as measured by a decrease in the incidence of nongonococcal urethritis to no more than 170 cases per 100,000 people. 1995 progress toward goal: approximately −35 to −40 percent
- Reduce gonorrhea to an incidence of no more than 225 cases per 100,000 people. 1995 progress toward goal: 171 percent
- Reduce the rate of repeat gonorrhea infection to no more than 15 percent within the previous year. 1995 progress toward goal: approximately 50 percent
- Reduce primary and secondary syphilis to an incidence of no more than 10 cases per 100,000 people. 1995 progress toward goal: approximately 90 percent
- Reduce cogenital syphilis to an incidence of no more than 50 cases per 100,000 live births. 1995 progress toward goal: approximately 30 percent
- Reduce genital herpes and genital warts, as measured by a reduction to 142,000 and 385,000, respectively, in the annual number of first-time consultations with a physician for the conditions. 1995 progress toward goal: approximately −35 percent away from target goal for genital herpes; 238 percent of target goal for genital warts
- Reduce sexually transmitted hepatitis B infection to no more than 30,500 cases. 1995 progress toward goal: approximately 75 percent
- Reduce the incidence of pelvic inflammatory disease, as measured by a reduction in hospitalizations for pelvic inflammatory disease to no more than 250 per 100,000 women aged 15 to 44. 1995 progess toward goal: 283 percent
- Confine annual incidence of diagnosed AIDS cases to no more than 98,000 cases. Revised goal: Confine annual incidence of diagnosed AIDS cases to no more than 43 per 100,000 population. 1995 progress toward goal achieved: cannot be displayed as a percentage of target achieved, based on the new case definition of AIDS
- Confine the prevalence of HIV infection to no more than 800 per 100,000 people. 1995 progress toward goal: data unavailable
- Reduce the proportion of adolescents who have engaged in sexual intercourse to no more than 15 percent by age 15 and no more than 40 percent by age 17. 1995 progress toward goal: approximately −150 percent in females and −75 percent in males aged 15
- Increase to at least 50 percent the proportion of sexually active, unmarried people who used a condom at their last sexual intercourse. 1995 progress toward goal: approximately 30 percent of goal met for females and 40 percent of goal met for males
- Reduce to no more than 1 per 250,000 units of blood and blood components the risk of tranfusion-transmitted HIV infection. 1995 progress toward goal: approximately 75 percent
- Increase to at least 80 percent the proportion of HIV-infected people who have been tested for HIV infection. 1995 progress toward goal: approximately 50 percent
- Provide HIV education for students and staff in at least 90 percent of colleges and universities. 1995 progress toward goal achieved: data unavailable
- Increase to at least 40 percent the proportion of ever sexually active adolescents aged 17 and younger who have not had sexual intercourse for the previous 3 months

human papilloma virus, cytomegalovirus, hepatitis B, vaginitis, and others. Nearly 12 million cases of STDs occur in the United States each year with two-thirds of all STDs occurring in persons younger than 25 years of age. The southern states have the highest STD rates in the United States.

It is imperative that you know about the most common STDs and especially how to prevent them. Asking questions and seeking information is not equated with being sexually active. In fact, once you are informed, you may decide to be abstinent to avoid unintended pregnancy and STDs. Abstinence is the first line of protection against future sterility, PID, and problem pregnancies and the only way to prevent unintended STDs and pregnancies. (See *Viewpoint:* "STDs.") If you intend to be sexually active, responsible behavior is important. (See *Assess Yourself:* "Assess Your STD Risk.") You need to know the risks associated with STDs and you need assertive skills to prevent unprotected sex. This chapter provides the information necessary to make informed choices and to protect yourself from unwanted risks.

Viewpoint

STDs: A Moral or Medical Issue?

The United States has one of the highest STD rates of industrialized countries, with teenagers accounting for 25 percent of all STDs. In fact, two-thirds of all STDs occur in persons younger than 25 years. Statistics suggest that 27 percent of females have had sexual intercourse by age 15, and half of all females have had sexual intercourse by age 17.[3] Healthy People 2000 has set a goal to reduce the proportion of adolescents who have engaged in sexual intercourse to no more than 15 percent by age 15 and to no more than 40 percent by age 17. Another goal was to increase to at least 50 percent the proportion of sexually active, unmarried people who used a condom at their last sexual intercourse.

Young men and women, particularly those at greatest risk for contracting HIV or other STDs, need to hear the message of postponement of sexual behavior and proper protection. A 1993 assessment of sexuality education by the Sex Information and Education Council of the United States (SIECUS) found forty-eight states either recommend or require sexuality education through state law or policy. The primary focus has been abstinence education. A review of thirty-five studies of sex education in schools found that sex education is most effective when given before a young person becomes sexually active and programs that promote both postponement of sex and protected sex are more effective than those that promoted abstinence alone.[4]

Abstinence-only curricula are supported by parents and community members who do not want teachers to address birth control, contraceptives, and sexual behaviors. For many of them, it is a moral issue. The debate regarding the moral versus medical aspects of teaching sex education, particularly reproductive health, continues to be waged. What do you think about the moral and medical arguments? Are schools, parents, churches, and communities doing everything they can do to prevent unintended pregnancies and STDs? What else could be done?

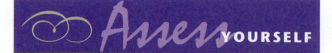

Assess Your STD Risk

Answer the following questions by checking yes or no on the appropriate line.

Yes	No	
____	____	Are you sexually active?
____	____	Is it very important to you *not* to get pregnant in the near future?
____	____	Do you find it difficult to always use your current birth control method?
____	____	Has the recent change in a relationship caused a change in your method of birth control?
____	____	Do you wonder if your partner has ever had a STD?
____	____	Do you have difficulty discussing STDs with your partner?
____	____	Have you or your partner had sex with more than one person over the past several months?
____	____	Do you use alcohol or drugs?
____	____	Does it surprise you that some STDs have no symptoms?

Having unprotected sex, even once, can put you at risk for sexually transmitted diseases or unintended pregnancy. If you are sexually active and answered yes to any of the previous questions, you may want to discuss prevention and protection with your health-care provider.[5]

DISCUSSING COMMON SEXUALLY TRANSMITTED DISEASES

Chlamydia

Chlamydia infection is the most common sexually transmitted disease in the United States with an estimated 4 million infections annually. In 1995, the Centers for Disease Control and Prevention (CDC) stated that the total number of reported chlamydia infections in the United States was 447,638 cases with females outnumbering males by six to one. The number of reported cases in females has risen steadily as states have focused their efforts on screening women, particularly those who are asymptomatic. And, changes in diagnostic testing allow direct measurement of chlamydia infection. In 1994, chlamydia became nationally notifiable through the efforts of the Council of State and Territorial Epidemiologists. In 1995, forty-eight states had implemented legislation mandating the reporting of cases to CDC. Chlamydia cases are likely to rise as better screening techniques, direct measurement, and national reporting efforts continue. In 1994 and 1995, the reported rate rose from 260.2 per 100,000 population to 290.3, reflecting the trend toward better screening.[6]

The bacterium *Chlamydia trachomatis* causes chlamydia infection and can persist for long periods of time without causing symptoms. The exposure to chlamydia is usually sexual intercourse and the site of infection is typically the cervix. Nearly 70 to 80 percent of women with chlamydia are asymptomatic until they experience the fever and pain associated with pelvic inflammatory disease. Twenty to 40 percent of women infected with chlamydia will develop PID if not adequately treated.[7] Symptomatic women may experience unexplained vaginal discharge, burning during urination, lower abdominal pain, bleeding between menstrual periods, fever, and nausea.[8,9]

Recurrence rates can be particularly disturbing. One research study estimated that the rate of recurrence of chlamydia infection was 42 percent for girls aged 10 to 14 and 25 percent for young women aged 15 to 19. This study also found that the recurrence rate for African American young women was twice that of white women.[10] Recurrence increases the risk of infertility with scarring of the fallopian tubes.

The CDC recommends that all sexually active, single women under age 24, and all women with **cervicitis** should be screened routinely for chlamydia infection because of the high morbidity associated when left untreated. Asymptomatic women with chlamydia infections as well as their partners should be treated. If the partner's infection goes untreated, the risk of recurrence through a repeat transmission exists. If the woman's infection goes untreated, serious complications including hospitalization for PID may result. Complications associated with chlamydia infection include cervicitis, infertility, chronic pain, salpingitis (inflammation of the fallopian tubes), increased risk of ectopic pregnancy, stillbirth, reactive arthritis, and neonatal **conjunctivitis** and pneumonia.[11]

Indicators such as nongonococcal **urethritis,** PID, and cervicitis are helpful in determining the incidence of chlamydia infections, but new diagnostic technology has allowed for more widespread screening. In the past, CDC used the incidence of nongonococcal urethritis (NGU) as an indicator of chlamydia infections. Today, a variety of tests including cell culture, antigen detection tests, nucleic acid hybridization tests, and nucleic acid amplification tests are used to diagnose chlamydia infection. Cell culture remains the gold standard for detecting chlamydia infection and is the diagnostic procedure of choice for women who have been raped or experienced incest. Many clinics routinely use nonculture tests because they are less expensive, provide quicker results, and have fewer handling requirements than cell cultures. However, these nonculture tests also have lower sensitivity for detecting chlamydia infections than cell cultures (40 percent versus 75 percent).[12,13]

The treatment of chlamydia is relatively simple. Antibiotics are given to treat chlamydia, either in a 7-day or single dose regimen, depending on the woman's compliance history and ability to pay. The single dose of azithromycin is three to five times more expensive than a 7-day regimen but has the advantage of one application.

Many women who test positive for chlamydia infection do not comply with the treatment protocol. One research study found that between 25 and 50 percent of the women who tested positive did not seek adequate treatment.[14] Despite better screening procedures, treatment compliance is difficult to ensure.

Pregnancy The CDC recommends that all pregnant women be tested for chlamydia infection during their third trimester, and erythromycin (or amoxicillin for women with intolerance to erythromycin) is the treatment of choice for women who test positive. Infants can be protected if this treatment is completed before delivery.[15,16] Some studies suggest that nearly two-thirds of infants become infected if born vaginally to mothers with chlamydia infection. Infants born with chlamydia respond readily to treatment. A woman who tests positive for chlamydia infection risks severe complications if treatment isn't administered promptly. The CDC estimates that 30 percent of women without treatment will become sterile.[17]

---

chlamydia (kla **mid** ee uh)—most common sexually transmitted disease found in U.S. women; caused by microorganisms that live as parasites within cells.

cervicitis (sir vuh **cy** tis)—acute or chronic inflammation of the uterine cervix.

conjunctivitis—swelling in the front of the white of the eye, caused by infection, allergy, or outside factors.

urethritis (yur ee **thri** tis)—inflammation of the urinary opening often caused by infection in the bladder or kidneys.

Gonorrhea

The incidence of **gonorrhea,** caused by the *Neisseria gonorrhea* organism, continues to decline and the CDC reports rates of 140.3 in 100,000 women annually. Gonorrhea rates have decreased dramatically since the mid-1970s for all groups except teenagers and some minority groups.[18] A large disparity in gonorrhea cases exists between white and African American men. African American teenagers (aged 15–19) have approximately a twenty-six times greater rate of reported gonorrhea than white teenagers. (See *FYI:* "Race and Ethnicity Discrepancies in STD Rates.") Adequate contraceptive protection is important in all sexual encounters, especially when one's risk is higher.[19,20] Figure 18.1 shows the decrease in rates of gonorrhea from 1981 until 1995 for males and females. It also shows the revised goal for the year 2000, which is 100 cases per 100,000 people. The current rates are slightly higher for men than women, although the disparity in rates has narrowed.

Gonorrhea can affect any of the mucous membranes including the vagina, cervix, anus, throat, and eyes. Symptomatic women may experience a thick yellow or white vaginal discharge, burning during urination, intercourse, and bowel movements, and

severe menstrual or abdominal cramps. The bacteria can move from the cervix, the site of first infection, into the uterus and fallopian tubes. Here it can remain indefinitely without causing symptoms and can begin to cause scarring and resultant chronic pain, ectopic pregnancy, or infertility. Nearly 50 percent of women who contract gonorrhea are initially asymptomatic. The first expressed symptoms may be those of pelvic inflammatory disease, rather than gonorrhea. Ten to 40 percent of women infected with gonorrhea develop PID if inadequately treated.[21]

A secretion is taken from the cervix, rectum, and throat for culturing to determine whether a person has been infected. Lab results of the culture take approximately a week to obtain. If a woman is infected, she and her partner must be treated concurrently to avoid reinfection, and they should abstain from intercourse during the treatment. Fortunately, most symptomatic men seek treatment quickly after gonococcal urethritis occurs because of pain with urination, and his partner(s) will be informed. A large increase in resistant strains to first-line antibiotics such as ampicillin, penicillin, and tetracycline has caused a change in CDC treatment recommendations. Uncomplicated gonorrhea can be treated with a single injection of ceftriaxone or cefotaxime, with a 7-day course of another antibiotic to treat coexisting

FYI

Race and Ethnicity Discrepancies in STD Rates

STD statistics provided by CDC suggest wide discrepancies in STD rates based on race and ethnicity. Gonorrhea rates among African American adolescents (15–19) are more than twenty-six times greater than the rate among white adolescents. Primary and secondary syphilis rates for African Americans are nearly sixty times than in whites; Hispanics have rates nearly four times than in whites. In 1995, of the 1,543 reported cases of congenital syphilis in which race and ethnicity were known, African American and Hispanic women accounted for 91 percent of all reported cases, whereas they account for only 21 percent of the female population. Race and ethnicity correlate with other determinants of health status including socioeconomic status, access to quality health care, and health-care-seeking behavior. Reporting biases may also contribute to the different rates of reported STDs.

FIGURE 18.1 Although the rates for gonorrhea in men and women have declined since the early 1980s, the CDC goal is to achieve a rate of a hundred cases in men and women annually.

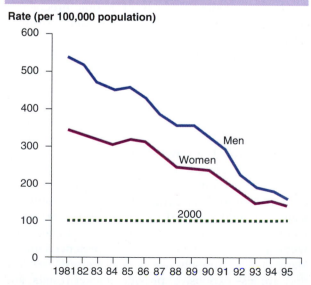

chlamydia infection. Cefotaxime is considerably cheaper and demonstrates comparable patient tolerance and treatment efficacy.[22]

Untreated, acute gonorrhea can result in systemic, disseminated infection. Nearly 80 percent of disseminated gonococcal infection occurs in young women. The three common features include arthritis, dermatitis, and tenosynovitis.[23]

Pregnancy and Infancy Gonorrhea results in adverse outcomes of pregnancy, including neonatal ophthalmia. This disease can be prevented with topical prophylaxis at delivery.

Syphilis

Syphilis is caused by the spirochete, *Treponema pallidum,* which spreads throughout the body within hours of infection. It is primarily transmitted through sexual contact, but can also be passed from the infected mother to a fetus. The number of reported cases (16,500) of syphilis in 1995 was the fewest reported cases since 1960. The current rate of 6.3 cases per 100,000 persons is low compared to other STDs and cases are primarily concentrated in the South. Thirteen of eighteen states or areas with syphilis rates above 4 per 100,000 are in the South. One of the largest increases in incidence has been among urban, African American heterosexuals. The rate among African Americans is nearly sixty times that in whites, and the rate for Hispanics is nearly four times that in whites.[24]

Syphilis is characterized by active and latent phases, called primary, secondary, latent, and tertiary. Primary syphilis occurs within 1 to 3 months of contact with an infected partner. The first symptom is a painless, red or brown sore (chancre) or sores on the mouth, reproductive organs, or fingers. This chancre will last from 1 to 6 weeks. In women, the chancre commonly appears on the labia, but may develop on the cervix, making detection difficult or impossible. Even though the sore disappears, the person still has syphilis, with half moving to the secondary phase and half to the latent phase.[25,26]

Symptoms of the secondary phase appear within 1 week to 6 months after the sore heals. The hallmark of this phase includes a rash that appears on the palms or soles and flu-like symptoms that disappear within 2 to 12 weeks. Some call secondary syphilis the great imitator, because it may be mistaken as a rash for eczema, cutaneous drug reactions, psoriasis, measles, or even sunburn. The flu-like symptoms may be mistaken for influenza of infectious mononucleosis.[27]

Those who progress to the latent phase, the period of time between the secondary and tertiary phase, have no clinical signs or symptoms. They may remain asymptomatic; however, one-third will move to the tertiary phase. The untreated persons still have syphilis.

Today, few women progress to the tertiary phase due to penicillin therapy. The tertiary phase is characterized by destructive lesions, lymph node involvement, and organ destruction. The central nervous system may be involved, causing meningitis, spinal lesions, or cerebral vascular syphilis. Cardiac lesions may cause destruction to the cardiovascular system.[28,29]

Syphilis has also been linked to increased susceptibility to HIV infection, because the open sores remove the virus barrier and carry mononuclear cells that easily draw HIV. The symptoms of syphilis may manifest differently for HIV-infected persons, so experts suggest that women testing positive for syphilis be advised to seek HIV testing. They should also be counseled about their increased risk for HIV infection and the importance of condom use.[30,31]

Any woman with genital lesions should be tested for syphilis. Most primary, secondary, and early latent syphilis cases are treated with one injection of penicillin, which is the drug of choice. Women who are allergic to penicillin can be treated with alternative drugs. Those with tertiary syphilis will need a longer regimen of treatment. All persons must be monitored to determine the efficacy of the treatment.[32]

Pregnancy Congenital syphilis is transmitted to the infant during pregnancy and has a devastating impact on the neonate. It accounts for 40 percent of fetal and perinatal deaths in affected infants, and morbidity is even higher with physical and mental developmental disabilities. Most cases of congenital syphilis are preventable if the pregnant woman is treated properly through early prenatal care. In 1988, the surveillance case definition for congenital

---

gonorrhea—a sexually transmitted disease caused by the bacterium *Neisseria gonorrhoea.*

syphilis—a sexually transmitted disease caused by the bacterium (spirochete) *Treponema pallidum.*

syphilis changed, causing an increase in reported cases of congenital syphilis. As syphilis rates increased in women, the number of cases of congenital syphilis also rose. Peaks in congenital syphilis usually occur 1 year after peaks in primary and secondary syphilis in women. The CDC recommends expanded screening to all childbearing age women in cities with high incidence and improving educational and service outreach for prenatal care to women in high incidence environments.[33]

Herpes Simplex Virus (HSV)

Herpes simplex is one of a family of common viruses including varicella zoster virus (chicken pox and shingles) and Epstein-Barr virus (mononucleosis). Herpes simplex virus (HSV) is a contagious viral infection and spreads from direct skin to skin contact of an infected partner to the other partner, particularly in the oral and genital areas. The two primary types of herpes simplex viruses are HSV-1 and HSV-2. HSV-1 usually manifests as cold sores or fever blisters, primarily around the mouth, and affects four in five adults or approximately 80 percent of all adults. HSV-2, commonly referred to as genital herpes, infects one in six adults or nearly 40 million American men and women.[34] HSV-1 and HSV-2 can manifest anywhere on the body, despite the common belief that HSV-1 is found only above the waist, and HSV-2 exists only below the waist.

The symptoms of genital herpes vary from one individual to another. Most infected women may not recognize the signs of genital herpes and many who experience an initial outbreak will never have additional outbreaks. Symptomatic persons may experience the first episode within 2 to 21 days of contact with an infected partner. The first symptoms of the active phase may include itching, burning, and swelling. A woman can experience symptoms common to all viral infections: fever, headaches, muscle aches, and chills. Eventually, small painful blisters (lesions) appear on the genitalia (sometimes the mouth), then rupture, crust over, and heal. The blisters disappear within 1 to 3 weeks but some of the herpes simplex virus remains. The virus travels down a nerve to the ganglia (a cluster of nerve cells) near the spine, and remains dormant until another outbreak occurs. Then the virus travels back down the nerve to the surface of the skin.[35]

Control efforts for HSV-2 are difficult because nearly 75 percent of individuals who transmit the virus are unaware of their infection. If a woman suspects that she has been exposed to HSV-2 she should consult a health-care provider during the active phase of the virus. The health-care provider will take a sample from the lesion and request a culture to determine if HSV-2 is present.

There is no cure for herpes simplex but the drug acyclovir (Zovirax) has effectively reduced the frequency and duration of recurrences in most people. Although acyclovir, an antiviral drug, prevents the multiplying of the herpes virus, it does not appear to reduce the transmission of the virus to one's partner. Acyclovir is available in pills, ointment, or injectable forms. The recommended regimen for the first episode of genital herpes is oral acyclovir taken five times a day for 7 to 10 days or until the active virus disappears.[36] Valacyclovir (Valtrex) and famciclovir (Famvir) are experimental versions of acyclovir that absorb more readily.[37]

Prevention Herpes has no cure, so prevention depends upon the management of outbreaks and preventing its spread to a partner (See *Her Story:* "Kristin.") A young woman with herpes can prevent recurrences by maintaining a healthy diet, exercising regularly, getting plenty of rest, and managing her stress level. Intimate contact remains the primary mode of transmission and there is no way to ensure that a partner will remain unaffected, because the virus can be present on the skin without recognizable symptoms. If the infected partner notices itching or tingling at the primary site of the infection or has blisters, she should avoid sexual contact or use additional precautionary measures. Sexual contact should also be avoided when sores are active, during the healing process, and for several days after the healing has occurred. Combining the condom with a contraceptive foam reduces the risk of transmission of HSV-2. Spermicide containing nonoxynol-9 has been shown to kill the herpes virus and other germs that cause STDs.[38]

A woman can spread herpes to other parts of her body. This transfer is referred to as **autoinoculation** and occurs by touching an area of shedding active cells and then touching another susceptible area. To prevent autoinoculation a woman should avoid touching active lesions or letting others touch the lesions. If her hands accidentally touch an active sore, she would wash them immediately to avoid spreading the virus to other susceptible parts. Towels are often a primary mode of autoinoculation transmis-

Her Story

Kristin

Kristin, a 19-year-old college sophomore, recently went to see Dr. Cox, a physician at the student health center. When Dr. Cox entered the room, she sat down and asked Kristin, "What brings you here today?" Kristin hesitated to answer and Dr. Cox began to sense that something was bothering Kristin, so she waited for her to speak. Finally, Kristin began, "Well, basically, I'm here to get some information from you. It is kind of hard to talk about it. I have been dating this really great guy for a long time now and, well, he is just so nice and considerate, and we really like each other. I have been thinking for awhile that we might be ready to start getting sexually involved. I guessed he felt the same way so when we went out the other night I brought it up. Ben's reaction surprised me. He just looked down at the table and didn't say anything, and that is not like him, he usually is very willing to talk, even about hard things. I kept encouraging him to share his feelings. Finally, he did. And that is why I am here with you today. You see, Ben has herpes. I want to continue to be involved with Ben, but I am scared. Dr. Cox, I don't want to get herpes and I don't want to overreact. So, what can I do?"

- Knowing the risks involved, is this a good time for Kristin to become sexually active?
- If Kristin chooses to become sexually active, what precautionary methods should she practice?

sion when she wipes over an active lesion and then spreads the shedding cells to another area. Towels should be laundered after every use to prevent this occurrence.[39]

Pregnancy   A pregnant woman with recurrent HSV-2 diagnosed before pregnancy has a relatively low risk of transmitting the virus to her neonate. Pregnant women with undiagnosed primary HSV-2 have a higher risk of transmission to the neonate, causing serious infections that can result in nerve damage and even death. Previously, cesarean sections were recommended for women with HSV-2 in an effort to prevent transmission of the virus to the neonate. Most women who had cesarean section births had recurrent lesions rather than primary lesions (a first or initial outbreak). Recently, some researchers have suggested that maternal morbidity and mortality from cesarean section procedures may

be actually higher than neonatal deaths prevented. Cesarean deliveries increase the hospital stay, require longer recuperation, increase the number of follow-up visits, and greatly increase the delivery costs. Cesarean sections are not completely effective in preventing transmission to neonates. An analysis of cost effectiveness showed a $2.5 million cost for each case of HSV-2 prevented.[40]

In another study evaluating the risk of pregnancy exposures to acyclovir, researchers found no increased risk for birth defects among infants exposed to acyclovir during pregnancy. However, the CDC recommends that acyclovir be administered intravenously only in life-threatening maternal infections and not systemically near term. The safety in human pregnancies has not been determined and the risk with drug exposure to the fetus is unclear.[41]

Human Papilloma Virus

Human papilloma virus (HPV) refers to a group of over seventy different types of viruses, one-third of which cause genital problems. Nearly 12 million Americans have HPV, with 750,000 new cases occurring each year. HPV can be found in nearly 40 percent of sexually active women in their twenties. A small percentage of infected persons develop genital warts, and an even smaller percentage develop a precancerous condition that shows up on an abnormal Pap smear.[42] Warts are the outward manifestation of HPV in symptomatic persons; some types appear on the hands and feet, and others, like types 6 and 11, on the genital area. Asymptomatic persons have the virus but no appearance of outward manifestations and may unknowingly transmit the virus to their partner(s).

---

herpes simplex—a viral infection that attacks the skin and nervous system, usually producing short-lasting, fluid-filled blisters on the skin and mucous membranes.

autoinoculation—self-spread of a disease from one part of the body to another.

human papilloma virus (HPV)—(pap ill **oh** ma)—a group of over seventy different types of viruses including genital warts; some increase the risk of cancer.

Genital warts, or condyloma, are usually spread by direct skin to skin contact with an infected person. The symptoms of genital warts include small, bumpy warts on the vaginal or anal area. These warts vary from small to large, raised to flat, or single to clustered. Warts can appear several weeks to several months after contact with an infected person. The warts may remain undetected when located inside the vagina, on the cervix, or in the anus. Most warts are painless and flesh colored, and will not disappear without medical attention. Some partners carry the virus without experiencing warts; others experience itching, pain, or bleeding.[43]

You should notify your health-care provider if you detect any unusual growths, bumps, or skin changes in the vaginal or anal areas or if your partner tells you he or she has HPV. A health-care provider diagnoses HPV by placing a drop of acetic acid on the infected area. This drop causes abnormal tissue to turn white and the HPV virus can then be detected through a colposcope, a magnifying lens.[44]

There is no cure for HPV although lesions can be removed with proper treatment and follow-up. Usually, several treatments are needed to remove visible warts. The type of treatment prescribed by the health-care provider depends on the location and size of the warts and the woman's preference of treatment. Current treatments of HPV include a conservative approach using cryotherapy with liquid nitrogen or a cryoprobe. Other treatments include chemicals such as podophyllin or trichloracetic acid (TCA), and laser surgery. Podofilox, an approved prescription drug, has the advantage of being a topical application that can be administered at home. Interferon has been used as a treatment but is not usually recommended because of its low efficacy, a high risk of toxicity, and overall expense.[45,46]

The decision to remove lesions located on the cervix depends on the severity and the risk of sexual transmission. They are usually removed by cryotherapy, laser, or loop excision. The goal of HPV treatment is the removal of external warts and the amelioration of signs and symptoms, not to cure the individual. Podophyllin and podofilox are not recommended treatment for pregnant women. Genital warts tend to proliferate during pregnancy, so experts recommend only the removal of visible warts.[47]

Risk of Cancer Approximately one-third of the estimated seventy types of HPV are associated with infections of the genital area, and six are associated with cervical cancer. Some types of HPV, such as types 16, 18, 31, 33, and 35, cause cervical cancer (CIN) or cervical dysplasia.[48] These cervical cell changes must be monitored closely, because they are linked to an increased risk of cervical cancer. The only effective treatment of cervical cancer is surgical removal of all or part of the cervix. In Third World countries, cervical cancer surpasses breast cancer in mortality in women. The United States has reduced the mortality due to cervical cancer through early detection (Pap smear). It is recommended that women with HPV monitor their condition closely and have Pap smears every 6 months. Other types of HPV, types 6 and 11, have been linked to cancers of the oral cavity, larynx, pharynx, and lungs.[49]

Pregnancy and Infancy HPV types 6 and 11 not only increase a woman's risk of cancer, they are also associated with potential disease in infants. Infants of childbearing women with HPV types 6 and 11 can contract laryngeal papillomatosis.

Hepatitis B Virus

An estimated 300,000 new cases of **hepatitis B** (HBV), a viral infection causing inflammation of the liver, are reported each year in the United States. Approximately one in ten infected persons will die of HBV-related complications such as fulminant hepatitis, cirrhosis, or liver cancer. HBV transmission is similar to HIV, through exposure to infected blood and unprotected sexual intercourse, but HBV is more easily transmitted than HIV. In fact, HBV is a hundred times more contagious than HIV.[50] Persons at highest risk for contracting HBV include **hemodialysis** patients, injectable drug users, health-care workers exposed to blood, infants born to HBV-positive women, gay men, and sexually active heterosexuals. Groups at highest risk for contracting HBV include Alaska Natives, Pacific Islanders, Asians, and other emigrating from high incident areas. International travelers to high incidence areas may also choose to receive the hepatitis B vaccine.[51] In women, heterosexual activity is the most common risk factor, followed by injectable drug use. The modes of transmission often overlooked by individuals include tattoos, ear piercing, nonmedication injections of vitamins, minerals, or steroids, and acupuncture treatments.[52]

Recognizing the risk factors for HBV is important; however, more than one-third of adults with acute hepatitis B have no identified risk factors. Sexually active women can reduce their risk of contracting hepatitis B virus by using vaginal contraceptives (spermicides containing nonoxynol-9) and refraining from anal intercourse. The CDC recommends that prostitutes, women with multiple partners, and women with a history of STDs receive hepatitis B vaccinations.[53] Symptoms of acute hepatitis B include **jaundice** and a tender liver upon palpitation. Hepatitis B follows a predictable course through four phases: incubation, prodrome, icteric, and convalescence phase. The prodome phase is characterized by generalized symptoms such as fever, fatigue, and discomfort. The icteric phase is recognized by jaundice and swelling of the liver, and the symptoms disappear during the convalescence phase.[54]

Nearly 95 percent of persons with hepatitis B recover, although a few persons contract fulminant hepatitis or experience persistent infections. The type of hepatitis (whether A, B, C, or E) can only be determined through serologic testing. The hepatitis B virus is present in all body fluids and can contain three antigens.[55]

Vaccination for Hepatitis B The incidence of HBV has increased steadily during the past decade despite access to a vaccine. The American College Health Association has recommended that all college students be vaccinated against HBV, because HBV strikes healthy, young people. One-third of infected persons are college age and more than one-third of infected persons do not have known risk factors. College women who are sexually active and have multiple partners, engage in any unprotected sex, have had another STD such as chlamydia or gonorrhea, or are studying for careers that involve exposure to blood should be vaccinated for HBV.[56]

Pregnancy and Infancy An estimated 22,000 infants are born to women with chronic HBV infection each year. These infants may not show early symptoms of infection, but they are at risk for chronic liver disease (hepatitis, cirrhosis, and carcinoma) and resulting death as adults. This risk prompted the American College of Obstetrics and Gynecology, the American Academy of Pediatrics, and the American Academy of Family Practice to recommend screening for hepatitis B surface antigen (HBsAg) in all pregnant women. They also recommended universal hepatitis B vaccination of infants in 1992. The Childhood Immunization Initiative set a goal of vaccinating 70 percent of all children 2 years old and younger with three or more doses of hepatitis B vaccine by 1996. At this time, it appears that the goal has not been reached because some health-care providers felt the guidelines were premature.[57,58]

REPRODUCTIVE TRACT INFECTIONS

Pelvic Inflammatory Disease

Pelvic inflammatory disease (PID) is one of the most severe outcomes of STD infections. PID is an infection of the upper portion of the female reproductive tract beyond the cervix. Common symptoms of PID include severe pelvic pain, high fever, chills, nausea, and vomiting. Spotting or pelvic pain can occur between menstrual periods and abnormal vaginal discharge is possible.

Women bear an inordinate burden from contracting STDs, with PID being one of the most serious consequences. Nearly 15 percent of women between ages 15 and 44 experience one incident of PID in their lifetime, and almost 1 million new cases of PID are diagnosed annually. Nearly 25 percent (250,000) of these women need costly hospitalization and although the antibiotics used to treat PID cure most women, approximately 200,000 women will continue to experience chronic pelvic pain and 150,000 women will become infertile. One estimate suggested that the direct and indirect costs of PID was $4.2 billion in 1990.[59]

Accurate estimates of PID rates are difficult to obtain, particularly because complex and invasive procedures are needed to diagnose it correctly.

---

hepatitis B—a viral infection causing inflammation of the liver; may be severe and result in prolonged illness or death.

hemodialysis—procedure that removes impurities or wastes from the blood.

jaundice—yellowing of the skin, mucous membranes, and eyes caused by too much bilirubin in the blood.

pelvic inflammatory disease (PID)—any inflammation of the female reproductive tract, especially one caused by bacteria.

FIGURE 18.2 Hospitalizations for PID from 1980–1993.

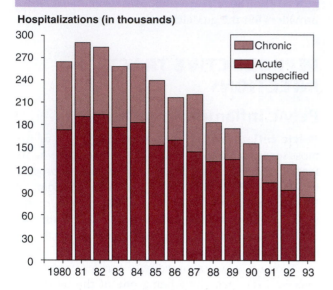

Interpretations of clinical findings are often used when reporting PID and these interpretations vary depending on the health-care provider. Figure 18.2 shows the decline in the rate of PID-related hospitalizations of women 15 to 44 years of age from 1980–1993. The graph demonstrates the trend toward a decline in PID hospitalizations throughout the 1980s and 1990s. These declines do not indicate a decrease in the incidence of PID, rather they point to a change in treatment protocol from inpatient to outpatient and better screening for chlamydia infections. More women are being treated for PID on an outpatient basis, thus the revised Healthy People 2000 goal has been expanded to track and reduce outpatient visits for PID.

PID is diagnosed by a health-care provider through a pelvic examination, or through analysis of cervical or vaginal secretions. If diagnosed, treatment includes antibiotics, rest, and sexual abstinence. Surgery may be required to remove any scars or abscesses or to repair injured reproductive organs.

Vaginitis

One in ten women who visit their health-care provider complain about vaginal discharge, a sign of **vaginitis.** Over 90 percent of vaginitis in women of reproductive age is classified as trichomoniasis, bacterial vaginosis (BV), or candidiasis. Nearly 45 percent have BV, 25 percent have trichomoniasis, and

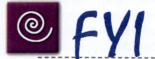

What to Tell Your Health-Care Provider

- When the symptoms started
- Texture, color, and odor of discharge
- Burning, itching, pain, or redness
- Change in bowel movements such as diarrhea
- Recent change in sexual partner or symptoms in current partner
- Problems in sexual intercourse such as pain with penetration during intercourse
- Anal intercourse
- Type of contraceptive used
- Use of home remedies or over-the-counter medications
- Number of pregnancies
- Previous pelvic infections, including during pregnancy

25 percent have candidiasis.[60] Your health-care provider will ask a number of questions to determine whether you have vaginitis or some other infection. The information provided in *FYI:* "What to Tell Your Health-Care Provider" will help to prepare you for the visit to your health-care provider.

Bacterial Vaginosis (BV) Bacterial vaginosis, formerly called nonspecific vaginitis, Gardnerella-associated vaginitis, or Haemophilis-associated vaginitis, is the most common cause of vaginal discharge and malodor. It frequently affects women with multiple sexual partners and is sexually associated, but not sexually transmitted. It is recognized by a homogeneous, white, noninflammatory discharge with a fishy odor, either before or after a vaginal sample is treated with a drop of potassium hydroxide (KOH) solution.

Bacterial vaginosis is associated with a number of possible severe consequences including cervicitis, PID, postpartum endometritis, premature labor, and recurring urinary tract infections. BV occurs when bacteria usually found in the vagina multiply and replace the prevailing bacteria, changing the balance of the vaginal flora.[61]

Symptomatic women need treatment, but studies have not supported treating asymptomatic women. There is no recognized equivalent in male partners, and treatment appears contraindicated for preventing recurrences. The CDC recommends treating BV with a 7-day regimen or a single dose of antibiotics, or the option of two topical agents. The topical agents are more expensive but appear to be equally effective for managing BV. Some health-care providers prefer the intravaginal administration over the systemic agents because of fewer possible side effects. Pregnant women are treated with topical agents because the oral antibiotic metronidazole is contraindicated.

Trichomoniasis Trichomonas, a one-celled parasite, is found in both men and women. It remains dormant in many asymptomatic women and causes vaginal irritation, itching, and diffuse, malodorous discharge in symptomatic women. The discharge varies but typically is thin, frothy, homogeneous, and yellow-green or grey. Most women experience red spots on the vaginal walls or a strawberry uterus, whereas most infected men are asymptomatic.[62]

Both partners need treatment for T vaginalis to be effectively cured because T vaginalis is sexually transmitted. **Trichomoniasis** is confirmed by the presence of trichomonads and a pH of 5 or more. If confirmed, an oral antibiotic (metronidazole) is usually prescribed for the woman and her partner.[63]

Candidiasis Vulvovaginal candidiasis, yeast infection, is not a sexually transmitted disease, but may co-exist with STDs. Candida is the term for a single-celled fungus often present in the human body. Candida and other yeasts are found in the vagina of nearly 20 percent of all women, many who are asymptomatic and do not need treatment. Symptomatic women will experience itching, with vaginal discharge, burning, or irritation in the vulvovaginal area. Pregnant women commonly experience yeast infections. Other common causes of yeast infections include significant changes in diet, some type of immune suppression, and/or the use of broad-spectrum antibiotics.

Many women use approved OTC medications to cure yeast infections, including vaginal topical creams, tablets, suppositories, and combination packs. Familiar trade names include Monistat 7, Gyne-Lotrimin, Mycelex-7, Fem Care, and others. Unfortunately, some women who self-diagnose a yeast infection may actually experience BV or another infection that cannot be cured by OTC medications. Women with pelvic pain, first-time infections, multiple sexual partners, or unprotected sexual encounters and pregnant women should see a health-care provider. Treatment of partners does not appear to reduce the incidence of yeast infections.[64]

Some women are more predisposed to recurrent yeast infections. The factors most often associated with repeat infections include diabetes, obesity, suppressed immunity, pregnancy, using broad-spectrum antibiotics, corticosteroids, or birth control pills. Self-care is appropriate for women who have recurrent yeast infections. If a self-diagnosed infection does not appear to respond to treatment, a health-care provider should be consulted.[65,66] When recurrent yeast infections occur without another cause, the health-care provider should suspect or rule out HIV. (See *Health Tips:* "Preventing Recurring Yeast Infections" for suggestions to help prevent yeast infections.)

---

health tips

Preventing Recurring Yeast Infections

- Use mild soaps and perfumes
- Use unscented toilet paper and sanitary pads
- Avoid feminine hygiene sprays
- Double rinse undergarments washed in harsh irritants
- Use 100 percent cotton undergarments to keep the genital area dry
- Wear loose rather than restrictive clothing
- Limit hot tub episodes
- Change swimsuits immediately after a hot tub or swim to reduce exposure to the genital area to moisture
- Wipe from front to back after a bowel movement to reduce possible infections
- Male partners must wash their penis or change condoms when moving from anal to vaginal intercourse
- Avoid sugar binges
- Monitor changes in dietary patterns

---

vaginitis (vaj in eye tis)—an infection of the vaginal area with discharge and itching.

trichomoniasis (trick oh mon **eye** ah sis)—a sexually transmitted disease caused by the protozoan (parasite) *Trichomonas vaginalis.*

AIDS

AIDS is the third leading cause of death among all women between the ages of 15 to 44, and the leading cause of death for African American women between ages 15 to 44. Figure 18.3 shows that 13,764 cases of AIDS were reported in 1995 for adolescents over age 13 and adult women. The majority of these cases were in younger women. Each year the number of HIV cases of women has grown—from 7 percent of all cases in 1985 to 18 percent in 1994.[67] The majority of women who contract AIDS are heterosexual or injecting drug users (IDUs). Figure 18.4 shows the AIDS cases among women by risk factor, as well as the cumulative percentages since 1981 and the current percentages in 1995. In 1995, there were 13,764 cases of AIDS reported in U.S. women with 38 percent occurring among IDUs and 38 percent among heterosexual women. Since 1981, there have been 71,818 cases of AIDS reported in U.S. women with 47 percent occurring among IDUs and 37 percent occurring among heterosexual women. Table 18.1 shows that minority women are disproportionately represented with African American and Hispanic women accounting for 77 percent of all reported AIDS cases (while constituting 21 percent of the female population).[68] Worldwide, women constitute 40 percent of all HIV-positive cases (approximately 10–12 million).

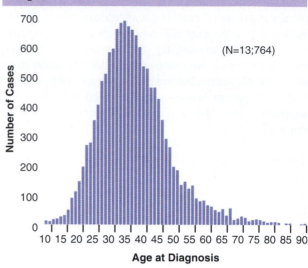

FIGURE 18.3 Women with AIDS by age at diagnosis, 1995.

Susceptibility to HIV

In 1992, the World Health Organization (WHO) changed its strategy for fighting AIDS and projected that by the year 2000, more women than men will have the disease. Women have a greater chance of becoming infected with HIV by heterosexual contact and often serve as the primary caregivers when

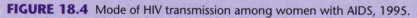

FIGURE 18.4 Mode of HIV transmission among women with AIDS, 1995.

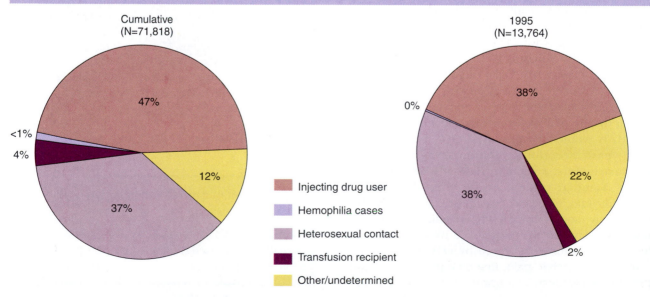

Table 18.1

Women with AIDS by Race/Ethnicity per 100,000 Women, United States, Reported in 1995			
Race/Ethnicity	No.	(%)	Rate/ 100,000 women
Black	7,680	(56)	59
White	3,106	(23)	4
Hispanic	2,847	(21)	25
Asian/Pacific Islander	74	(<1)	2
American Indian/ Alaska Native	38	(<1)	5
Total*	13,764	(100)	12

*Includes 19 women of unknown race/ethnicity.

relatives become infected. The WHO suggests that biologic factors, epidemiologic factors, and social vulnerability cause women to be more susceptible to HIV. Women have increased biologic risk due to greater mucosal surface exposed during intercourse and higher concentrations of HIV in seminal fluids.

The increased epidemiologic risk occurs because women date or marry older men who have often been with multiple partners. For instance, most teenage women date older males (sometimes in their twenties). These males are more likely to have had several sexual partners. The more partners, the greater the risk of contracting HIV or another STD.

Social vulnerability becomes a risk factor when passive women are afraid to demand the use of a condom. They rely on their partner to determine whether a condom will be used, and if the partner refuses to use one, she may acquiesce to his desires. She must also rely on the fidelity of her partner, although extramarital relationships are common. This behavior also increases her risk of HIV and other STDs.[69] (See *Her Story:* "Rebekka.")

Defining HIV/AIDS

AIDS stands for *acquired immune deficiency syndrome* and is a group of signs or symptoms that occur when the immune system does not function properly. Human **immunodeficiency** virus (HIV) is the organism that causes the disease. In the vast majority of full blown AIDS, the person eventually dies, although the length of life for a person with AIDS continues to increase with new drug therapies and more aggressive, early treatment.

Her Story

Rebekka

Rebekka had a dream. She wanted to be a famous model. Few women achieve success in this career, but Rebekka's dream came true. She was *Playboy* magazine's "Miss September of 1986." Rebekka now speaks at schools and shares her life story with children but she is not at the school to talk about being a model. Rebekka is speaking out about something that changed her life forever; she has AIDS. While living in the fast lane of her modeling career, she had unprotected sex with one man. She is now educating young people about the perils of promiscuity. When her AIDS test first came back positive she began abusing drugs and twice tried suicide. Now she has found new meaning in her life. She said, "Right now, my career move is living, it's a full-time job. I'm still a Playmate, and I'm really glad, because *Playboy* gave me a voice. And I'm using my voice to fight AIDS."

- What do you think of Rebekka's message?
- Do you think she is making a difference in her audience's lives?
- What makes Rebekka more effective in giving her message when compared with other individuals?

In 1993, the Centers for Disease Control issued the Revised Classification System for HIV infection and Expanded Surveillance Case Definition for AIDS Among Adolescents and Adults.[70] The surveillance case definition expanded to include all HIV-infected persons with less than 200 CD4+ T-lymphocytes/μL or a CD4+ percentage of less than 14. The definition of AIDS was further expanded to include pulmonary tuberculosis (TB), recurrent pneumonia, and invasive cervical cancer. Invasive cervical cancer can be prevented if detected early, which makes gynecologic exams an important screening component of medical treatment for women. (See *FYI:* "Revised AIDS Surveillance Case Definition" for a list of conditions included in the AIDS surveillance case definition.)

immunodeficient—an abnormal state of the immune system in which the body's defense system does not work properly to fight foreign substances in the body.

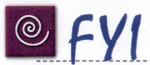

Revised AIDS Surveillance Case Definition

Candidiasis of bronchi, trachea, or lungs
Candidiasis, esophageal
Cervical cancer, invasive*
Coccidiodomycosis, disseminated or extrapulmonary
Cryptococcosis, extrapulmonary
Cryptoporidiosis, chronic intestinal (greater than 1 month's duration)
Cytomegalovirus disease (other than liver, spleen, or nodes)
Cytomegalovirus retinitis (with loss of vision)
Encephalopathy, HIV-related
Herpes simplex: chronic ulcer(s) (greater than 1 month's duration); or bronchitis, pneumonitis, or esophagitis
Histoplasmosis, disseminated or extrapulmonary
Isosporiasis, chronic intestinal (greater than 1 month's duration)

Kaposi's sarcoma
Lymphoma, Burkitt's (or equivalent term)
Lymphoma, immunoblastic (or equivalent term)
Lymphoma, primary, of brain
Mycobacterium avium complex or M. kansaisii, disseminated or extrapulmonary
Mycobacterium tuberculosis, any site (pulmonary* or extrapulmonary)
Mycobacterium, other species or unidentified species, disseminated or extrapulmonary
Pneumocystis carinii pneumonia
Pneumonia, recurrent*
Progressive multifocal leukoencephalopathy
Salmonella septicemia, recurrent
Toxoplasmosis of brain
Wasting syndrome due to HIV

Contracting AIDS

HIV is carried from one person to another through blood, semen, and vaginal secretions. It can be transferred through sexual contact, sharing injecting drug needles, from mother to infant before or during childbirth and occasionally through breast-feeding, and through receiving blood or blood products from someone infected with HIV. In the United States, all blood banks began screening for HIV in 1985 so anyone receiving a transfusion after this date is virtually free from the possibility of transmission. The most common way for heterosexual women to contract AIDS is through injecting drug use, although heterosexual women are facing an ever-increasing risk from contact with bisexual or heterosexual men. HIV is not transmitted through casual contact, tears, or saliva.

Symptoms of HIV

Symptoms of AIDS may be similar to other diseases, however they take longer to disappear and/or may recur. Common early symptoms of AIDS include recurring fever including "night sweats"; rapid weight loss without diet or exercise; diarrhea lasting longer than several weeks; white, thick spots or coating in the mouth; a dry cough and shortness of breath; or purple bumps on the skin, inside the mouth and in the rectum.

Diagnosis of HIV

If a woman believes she has been infected or exposed to the HIV virus through sex, injecting drug use, or other contact with contaminated blood, she should request an HIV antibody test. Because women can be infected more easily than men, they should request testing if they have the slightest suspicion of exposure. If a woman selects a testing center, it should offer pre- and post-test counseling, as well as confidentiality from employers and health insurance. If possible, she should choose a center that offers anonymous testing. Two tests are used for diagnosis: the **ELISA test** (enzyme-linked immunosorbent assay), a general screening test with high sensitivity, and the **Western blot test,** a less sensitive, more expensive but more specific test for the HIV antibody. If a person tests positive for the HIV antibody with the ELISA test, a second ELISA test is conducted on the same sample. If this test is positive, the Western blot test is conducted. If the Western blot test is positive, the person is said to be HIV-positive. Nearly 90 percent of low-risk persons who test positive on the ELISA test will test negative on the Western blot test. Results for each test often takes up to a week for reporting.

A woman must wait nearly a month from the time of the suspected exposure before getting tested. It takes approximately 45 days between the time of initial exposure and the body's building of enough antibodies for detection. This period between infection and antibody development is called the window period. This period will usually take between 2 weeks and 6 months, and can occur up to 18 months later. Experts recommend two sets of tests, approximately 6 months apart, be conducted for conclusive results. If a woman is unsure of where to go for HIV counseling and testing, she can contact the National AIDS Hotline.

Pneumocystis carinii **pneumonia (PCP)** is the leading AIDS-defining diagnosis among women reported with AIDS through June 1993 even though the AIDS case surveillance definition has been expanded to include invasive cervical cancer. The addition of invasive cervical cancer to the definition serves as a reminder to physicians that women with and at risk for HIV infection should have a Pap smear annually.[71]

Home HIV Tests

In 1996, the FDA approved new home HIV tests. These tests are accurate when used properly. When the first tests for HIV were conducted in the early 1980s, health-care providers believed that all HIV-positive persons needed immediate professional counseling. However, many people refused to be tested because of concerns about lack of anonymity and potential loss of health insurance benefits. The process of testing also prevented many people from seeking HIV-testing services. The CDC estimates that nearly 60 percent of Americans at risk for contracting HIV have not been tested. These home tests may encourage people at risk for HIV to seek testing.

Today, women who may be HIV-positive need to be diagnosed early because early detection leads to early treatment. Early treatment for an HIV-positive woman can ensure a longer life, and may delay symptoms of AIDS indefinitely. Two home tests are currently FDA approved and marketed. Confide HIV Testing Service (TM) is marketed by Direct Access Diagnostics, a subsidiary of Johnson and Johnson. It is available through a toll-free number, 1–800–THE–TEST. Home Access Express (TM) is marketed by Home Access Health Corporation of Hoffman Estates, Illinois, and is available through a toll-free number, 1–800–HIV–TEST. Test kits also are available through pharmacies nationwide.

Treatment of HIV

Drug treatment typically focuses on reducing the viral load or reinforcing the immune system. The viral load

JOURNAL ACTIVITY

Browsing the Internet for AIDS Research

Browsing the Internet can be an effective way to keep updated on recent AIDS research advances. The National Institute for Allergies and Infectious Diseases has a web page of recent news releases. News releases like the following are provided: ACTG 315 Preliminary Results: Drug Cocktail Restores Partial Immune Function, Primary Immune Response to HIV Predicts Disease Progression, and Study Finds No Gender Difference in Chlamydia Transmission Rates. Check the web page at www.niaid.nih.gov for the most recent news releases. Which news releases are of interest to you? Share your findings with classmates.

can be lowered or kept low by "blocking HIV attachment to the CDR cell, blocking antigens on the virus envelope, interfering with the uncoating of the virus as it enters the cell, disrupting the translation of virus RNA to cell DNA, and disrupting the assembly and maturation of virus particles in the CDR cell, and their release as a free-floating virus in the body."[72] Combinations of drugs are often used to impact the HIV virus at its various stages. Familiar drugs include AZT, ZDV, ddI, ddC, and the newer protease inhibitors like Invirase and Viracept. Also, complete *Journal Activity:* "Browsing the Internet for AIDS Research" and see *Viewpoint:* "Discrimination in AIDS Research."

HIV and Children

Cases of HIV in young children continue to rise as the rate of infection among heterosexual women of childbearing age rises. Most of these cases result

ELISA test—abbreviation for enzyme-linked immunosorbent assay screening test for the HIV antibody.

Western blot test—laboratory test used to detect the presence of HIV antibody; regarded as more accurate than the ELISA test.

pneumocystis carinii **pneumonia (PCP)**—a protozoal infection of the lungs; the most common cause of death of people with HIV.

Viewpoint

Discrimination in AIDS Research

Maureen Perry, in the spring issue of *Women Being Alive Newsletter,* wrote: "Fourteen of the 21 oncology/cancer trials currently in the ACTG's are studying treatments for Kaposi's Sarcoma, a cancer occurring almost exclusively in men. The exclusion of women from trial #216, though unethical, is not surprising. The ACTG's have continuously ignored women in the epidemic, as well as minorities."[74]

The issue at hand was the handling of trial #216, a study originally designed to study the effects of isotretinoin and interferon in the prevention of anal and cervical neoplasia, precursors to cancer, related to anogenital human papilloma virus (HPV). The ACTG funded a project to address the drugs' potential to prevent recurrent cervical neoplasia (AIN), ignoring the drugs potential to prevent recurrent cervical neoplasia (CIN). Under public scrutiny, the ACTG funded a second study to address CIN. This is just one example of the limited (almost nonexistent) focus on women's signs, symptoms, and treatment for HIV infections. In 1994, women accounted for 18 percent of the participants in the ACTG trials compared to 10 percent in 19091 and 7 percent in 1988.[75] What can you do to ensure that women receive fair and ethical treatment in medical research? What additional information do you need? What actions will you take?

from the passing of the HIV virus from infected mothers in utero or during childbirth, and occasionally, through breast-feeding. A study by the AIDS Clinical Trials Group (ACTG) found that infants born to HIV-positive women have an 8.3 percent chance of contracting the disease during the fetal stage or birth if both mothers and their babies receive AZT compared to a 25.5 percent chance of contracting the disease when administered a placebo. The findings led to the discontinuation of the trial so all HIV-positive pregnant women in the study were administered AZT as well as their infants for the first 6 weeks after birth.[73]

Determining an infant's HIV status after birth is difficult because a mother's antibodies may remain in the infant's system for several months. If a woman discovers her HIV-positive status upon becoming pregnant, she faces the shock of her own positive test concurrently with the possibility of transmitting the virus to her newborn. If the child tests negative, the mother still faces her own disease and the likelihood that she won't be able to raise her child.

PREVENTION STRATEGIES

STD infections have special implications for women because women are less symptomatic, more difficult to diagnose, less frequently tested, and suffer more severe consequences. Also, the transmission of STDs is easier from men to women. One study found that men infected with HIV are nearly twice as likely to infect their female partners as conversely.[76] These factors make prevention efforts extremely important. What prevention strategies are available for women? What behaviors are considered safer? This section reviews some of the available options for women.

Abstinence

Sexual abstinence is the only 100 percent effective method to prevent sexually transmitted diseases. Abstinence means no exchange of body fluids and no skin to skin exposure of the genital areas. Young people need to understand that being physically developed does not necessarily equate with psychological readiness for a sexual relationship. When is abstinence appropriate? *ANYTIME YOU CHOOSE!* Abstinence is certainly an appropriate choice for women when they are not psychologically ready, when they have been drinking, if they have had unprotected sex with a different partner without subsequent testing, or if they don't have adequate protection (condoms). Can you think of other times when a woman might choose abstinence?

Monogamy

More young women today are choosing to delay sexual intimacy until they have a committed relationship or until they are married. A committed relationship is not synonymous with "serial monogamy." Serial monogamy means having several relationships over time, with just one partner in each relationship. For teenagers, serial monogamy may mean having only one partner; however, the length of time for the relationship can vary from several days to several months. Reducing the number of sexual partners over one's lifetime and choosing a partner who has had fewer sexual partners translates into less exposure to the risk of contracting a STD.

Engaging in Less Risky Behaviors with Partners

The American College Health Association provides a list of sexual behaviors that encourage safer sex. Sexually transmitted diseases are not dependent on who the person is, but rather on what the person does. Sexual behaviors can be considered safe (dry kissing) to dangerous (unprotected vaginal or anal sex). Review the list provided in *FYI:* "Playing It Safe with Sexual Behaviors." Are there other behaviors you would add to the list? Where would you place these behaviors? Then complete *Journal Activity:* "Reasons for Unprotected Sex."

Oral Contraceptives

Oral contraceptives are not effective in preventing sexually transmitted diseases. They appear to reduce the risk of PID, but increase the risk of STDs. With

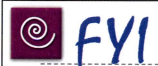

Playing It Safe with Sexual Behaviors

SAFE

Dry kissing
Mutual masturbation on healthy skin
Oral sex on a man with a latex condom
Touching, massage, fantasy

LESS RISKY

Vaginal intercourse with a latex condom and
    nonoxynol-9
Wet kissing
Anal intercourse with a latex condom with
    nonoxynol-9

RISKY

Oral sex on a man without a condom
Masturbation on open-broken skin
Oral sex on a woman

DANGEROUS

Vaginal intercourse without a condom
Anal intercourse without a condom
Sharing a needle or blood contact
Semen or urine in the mouth

JOURNAL ACTIVITY

Reasons for Unprotected Sex

As a class assignment or an assignment with friends, brainstorm all the reasons that college women may give for putting themselves at risk for having unprotected sex with a partner. For each reason, write an alternative positive response in your journal.

Example

Reason: If I carry a condom with me, he could think that I'm planning to have sex.
Alternative response: I have a right to protect myself and the right to choose when and with whom I have sex.

---

the rise in HIV infections in heterosexual women, young women need contraceptive methods that increase their protection from sexually transmitted diseases, as well as unwanted pregnancies. These young women may be lured into a false sense of protection by focusing on pregnancy, not HIV and STD prevention. Most health-care providers recommend using oral contraceptives and condoms with spermicide to reduce the risk of unwanted pregnancies *and* STDs.

Male Condoms

Male condoms are one of the most effective methods available for preventing STDs. Most viruses do not pass through the latex condom when properly used. The problem for many young women is their difficulty in insisting that their male partner use condoms, and also requesting that the condom be latex with nonoxynol-9. If the male partner refuses to use a condom, she is faced with additional decisions. If her partner consents to using a condom, she cannot ensure that this young man will use the condom properly so she may want to consider an additional alternative.

The FDA monitors condom safety and each manufactured condom is tested electronically for holes before packaging. Condom breakage during intercourse is estimated at less than 2 per 100 condoms. Although condoms are not 100 percent effective, the overall failure is seldom due to the condom itself, but rather results from inconsistent or incorrect use. Condoms should never be used with lubricants made from mineral oil, vegetable oil, or petroleum-based products. Vaginal creams may have mineral oil components and massage oils may have a vegetable oil base, and these components can destroy the integrity of the condom. (See *Health Tips:* "Condom Do's and Don'ts.")

> ## h e a l t h   t i p s
>
> ### *Condom Do's and Don'ts*
>
> ### DO
>
> - Use a condom every time you have vaginal and/or anal intercourse.
> - Use a safe lubricant to reduce the chance of the condom tearing or breaking during vaginal and/or anal intercourse.
> - Use a latex condom with a receptacle tip and nonoxynol-9, and squeeze the air out of the tip before using it.
> - Condoms need to be rolled down an erect penis before any sexual activity and worn until the man has an ejaculation.
> - Hold on to the condom at the base of the penis while the man withdraws from the woman's vagina.
>
> ### DO NOT
>
> - Do not reuse the condom.
> - Do not use Vaseline, baby oil, or hair grease for lubrication because they will weaken the condom.
> - Do not store condoms in glove compartments or wallets. Heat can cause condoms to decay and break easily.

Female Condoms

The female condom, Reality™, offers a woman another alternative contraceptive method and allows her to have more control over the sexual experience. She can insert it before intercourse, unlike the male condom that requires an erect penis before it can be applied. The female condom protects the outer labia, thus offering better protection against HPV or HSV. Reality is made of polyurethane, a more effective protection than latex. The disadvantages include its higher price and the need to communicate openly between the partners. The female condom has a closed end that is inserted into the vagina and covers the cervix, and an open end that rests against the vulva and covers the labia. It acts as a barrier to prevent semen from entering the vagina and can be used with a spermicide. Current data suggests that this method has a failure rate of between 11 and 15 percent, similar to other barrier methods. The efficacy of this method in preventing HIV or other STDs still remains uncertain.[77,78] You have a variety of strategies available to prevent unwanted STDs and unintended pregnancies, from abstinence to proper protection. Keep informed! Stay assertive! ∽

Chapter Summary

- Nearly fifty different STD-related organisms and syndromes are recognized today.
- The United States has one of the highest STD rates of industrialized countries.
- Teenagers account for 25 percent of all STDs.
- Chlamydia is the most common sexually transmitted disease in the United States and must be reported by all fifty states.
- Chlamydia is treated with antibiotics, either in a 7-day or single dose regimen.
- Gonorrhea has declined since the 1970s except in teenagers and some minority groups. A large discrepancy in cases exists between African American and white teenagers.
- Syphilis is caused by the spirochete, *Treponema pallidum.* The number of cases reported in 1995 was the fewest reported cases since 1960.
- Syphilis has four phases: primary, secondary, latent, and tertiary. Congenital syphilis is transmitted to the infant during pregnancy.
- Genital herpes is incurable and difficult to control. Autoinoculation is the self-spread of the virus from one body part to another. Acyclovir has some effectiveness in preventing a herpes outbreak.
- Several types of human papilloma viruses, genital warts, are associated with cancer.
- Hepatitis B is a viral infection causing inflammation of the liver. HBV is transmitted through exposure to infected blood and unprotected sexual intercourse. A vaccine exists to prevent HBV.
- Pelvic inflammatory disease causes chronic pelvic pain, infertility, and ectopic pregnancies.
- Most vaginitis is classified as trichomoniasis, bacterial vaginosis, or candidiasis.
- AIDS is the third leading cause of death in women between the ages of 15 and 44, and the leading cause of death in African American women between the ages of 15 and 44.
- Invasive cervical cancer has been added to the list of AIDS-defining diseases. Invasive cervical cancer can be prevented with early detection.
- The National AIDS Hotline number is 1-800-342-AIDS.

Review Questions

1. Which STD has the highest incidence? What complications are associated with this STD?
2. Describe the four stages of syphilis.
3. What are the demographic characteristics that make a person more susceptible to STDs and/or AIDS?
4. Which individuals and groups are most susceptible to hepatitis B virus?
5. What complications can occur when pelvic inflammatory disease remains untreated?
6. What is the length of the window period for determining the presence of HIV antibodies?
7. What are the known modes of transmission of HIV?
8. What measures can you take to prevent AIDS and other STDs?

Resources

Organizations and Hotlines

CDC National AIDS Clearinghouse
P.O. Box 6003
Rockville, MD 20849-6003
Telephone: (800) 458-5231

CDC National STD Hotline
Telephone: (800) 227-8922
Monday–Friday, 8 A.M. to 11 P.M. (Eastern)

National Herpes Hotline
Telephone: (919) 361-8488
Monday–Friday, 9 A.M. to 7 P.M. (Eastern)

American Social Health Association
P.O. Box 13827
Research Triangle Park, NC 27709

Vaccination Information for International Travellers
Centers for Disease Control
Telephone: (404) 332-4559

CDC National AIDS Hotline
English service (800) 342-AIDS (2347)
 (7 days a week, 24 hours a day)
Spanish service (800) 344-7432
 (7 days a week, 8 A.M. to 2 A.M. EST)
TDD service for the deaf (800) 243-7889
 (Monday through Friday, 10 A.M. to 10 P.M. EST)

Websites

National Institute for Allergies and Infectious Diseases
www.niaid.nih.gov

Centers for Disease Control and Prevention
www.cdc.gov

Journal of the American Medical Association
www.ama-assn.org

GENA/aegis-International Hub
gopher.hivnet.org

Food and Drug Administration
www.fda.gov

Planned Parenthood Federation of America
www.ppfa.org

Suggested Readings

CDC National AIDS Clearinghouse. February, 1995. *Guide to selected HIV services and materials for women.* Rockville, Md. Department of Health and Human Services.
The Helper (a quarterly newsletter for people with herpes). Herpes Resource Center, P.O. Box 13827, Research Triangle Park, NC 27709.

References

1. Washington, A. E., P. S. Arno, and M. A. Brooks. 1986. The economic costs of pelvic inflammatory disease. *JAMA*, 255:1735-38.
2. U.S. Public Health Service. 1991. Curbing the increase in rates of STDs. *Aids Weekly:* 9-11.
3. *Healthy People 2000: National health promotion and disease prevention objectives.* 1991. U.S. Department of Health and Human Services, DHHS Publication No. (PHS) 91-50212, p. 193.
4. Howard, M., and J. B. McCabe. 1990. Helping teenagers postpone sexual involvement. *Family Planning Perspectives,* 22 (1): 21-26.
5. U.S. Public Health Service, Curbing the increase in rates of STDs.
6. Division of STD Prevention. September, 1996. Sexually transmitted diseases surveillance, 1995. U.S. Department of Health and Human Services, Public Health Service. Atlanta: Centers for Disease Control and Prevention.

7. Ibid.
8. Chlamydia prevalence and screening practices—San Diego County, California, 1993. May, 1994. *Morbidity and Mortality Weekly Report:* 366-70.
9. Update: New weapons in the war against chlamydia trachomatis infection. 1994. *Consultant,* 34: 103-5.
10. Hillis, S. D., A. Nakashima, P. A. Marchbanks, and others. 1994. Risk factors for recurrent Chlamydia trachomatis infections in women. *American Journal of Obstetrics and Gynecology,* 170: 801-6.
11. Ibid.
12. Hook, E. W., C. Spitter, C. A. Reichart, and others. 1994. Use of cell culture and a rapid diagnostic assay for Chlamydia trachomatis screening. *JAMA,* 272: 867-70.
13. Hillis, Nakashima, Marchbanks, and others. Risk factors for recurrent Chlamydia trachomatis infections in women.
14. Hook, Spitter, Reichart, and others. Use of cell culture and a rapid diagnostic assay.
15. Majeroni, B. A. 1994. Chlamydia cervicitis: Complications and new treatment options. *American Family Physician,* 49: 1825-30.
16. Randall, T. 1993. New tools ready for chlamydia diagnosis, treatment, but teens need education most. *JAMA,* 269: 2716-17.
17. Division of STD Prevention, Sexually transmitted disease surveillance, 1995.
18. Gonorrhea increase may spur HIV spread among teenagers. 1994. *AIDS Alert,* 9: 139-40.
19. Division of STD Prevention, Sexually transmitted disease surveillance, 1995.
20. Divergence in trends of syphilis and gonorrhea. 1992. *American Family Physician,* 45: 852.
21. Division of STD Prevention, Sexually transmitted disease surveillance, 1995.
22. Cefotaxime vs. ceftriaxone in the treatment of gonorrhea. (Adapted from the Southern Medical Journal, April 1994.) 1994. *American Family Physician,* 50: 1126.
23. Kerle, K. K., J. R. Mascola, and T. A. Miller. 1992. Disseminated gonococcal infection. *American Family Physician,* 45: 209-14.
24. Division of STD Prevention, Sexually transmitted disease surveillance, 1995.
25. Goens, J. L., C. K. Janniger, and K. DeWolf. 1994. Dermatologic and systemic manifestations of syphilis. *American Family Physician,* 50: 1013-20.
26. Bolan, G., C. Fontenot, and others. 1993. Syphilis: Are you missing it? *Patient Care,* 27: 126-42.
27. Ibid.
28. Goens, Janniger, and DeWolf, Dermatologic and systemic manifestations of syphilis.
29. Bolan, Fontenot, and others, Syphilis.
30. Goens, Janniger, and DeWolf, Dermatologic and systemic manifestations of syphilis.
31. McCabe, E., L. R. Jaffe, and A. Diaz. December 1993. Human immunodeficiency virus seropositivity in adolescents with syphilis. *AIDS Weekly:* 24. (Abstract)
32. Bolan, Fontenot, and other, Syphilis.
33. Division of STD Prevention, Sexually transmitted disease surveillance, 1995.
34. Herpes: questions and answers. 1994. Research Triangle Park, N.C.: American Social Health Association.
35. Ibid.
36. Division of STD Prevention, Sexually transmitted disease surveillance, 1995.
37. Herpes: GMHC Treatment Issues Fact Sheet. http://www.gmhc.org/living/medcare/herpes.html
38. Genital herpes information page. http://www.missouri.edu/shape/specinfs/hsv-ii.html
39. Ibid.
40. Randolph, A. G., A. E. Washington, and C. G. Prober. 1993. Cesarean delivery for women presenting with genital herpes lesions: Efficacy, risks, and costs. *JAMA,* 270: 77-82.
41. Pregnancy outcomes following systemic prenatal acyclovir exposure—June 1, 1984-June 30, 1993. 1993. *Morbidity and Mortality Weekly Report,* 42: 806-9.
42. HPV grown in tissue culture. August, 1992. *Cancer Weekly:* 3-4.
43. Some questions and answers about HPV and genital warts. 1994. Research Triangle Park, N.C.: American Social Health Association. (pamphlet)
44. Ibid.
45. Ibid.
46. Bowie, W. R., M. R. Hammerschlag, and D. H. Martin. 1994. STDs in '94: The new CDC guidelines. *Patient Care,* 28: 29 -39.
47. Ibid.
48. Becker, T. M., C. M. Wheeler, and others. 1994. Sexually transmitted diseases and other risk factors for cervical dysplasia among southwestern Hispanic and non-Hispanic white women. *JAMA,* 271: 1181-88.
49. Kozel, R., B. McGregor, and P. Manalo. February, 1993. Use of polymerase chain in detecting human papilloma virus in dual primary tumors of the upper aerodigestive tract. *Cancer Weekly:* 17-18.
50. Students at risk from hepatitis B. January, 1994. *USA Today,* 122: 8.
51. *AIDS Weekly.* December 9, 1991.
52. Study links types of sexual behavior in women to hepatitis B transmission. May, 1992. *Cancer Weekly:* 10-11.
53. Rosenblum, L., W. Darrow et al. May 13, 1992. Sexual practices in the transmission of Hepatitis B virus and prevalence of Hepatitis Delta virus infection in female prostitutes in the United States. *JAMA,* 267 (18): 2477-81.

54. Bazzi, M. N. 1994. Hepatitis or not? (Case and Comment). *Patient Care,* 28: 179–85.

55. Ibid.

56. Students at risk.

57. Brown, E. A., H. Kawanishi, and E. R. Schiff. 1994. Hepatitis C & E: How much of a threat? *Patient Care,* 28: 105–12.

58. Vaccination coverage of 2-year-old children—United States, 1993. 1994. *Morbidity and Mortality Weekly Report,* 43: 705–9.

59. *AIDS Weekly.*

60. Eschenbach, D. A., and P. B. Mead. 1992. Managing problem vaginitis. *Patient Care,* 26: 137–45.

61. Deutchman, M. E., D. J. Leaman, and J. L. Thomason. 1994. Vaginitis: Diagnosis is the key. *Patient Care,* 28: 39–53.

62. Ibid.

63. Ibid.

64. Ibid.

65. Ibid.

66. Ibid.

67. Segal, M. October, 1993. Women and AIDS. *FDA Consumer* (Revised 1995). http://www.fda.gov

68. 1995 AIDS Surveillance. http://www.cdc.gov

69. Women and children: Increasingly targeted by HIV. 1994. *UN Chronicle,* 31: 56–57.

70. 1993 Revised Classification System for HIV Infection and Expanded Surveillance Case Definition for AIDS Among Adolescents and Adults. *MMWR* 41 (RR-17), December 18, 1992.

71. Division of STD Prevention, Sexually transmitted disease surveillance, 1995.

72. Media Guide: XI International Conference on Aids, Vancouver, B.C. http://www.asi.bc.ca/bcba/kingsley/inf-diseases.html

73. Clinical alert: Important therapeutic information on the benefit of Zidovudine (AZT) for the prevention of the transmission of HIV from mother to infant. National Institute of Allergy and Infectious Diseases. www.niaid.nih.gov

74. Perry, M. Spring, 1994. AIDS clinical trials and tribulations: Research discriminates against women. *Women Being Alive Newsletter.* http://gopher.hivnet.org

75. Segal, M. October, 1993. Women and AIDS. *FDA Consumer* (Revised September 1996.)

76. European Study Group on Heterosexual Transmission of HIV. March 28, 1992. Comparison of female to male and male to female transmission of HIV in 563 stable couples. *British Medical Journal,* 304: 809–13.

77. A condom for women. 1992. The University of California, *Berkeley Wellness Letter* 8: 6–7.

78. Vaginal pouch gets advisory panel nod. 1992. *FDA Consumer,* 26: 5.

Nineteen

Managing Cardiovascular Health and Other Chronic Conditions

◼ chapter objectives

When you complete this chapter you will be able to:
- Describe how the cardiovascular system functions.
- Differentiate among the types of heart disease.
- Compare and contrast the various chronic conditions.
- Determine risk factors for heart disease and other chronic conditions.
- Describe ways to increase the protective factors that prevent heart disease and other chronic conditions.
- Identify the early warning signals for heart disease and other chronic conditions.
- Explain the current treatment protocols for heart disease and other chronic conditions.

LEADING CAUSE OF DEATH IN WOMEN

Cardiovascular diseases kill more women than any other disease, including lung or breast cancer. In 1995, 479,359 women (51.8 percent of all cardiovascular deaths) died from cardiovascular diseases, nearly one-third of deaths from all causes in women and more than cancer, accidents, and diabetes combined. The American Heart Association states that one in eight women aged 45 and over have had a heart attack or stroke and one in three women over age 65 suffer from some form of heart disease. Although heart disease is more prevalent in men, it is infinitely more deadly in women, with 39 percent of women dying within one year of a heart attack compared to 31 percent of men. (See *Her Story:* "Danielle.") African American women have a greater risk for coronary artery disease (CHD) than white women, and are 68.9 percent more likely to die. Likewise, Hispanic and Native American women have an increased risk of coronary artery disease.[1]

Until recently, men received nearly all the media, medical, and research attention concerning heart disease, even though one-half of all deaths from heart attacks occur in women. The Framingham Heart Study, a landmark longitudinal study of heart disease, initially focused on premature heart disease and fatal heart attacks that occurred mainly in men. These researchers did not discover until decades later that compared to men, women died in equal numbers from CHD; they just developed heart disease seven to ten years later! So, by age 65, the number of deaths from ischemic heart disease is actually higher in women.

HEALTHY PEOPLE 2000 OBJECTIVES

- Reduce coronary heart disease deaths to no more than 100 per 100,000 people. 1995 progress toward goal: 55 percent
- Reduce stroke deaths to no more than 20 per 100,000 people. 1995 progress toward goal: 35 percent
- Reverse the increase in end-stage renal disease (requiring maintenance dialysis or transplantation) to attain an incidence of no more than 13 per 100,000. 1995 progress toward goal: -286 percent
- Increase to at least 50 percent the proportion of people with high blood pressure whose blood pressure is under control. 1995 progress toward goal: 25 percent
- Increase to at least 90 percent the proportion with high blood pressure who are taking action to help control their blood pressure. 1995 progress toward goal: 10 percent
- Increase to at least 90 percent the proportion of adults who have had their blood pressure measured within the preceding two years and can state whether their blood pressure was normal or high. 1995 progress toward goal: 50 percent

- Reduce to no more than 8 percent the proportion of people who experience a limitation in major activity due to chronic conditions. 1995 progress toward goal: -90 percent
- Reduce diabetes-related deaths to no more than 34 per 100,000 people. 1995 progress toward goal: no progress
- Reduce the most severe complications of diabetes, including end-stage renal disease, blindness, lower extremity amputation, perinatal mortality, and major congenital malformations. 1995 progress toward goal: -500 percent
- Reduce diabetes to an incidence of no more than 2.5 per 1,000 people and a prevalence of no more than 25 per 1,000 people. 1995 progress toward goal: 25 percent
- Increase to at least 90 percent the proportion of perimenopausal women who have been counseled about the benefits and risks of estrogen replacement therapy (combined with progestin, when appropriate) for prevention of osteoporosis. 1995 progress toward goal: data unavailable

Her Story

Danielle

Grandma had her first heart attack when she was 67, six months after my grandfather died. Actually, Dr. Sawyer said that she must have had several previous heart attacks based on the scar tissue, but she never went in for treatment. Grandma resisted going to the doctor, but this time was different. She knew something was terribly wrong. Going to the doctor might mean staying in the hospital and she believed that only people who were dying went to the hospital. She wasn't ready to die, or if she was going to die, she would rather be at home.

I was a 20-year-old college student at the time and had just come home for a holiday break. I offered to stay with Grandma those first few days after her release from the hospital. The doctor said that nothing more could be done for her. I was scared; she was scared! What if she had another one? What if she died in her sleep or was too weak to call for help?

The first event that demonstrated her overall weakness was when she kneeled to retrieve a cooking pan from the cupboard and couldn't even stand up without help. She needed my assistance, and as we edged slowly

to the chair, we both had tears. This strong, independent woman whose first husband had died and left her to raise six children was so weak she couldn't kneel and get back up. Grandma died two months later from her final heart attack.

At the funeral, the family kept saying, "It isn't fair. She was too young and energetic to die. If only she hadn't smoked those cigarettes." For years, I've believed that cigarettes alone were the cause. After all, men, not women, died from heart attacks. Heart attacks in women were the exception, not the rule.

Cigarettes are certainly harmful, but Grandma had a number of risk factors, particularly age and cigarette smoking. She was a prime target for heart disease; we just didn't know enough about the additional risks.

As you read this chapter, think about those in your life who have a number of risk factors.
- What can they do to live life more fully?
- What are their risk factors?
- What can you do to reduce your risks of having a heart attack?

FIGURE 19.1 The cardiovascular system.

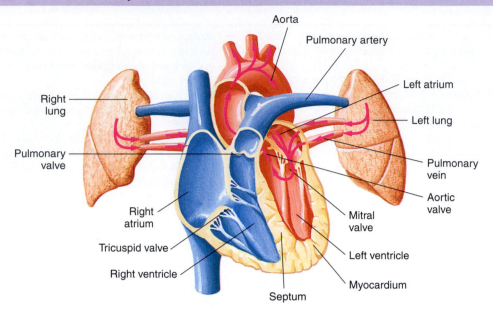

Aorta

Pulmonary artery

Right lung

Left atrium

Left lung

Pulmonary valve

Pulmonary vein

Aortic valve

Right atrium

Mitral valve

Tricuspid valve

Left ventricle

Right ventricle

Myocardium

Septum

The first conference related to women's heart health, sponsored by the American Heart Association, was held in 1964. Its main focus was *how women could help protect their husbands' hearts.* It isn't surprising that the focus was on husbands because heart research often studied only male subjects, and when females were included, they were underrepresented. The findings and recommendations of heart research involving men were then projected to include women. Not recognizing the impact of heart disease in women was an unfortunate mistake. Even today, women's warning signs and symptoms are taken less seriously, treatment is less aggressive, and research on heart disease is limited in number or excludes women altogether. Clinical trials often excluded women because researchers worried about conducting tests on women of childbearing age. Hormonal fluctuations in these women might influence drug trials and if they unknowingly became pregnant, drug exposure might harm the fetus. Women over age 65 with comorbidities were often excluded in clinical trials because their illnesses might produce inaccurate results. Thus, research regarding risk and protective factors for heart disease remains incomplete despite the knowledge that women continue to be more likely to die from heart attacks than men.

CARDIOVASCULAR DISEASES

Normal Cardiovascular Functioning

The **cardiovascular system** includes the heart and blood vessels. (See Fig. 19.1.) The heart is a four chamber pump composed of cardiac muscle. This muscular pump sends blood throughout the body from early conception until death. The heart is located in the middle of the chest, below the sternum, and is about the size of a clenched fist. The two upper chambers, called atria, receive blood. The right atrium receives deoxygenated blood from all parts of the body and the left atrium receives oxygenated blood from the lungs. The two lower chambers, called ventricles, send blood. The right ventricle pumps deoxygenated blood into the lungs and the left ventricle pumps oxygenated blood to the entire body. The blood in the heart passes through valves that separate these chambers. The opening and closing of the valves (tricuspid, pulmonic, mitral, and aortic) cause the familiar pumping sound heard in a stethoscope. If these valves fail to function properly, blood may flow back into a chamber and cause a murmur.

The Vascular System The vascular system is composed of arteries, veins, capillaries, arterioles,

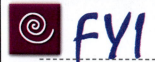

Coronary arteries

The heart muscle has arteries to provide oxygen to itself. These arteries are the right coronary, left anterior descending, and the left circumflex. The right coronary artery nourishes the back of the heart. The left anterior descending artery nourishes the front part of the heart and septum. The left circumflex nourishes the side of the heart. Smaller coronary arteries called corollary arteries connect to larger arteries and help nourish the heart and may replace the function of larger arteries if they malfunction. Because women's arteries are smaller than men's, it takes less plaque to cause an obstruction or occlusion. ∽

and venules. The **arteries** carry blood away from the heart and are larger closest to the heart. As the arteries move further from the heart, they become the arterioles that feed the **capillaries.** The capillaries filter the blood, taking food and oxygen from the arterioles and sending waste products and carbon dioxide to the venules. The venules carry blood into increasingly larger **veins** as blood flows to the heart. Problems with the arteries can cause a myocardial infarction, and problems with the veins can lead to congestive heart failure. Because a woman's heart and blood vessels are typically smaller than a man's, she often has more difficulties being treated and less plaque buildup is needed to block an artery.

Types of Heart Disease

The development of heart disease and the progression of atherosclerosis are influenced by a number of factors including genetic predisposition, gender, race, advancing age, and lifestyle choices. Heart disease develops gradually as narrowing of the coronary vessels causes changes in the blood flow to the heart. The changes to the coronary vessels evolve into lesions that further obstruct blood flow. Initially, partial obstruction of a major vessel or its branches may occur. However, over time, a blood clot from somewhere above the obstruction may break free and lodge in the obstruction, thus causing a total occlusion of the vessel.

Atherosclerosis Atherosclerosis is a gradual process of artery breakdown caused when circulating fats (cholesterol and others) penetrate the lining of the arterial wall. Although heredity is often implicated, the primary factor is excess cholesterol circulating in the bloodstream. When excess cholesterol bombards the arteries over a prolonged period, several reactions may develop: fat permeates the tissue macrophages, artery walls breakdown, and muscle tissue is replaced with less elastic material, plaque (accumulated platelets and red blood cells) forms and begins to occlude the artery.[2] (See Fig. 19.2.)

The primary risk factors for developing atherosclerosis are dietary intake of saturated fatty acids, elevation of systemic blood pressure, cigarette smoking, and glucose intolerance.

Angina Pectoris Chest pain is a common complaint heard by health-care providers. **Angina,** a derivative from the Greek language, means "to strangle" and describes a cluster of symptoms associated with oxygen deprivation. All attacks of angina begin as **ischemia** of the working heart muscle, forcing the

---

cardiovascular system—body system that includes the heart and blood vessels.

arteries—blood vessels that carry oxygenated blood to the body and the heart.

capillaries—blood vessels that have thin membranes that allow for the exchange of carbon dioxide and waste by-products for oxygen and food.

veins—blood vessels that carry deoxygenated blood and waste by-products to the heart and lungs.

atherosclerosis (ath er oh scler **oh** sis)—common disorder of arteries in which yellowish plaque, caused by circulating fats, penetrates the inner walls of arteries.

angina (an **jie** nuh)—cluster of symptoms associated with oxygen deprivation.

ischemia (iss **key** me ah)—lack or absence of oxygen.

FIGURE 19.2 Progression of atherosclerosis.

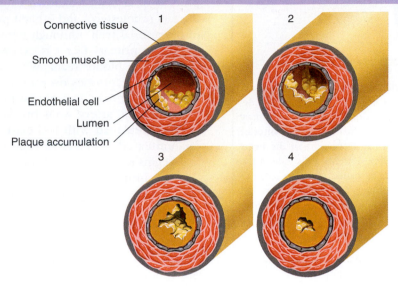

Connective tissue

Smooth muscle

Endothelial cell

Lumen

Plaque accumulation

heart to work in the absence of oxygen. Chemical substances accumulate in the anaerobic state and these substances are believed to initiate the pain associated with angina.

Women, older women in particular, appear to have a higher incidence of angina than men, and for many, it may be the first warning sign of coronary heart disease (CHD). It results when the heart does not get enough oxygen, often because a spasm causes temporary narrowing of a coronary artery or atherosclerosis blocks a portion of the artery. Angina is not a heart attack, and once the pain passes (usually in less than a minute), blood returns to the heart muscle and the cells function normally. Even though angina occurs more often in older women, CHD tends to manifest similarly in women and men with approximately 50 percent of patients having a **myocardial infarction** (MI), 30 percent having angina, and 20 percent experiencing sudden death.[3]

Classic angina manifests as a feeling of heaviness, pressure, or burning in the chest, with pain radiating into the back, neck, and sometimes the inner part of the left arm. Feelings of suffocation and impending death are quite common. Women who experience angina often exhibit signs dissimilar to classic angina symptoms. In fact, the signs are often more subtle in women and can be very confusing. Women frequently experience inconsequential chest pains and fleeting rhythm disturbances when they are young. Therefore, they may be more likely to mistake angina for heartburn, gastric disorders, asthma, allergies,

and bronchitis because they mimic the symptoms of angina. Some women describe a feeling of weakness and lethargy, others as back pain. However angina manifests itself, women need to inform their health-care providers when they experience chest pain.

Angina is *not* a minor symptom, and should be taken seriously by a woman and her health-care provider. Although nearly 80 percent of angina pains will not develop into heart attacks, these pains may be a precursor to heart disease and may precede a full-blown heart attack. Physical exertion, emotional stress, or exposure to intense cold often induce angina. If necessary, rest and vasodilation of the coronary arteries by using drugs can alleviate the pain.

The factors that may reduce or control angina include quitting smoking, regular exercise and weight management, avoiding high altitudes and cold air, avoiding excessive alcohol, salt, or heavy meals, and decreasing emotional stress and physical exertion.[4]

The primary objective for treatment of angina is to improve coronary blood flow, and secondarily, to reduce the amount of oxygen needed by the heart. Health-care providers may prescribe nitroglycerine, beta blockers, or calcium channel blockers for angina.

Medications reduce the cardiac need for oxygen but do not increase coronary blood flow. Surgical procedures such as coronary artery **bypass** grafting (CABG) or percutaneous transluminal coronary **angioplasty** (PTCA) are designed to increase coronary blood flow.[5] Previously, many women suffered

FIGURE 19.3 Angioplasty. (*A*), A "balloon" is surgically inserted into the narrowed coronary artery. (*B*), The balloon is inflated, compressing plaque and fatty deposits against the artery walls.

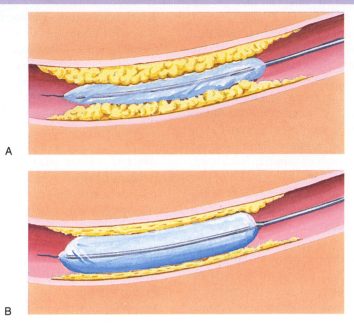

A

B

complications during angioplasty from tears to the arteries caused by larger balloons. Today's smaller and finer balloons have improved the prognosis for women. (See Fig. 19.3.)

Myocardial Infarction

When myocardial infarction (MI) occurs, blood flow to the affected heart area ceases. This condition is commonly created when a moving blood clot (embolism) lodges in a coronary vessel and causes complete occlusion of the vessel. Occlusion occurs at a point where the vessel is too small for the clot to pass through. The heart tissue normally served by this vessel begins to experience almost immediate ischemia, and tissue death occurs unless corollary vessels provide the needed oxygen.

Angina pain occurs immediately and intensely in most MI cases. The difference between angina and MI is that the pain with MI cannot be alleviated by drugs because the tissue is depleted of blood flow. Some tissue death occurs with all MIs but the extent of damage is dependent on the size and location of the artery supplying oxygen and the degree to which the tissue area remains deprived of oxygen. If corollary arteries can supply the oxygen, the extent of the damage may be minimal.

Regardless of age and treatment, MI is often more lethal for women than men. Women are more likely to die within a year of the first heart attack or to have a second MI within five years. Women experience more in-hospital mortality, more recurrent angina, and more congestive heart failure after discharge.[6]

Congenital Heart Disease

Heart disease is **congenital** when you are born with it. Advances in medical treatment have dramatically altered the outlook for children with congenital heart disease. Many, who previously would have died as children, can expect to live a full adult life. In the United States, the number of women living with congenital heart disease is growing. These women need healthcare providers who understand the nuances of this

---

myocardial infarction (in **fark** shun)—a heart attack.

bypass—any one of many types of surgery that allows blood to travel past or around a blockage.

angioplasty (an gee oh **plas** tee)—procedure that widens a narrow artery.

congenital heart disease—defect of the heart or great vessels existing from birth.

disease. Many had surgery as children, but they seldom completely recovered. Thus, as adults, they face the possibility of long-term medical surveillance and further treatment.

Adolescents face numerous dilemmas and deal with many questions, such as scars, chronic illness, types of exercise, sexual activity, type of contraception, and so on. Young women with congenital heart disease have further considerations. If they are considering having children, they need adequate family planning counseling. In some cases, pregnancy is strongly discouraged. These young women need advice from health-care providers familiar with their particular disease.

A major dilemma for many young adults is the issue of health insurance once coverage under their parent's policy ends. Insurance companies routinely deny coverage for various congenital lesions that have a low morbidity and mortality rate. Studies by the National Heart, Lung, and Blood Institute (NHLBI) and the Mayo Clinic confirm that many of these individuals have normal longevity and minimal mortality. Yet, insurance companies still deny or limit coverage to these individuals.[7]

Arrhythmia Arrhythmia, known as irregular heartbeats, can manifest as loss of sinus rhythm or tachyarrhythmia. Atrial fibrillation occurs when the right and left atria lose their rhythm and the heart beat can increase to several hundred beats per minute. If left unchecked, this arrhythmia can cause dizziness, chest pain, and even blood clots. Ventricular fibrillation causes the ventricles to lose their rhythm and makes them unable to circulate blood properly. If left unchecked, this arrhythmia can cause death. Arrhythmia is the most frequent medical problem for children with congenital heart disease.[8]

Congestive Heart Failure **Congestive heart failure** (heart failure or cardiac failure) occurs when the heart is too weak to pump blood to the body. It is more common in women, particularly older women, and results from cumulative damage to the heart. The best treatment is prevention of further damage. However, as the heart loses its ability to pump blood throughout the system, it compensates by enlarging and then beating more rapidly. The heart works harder and more inefficiently. Medications, particularly ACE inhibitors, can prevent the onset of symptoms. Common symptoms include shortness of breath and labored breathing, and

edema (swelling that leaves a white mark when pressed) in later stages.

Endocarditis **Endocarditis** is a cardiac infection with symptoms of fever. This condition is a risk for all women with congenital heart disease and, particularly those with bicuspid aortic valve disease and **mitral valve prolapse (MPV).** Adolescents with congenital heart disease and women with undiagnosed MPV are typically at greater risk because of decreased compliance with antibiotic treatment.

Mitral valve prolapse Approximately 5 to 10 percent of all women have this apparently hereditary disorder. A prolapsed valve means that it is enlarged (floppy) and may not close securely as blood is pumped from the left atrium to the ventricle. MVP is usually not life-threatening but causes great anxiety for a woman who experiences the stabbing pain, dizziness, palpitations, and other symptoms that mimic a panic attack. All women with MVP should be under health-care supervision because of greater risk for bacterial endocarditis. They also should receive an antibiotic before any dental work is attempted.[9]

Silent ischemia With this condition the heart is deprived of oxygen but a woman may not know it. Sometimes this problem can be diagnosed with a stress test or ECG. Silent ischemia is most common in diabetics, particularly those who suffer from a sensory disturbance (not feeling body sensations). Medication or angioplasty may help alleviate the problem.[10]

Risk Factors

The primary unchangeable risk factors for heart disease in women include increasing age, race, postmenopausal status, and a family history of heart disease. (See *FYI:* "The Protective and Risk Factors for Cardiovascular Disease.") Changeable risk factors include smoking cigarettes, high blood pressure, high LDL or low HDL cholesterol levels, and lack of exercise. Contributing risk factors include high triglycerides, obesity, stress, and diabetes or glucose intolerance. Researchers, over the past five years, have begun to examine the difference between men and women regarding risk factors for heart disease. For example, low levels of HDL and high levels of blood lipid lipoprotein(s) are more predictive of heart disease in women than in men. According to

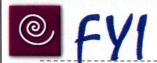

The Protective and Risk Factors for Cardiovascular Disease

Unchangeable Risk Factors
Family history
Race
Age
Postmenopausal status
Changeable Risk Factors
Cigarette smoking
High blood pressure
Sedentary lifestyle
High LDL level
Low HDL level
Contributing Factors
High triglycerides
Diabetes
Obesity
Stress
High sodium intake
Protective Factors
High HDL cholesterol
Regular exercise
Hormone replacement therapy
Low-fat diet
High total/HDL cholesterol ratio
Moderate alcohol consumption
Possible Protective Factors
Vitamin E
Aspirin
Foods high in beta-carotene

Association states that African American women aged 35 to 84 have 1.4 times the death rate from heart attack than white women.

Postmenopausal Status Women who experience premature menopause (before age 40) are at greater risk for heart disease. Estrogen protects a woman from heart disease by keeping total cholesterol levels low. Once estrogen levels drop (either from menopause or hysterectomy), a woman's risk of heart disease increases. In fact, after ten to fifteen years, a woman's risk is comparable to a man's risk of heart attack.

Changeable Risk Factors

Cigarette smoking As stated in chapter 9, cigarette smoking is decreasing in all groups except young teenage women. Smoking is a major cause of coronary heart disease and stroke in women. Smoking accounts for nearly 40 percent of all heart disease deaths and counteracts the benefits of estrogen. Research from the Nurses Health Study (see chap. 1) showed that risk for coronary heart disease was greatest for women who started smoking before age 15. Once a woman has stopped smoking, her risk for heart disease is reduced by one-third within two years and continues to decrease during the next ten to fourteen years to a level comparable to the nonsmokers.[12]

High Blood Pressure **Hypertension,** often called the silent killer, remains a major risk factor in heart attack, stroke, congestive heart failure, and kidney failure. Essential or primary hypertension, the most common type, has no known underlying cause. Although the causes of hypertension in 90 percent of

Dr. S. Ward Casscells, "We know the coronary death rate is falling faster for men than for women, and that may be due in part to a lack of recognition and treatment of these risk factors."[11]

Unchangeable Risk Factors

Increasing Age One in nine women between ages 45 and 64 and one in three women aged 65 and over have some form of cardiovascular risk. As you age, your risk for heart disease increases.

Family History Your chances of developing heart disease are increased if members of your family have heart disease.

Race African American women have a greater risk of heart disease than whites. The American Heart

congestive heart failure—circulatory congestion caused by heart damage that inhibits adequate blood flow to the body.

endocarditis (en doe car **die** tis)—defect in which the lining of the heart and heart valves become inflamed.

mitral valve prolapse (MVP)—one or both flaps of the mitral valve protrude into the left atrium during narrowing of the lower chamber.

hypertension—common disorder marked by high blood pressure.

the cases are not known, the contributing factors of uncontrolled hypertension are understood. Secondary hypertension, caused by an underlying disease and less common overall, is more common in women than men.

Hypertension occurs when the heart is forced to exert more pressure to pump blood through the arteries to the body, thus causing a rise in blood pressure. Blood pressure is measured with a sphygmomanometer. Using a rubber cuff to exert pressure on the arm, blood flow is temporarily stopped to the brachial artery and a stethoscope is used to listen for blood flow as it begins to flow through the brachial artery. **Systolic blood pressure** (numerator) is the amount of pressure the blood exerts against the arteries while the heart is contracting. **Diastolic blood pressure** (denominator) is the amount of pressure the blood exerts against the arteries while the heart is filling and resting between beats. Normal blood pressure is 120 mm Hg systolic or lower and 80 mm Hg diastolic or lower (120/80). High blood pressure in adults has been defined as blood pressure equal to or greater than 140 mm Hg systolic and/or 90 mm Hg diastolic and/or taking antihypertensive medication.[13] Systolic hypertension, a systolic reading over 160, is common in women, particularly the elderly.

Thirty million American women have high blood pressure. After age 65, 66 percent of all women and 83 percent of African American women suffer from hypertension. Hypertension develops earlier in life in African Americans and is usually more severe. More than one in every three African Americans over age 18 is estimated to have high blood pressure.[14] Nearly one-half of the women with hypertension are not on therapy and only 20 percent of treated women are on adequate therapy.

High blood pressure tends to run in families, but has no known cause and appears without symptoms. Other uncontrollable factors include age, race, and gender. Obesity, diabetes, and regular alcohol use increase the likelihood of having high blood pressure. A Mayo Clinic study found that women, ages 40 to 59, with high blood pressure can expect to encounter five times the normal rate of angina, heart attack, or sudden death. Losing weight, reducing sodium intake, exercise, and medications can act as protective factors. However, controlled hypertension by drug therapy remains a risk factor because it does not decrease the risk of CHD.

High Blood Cholesterol The message of high-fiber, low-fat, low-cholesterol, low-sodium eating habits may be circulating, but it still hasn't translated into improved eating patterns. A recent Gallup poll found that 90 percent of the women interviewed believed they ate a healthful diet, yet only 20 percent met the new dietary guidelines. Women may think they are reducing their risks of CHD by switching from animal fats (butter) to vegetable fats (margarine). However, the Nurses Health Study found that intake of trans-fatty acids, found in vegetable sources (particularly partially hydrogenated vegetables oils such as margarine, shortening, cookies, and white bread) definitely increased a woman's risk of CHD.[15] Saturated fats should be replaced with mono-unsaturated fats. Polyunsaturated fats reduce HDL levels and total cholesterol levels, whereas monounsaturated fats have less effect on reducing HDL levels and total cholesterol.

Cholesterol, a fatlike substance, enters the blood in two ways, through absorption in the small intestine of animal products we consume and the production in the liver from other dietary fats we eat.

Women have average blood cholesterol levels of approximately 215 mg/dL, but should be striving for LDL levels below 130 and HDL levels above 55. Because LDL is difficult to measure, the National Institutes of Health recommend that women know their total cholesterol/HDL ratio, for example 240/40 would be six to one or simply 6. A ratio below 3.5 is recommended, between 3.5 and 6.9 constitutes moderate risk, and over 7.0 is dangerous.

Younger women appear to have higher HDL than men, particularly during childbearing years. However, by age 55, women tend to have higher total cholesterol as well. Their protective advantage remains if the HDL stays high. Reducing cholesterol through diet, exercise, and stress reduction can slow the development of heart disease, and some studies even suggest that atherosclerosis can be reversed. (See *FYI:* "Different Screening for Women Recommended.")

Physical Inactivity Women who are inactive have twice the risk of heart disease. Exercise reduces triglycerides and enhances one's sense of well-being.

Contributing Factors

Diabetes The Nurses Health Study found that women with diabetes lose their protective factor for CHD. These women, when compared to women without diabetes, are significantly more at risk for CHD than men with diabetes compared to men without diabetes. In fact, diabetic women

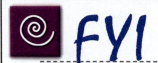

Different Screening for Women Recommended

A news release on February 14, 1996, by the University of Texas Health Science Center at Houston stated that they would immediately begin to screen women differently for heart disease. In addition to the traditional risk factors, they began to monitor lipoprotein a (LP(a)), fibrinogen, homocysteine, and serum magnesium levels. They stated that research shows high levels of LP(a) are more predictive of coronary disease in women than men. Fibrinogen, a clotting precursor, tends to be higher in women than men. High levels of homocysteine, a metabolite of the amino acid methionine, can decrease the production of clot-preventing and clot-dissolving substances. Research suggests that high levels of homocysteine are as predictive of coronary disease as high blood pressure, smoking, and high cholesterol. Magnesium decreases blood pressure, glucose intolerance, arrhythmias, and the risk of cardiac death. Lower levels of magnesium can be found in pregnant and postmenopausal women. Low levels of magnesium are associated with low levels of folic acid that normalizes homocysteine levels.[16]

have comparable levels of CHD to diabetic men. Diabetic women need to receive strong encouragement to maintain low body fat.

Obesity Estimates suggest that more than 50 percent of Hispanic and African American women and 35 percent of white women are overweight. Overweight is defined as body mass index (BMI) equal to or greater than 23.4 for females aged 12 to 14, 24.8 for females aged 15 to 17, 25.7 for females aged 18 to 19, and 27.3 for females over age 20. Although obesity, not overweight, is recognized as a risk factor for heart disease, overweight is a precursor to obesity. Obesity is recognized as a BMI over 30. The risk of chronic disease such as heart disease increases with an increase in BMI. The Nurses Health Study found that 40 percent of heart attacks in premenopausal women were related to obesity. Obesity and overweight can contribute to an increase in high cholesterol, hypertension, and diabetes. You can determine your body mass index by using the formula found in figure 8.6.

Stress The relationship between stress and coronary disease in women remains elusive. Although type A behavior has been linked to heart disease in men, there is no link between type A behavior in women and heart disease.[17] Studies show that women who hold in anger are more susceptible to heart attacks. The bleakest survival prognosis for women with CHD is for women who are divorced, work full time, lack a college education, and earn less than $20,000 a year. These women tend to suppress anger, resentment, and loneliness. However, women who work outside the home do not exhibit differing rates of heart disease when compared to women who do not work outside the home.

A 20-year follow-up of the Framingham data found that perceived financial status was a risk factor among employed women. Women who perceived themselves to have a lower financial status compared to their peers were at greater risk for heart disease. The risk factor for homemakers included symptoms of tension and anxiety, loneliness, difficulty sleeping, infrequent vacations, and perception of susceptibility to CHD. Women with low educational level, tension, and lack of vacations, regardless of employment status, were risk factors for both groups.[18]

Now complete *Assess Yourself:* "RISKO for Women" to determine your risk for heart disease.

Protective Factors Against Heart Disease

Protective factors against heart disease include estrogen, high HDL levels, moderate alcohol consumption, exercise, and dietary changes. These factors have been identified as reducing the risk of heart disease.

Estrogen The Nurses Health Study found that women on estrogen replacement therapy (ERT) reduced their risk of heart disease by nearly 50 percent. Estrogen enhances the cholesterol profile in women with total cholesterol lowered, HDL choles-

systolic blood pressure (sis **tol** ick)—amount of pressure the blood exerts against the arteries while the heart is contracting.

diastolic blood pressure (die **ah** sto lick)—amount of pressure the blood exerts against the arteries while the heart is relaxing.

Assess Y O U R S E L F

RISKO for Women

Add up your total number of points for each of the risk factors that follow. Then see what your score means below.

1. Systolic Blood Pressure

If you *are not* taking antihypertensive medications and your blood pressure is . . .

125 or less	0 points
between 126 and 136	2 points
between 137 and 148	4 points
between 149 and 160	6 points
between 161 and 171	8 points
between 172 and 183	10 points
between 184 and 194	12 points
between 195 and 206	14 points
between 207 and 218	16 points

If you *are* taking antihypertensive medications and your blood pressure is . . .

117 or less	0 points
between 118 and 123	2 points
between 124 and 129	4 points
between 130 and 136	6 points
between 137 and 144	8 points
between 145 and 154	10 points
between 155 and 168	12 points
between 169 and 206	14 points
between 207 and 218	16 points

Your points: _____

2. Blood Cholesterol

Locate the number of points for your total and HDL cholesterol in the table below.

		HDL							
		25	30	35	40	50	60	70	80
	140	2	1	0	0	0	0	0	0
	160	3	2	1	0	0	0	0	0
	180	4	3	2	1	0	0	0	0
Total	200	4	3	2	2	0	0	0	0
cholesterol	220	5	4	3	2	1	0	0	0
	240	5	4	3	3	1	0	0	0
	260	5	4	4	3	2	1	0	0
	280	5	5	4	4	2	1	0	0
	300	6	5	4	4	3	2	1	0
	340	6	5	5	4	3	2	1	0
	400	6	6	5	5	4	3	2	2

Your points: _____

3. Cigarette Smoking

If you . . .

do not smoke	0 points
smoke less than a pack a day	2 points
smoke a pack a day	5 points
smoke two or more packs a day	9 points

Your points: _____

4. Weight

Locate your weight category based on the table below.
Categories:

weight category A	0 points	weight category C	2 points
weight category B	1 point	weight category D	3 points

		CATEGORY			
FT	IN	A	B	C	D
4	8	up to 139	140–161	162–184	185+
4	9	up to 140	141–162	163–185	186+
4	10	up to 141	142–163	164–187	188+
4	11	up to 143	144–166	167–190	191+
5	0	up to 145	146–168	169–193	194+
5	1	up to 147	148–171	172–196	197+
5	2	up to 149	150–173	174–198	199+
5	3	up to 152	153–176	177–201	202+
5	4	up to 154	155–178	179–204	205+
5	5	up to 157	158–182	183–209	210+
5	6	up to 160	161–186	187–213	214+
5	7	up to 165	166–191	192–219	220+
5	8	up to 169	170–196	197–225	226+
5	9	up to 173	174–201	202–231	232+
5	10	up to 178	179–206	207–238	239+
5	11	up to 182	183–212	213–242	243+
6	0	up to 187	188–217	218–248	249+
6	1	up to 191	192–222	223–254	255+

Your points: _____

WHAT YOUR SCORE MEANS

Note: If you're diabetic, you have a greater risk of heart disease. Add 7 points to your total score.

0–2	You have a low risk of heart disease for a person of your age and sex.
3–4	You have a low-to-moderate risk of heart disease for a person of your age and sex. That's good, but there's room for improvement.
5–7	You have a moderate-to-high risk of heart disease for a person of your age and sex. There's considerable room for improvement in some areas.
8–15	You have a high risk of developing heart disease for a person of your age and sex. There's lots of room for improvement in all areas.
16 & Over	You have a very high risk of developing heart disease for a person of your age and sex. You should act now to reduce all your risk factors.

h e a l t h   t i p s

Choose Foods to Reduce Your Risk of Heart Disease

- Increase folic acid. Choose from green leafy vegetables, breads, seeds, and fortified products. This helps to normalize homocysteine levels.
- Increase B(6). Choose from green leafy vegetables, bananas, beans, animal sources, and potatoes. This helps to normalize homocysteine levels.
- Reduce body weight by decreasing caloric intake and use olive oil. This helps to lower fibrinogen levels.
- Increase intake of fruits and vegetables. This helps to lower LP(a) levels.
- Increase niacin. Choose foods high in protein (meat, fish, cheese), mushrooms, asparagus, leafy green vegetables, fortified grains, breads, and cereals. Niacin is water soluble so the vitamin will leach out if you cook them in water. This helps to lower LP(a) levels.
- Increase vitamin E levels. Wheat germ, corn and soybean oil, nuts and seeds, green leafy vegetables,

and fortified cereals are good sources. Vitamin E is fat-soluble so it can be destroyed by heat. Don't fry these foods; just lightly drip oil onto foods.
- Increase magnesium levels. Magnesium levels are closely associated with folic acid levels. Foods high in magnesium include dark green leafy vegetables, nuts, legumes, and seafood.
- Reduce saturated fats to less than 10 percent of total calories. Found mainly in animal products, limit your intake of whole milk dairy products like butter, cheese, milk, and ice cream, meat and poultry skin, and coconut and palm oil.
- Reduce your cholesterol intake to less than 300 mg each day. Cholesterol is found only in animal products. This helps to lower cholesterol levels.

---

terol elevated, and LDL cholesterol lowered. Estrogen also seems to relax the coronary arteries, thus reducing the likelihood of spasm and high blood pressure. ERT is contraindicated for women with a family history of breast cancer or endometrial cancer.

Most hormone replacement therapy today includes the use of progestin to reduce the risk of breast and uterine cancer. The impact of this combination therapy on heart disease is still unknown. Wyeth Labs began the HERS Study (Heart and Estrogen/Progestin Replacement Study) in January 1993 to determine the effects of hormone replacement therapy on women who already have heart disease. This randomized study will answer some of the questions regarding the benefits and risks of HRT. However, the focus of this study is secondary prevention, so the cost/benefit of HRT as primary prevention will remain unanswered until further randomized tests are conducted.

Diet During the next decade, the Women's Health Study will be evaluating the effect of beta-carotene, vitamin E, and other antioxidants as protective factors for CHD. The effect of these nutrients on the slowing of atherosclerosis will determine their contribution to reducing the risk of stroke and heart attacks. (See *Health Tips:* "Choose Foods to Reduce Your Risk of Heart Disease.") The Nurses Health Study found that women with the highest intake of vitamin E (at least 100 IU for two or more years) had a lower risk of

heart disease. Women who took vitamin E supplements for two years reduced their risk of heart disease, whereas those who took supplements for a shorter length of time were not found to reduce their risk significantly. Researchers suggested that vitamin E may prevent the oxidation of LDL cholesterol, thus reducing the development of atherosclerosis.[19]

Alcohol Consumption Women who consume alcohol appear to reduce their risk of ischemic heart disease by approximately 20 percent when compared to abstainers. Women who moderately consume alcohol (defined as one-half to two drinks daily, but never more than two drinks) decreased their risk of heart disease by 36 to 39 percent compared to abstainers.[20]

Exercise The positive effects of exercise include increases in HDL cholesterol levels, reduction in blood pressure, and caloric consumption.[21] Women who have an HDL cholesterol level greater than 60 have an added protective factor for CHD.

Aspirin The Nurses Health Study found that women who took one to six aspirins per week had a 30 percent lower risk of heart disease.[22] The use of aspirin is supported by health-care providers for women to control unstable angina and to reduce the risk of a second heart attack.

Viewpoint

Gender Bias in Diagnosis and Treatment

Studies have found conflicting results regarding the effect of gender bias on the diagnosis and treatment of heart disease. Some studies showed that women received fewer diagnostic tests for heart disease, fewer referrals for exercise rehabilitation, had a greater risk of death, cardiac distress, and reinfarction within one year of MI, and had treatment withheld or delayed.[23,24] Others found no bias in referral for cardiac catheterization and suggested that differential treatment resulted because women delayed medical care, were older, and had more complications at the time of diagnosis.[25,26] A review of current strategies for angioplasty and coronary artery bypass surgery suggested that the research remains ambiguous regarding gender bias in treatment and stressed the need for future randomized tests.[27]

Many family physicians are unaware that diagnostic tests to determine heart disease differ for men and women. The most effective diagnostic tool for men is the treadmill test but women need the treadmill combined with an echocardiogram or nuclear imaging. Do you think a gender bias exists?

health tips

Warning Signs of Stroke

- Sudden weakness or numbness on one side of the body, usually the face, arm, or leg
- Sudden blurred or dimness in vision, often on one side
- Loss of speech or difficulty comprehending speech
- Sudden and severe headaches with no known cause
- Dizziness and lack of balance, with possibility of sudden, unexplained falls
- Recurring TIAs or mini-strokes that last several minutes

Screening and Diagnosis

Women who suspect they have heart disease should be assertive in getting a proper diagnosis. Many of the traditional tests used for screening for heart disease were developed for men. For example, women often have false positive results from the traditional stress test, which is a treadmill test. Women can receive better results from a stress-echocardiogram. A stress-echocardiogram is a noninvasive technique using a treadmill test and ultrasound pictures of the heart. The ultrasound pictures allow the cardiologist to view the heart muscle contractions at peak exercise. Other advantages of the stress-echocardiogram are its lower cost and better diagnostic results. (See the *Viewpoint:* "Gender Bias in Diagnosis and Treatment.")

STROKE

Stroke is the third leading cause of death in women and the leading cause of adult disability, yet few women know the warning signs. (See *Health Tips:* "Warning Signs of Stroke.") More than 88,000

women die every year of stroke and African American women have an 83 percent higher death rate from stroke than white women.

Stroke is a form of vascular disease with many causes and levels of severity. An artery carrying **oxygen-rich** blood to the brain may suddenly become clogged or burst, preventing blood flow to the brain. The two primary types of stroke include hemorrhagic and ischemic stroke. Hemorrhagic strokes are further subdivided into subarachnoid or intracerebral stroke, depending on the location in the brain of the burst blood vessel. Hemorrhagic strokes, about 20 percent of all strokes, are more common in young women, and 67 percent of all subarachnoid strokes occur in women. Ischemic stroke, which is about 80 percent of all strokes and is more common in older women, occurs when a blood vessel is blocked and oxygen is prevented from flowing to the brain. Ischemic stroke results from an embolism, large artery thrombosis, or small penetrating artery thrombosis.[28] (See Fig. 19.4.)

Risk Factors for Stroke

The risk factors for stroke include those that cannot be changed, those that can be reduced with medical treatment, and those that can be reduced with lifestyle changes. The risk factors that cannot be altered include: age (older women are at increased risk), race (African American and Hispanic women are at increased risk), heredity, diabetes, and the experience of a prior stroke.

The risk factors that can be altered with medical treatment include hypertension, heart disease, and transient ischemic attacks (TIAs). These factors can

FIGURE 19.4 Causes of stroke.

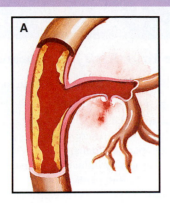

Hemorrhage
The sudden bursting
of a blood vessel.

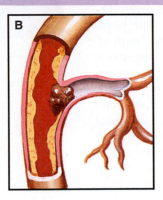

Embolus
A clot that moves through
the circulatory system
and becomes lodged at
a narrowed point within
a vessel.

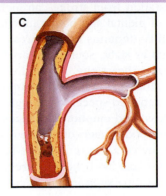

Thrombus
A clot that forms within
a narrowed section of a
blood vessel and remains
at its place of origin.

be altered with small doses of aspirin. Another risk factor that can be altered with medical treatment is atrial fibrillation, or irregular heartbeat. Atrial fibrillation increases the risk of a blood clot breaking free and moving to the brain. Recent research suggests that blood thinners can dramatically reduce the risk of stroke from atrial fibrillation by reducing potential clotting.

The risk factors that can be modified with lifestyle changes include reducing blood cholesterol and lipids, quitting cigarette smoking, limiting alcohol intake to no more than two drinks a day, exercising regularly, practicing relaxation techniques, and maintaining a desirable weight.

Two studies may be of particular interest regarding risk factors in women. The first study found that hormone replacement therapy was associated with a decrease in risk of stroke incidence and mortality.[29] The second study found a significant dose-response relationship between daily cigarette consumption and ischemic stroke. Women who smoked more cigarettes and for more years had a greater risk of stroke. Women who stopped smoking, regardless of their age at starting smoking or the number of cigarettes smoked, experienced significant reduction in stroke risk within two to four years.[30]

Treatment

Whenever a warning signal occurs, a woman should consult her health-care provider. Knowing the warn-

ing signs is important because new drugs can break up clots and limit damage to the brain if administered promptly. Treatment approaches differ depending on the type of stroke a woman experiences. Health-care providers find it far easier to predict survival than functional outcome. Level of consciousness is the best predictor of short-term survival, whereas recovery during the first thirty to sixty days predicts potential functional outcome.

A new procedure, carotid endarterectomy, has prevented thousands of strokes. This surgery removes fatty buildup (atherosclerosis) in the carotid arteries (blood vessels in the neck that supply oxygen to the brain). This procedure was shown to benefit men who suffered strokes or showed symptoms, but women did not benefit equally. A study of 1,662 men and women aged 40 to 79 with 60 percent or more blockage found that men experienced a 69 percent reduction in risk, whereas women showed only a 16 percent change.[31] The reason for this discrepancy is unknown, and further research is needed to elucidate the gender differences.

stroke—a vascular disease caused when a blood vessel bursts or becomes clogged in the brain; a brain attack.

Disability from Stroke

The devastation from stroke can include severe impairment of mental and bodily functions. The physical disability depends on the area of the brain affected such as sight, sound, motor skills, autonomic body systems (heart rate, respiration, body temperature), or language. Physical changes (permanent paralysis, impaired speech or thought processes, and memory loss) and emotional changes (loss of sexual desire, poor body image, depression) are common.

The rehabilitation of a stroke patient begins as soon as possible with health-care staff and family members offering support and encouragement. Over 70 percent of all stroke patients regain independent living, and nearly 33 percent return to work. The key to helping a woman recover from a stroke is access to rehabilitation. If she has private insurance to cover the cost of rehabilitation, her prognosis for recovery is better. Many elderly women rely on Medicare for insurance, either being too poor to purchase additional insurance or losing the private insurance when a spouse dies.

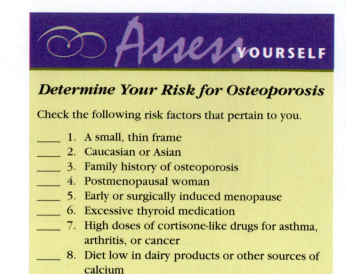

Assess YOURSELF

Determine Your Risk for Osteoporosis

Check the following risk factors that pertain to you.

_____ 1. A small, thin frame
_____ 2. Caucasian or Asian
_____ 3. Family history of osteoporosis
_____ 4. Postmenopausal woman
_____ 5. Early or surgically induced menopause
_____ 6. Excessive thyroid medication
_____ 7. High doses of cortisone-like drugs for asthma, arthritis, or cancer
_____ 8. Diet low in dairy products or other sources of calcium
_____ 9. Sedentary lifestyle
_____10. Cigarette smoker
_____11. Excessive alcohol intake

The more items you have checked, the greater your risk for developing osteoporosis. What can you do to increase your protective factors and reduce your risks?

OSTEOPOROSIS

Osteoporosis (porous bone), a bone-weakening disorder, results in bone mineral loss and increases the risk of skeletal frailty and fracturing. Although perceived as a disease of old age, osteoporosis starts in childhood. It has been described as a "pediatric disease with a geriatric outcome."[32] Genetics, diet, and exercise play a major role in determining peak bone mass, an indicator of future bone density. Primary prevention focuses on increasing peak bone mass, reached between the ages of 30 and 35 years, and reducing bone loss in later life. The greatest loss in bone density occurs in women during the first five years after menopause, but continues for eight to ten years before leveling to approximately 1 percent a year.

Osteoporosis affects approximately 25 million Americans, predominately women. Age is the predominant risk factor for osteoporosis. An estimated 50 percent of women over age 45, and 90 percent of women over age 75 have osteoporosis.[33] Half of these women may experience a fracture related to osteoporosis, nearly 1.3 million fractures a year.[34] The average age for a hip fracture is 80 years. Because 25 percent of hip fracture patients die within

one year, 15 to 25 percent remain in long-term care for at least one year, and half never walk independently again.[35,36]

Heredity also influences the risk of osteoporosis. Common genetic differences have been found to account for 7 to 10 percent of the difference in bone density, particularly at the hip and spine.

Young women who are at increased risk for osteoporosis include highly trained female athletes with amenorrhea and those suffering from anorexia and bulimia nervosa. (Refer to chapter 7 for a discussion of anorexia and bulimia nervosa.) Complete *Assess Yourself:* "Determine Your Risk for Osteoporosis."

Protective Factors Against Osteoporosis

Exercise Exercise, particularly weight-bearing activities, acts as a protective factor against bone loss and fracture. Weight-bearing activities such as running, brisk walking, hiking, weight lifting, and aerobics increase bone mineral density. Swimming, biking, and other weight-supported activities have less benefit. The greatest increase in density occurs at the site of maximum stress and repetition.[37] For instance, a tennis player's dominant arm is considerably larger than her nonplaying arm. Exercise provides the added benefit of muscle strength, tone, and balance, all important factors in reducing the likelihood of falls and fractures in older women.

Diet Calcium and vitamin D are two major nutrients needed to prevent osteoporosis. Studies have found that peak bone mass can be increased by drinking milk during childhood and adolescence and increasing calcium intake beyond the current RDA standards.

Calcium plays a variety of roles in body functioning besides increasing bone density. When blood levels of calcium drop, the heart, muscles, and nerves deplete the calcium from bones to function properly. Vitamin D, essential for building bone, must be present for calcium to be adequately absorbed through the small intestine. Vitamin D is synthesized by skin exposed to sunlight, and with increased age, the skin seems to lose the ability to produce adequate amounts of vitamin D. Thus, milk and vitamin supplements are important sources of vitamin D in later years.

Hormone Replacement Therapy The loss of estrogen during menopause contributes to loss in bone mass. Estrogen has been approved for preventing osteoporosis, with studies finding that estrogen reduces hip-fracture rates. Estrogen improves calcium absorption and reduces calcium lost in the urine. When a woman stops taking estrogen, she eventually reaches the level of bone loss of those who never took estrogen.

Risk Factors for Osteoporosis

Hypogonadism Hypogonadism is a secondary characteristic occurring with excessive exercise, or anorexia and bulimia nervosa. Exercise can be a risk factor for competitive female athletes, particularly distance runners, gymnasts, and dancers. These athletes commonly experience exercise-induced amenorrhea due to intense training regimens and extreme restricted caloric intake. Although the exact cause of amenorrhea is unknown, reduced body fat appears to be a major factor. These athletes, whether young girls or mature women, experience a reduction in bone density despite intense weight-bearing activity. The effects of short-term amenorrhea seem to be reversible; however, research has not determined the impact of long-term amenorrhea (two to three years)

on future bone density. If bone density loss is irreversible, the likelihood of osteoporosis would increase.[38]

Exercise-induced amenorrhea is not a minor problem. Any female athlete who experiences more than six months of amenorrhea should be evaluated for loss of bone density, and strongly encouraged to reduce training to a level at which menstruation occurs.[39] Health-care providers may prescribe oral contraceptives to induce menstruation and increase estrogen levels.

Anorexia and bulimia nervosa can also contribute to rapid bone loss and fracture. Estrogen deficiency, malnutrition, and glucocorticoid excess may be experienced in these conditions. One study found that calcium supplementation, resumed menstrual function, and exercise did not significantly restore skeletal mass within two years.[40] However, longitudinal studies suggest that bone mass may return within a longer time frame. Women who have exercise induced amenorrhea or anorexia nervosa should be encouraged to gain weight to a level at which menstruation occurs naturally. Oral contraceptives can be prescribed for estrogen deficiency but are ineffective until weight gain and full endocrine function are restored.[41]

Smoking and Excessive Alcohol Intake Smoking affects the processing of vitamin D and reduces the calcium absorption necessary for maintaining bone density. One study found that bone density in men and women over age 60 varied directly with the number of cigarettes smoked. Women were especially impacted by the number of cigarettes they smoked.[42] Thus, quitting smoking at any age may reduce bone loss.

Studies related to excessive alcohol consumption, more than three drinks a day, and bone loss were mixed. Some studies suggested that excessive drinking interfered with calcium and vitamin D absorption, and others found no relationship between alcohol intake and osteoporosis. (See the *FYI:* "Protective and Risk Factors for Osteoporosis" for a summary of such factors.)

---

osteoporosis—a bone-weakening disorder in which normal bone density is lost and is marked by thinning of bone tissue and growth of small holes in bone.

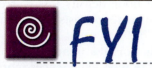

FYI *Protective and Risk Factors for Osteoporosis*

Unchangeable Risk Factors
Female gender
Advanced age
Early menopause
Heredity
Thin body type
Changeable Risk Factors
Hypogonadism (secondary to exercise-induced amenorrhea or anorexia or bulimia nervosa)
Cigarette smoking
Excessive alcohol intake

Protective Factors
Calcium
Vitamin D
Weight-bearing exercise
Hormone replacement therapy

Measuring Bone Density

The bone density of female athletes, women with eating disorders, women 60–70 years of age with fracture experience, and peri-menopausal women debating about HRT should be assessed. Densitometry, measuring bone density, determines a woman's risk for osteoporosis.

DIABETES MELLITUS

Insulin-Dependent Diabetes Mellitus (IDDM)

Insulin-dependent diabetes mellitus (IDDM) is now called Type 1 diabetes, and in the past was referred to as juvenile diabetes because it occurred primarily in young children and adolescents. Type 1 diabetes accounts for one in ten of all types of diabetes, or approximately 300,000 cases. It is known as insulin-dependent because the pancreas either stops producing insulin or makes too little for the body to convert glucose to energy.

Because the body cannot convert glucose, the level of sugar in the blood stream rises to dangerous levels. The only way to lower the level of blood sugar is to inject insulin under the skin.

The cause of Type 1 diabetes is unknown, however, heredity and environment seem to play a role. Type 1 diabetes can be triggered by an autoimmune response to a variety of viruses (much like arthritis, multiple sclerosis, etc.). Some studies have linked it with a defect in the immune system that triggers the body to destroy its own insulin-producing cells. Type 1 diabetes is treated by daily insulin injections, exercise, and a diet low in sugar intake.

Non-Insulin-Dependent Diabetes Mellitus (NIDDM)

Non-insulin-dependent diabetes mellitus (NIDDM) is now referred to as Type 2 diabetes, or adult-onset diabetes. Risk factors for women include being over age 40, being overweight, having a family member with diabetes, giving birth to a baby over 9 pounds, having frequent miscarriages, and race (African American, Hispanic, or Native American). African American women have 50 percent more risk than white women for developing Type 2 diabetes. As stated earlier, African American women are at greater risk for obesity, which seems to be the primary factor for the increased risk of Type 2 diabetes.[43] In addition, some studies found that women who smoke have a higher risk of developing Type 2 diabetes than women who never smoked or quit smoking. And, the risk of Type 2 diabetes appears to be dose-related: the more cigarettes she smokes, the greater her risk.[44] (See *Health Tips:* "Warning Signs of Diabetes.")

Of all diabetics 90 percent have Type 2 diabetes, a condition in which the body either produces too little insulin or cannot use insulin properly. Blood sugar increases in the blood stream and causes complications. Type 2 diabetes can be prevented by avoiding obesity and staying physically active throughout life. Women with Type 2 diabetes should

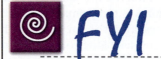

A New Drug for Type 2 Diabetics?

The FDA has recommended approval for the drug Rezulin for treating the underlying cause of Type 2 diabetes, the gradual loss of natural insulin's ability to work. Rezulin is believed to work by resensitizing the body to insulin. Those persons who are unable to control the production of insulin through diet, exercise, and other medications may be considered for Rezulin treatment. A preliminary study funded by Parke Davis, the pharmaceutical company that produces Rezulin, found that 58 percent of participants reduced their daily insulin dose and 15 percent stopped taking insulin altogether. Further research and study are needed into this promising approach to treating Type 2 diabetes.

reduce weight and maintain a healthy diet. Sometimes, women can use these measures alone to control it, whereas other women will need medication or insulin shots. (See *FYI:* "A New Drug for Type 2 Diabetics?")

Gestational Diabetes

Gestational diabetes occurs in 3 to 5 percent of all pregnancies, about 100,000 cases each year. The definition of gestational diabetes is controversial. Pregnant women with high blood glucose levels during pregnancy who had no previous signs of diabetes are said to have gestational diabetes. It is recognized by carbohydrate intolerance with an onset or first recognition during pregnancy. Some health experts believe all women should be screened between weeks 24 and 48, whereas others would screen only pregnant women over age 30. Perinatal mortality of women with gestational diabetes is similar to that of nondiabetic women. Yet, these women often choose to deliver by 40 weeks because they fear macrosomia (fat babies) and fetal distress (particularly broken shoulders). Recent studies suggest that women with gestational diabetes can go past term if rigorous testing and monitoring is conducted during the term. These women must comply with the instructions given by the health-care provider.

Many women who experience gestational diabetes will experience a return to normal blood sugar levels after the pregnancy. However, studies show that they remain more susceptible to gestational diabetes in future pregnancies and Type 2 diabetes, thus they should be strongly encouraged to maintain a healthy diet and exercise frequently.

EPILEPSY

Epilepsy, a chronic brain disorder characterized by recurrent seizures, affects 1 to 3 percent of the population. Epilepsy is a general term for more than twenty different types of seizure disorders and occurs when a brief, temporary increase in electrical energy passes between cells. The sudden overload may effect a small part of the brain, or the whole

insulin-dependent diabetes mellitus (IDDM)—now called Type 1 diabetes, the body cannot convert glucose so injections of insulin are necessary.

non-insulin dependent diabetes mellitus (NIDDM)—now referred to as Type 2 diabetes, a condition in which the body produces too little or cannot use insulin properly.

epilepsy—a group of nervous system disorders caused by uncontrolled electrical discharge from nerve cells of the surface of the brain marked by recurrent seizures.

system. (See *Health Tips:* "First Aid for Seizures.") Initially, controlling the seizures is the primary concern of health-care providers and the person with epilepsy. However, it doesn't take long to realize that the social stigma connected with epilepsy is often more difficult to overcome.

Psychosocial and Economic Considerations

The person with epilepsy and her caregiver (if dealing with a child) may know a lot about the illness, including what seizures are, what to do when one occurs, what medications do, how they should be taken, and their potential side effects. But what about the psychosocial, legal, and economic aspects of epilepsy? How are these addressed? Many questions arise such as: Should I tell my instructors? Is it safe to drive a car? Can I drink alcohol? What will my friends think, how will they act? Is it safe to get pregnant?[45]

Educating the person with epilepsy and her caregiver is important, but so is educating the public. Education is the only way to reduce or eliminate the stigma associated with epilepsy. Employers, family, and friends of persons with epilepsy need to educate themselves about the disorder.

Over 70 percent of persons with epilepsy achieve good control through drug therapy. The choice of drug therapy for each woman must be individualized, and new drugs are continually being researched and marketed. Unfortunately, these drugs sometimes have unwanted side effects.

Pregnancy and Antiseizure Drugs

A woman with epilepsy has an increased risk of delivering a baby with birth defects, but researchers have not determined whether the risks result from medications or genetic influences. Studies regarding antiseizure drugs during pregnancy have produced conflicting results. Some studies found that women taking antiseizure drugs had a 15 percent increased risk of having a baby with birth defects. Other studies found that the type of medication determined the risk, with some drugs showing only 1 to 2 percent increased risk factors. Adverse outcomes may include prematurity, increased risk of epilepsy in the child, and fetal malformations.[46]

No anticonvulsant or neuroleptic is without risk when used during pregnancy. Yet, the risk of birth defects from medication is greatly outweighed by the risk to the fetus of uncontrolled seizures. The oxygen supply can be cut off to the fetus causing serious damage if a pregnant woman suffers a grand mal seizure. A woman with a history of epilepsy should continue medication during pregnancy under the supervision of her health-care provider.

ARTHRITIS

Arthritis is an inflammatory condition of the joints, characterized by swelling, pain, and/or difficulty moving that persists for more than two weeks. (See *Health Tips:* "SERIOUS.") Over a hundred types of arthritis and related diseases (known as rheumatic diseases) have been classified, with consequences ranging from mild to debilitating. The variety of arthritis and related diseases that women often

---

health tips

First Aid for Seizures

What to Do:
- Look for medical identification.

- Loosen collars and ties.

- Protect the head from injury.

- Protect the person from nearby hazards.

- Turn person on side to keep airway clear.

- Call for aid.

What Not to Do:
- Do not place anything in the mouth. (The tongue cannot be swallowed.)

- Do not provide any liquids during or immediately after the seizure.

- Do not give artificial respiration.

- Do not restrain the person.

---

health tips

SERIOUS: The Warning Signs of Arthritis

Swelling in one or more joints

Early morning stiffness

Recurring pain or tenderness in any joint

Inability to move a joint normally

Obvious redness and warmth in a joint

Unexplained weight loss, fever, or weakness combined with joint pain

Symptoms like these persisting for more than two weeks

encounter include carpal tunnel syndrome, gout, Marfan syndrome, scleroderma, and fibrositis. If you experience arthritis, you need to know which type because treatment protocols vary.

Arthritis affects approximately 43 million U.S. women and rates are similar in African American women and white women, but lower in Hispanic women.[47] Arthritis is a leading cause of work-related disability with nearly one-half of persons aged 65 and over reporting some degree of arthritis. The estimated prevalence of arthritis has risen over the past ten years, along with reported activity limitation at increasing ages.

Treatment can include rest, relaxation, exercise, the use of heat or cold, medications, and surgery. Many traditional or alternative therapies exist that can be beneficial to a person suffering from arthritis, but as a consumer, you need to be informed and watch carefully for quackery.

Osteoarthritis

Osteoarthritis occurs when tissues that allow joints to move smoothly break down from overuse or some other cause. It is the most common kind of arthritis and affects the weight-bearing joints, particularly the knees, hips, and ankles, but it can also affect the hands.

Rheumatoid Arthritis

Rheumatoid arthritis is an autoimmune, chronic inflammatory disease of unknown cause. Some scientists speculate that a slow bacterial infection may be implicated. It affects three times more women than men and is most prevalent in postmenopausal women. Symptoms often begin in women between the ages of 30 and 50. If left untreated, joint destruction can occur quickly, often affecting finger joints first. They become swollen and inflamed, and this condition lasts for an extended period of time. A pattern of flare-ups and remissions begins, and, eventually, the cartilage between the joints disappears and bone-to-bone irritation and pain ensues.

Treatment The treatment approach to RA has changed dramatically over the past several years. The traditional pyramid approach to treatment involved a first-line therapy, consisting of nonsteroidal anti-inflammatory drugs, bed rest, and physical therapy. As joint pain increased, second-line therapy was added. This approach has been replaced by an ear-

lier, more aggressive intervention. Health-care providers now begin treatment efforts aimed at preventing early joint injury. Second-line therapy, using a variety of drugs, begins at the first sign of clinical or functional deterioration.[48] In addition to drug therapy, treatments such as ultrasound, exercise in warm water, and applications of heat may be used.

The medications used for first- and second-line therapies have remained the same for some time. The change in treatment has been the accelerated intervention. New breakthroughs in research during the past several years hold promise for an eventual cure. Scientists are currently studying the effect of immune responses in maternal-fetal relationships (pregnant women often experience remission of RA) and gene therapy to treat and understand arthritis.

Systemic Lupus Erythematosus (SLE)

Systemic **lupus** erythematosus is a chronic, autoimmune disease that causes inflammation and affects the vital organs, especially the skin, kidneys, heart, lungs, brain, and CNS. One of the three types of lupus, it is the most common and is recognized by the red, butterfly rash found across the bridge of the nose. Lupus is not infectious or rare. A 1994 research study showed that between 1.4 and 2 million people, or 1 in every 185 Americans, were diagnosed with lupus.

SLE afflicts primarily women of childbearing age, and nearly 50,000 new cases are diagnosed each year. Women of African American, Native American, and Asian origin are believed to be at greater risk for developing SLE although the research is inconclusive. The cause is unknown; however, genetic and environmental factors have been implicated in this autoimmune disease.

Signs and symptoms The most commonly reported symptoms of SLE are found in *FYI:* "The Most Common Symptoms of Lupus." The pattern of remission and flare-ups is common and can be fatal if left

---

arthritis—an inflammatory condition of the joints characterized by pain and swelling.

lupus—systemic lupus erythematosus is a chronic, autoimmune disease that causes inflammation and affects vital organs.

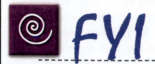

The Most Common Symptoms of Lupus

- Achy joints (arthralgia)
- Fever over 100° F
- Prolonged or extreme fatigue
- Arthritis (swollen joints)
- Skin rashes
- Anemia
- Kidney involvement
- Pain in the chest on deep breathing (pleurisy)
- Butterfly-shaped rash across the cheeks and nose
- Sun or light sensitivity (photosensitivity)

untreated. Flare-ups are often precipitated by exposure to sunlight, an infection, or a drug reaction.

Diagnosis and Treatment The immunofluorescent antinuclear antibody (ANA) test is a screening test for the presence of autoantibodies and is used to diagnose SLE. Determining whether a woman has SLE depends on the results of the ANA test and a minimum of four supporting symptoms. With fewer symptoms, additional laboratory tests will be conducted to diagnose SLE.

Treatment for SLE is similar to arthritis and the prognosis for women who follow treatment protocol is excellent. Preventive measures are equally important, including avoidance of excessive sun exposure, use of sunscreens, regular exercise, stress management, no smoking, limited or no alcohol consumption, proper use of prescribed medications, and maintaining proper nutrition. Nearly 80 to 90 percent of women with SLE can expect to live a normal lifespan.

MULTIPLE SCLEROSIS

Multiple sclerosis is a progressive, debilitating disease of the central nervous system. It is characterized by the loss of myelin, a fat protein substance that surrounds nerve fibers in the brain, spinal cord, and optic nerve, and enhances conduction of nerve impulses. Although the cause remains unknown, scientists speculate that the autoimmune system is in-

volved in the demyelation of nerve cells and MS may be triggered by a number of factors including viral infections, allergic reactions, nutritional deficiencies, or toxins. No association between trauma and MS has been found through research, although many people still believe trauma causes onset or exacerbates MS.

Multiple sclerosis affects primarily young white adults, often between the ages of 30 and 40. Women comprise 60 percent of all MS cases. Many ethnic groups, such as African Americans, Eskimos, and Asians, seldom if ever develop MS. Studies have demonstrated high rates among identical twins and increased incidence in temperate climates zones.

Signs and Symptoms

The most common symptoms of MS are gait disturbances and loss of sensation and vision. Symptoms may include fatigue, headaches, memory loss, numbness of body parts, and falling or tripping. Overall, diagnosing MS by the presenting symptoms is difficult. Many women endure years of tests before an accurate diagnosis is made.

Diagnosis and Treatment

The diagnosis of MS is primarily determined by clinical evidence (the presence of a lesion or multiple lesions in the white matter of the brain) and symptoms that occur on several occasions. Magnetic resonance imaging (MRI) has facilitated earlier diagnosis, but nearly 50 percent of all cases need further diagnostic tests to confirm MS.

There is no cure for MS, a disease with a relapsing and remitting course. In 1993, the FDA approved the use of Betaseron for the treatment of relapsing/remitting MS. The drug was distributed directly from the manufacturer, Berlex Laboratories, to patients through the local pharmacists (an unprecedented procedure designed to keep costs low). Because quantities were limited initially, individuals interested in receiving the drug participated in a national lottery to determine access. A month's supply of Betaseron costs approximately $1,000 and by the end of 1995, nearly 100,000 persons were receiving treatment. Berlex provides a sliding fee scale for those individuals who are uninsured.

Research efforts focus on cell biology, immunology, and virology. Each research avenue provides hope for arresting further disease progression and providing an eventual cure.

ALZHEIMER'S DISEASE

Alzheimer's disease (AD), the most common dementia, is characterized by confusion, memory failure, behavioral disturbances, progressive deterioration with plateaus, and eventually death (often from bronchopneumonia). There are no specific tests for AD, and the only definitive confirmation is at autopsy. The AD diagnosis is made from the clinical history and assessment of cognitive function. The primary feature is sufficient cognitive impairment that daily functioning becomes impossible. One in twenty-six persons between ages 65 and 76 have AD, and nearly one in two persons over age 85.

The causes of AD are unknown. Some researchers suggest AD is related to a genetic component and point to apoE4 genes that failed to bind to specific proteins. Others dispute this finding and suggest that other proteins are converted into insoluble senile plaque.[49] Others suggest that multiple processes, in various combinations, lead to AD.

Signs and Symptoms

A key component of AD is memory loss, exhibited by forgetfulness. Actions such as missed appointments, unreturned telephone calls, trouble finding the right word, and difficulty understanding conversation may be signs to watch. Failing to recognize people, getting lost while alone, relinquishing important responsibilities (such as paying the bills), or reducing social circles may also be signs. The Alzheimer's Disease Association provides a list of ten warning signs to recognize AD (see *Health Tips:* "Ten Warning Signs to Recognize AD").

▶ h e a l t h   t i p s

Ten Warning Signs to Recognize AD

- Recent memory loss that affects job performance.
- Difficulty performing familiar tasks.
- Problems with language such as forgetting simple words or using words inappropriately.
- Time and space disorientation.
- Poor judgment.
- Problems with abstract thinking.
- Misplacing items.
- Changes in mood or behavior. Rapid mood swings.
- Changes in personality.
- Loss of initiative.

Risk and Protective Factors

A large study at USC found that women who had used estrogen replacement therapy were 40 percent less likely to have AD than women who died of other causes. However, some researchers cautioned that the increased prevalence of AD in women may be due to factors other than decreased estrogen after menopause.

Reports on aluminum as a cause of AD have not been confirmed. Results suggest that high levels of aluminum in the brains of persons with AD may be a marker rather than a cause. And, studies using more sensitive equipment have failed to replicate initial studies of aluminum and AD.

Treatment

Alzheimer's disease has no cure, so drug therapy consists of managing the symptoms including AD-related depression, sleep/wake cycle alterations, and aggressive behaviors. Tacrine (Cognex) was the first drug approved by the FDA for AD and has been somewhat effective in delaying AD symptoms in individuals with mild to moderate cognitive deficits. A second drug, recently approved by the FDA, is donepezil (Aricept). It is said to have fewer side effects and offers women the choice of taking one pill a day, as opposed to four Cognex tablets daily. Both drugs ease the symptoms but neither slows the progression of AD.

Nondrug therapies include providing the AD patient with a stable and familiar environment. Often, the family attempts to provide a supportive environment during the mild to moderate stages of AD. The person with AD should be encouraged to function independently, and the daily routine should become familiar. A consistent schedule for daily activities reduces agitation and safety can be enhanced by placing locks on doors.

Nursing homes that accept persons with AD often provide alarms and codes to secure doors, visual pictures for communicating and stimulating memory, and measures to prevent wandering.[50] Col-

---

multiple sclerosis—a disease of the central nervous system characterized by loss of the protective myelin covering of the nerve fibers.

Alzheimer's disease—a form of brain disease characterized by dementia.

lecting and sharing personal items helps to stimulate the memory of persons with AD.

Role of Caregiver

AD seriously impacts caregivers as well as persons with AD. Caregivers suffer from anxiety, depression, and anger. They can receive needed assistance by joining a support group. These support groups offer emotional support and current information about additional home health services, the behavior of persons with AD, and help in nursing-home placement. Recent studies suggest that a person with AD can stay home nearly a year longer if caregivers have a support system that offers emotional and informational support. Most urban areas provide support groups for caregivers and the national office of the

> ### JOURNAL ACTIVITY
>
> #### Your Family Tree and Chronic Disease
>
> Now that you have finished this chapter, create a family tree that includes siblings, parents, grandparents, and great-grandparents. Under each name, include the diseases or conditions that each person has or had. Select one disease or condition and write all the protective factors that you can practice to reduce your risk of contracting this disease.

Alzheimer's Association provides information regarding the location of your local chapter. Now complete *Journal Activity:* "Your Family Tree and Chronic Disease."

Chapter Summary

- More women die from cardiovascular disease than any other disease.
- African American women are at greater risk than white women for coronary artery disease.
- Atherosclerosis is a gradual process of artery breakdown that causes plaque to accumulate and form occlusions.
- Heart attacks are more lethal for women than men.
- High blood pressure is defined as a systolic pressure of 140 mm Hg and/or diastolic pressure of 90 mm Hg and/or taking antihypertensive medication.
- A total cholesterol/HDL ratio below 3.5 is recommended for heart health.
- Estrogen replacement therapy reduces the risk of heart disease.
- Stroke is the third leading cause of death and the leading cause of disability in women.

- Osteoporosis is a bone-weakening disorder causing bone mineral loss and skeletal frailty.
- African American women compared to white women are 50 percent more likely to develop Type 2 diabetes.
- The best way to overcome the stigma of epilepsy is by educating the public.
- Arthritis, an inflammatory condition of the joints, is the leading cause of work-related disability.
- Systemic lupus erythematosus affects primarily women of childbearing age.
- Multiple sclerosis affects primarily young white women, often between the ages of 30 and 40.
- Alzheimer's disease is the most common dementia and a key component is memory loss.

Review Questions

1. What is the leading cause of death in women?
2. What is atherosclerosis?
3. What are the signs and symptoms of angina?
4. What is the difference between a heart attack and congestive heart failure?
5. What are the primary risk and protective factors for heart disease?
6. How can hypertension be controlled?

7. What are the warning signs of stroke? Type 2 diabetes? Arthritis?
8. What are the risk and protective factors for osteoporosis?
9. What causes lupus? Multiple sclerosis? Alzheimer's disease?
10. What can you do to protect yourself against chronic conditions?

Resources

Organizations and Hotlines

American Heart Association
7272 Greenville Avenue
Dallas, TX 75231
Telephone: (800) 242-8721
Referrals to local chapters and current information on heart conditions

National Heart, Lung, and Blood Institute (NHLBI)
P.O. Box 30105
Bethesda, MD 20824-0105
Telephone: (301) 251-1222

National Osteoporosis Foundation
2100 M Street N.W., Suite 602-B
Washington, D.C. 20037
Telephone: (800) 223-9994
Free information is available upon request

Epilepsy Foundation of America (EFA)
Information and Referral Department
4351 Garden City Drive
Landover, MD 20785
Telephone: (800) EFA-1000

Arthritis Foundation Information Line
P.O. Box 19000
Atlanta, GA 30326
Telephone: (800) 283-7800
Provides information regarding local chapters and physician referrals, general information on arthritis, and supports research regarding a cure and prevention of arthritis

Alzheimer's Association (National Office)
919 N. Michigan Ave. Suite 1000
Chicago, IL 60611-1676
Telephone: (800) 272-3900
This resource will prove most beneficial to families of persons with AD. Literature and information about support groups can be obtained

National Stroke Association
8480 East Orchard Road, suite 100
Englewood, CO 80111
Telephone: (800) STROKES

Lupus Foundation of America, Inc.
4 Research Place, Suite 180
Rockville, MD 20852-3226
Telephone: (800) 558-0121
For information about various aspects of lupus. A grassroots, volunteer-driven organization

American Diabetes Association
1660 Duke Street
Alexandria, VA 22314
Telephone: (800) 232-3472
Professional association and a voluntary organization with state and local affiliates and chapters. Serves people with diabetes and their family and friends, as well as health professionals and research scientists

National Multiple Sclerosis Society
Telephone: (800) Fight-MS
Telephone: (800) 334-4867

Websites

National Heart, Lung, and Blood Institute
www.nhlbi.nih.gov

National Multiple Sclerosis Society
www.nmss.org

American Heart Association
www.amhrt.org

Arthritis Foundation
www.arthritis.org

Suggested Readings

Diethrich, E. B., and C. Cohan. 1992. *Women and heart disease.* New York: Ballantine Books, Random House Inc.

Ross, E., and J. Sachs. 1996. *Healing the female heart: A holistic approach to prevention and recovery from heart disease.* New York: Pocket Books, Simon & Schuster Inc.

Thorsheim, H. I., and B. B. Roberts. 1990. *Reminiscing together.* Minneapolis, MN: CompCare Publishers. (800-328-3330)

(A book for assisting caregivers with tools for reminiscing and stimulating memory in persons with AD)

References

1. American Heart Association. 1996. Heart and stroke facts: 1995 statistical supplement. Dallas, Tx.: American Heart Association.
2. Waters, W. 1992. Pathophysiology and treatment of angina pectoris. *Drug Topics,* 136: 102.
3. Cody, R. J., C. R. Conti, and P. Samet. 1993. Managing angina and concomitant disease. *Patient Care,* 27: 45–72.
4. Ibid.
5. Pandora's angina. 1992 (Editorial.) *The Lancet,* 339: 782–83.
6. Amsterdam, E. A., and M. J. Legato. 1993. What's unique about CHD in women? *Patient Care,* 27: 21–61.
7. Cotton, P. 1991. Insurance loss threatens medical gain. *JAMA,* 266: 2158.
8. Ross, E., and J. Sachs. 1996. *Healing the female heart.* New York: Pocket Books.
9. Ibid.
10. Ibid.
11. Women need to be screened differently than men for heart disease. April, 1996. University of Texas, Houston Health Science Center, *Lifestyle Health Letter,* 8 (4): 1–2.
12. Kawachi, I., G. A. Colditz, and others. 1994. Smoking cessation and time course of decreased risks of coronary heart disease in middle-aged women. *Archives of Internal Medicine,* 154: 169–75.
13. National Heart, Lung and Blood Institute. 1985. Hypertension prevalence and the status of awareness, treatment, and control in the United States. Final report of the subcommittee on definition and prevalence of the 1984 joint national committee. *Hypertension,* 7 (3): 457–68.
14. American Heart Association, Heart and Stroke Facts.
15. Willett, W. C., M. J. Stampfer, J. E. Manson, and others. 1993. Intake of transfatty acids and risk of coronary heart disease among women. *The Lancet,* 341: 581–85.
16. Gender-based screening for heart disease starts at UT Houston. February, 1996. Office of Public Affairs, The University of Texas-Houston Health Science Center, 7000 Fannin, Suite 1200, Houston, TX.
17. Facts about heart disease and women: Are you at risk? National Heart, Lung, and Blood Institute. www.fido.nhibi.nih.gov
18. Myocardial infarction and coronary death among women: Psychosocial predictors from a 20-year follow-up of women in the Framingham Study. 1992. *American Journal of Epidemiology,* 135: 854–64.
19. Stampfer, M. J., C. H. Hennekens, J. E. Manson, and others. 1993. Vitamin E consumption and the risk of coronary disease in women. *New England Journal of Medicine,* 328: 1444–49.
20. Garg, R., D. K. Wagener, and J. H. Madans. 1993. Alcohol consumption and risk of ischemic heart disease in women. *Archives of Internal Medicine,* 153: 1211–16.
21. Blari, S. N., H. W. Kohl, R. S. Paffenbarger, and others. 1989. Physical fitness and all-cause mortality: A prospective study of healthy men and women. *JAMA,* 262: 2395–401.
22. Manson, J. E., M. J. Stampfer, G. A. Colditz, and others. 1991. A prospective study of aspirin use and primary prevention of cardiovascular disease in women. *JAMA,* 266: 521–27.
23. Young, R. F., and E. Kahana. 1993. Gender, recovery from late life heart attack and medical care. *Women & Health,* 20: 11–31.
24. Eysmann, S. B., and P. S. Douglas. 1992. Reperfusion and revascularization strategies for coronary artery disease in women. *JAMA,* 268: 1903–7.
25. Mark, D. B., L. K. Shaw, and others. 1994. Absence of sex bias in the referral of patients for cardiac catheterization. *The New England Journal of Medicine,* 330: 1101.
26. Fiebach, N. H., C. M. Viscoli, and R. I. Horwitz. 1990. Differences between women and men in survival after myocardial infarction. *JAMA,* 263: 1092–96.
27. Eysmann and Douglas, Reperfusion and revascularization strategies.
28. Stroke diagnosis and treatment. 1992. *American Family Physician,* 45: 1886–88.
29. Finucane, F. F. 1993. Decreased risk of stroke among postmenopausal hormone users: Results from a national cohort. *JAMA,* 269: 2730. (Abstract.)
30. Kawachi, I., G. A. Colditz, M. J. Stampfer, and others. 1993. Smoking cessation and decreased risk of stroke in women. *JAMA,* 269: 232–36.
31. Fackelmann, K. A. 1994. Artery surgery slashes risk of stroke. *Science News,* 146: 228.
32. McBean, L. D., T. Forgac, and S. C. Finn. 1994. Osteoporosis: Visions for care and prevention—A conference report. *Journal of the American Dietetic Association,* 94: 668–71.
33. Iskrant, A. P., and R. Smith. 1969. Osteoporosis in women 45 years and older related to subsequent fractures. *Public Health Reports,* 84: 33–38.
34. National Institutes of Health. 1984. Consensus statement: Osteoporosis. *JAMA,* 252: 799–802.
35. McBean, Forgac, and Finn, Osteoporosis.
36. Kanis, J. A., and F. A. Pitt. 1992. Epidemiology of osteoporosis. *Bone,* 13: S7–15.
37. Wolman, R. L. 1994. Osteoporosis and exercise. *British Medical Journal,* 309: 400–3.

38. Ibid.

39. Ibid.

40. Rigotti, N. A., R. M. Neer, and others. 1991. The clinical course of osteoporosis in anorexia nervosa: A longitudinal study of cortical bone mass. *JAMA,* 265: 1133–38.

41. Carr, B. R., B. Dawson-Hughes, and B. Ettinger. 1993. A real-world approach to osteoporosis. *Patient Care, 27:* 31.

42. Hollenbach, K. A., E. Barrett-Conner, and others. 1993. Cigarette smoking and bone mineral density in older men and women. *American Journal of Public Health,* 83: 1265.

43. McNabb, W. L., M. T. Quinn, and L. Rosing. 1993. Weight loss program for inner-city black women with non-insulin-dependent diabetes mellitus: PATHWAYS. *Journal of the American Dietetic Association,* 93: 75–77.

44. Rimm, E. B., J. E. Manson, M. J. Stampfer, and others. 1993. Cigarette smoking and the risk of diabetes in women. *American Journal of Public Health,* 83: 211–14.

45. Cochran, J. W., E. S. Kessler, and R. Wittenborn. Neurologic disease: 5 scenarios to manage. *Patient Care,* 28: 32.

46. Gazaway, R. M., J. R. Niebyl, and others. 1993. Drugs in pregnancy: Epilepsy, cancer, and more. *Patient Care,* 27: 79.

47. Arthritis prevalence and activity limitations—United States, 1990. 1994. *Morbidity and Mortality Weekly Report,* 43: 433–38.

48. Laino, C. 1994. Rheumatoid arthritis: Rather than waiting months for a response to NSAIDs, rheumatologists are embracing an early, more aggressive use of second-line therapies at the first sign of clinical or functional deterioration. *Medical World News,* 35: 28–33.

49. Rossor, M. 1993. Alzheimer's disease. *British Medical Journal,* 307: 779–82.

50. Bloom, A., and A. Rulnick. 1994. AAHSA survey highlights similarities, variations in special care programs. *The Brown University Long-Term Care Quality Letter,* 6: 1.

Twenty

Reducing Your Risk of Cancer

■ chapter objectives

When you complete this chapter you will be able to:
- Identify the seven warning signs of cancer.
- Describe the classifications of cancers.
- Explain possible lifestyle and genetic causes of cancer.
- Identify the risk and protective factors for each cancer.
- Identify the primary cancers based on incidence and mortality.
- Describe the issues about tamoxifen for prevention of breast cancer.
- Compare and contrast medical and complementary treatment options.
- Explain the importance of social support in recovery from cancer.

THE BIG "C"

One in three women today can expect to have cancer in her lifetime, and nearly 50 percent of these cases involve the female reproductive system. Many women will someday hear the words, "Your pap smear was positive; we need to do further tests," or "You have a lump in your breast; we need to schedule a biopsy." Despite reassurance from the healthcare provider that there is no cause for concern at this time, a woman would probably experience a myriad of feelings. Two common reactions might be (1) to assume the worst, "It's CANCER and I'm going to die" or (2) to deny it, "There can't be anything wrong with me." It is because the word "cancer" is so stigmatized that it evokes such strong emotions.

This chapter provides information on the nature and sites of the most common cancers found in women, gives guidelines for early detection, suggests strategies for prevention and early intervention, and discusses various medical and complementary treatment protocols. This information can assist you to develop a realistic plan for cancer prevention and management.

DEFINING CANCER

Some women have the perception that all tumors are cancerous, that all cancers are the same, and that cancer is synonymous with death. However, most tumors are **benign** and many different types of cancer have

HEALTHY PEOPLE 2000 OBJECTIVES

- Reverse the rise in cancer deaths to achieve a rate of no more than 130 per 100,000 people. 1995 progress toward goal: approximately 25 percent
- Reduce the rise in lung cancer deaths to achieve a rate of no more than 42 per 100,000 people. 1995 progress toward goal: data unavailable
- Reduce breast cancer deaths to no more than 20.6 per 100,000 women. 1995 progress toward goal: approximately 60 percent
- Reduce deaths from cancer of the uterine and cervix to no more than 1.3 per 100,000 women. 1995 progress toward goal: approximately 8 percent
- Reduce colorectal cancer deaths to no more than 13.2 per 100,000 people. 1995 progress toward goal: approximately 95 percent
- Increase to at least 80 percent the proportion of women aged 40 and older who have ever received a clinical breast examination and a mammogram, and to at least 60 percent those aged 50 and older who have received them within the preceding one to two years. 1995 progress toward goal: approximately 85 percent
- Increase to at least 95 percent the proportion of women aged 18 and older who have ever received a Pap test, and to at least 85 percent those who received a Pap test within the preceding one to three years. 1995 progress toward goal: approximately 98 percent
- Ensure that Pap tests meet quality standards by monitoring and certifying all cytology laboratories. 1995 progress toward goal: data unavailable
- Ensure that mammograms meet quality standards by monitoring and certifying at least 80 percent of mammography facilities. 1995 progress toward goal: approximately 75 percent

health tips

CAUTION: Warning Signs of Cancer

Change in bowel or bladder habits.
A sore that does not heal.
Unusual bleeding or discharge.
Thickening or a lump in the breast or elsewhere.
Indigestion or difficulty in swallowing.
Obvious change in a wart or mole.
Nagging cough or hoarseness.

been isolated. Cancer is recognized as a **malignant neoplasm** characterized by uncontrolled growth of anaplastic cells that often invade surrounding tissue and **metastasize** to distant body sites.

The prognosis for a woman with cancer depends upon a variety of factors, including the nature of the tumor, its location, and its stage. The key to survival of cancer is early detection. The earlier cancer is diagnosed, the better the prognosis. If any of the seven warning signs for cancer are present, you are advised to see your health-care provider immediately. (See *Health Tips:* "CAUTION.")

In 1997, it was estimated that 596,600 women would be diagnosed with cancer and 265,900 would die (see Table 20.1). The highest incidence and mortality rates for reported cancer cases in women are for cancers of the breast, lungs, and colon and rectum. (See *FYI:* "Cancer Incidence by Race and Ethnicity.")

CLASSIFICATIONS OF COMMON MALIGNANCIES

Each cancer is distinguished by the nature, site, or clinical course of the lesion. Generally, cancers are classified according to the part of the body in which they originate or by the type of cell as seen under the microscope. The World Health organization has identified forty-six body sites and numerous types of cancer at each site; well over a hundred different cancers.

benign—not cancerous; harmless.

malignant—uncontrolled growth of a cell making exact multiple copies of itself.

neoplasm—abnormal development of cells that may be harmless or cancerous.

metastasis—the process by which cancer is spread to distant parts of the body.

Table 20.1

Leading Sites of New Cancer Cases and Death in Women, 1997 Estimates

CANCER CASES	CANCER DEATHS
Breast 180,200	Lung 66,000
Lung 79,800	Breast 43,900
Colon & rectum 64,800	Colon & rectum 27,900
Corpus uteri 34,900	Pancreas 14,600
Ovary 26,800	Ovary 14,200
Non-Hodgkin's lymphoma 23,300	Non-Hodgkin's lymphoma 11,400
Melanoma of the skin* 17,400	Leukemia 9,540
Urinary bladder 15,000	Corpus uteri 6,000
Cervix 14,500	Brain 6,000
Pancreas 14,200	Stomach 5,700
All Sites 596,600	All Sites 265,900

*Excluding basal and squamous cell skin cancer.

The four most common categories of cancer are carcinoma, sarcoma, lymphoma, and leukemia. (See Fig. 20.1.)[1] The reason for discussing these broad categories of cancers is to provide you with an understanding that all cancers are *not* the same. Carcinomas are by far the most common type of cancer found in the United States, a full 85 percent of all reported cancers. Carcinomas begin in the glandular or epithelial cells, which line the organs of the body. Sarcomas are cancers that begin in the connective tissues of the body, either the bone or soft tissues. Most tumors of bone and soft tissues are benign, and sarcomas are relatively rare in the United States. They account for less than 2 percent of all new cancer cases each year.

Lymphomas are cancers of the lymphatic system, and can be broadly subdivided into Hodgkin's disease and non-Hodgkin's lymphomas (a number of diseases).

Leukemia is a cancer of the blood-forming tissues and can be one of many types. Early symptoms may mimic other diseases, including mononucleosis, tonsillitis, mumps, and others. Therefore, blood tests and examination of the cells in the bone marrow are necessary for diagnosing leukemia.

In addition to the most common categories, it is important to understand the difference between in situ and invasive cancer. *In situ* refers to tumors that are usually early stage and localized. The survival rates are usually higher than *invasive* cancer that has

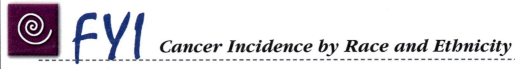

FYI *Cancer Incidence by Race and Ethnicity*

The rate of cancer among women varies by race. Alaska Native women have the highest reported rates of cancer, followed by white women. The leading cancer sites among Alaska Native women are breast, colon and rectum, and lung. In fact, they have the highest rates of colorectal and lung cancer among all women. White women have the highest rates of breast cancer among all women, whereas African American women have the highest rates of lung and colon and rectum cancer of any group except Alaska Natives. The leading cancer sites among African American women are breast, colon and rectum, lung, uterine, and cervical cancer. Asian and Pacific Island women experience higher rates of breast, lung, and colon and rec-

tum cancer than any other cancer. However, stomach cancer is the leading site for Japanese and Korean American women and cervical cancer is the leading site for Vietnamese American women. The leading cancer sites for Hispanic and Latino women are breast, lung, and colon and rectum. Hispanic women are second only to Vietnamese women in the high rates of cervical cancer. Reported cancer rates are lowest for Native American women from New Mexico and Korean American women. The data for Native American women from New Mexico, although showing the lowest overall reported cancer rates, are not known to be accurate. These women have been underrepresented in most studies.

FIGURE 20.1 Common classifications of cancer.

Carcinoma

A malignant epithelial neoplasm that tends to invade surrounding tissue and to metastasize to distant regions of the body. Carcinomas develop most frequently in the skin, large intestine, lungs, stomach, prostate gland, cervix, or breast. The tumor is firm, irregular, nodular, with a well-defined border.

Sarcoma

A malignant neoplasm of the soft tissues arising in fibrous, fatty, muscular, synovial, vascular, or neural tissue, usually first presenting as a painless swelling. About 40 percent of sarcomas occur in the lower extremities, 20% in the upper extremities, 20% in the trunk, and the rest in the head, neck or retroperineum. The tumor, composed of closely packed cells in a fibrillar or homogeneous matrix, tends to be vascular and is usually highly invasive.

Lymphoma

A neoplasm of lymphoid tissue that is usually malignant. Characteristically, the appearance of a painless, enlarged lymph node or nodes is followed by weakness, fever, weight loss, and anemia.

Leukemia

A malignant neoplasm of blood-forming tissues characterized by diffuse replacement of bone marrow with proliferating leukocyte precursors, abnormal numbers and forms of immature white cells in circulation, and infiltration of lymph nodes, the spleen, and the liver. Acute leukemia usually has a sudden onset and rapidly progresses from early signs, such as fatigue, pallor, weight loss, and easy bruising, to fever, hemorrhages, extreme weakness, bone or joint pain, and repeated infections. Chronic leukemia develops slowly, and signs similar to those of the acute forms of the disease may not appear for years.

spread to other tissues. A variety of systems are used to determine the stage of cancer according to the major factors influencing prognosis. The most common system for determining the stage of cancer is the **TNM** staging system, developed by the American Joint Committee on Cancer and the International Union Against Cancer. In the TNM system, T represents the tumor size and level of invasion ranging from 1 to 4. N represents the nodal involvement, the size, the number, and degree of spread to lymph nodes ranging from 1 to 4. And, M represents the absence or presence of distant metastases, denoted as X, 0, or 1. For example, Stage 0 for breast cancer refers to noninvasive or in situ cancers, whereas Stage 4 means the carcinoma extends beyond the breast to another part of the body such as bone, liver, or lung. Each cancer site has a different staging, unique to the site.[2] Gynecologic cancers are fre-quently classified according to the guidelines of the International Federation for Gynecologic Oncology (FIGO). This system divides the disease into five stages from Stage 0, a carcinoma in situ, to Stage IV, the metastasis to other sites. The stages were further subdivided into three grades with Grade 1 being well-differentiated with the best prognosis and Grade 3 being least-differentiated with the poorest prognosis.[3] For example, Stage I for endometrial cancer refers to carcinoma in situ, whereas Stage IV means the carcinoma extends beyond the pelvis and involves the bladder or rectum.

TNM—a system for staging cancerous tumor disease.

Table 20.2

The Probability of Developing Cancer

		Birth to 39	40 to 59	60 to 79	Birth to Death
All sites*	Female	1.96 (1 in 51)	9.12 (1 in 11)	22.48 (1 in 4)	38.33 (1 in 3)
Breast	Female	0.46 (1 in 217)	3.92 (1 in 26)	6.94 (1 in 14)	12.61 (1 in 8)
Colon & Rectum	Female	0.05 (1 in 2,000)	0.70 (1 in 143)	3.24 (1 in 31)	5.77 (1 in 17)
Lung	Female	0.03 (1 in 3,333)	1.05 (1 in 95)	3.83 (1 in 26)	5.48 (1 in 18)

*Excludes basal and squamous cell skin cancers and in situ carcinomas except bladder.

CAUSES OF CANCER

Scientists remain uncertain about the exact causes of cancer, although external (chemicals, radiation, and viruses) and internal (hormones, immune conditions, and inherited mutations) factors are recognized. Lifestyle and environmental factors account for most cancer risk and a number of known **carcinogens** have been identified. Cigarette smoking, exposure to carcinogenic chemicals, ionizing radiation, and ultra-violet rays account for more than 80 percent of all cancers. Several theories regarding the causes of cancer have been postulated during the past several decades. This section discusses some of the lifestyle and environmental factors contributing to cancer, and the biological changes that develop to increase the risk of contracting cancer.

Lifestyle Factors Implicated in Cancer

Cigarette Smoking Cigarette smoking is associated with cancers of the lung, larynx, pharynx, oral cavity, esophagus, pancreas, and bladder. Cigarette smoking accounts for 87 percent of lung cancer deaths and 29 percent of all cancer deaths. Passive (or secondhand) smoke causes disease, including lung cancer, in healthy nonsmokers. Nearly 25 percent of all adults in the United States still smoke, but the per capita consumption of cigarettes continues to decline. The smoking prevalence among white women has decreased from 30 percent to 23 percent and among African American women from 32 percent to 22 percent between 1983 and 1994. Smoking cigarettes remains the most significant factor in premature death of women, particularly in the areas of cancer and heart disease. Lung cancer mortality rates are eleven times higher for female smokers compared to females who had never smoked. In addition, secondhand smoke contributes to nearly 3,000 lung cancer deaths in nonsmoking adults each year.[4]

Diet Research suggests that approximately one-third of cancer deaths in the United States are due to dietary factors. The types of food consumed, the amount of fat consumed rather than the specific type of fat consumed, food preparation methods, and overall caloric balance are risk factors for some cancers in women, particularly cancers of the breast, colon, and rectum. Healthy People 2000 set a goal of reducing dietary fat intake to an average of 30 percent of calories among people aged 2 and older. Baseline data suggested that about 36 percent of calories came from total fat and 12 percent from saturated fat for women aged 19 through 50. In 1995, only about 20 percent of the adult population had achieved an average daily goal of no more than 30 percent of calories from fat and less than 10 percent calories from saturated fat.

Scientific studies suggest that fruits and vegetables (especially green and dark yellow vegetables, cruciferous vegetables, soy products, and legumes) are protective factors for preventing some types of cancer, particularly for cancers of the gastrointestinal and respiratory tracts.[5] The 5-A-Day program, a partnership of grocers, produce suppliers, and federal and state health agencies, have undertaken a nationwide campaign to encourage people to eat five or more servings of fruits and vegetables each day as part of a low-fat, high-fiber diet.

Age Cancer deaths are certainly age-related. Even though the age-adjusted death rate from cancer has been rising, much of the increase can be attributed to a rise in lung cancer death rates. Most other age-related cancers have leveled off and for people younger than 55, the cancer death rate has declined. Over 50 percent of all cancers occur in persons over the age of 65, and the age-related death rate for people aged 55 and older is still rising. Table 20.2 shows the probability of developing cancer for the age groups 1–39, 40–59, and 60–79. You can see that the probability for all sites increases with older age.

Viruses   A number of viruses have been linked to an increased risk of cancer, including hepatitis B, HTLV-1, HSV-2, Epstein-Barr, and some types of HPV. Hepatitis B has been linked to liver cancer, whereas HSV-2 and HPV have been associated with an increase in cervical cancer.

Alcohol Consumption   Heavy alcohol consumption, particularly in conjunction with cigarette use or chewing tobacco, contribute to an increased risk of cancer. These cancers include mouth, esophagus, liver, larynx, and stomach. Alcohol is associated with an increased risk of breast cancer among women, but the reason is unknown. Some studies suggest that drinking alcohol is related to changes in hormonal levels, particularly an increase in estrogen levels in women.[6] Further study of the relationship among alcohol intake, hormonal levels such as estrogen, and breast cancer is warranted.

It is important to recognize that cancer can occur in women who may not have any of the risk factors identified above. You need to know the warning signs and get regular cancer screening examinations by your health-care provider because early detection is extremely important.

Environmental Factors Implicated in Cancer

Radiation   Ionizing radiation (X rays, radon, etc.) has been linked to certain cancers including leukemia, breast cancer, and lung cancer. Low-dose levels have a negligible effect on cancer risk (medical and dental X rays), but limiting exposure is prudent.

Exposure to Sun   Ultraviolet rays (both UVA and UVB) have been linked to skin cancer. Healthy People 2000 set a goal to increase to at least 60 percent the proportion of people of all ages who limit sun exposure, use sunscreens and protective clothing when exposed to sunlight, and avoid artificial sources of ultraviolet light (such as sun lamps and tanning booths). UV radiation causes most cases of basal and squamous cell skin cancer and contributes significantly to skin melanoma. Levels of UV radiation may be increasing due to changes in the earth's ozone layer.[7]

Hair Dyes   Past research studies connected non-Hodgkin's lymphoma to the use of hair dyes by women. However, a more recent prospective study[8,9] of over 500,000 women found that those at risk had used dark (particularly black) hair dye for over twenty years. No association between hair dye and other types of cancer were found. Because more than one-third of adult American women use hair dye, this study demonstrates the importance of having adequate knowledge to make informed choices.

Electromagnetic Fields   The public continues to receive conflicting reports on the association between certain cancers and low-frequency electromagnetic fields (electric transmission lines, transformers, local household wiring). Researchers[10] have found no significant link between the increase in per capita power consumption and the incidence of different cancers. Studies continue regarding the association of electromagnetic fields and cancer.

Contributing Factors

A number of environmental and lifestyle factors continue to be studied. Oftentimes new research suggests that certain foods or environmental factors cause cancer. It is only after numerous studies have verified these findings that the factor can really be considered a carcinogen. A number of the following factors have been implicated after considerable study: Agent Orange, DES in pregnant women, a high-fat diet, tobacco, pesticides, sunlight, estrogen replacement therapy, worksite substances such as asbestos, formaldehyde, X rays, and some viruses. It is important to have adequate information before assuming that a particular substance causes cancer, or increases your risk of getting cancer. Now complete *Assess Yourself:* "What Is Your Cancer Risk?"

CURRENT RESEARCH REGARDING CAUSES AND TREATMENT

Molecular and Cellular Causes of Cancer

Most carcinogens are introduced into the body through air, water, or diet and then deactivated by the body's immune system. However, some foreign

---

carcinogens—substances that can cause the growth of cancer.

Assess YOURSELF

What Is Your Cancer Risk?

Check all of the following risk factors that apply to you.

Lung Cancer

_____ 1. Cigarette smoking
_____ 2. Living with a person who smokes
_____ 3. Exposure to chemicals that are known carcinogens
_____ 4. Radiation exposure
_____ 5. Radon exposure
_____ 6. Living in an area with heavy air pollution

Colon and rectal cancer

_____ 1. Family history
_____ 2. Physical inactivity
_____ 3. High-fat diet
_____ 4. Low-fiber diet

Breast Cancer

_____ 1. Family history
_____ 2. Early menarche—before age 12
_____ 3. Late menopause—after age 50
_____ 4. Lengthy exposure to cyclic estrogen
_____ 5. Never having children
_____ 6. First birth of a child at a later age
_____ 7. Obesity
_____ 8. High socioeconomic status
_____ 9. Higher education level

Cervical Cancer

_____ 1. First intercourse at early age
_____ 2. Multiple sex partners
_____ 3. Cigarette smoking
_____ 4. Low socioeconomic status

Endometrial Cancer

_____ 1. Estrogen
_____ 2. Tamoxifen
_____ 3. Early menarche—before age 12
_____ 4. Late menopause—after age 50
_____ 5. Never having children
_____ 6. History of infertility or failure to ovulate
_____ 7. Diabetes
_____ 8. Gallbladder disease
_____ 9. Hypertension
_____10. Obesity

Ovarian Cancer

_____ 1. Age (over 50)
_____ 2. Never having children
_____ 3. Family history of ovarian cancer
_____ 4. Breast cancer
_____ 5. Living in an industrialized country

Skin Cancer

_____ 1. Exposure to UV rays
_____ 2. Fair complexion
_____ 3. Family history
_____ 4. Occupational exposure to coal tar, pitch, etc.

What measures can you take to reduce your risks?

---

substances become activated within the body and bind to the genetic coding material, DNA. Altered DNA may be responsible for the growth in cancer cells. Once scientists delineate the causes of cancer and the mechanisms contributing to abnormal cell growth, the possibility for a cure increases. Several theories elucidate the causes of abnormal cell growth and are discussed in the following sections.

Cell Cycle Research

One avenue of cancer research is the study of the cell cycle. Cancer cells exhibit a loss of differentia-

tion, increased invasiveness, and a decrease in drug sensitivity compared to normal cells. A normal cell cycle requires the coordination of a variety of macromolecular syntheses, assemblies, and movement. Hartwell and Kastan[11] suggest that defects in the synthesis, assembly, or movement of DNA, the spindle, or spindle pole during replication may result in genetic instability that characterizes precancerous and cancerous cells. They conclude that if genomic instability contributes to cancer development, then finding procedures to reduce the instability may reduce the incidence and rate of cancer development. Cell biologists continue to explore the genetic changes that lead to cancer.[12]

Gene Mutation Research

Oncogenes play a role in normal cell growth, however, when oncogenes mutate, they can cause rapid cell division. Ras oncogene mutation is found in 50 percent of all colon cancers, 90 percent of pancreatic cancers[13], and is a major factor in many epithelial cancers and myeloid leukemias.[14] Easton and colleagues[15] found that the mutation of BRCA1 accounted for approximately 45 percent of families with significantly high breast cancer incidence and around 80 percent of families with increased incidence of both early-onset breast cancer and ovarian cancer. The presence of certain oncogenes may be used to diagnose the susceptibility of individuals to particular cancers and may provide a better understanding of cancer biology.

Some individuals may be more susceptible to mutations of genes, called suppressor genes. Although normal suppressor genes control cell growth, mutated ones allow rapid cell division. Researchers found mutations of the tumor suppressor gene p53 were common in soft tissue sarcoma patients who had a personal or family history of cancer, but not in patients without this background. The identification of these mutations may allow for genetic counseling.[16] Other researchers found that the overexpression of p53 protein strongly correlates with poor clinical outcome in patients with soft tissue sarcoma.[17] Science is beginning to unravel the mechanism of some cancers, and genetic engineers hope to one day have the capacity to eliminate mutated genes and replace them with normal genes.

Adjuvant Treatment

Adjuvant therapy, such as radiation therapy or substances to enhance the action of drugs to treat the cancer, refers to the use of other forms of treatment to supplement and/or enhance the primary treatment. The use of drugs pre- and postoperatively improve the survival rate with certain cancers. Neoadjuvant therapy is a term used to describe the use of drugs to shrink the cancer before surgical removal. This treatment is used with certain types of cancer, including later stage breast cancer and brain tumors. **Chemotherapy,** chemical systemic treatment, can cure some cancers, keep others from spreading, cause remission, or reduce large tumors before surgery. Researchers continue to seek the most effective combinations of treatments to increase the survival rate.

Immunotherapy Research

Immunotherapy enhances the body's own immune system to fight a disease. When the body is functioning effectively, the immune system controls cancer cells. T-helper cells and **macrophages** use their own chemicals, tumor necrosis factor, interleukin, and interferon, to prevent tumor growth or attack cancer cells. Interferon, interleukin-2, and other biologic response modifiers are being tested for effectiveness in boosting the immune system's ability to counter the malignant cell division. Gene therapy and vaccines are also being studied.

Bone Marrow Transplant Research

Women with breast cancer and other malignant tumors are turning to **autologous** bone marrow transplants for help. A woman's own marrow is removed before chemotherapy or radiation therapy and later restored. This procedure reduces the risk of rejection and allows the woman to tolerate larger doses of chemotherapy treatment.[18] Now see *Viewpoint:* "Are We Winning the 'War on Cancer'?"

CANCER AT SELECTED SITES: WHAT YOU NEED TO KNOW

Lung Cancer

Lung cancer surpassed breast cancer as the leading cause of cancer death in women in 1987. One decade later, an estimated 66,000 women will die from lung cancer, many of them needlessly. They are dying because they smoke cigarettes. Lung cancer death rates for women have increased 159 percent between 1973 and 1993, due primarily to the increase in cigarette smoking.[19] Also see *Viewpoint:* "Cancer Rates Rising in China."

---

oncogenes (on koe genes)—genes that may possibly cause a cell to be changed to cancer.

adjuvant therapy—treatment with substances that enhance the action of drugs to help the body produce antibodies.

chemotherapy—use of drugs to treat disease, most often cancer.

macrophage—any large cell that can surround and digest foreign substances in the body.

Viewpoint

Are We Winning the "War on Cancer"?

The fear of cancer has increased proportionately to the risk of contracting the disease, from one in six in the 1960s to one in three in the 1990s. In 1971, President Nixon declared a "war on cancer" and Congress passed the National Cancer Act, which included funding for the creation of the National Cancer Institute. Although NCI had many responsibilities assigned to it, one of its primary roles was to find a cure for cancer. In 1992, more than 10 percent of the nation's entire health-care expense was spent on treatment and research. The American public continues to receive mixed messages regarding the progress of cancer research. On the one hand, NCI and the American Cancer Society suggest that we are winning the war on cancer. Officials point to the improvement of "five-year survival rates" for many cancers. On the other hand, some researchers point out that the incidence of many cancers continues to increase. They suggest that the overall survival rate trends have only risen a few percentage points since the early 1970s. In fact, early detection accounts for most of the current success in treatment.

What are the facts? Some researchers suggest that we need to continue to spend our resources on finding a cure and better treatment for cancer. Others support more prevention, focusing primarily on lifestyle and environmental factors. What do you think? Which areas are most important to you?

Viewpoint

Cancer Rates Rising in China

China is the world's largest consumer of tobacco and, in 1993 alone, Chinese deaths from lung cancer rose nearly 5 percent. In 1992, coincidentally, the Chinese government earned more tax revenue from tobacco than from any other industry, collecting $30.5 million and they projected an even higher rate of revenue in the future. Three American tobacco companies have signed contracts for producing tobacco in China: Philip Morris, RJR Nabisco, and Rothmans.

The American Cancer Society reports that U.S. cigarette exports increased about 230 percent since 1987. This increase in exports to other countries includes Japan, South Korea, and the former Soviet Union.[22] What do you think about the American business involvement in the Chinese tobacco industry? What's the message to the people of China? What are your thoughts about the increase in exports to other countries?

Risk and Protective Factors The best advise for the prevention of lung cancer is: If you don't smoke, don't start. If someone close to you smokes, ask them to smoke somewhere else. If you smoke, QUIT! The incidence of lung cancer among women has continued to rise during the past twenty years, paralleling a previous increase in smoking. Passive or secondhand smoke is another primary risk factor for lung cancer. Avoiding smoke-filled areas, including the home of a smoker who smokes indoors, acts as a strong protective factor for not getting lung cancer.

Young teenage girls are being lured by the tobacco industry to assert their independence and charm by picking up the smoking habit. They also get the promise of weight control just by smoking cigarettes. Advertisements push cigarettes by promising independence, weight control, and romance. Unfortunately, what young women have to look forward to is premature aging, an increase in facial wrinkles, and becoming addicted to a powerful, cancer-causing product.

The overwhelming number of women who develop lung cancer are smokers or have lived with a smoker. However, some other factors have been implicated in increasing your risk of lung cancer including having asbestos lung disease, obstructive airway disease, exposure to radon, and exposure to a variety of occupational substances such as chromium, coal products, iron oxide, nickel, mustard gas, petroleum, and uranium.

Early Detection The signs and symptoms a woman needs to recognize are a persistent cough, blood in the sputum, chest pain, and recurring pneumonia or bronchitis. By the time these symptoms occur, lung cancer is often in its more advanced stages and has metastasized to other areas.

Screening None of the many screening tests that have been used to detect lung cancer has demonstrated a decrease in mortality, including X-ray films, fluoroscopy, tomography, bronchography, angiography, cytologic studies of sputum, bronchial washings, and needle **biopsy,** and more recently the **magnetic resonance imaging (MRI)** and **monoclonal antibodies.**[20,21] Because advanced-stage lung cancer causes such high mortality and screening has no effect on mortality rates, the best hope is prevention, and better techniques for detection and treatment. More effective imaging methods and increased emphasis on smoking cessation are necessary for reducing lung cancer mortality.

Treatment By the time a woman knows she has lung cancer, the cancer has likely metastasized to other areas of the body or to a greater portion of the lung. Epidermoid (squamous) cancers and adenocarcinomas account for 60 percent of lung cancers, 25 percent are small or oat cell carcinomas, and 15 percent are large cell anaplastic cancers. Adenocarcinomas are by far the most common lung cancer in women. The prognosis for survival from lung cancer is poor, with only 13 percent of women diagnosed with lung cancer managing to survive five years or more.[23] A combination of surgery, radiation, and chemotherapy are used to stop the spread of lung cancer.

Breast Cancer

Breast cancer is the leading cause of cancer death in African American women and the second leading cancer killer of all women. Even though white women have the highest incidence rate of breast cancer, African American women have the highest death rate. Some researchers speculate that the higher death rate is probably due to diagnosis at a later stage of the disease. These women wait longer, are less likely to practice breast self-examination, and have fewer mammograms.

The incidence of breast cancer has been increasing by approximately 2 to 4 percent per year since 1980 and accounts for 30 percent of all cancers in women. The cause for the continued rise in breast cancer remains speculative. Some of the recent rise in incidence has been attributed to increased emphasis on early detection, primarily through the use of mammograms. The American Cancer Society estimates that

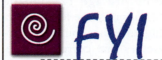

Abortion and Breast Cancer not Associated

A study conducted by researchers in Denmark found that there is no overall increase in breast cancer for women who had abortions between the 7th and 14th weeks of gestation. Women who had later term abortions may face a greater risk of breast cancer; however, other factors may have contributed to the increased risk.

180,200 women will get breast cancer and 43,900 women will die from breast cancer in 1997.[24] (See *FYI:* "Abortion and Breast Cancer not Associated.")

Risk and Protective Factors What do you think your risk for breast cancer is (high, medium, low)? Would you think it was low if your mother or grandmother didn't have breast cancer? Many women conclude that if their family history is free of breast cancer, they are free from risk. Not true! Although family history is a recognized risk factor, 85 to 95 percent of all women who develop breast cancer have no family history of the disease. In fact, 75 percent of all breast cancers occur in women with no known risk factors. All women are at risk because the two main risk factors are (1) being a woman and (2) getting older.

Identifiable risk factors, besides family history, include never having children; having your first child

autologous (**awe** tol la jis)—procedure in which bone marrow is removed from a person, stored, and then returned to the person's own system.

biopsy—surgical removal of tissue for microscopic examination diagnosis.

magnetic resonance imaging (MRI)—magnetic fields that absorb radio waves to produce images of organs and processes inside the body.

monoclonal antibodies—a group of identical antibodies made from a single antibody.

after age 30; menarche before age 12; starting menopause after age 55; history of some forms of benign breast disease, and higher education and socioeconomic status. Other factors that correlate somewhat with increased risk for breast cancer include eating a high-fat diet, heavy alcohol consumption, physical inactivity, and being 40 percent more than your desirable body weight.[25]

The best protection for a woman is early detection, that is, regular screening mammograms, (See *FYI:* "Guidelines for Breast Cancer Detection"), breast exams by a health-care provider, and monthly breast self-exams. (See *Viewpoint:* "FDA Approves Tamoxifen for Breast Cancer Prevention Trials.") A second protective factor is immediate treatment if breast cancer is diagnosed.

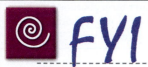 ## FYI *Guidelines for Breast Cancer Detection*

The American Cancer Society, the National Cancer Institute, and other medical groups recommend routine mammograms for all women over the age of 40. There is still some discrepancy for women in their forties. The American Cancer Society recommends mammograms *every year* for all women over the age of 40, and the National Cancer Institute recommends mammograms *every year or two* for all women over the age of 40. Both groups agree that mammograms should be conducted annually for women over age 50. Mammograms today can detect cancer in very early stages, well before physical symptoms can be detected by the woman or her health-care provider. Studies show that women in their forties who had regular mammograms compared to those who did not have periodic mammograms were less likely to die of breast cancer and had more treatment options.

The American Cancer Society still recommends breast self-examination for women aged 20 and over every month. (Refer back to chap. 14 for BSE instructions.) Breast clinical examinations are every three years for women aged 20 and over and every year for women aged 40 and over. ∽

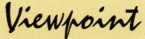
Viewpoint

FDA Approves Tamoxifen for Breast Cancer Prevention Trials

In April 1992, the FDA approved the use of tamoxifen (marketed as Nolvadex) for a five-year study by the National Cancer Institute (NCI) to determine whether it prevents breast cancer in *normally healthy* women. The Breast Cancer Prevention Trials began with the federal government soliciting the participation of 16,000 healthy women at a higher-than-average risk for breast cancer.

In 1993, the study was suspended as evidence was revealed that women taking tamoxifen had significantly higher rates of endometrial cancer. In two unrelated studies, breast cancer patients receiving tamoxifen for five or more years developed almost three times as many endometrial cancers as women receiving a placebo. A Dutch study also found four times greater rates of endometrial cancer in women who had taken tamoxifen, with duration of use being more important than dosage.[26] After reviewing the data and with the support of NCI, the FDA approved resumption of the study and warned women receiving tamoxifen to get regular gynecologic exams, report immediately any abnormal vaginal bleeding or discharge, and to avoid pregnancy due to possible fetal damage while taking tamoxifen. The FDA also recommended that women not take tamoxifen to prevent breast cancer unless they were among the 11,000 women enrolled in the NCI study. NCI believed the research study had merit and that the women currently enrolled in the study were at greater risk for breast cancer than uterine cancer.

The National Women's Health Network (NWHN)[27] was against the study from the beginning. They opposed the use of a toxic chemical, tamoxifen, with normally healthy women. And, with the increased information about endometrial cancer, they wanted the study to be discontinued and warnings sent to every woman who was prescribed tamoxifen for breast cancer therapy.

What do you think? Should the study continue? How should women be warned about the effects of tamoxifen?

Early Detection The two most common warning signs are lumps or thickening in the breast. Most lumps are benign, particularly lumps that are soft, round, smooth, or movable. Generally, an irregular, hard lump that feels attached to breast tissue is more likely to be malignant. Most breast cancers (70–80 percent) begin in the cells of the ducts, usually of the upper outer portion of the breast. This type of breast cancer is called ductal carcinoma. The other type of breast cancer begins in the lobes or lobules and is called lobular carcinoma.

Additional warning signs include a change in the size or shape of the breast, discharge from the nipple, or a change in the color or texture of the skin of the breast or around the areola. Any discharge from the nipple should be brought to the attention of your health-care provider!

Screening Early detection of breast cancer increases the likelihood of being cured. The best methods for detecting breast cancer are screening mammography, breast self-examination (BSE), and clinical breast examination (CBE). Lumps or changes discovered by BSE should be reported to your health-care provider immediately. The longer you wait, the worse the prognosis. Women who delayed less than one month have a death rate of 5 percent. Women who delayed a year or more have a death rate of 37 percent.[28]

Mammography Mammography allows health-care providers to detect breast cancer up to two years before a lump can be felt. Early detection increases the likelihood that the cancer hasn't spread. High-quality mammography, an X-ray technique to visualize the internal structure of the breast, helps health-care providers identify very small lumps, areas of calcification, or other tissue changes. Mammography is the best method for detecting breast cancer, but it is not perfect. Dense breast tissue, common in younger women, reduces the mammographic image and makes early diagnosis of breast cancer more difficult. Young women in particular may experience more false positives, that is, suspicious lesions found through mammography that when biopsied are shown to be benign. One of the reasons for the controversy regarding mammography for young women is the additional monetary cost and emotional turmoil of false positives. False-negative results are rare, particularly with better imaging techniques. However, because they can occur, breast-self examination and clinical breast examination are important.

Women with breast implants should know that mammographic images have limited effectiveness. They should inform the technician before the mammogram is taken. The facility needs to use special techniques designed for women with implants, and technicians need to be familiar with doing mammograms for women with breast implants.

In response to questions regarding the administration of mammography by untrained personnel and with substandard equipment, Congress passed Public Law 102–539, the Mammography Quality Standards Act (MQSA) of 1992. MQSA mandated the Department of Health and Human Services (DHHS) to develop uniform guidelines for quality assurance of mammography. The department gave the FDA authority to administer regulations, training, and oversight of facilities. In addition, the FDA established a National Mammography Quality Assurance Advisory Committee. The current guidelines require all mammography facilities to be accredited and inspected annually. Radiological equipment must be dedicated to mammography, technicians conducting and health-care providers interpreting the mammograms must be certified or licensed, and medical physicists must inspect the facilities annually. Also, facilities must maintain medical record keeping and disposition of written reports, not limiting access of women to their records.[29] The first report by the General Accounting Office (GAO) to Congress occurred in 1995. The GAO concluded that the impact of the law was positive and that the overall quality of mammography services was excellent with 80 percent of facilities having no violations or minor ones.[30]

Despite the known benefits of mammography, most women over the age of 40 have not had an initial screening mammogram and are unaware of its importance in early detection. It is frequently the fear of cancer that keeps a woman from seeking immediate treatment when she detects a change in her breast tissue.

Biopsies What happens if a lump is found? A second mammogram may be required if a positive result occurs. However, mammography cannot distinguish benign from malignant lesions with absolute certainty. The health-care provider may proceed with

mammography—imaging of the breast produced by low-dose X ray.

fine-needle aspiration, a procedure involving a very thin needle and a syringe. Fine-needle aspirations are most common in women who have large, palpable lesions. A needle is placed into the lump to determine if the lesion is solid or a fluid-filled **cyst.** If the lesion is fluid-filled, the health-care provider drains the fluid and the cyst collapses. If the cyst reappears, it can be drained again. No further treatment is necessary if the cyst does not reappear.

If the lesion is solid, the health-care provider may attempt to draw out some cells for microscopic analysis. Fine-needle aspiration biopsy of a solid mass lesion requires great skill by the health-care provider. It is important that cancerous cells be prevented from leaking out of the lesion into the body cavity.

Core needle biopsy requires local anesthesia and uses a larger needle with a special cutting edge. A small core of tissue is removed, which may cause some bruising, but rarely leaves a scar. This procedure is difficult, if not impossible, for hard or small lumps. Oftentimes, needle biopsies will be verified by surgical biopsies before further treatment is recommended.

A biopsy is the only method to determine if cancer cells are present. Whether surgical breast biopsy or needle aspiration is chosen by the health-care provider depends on the nature and location of the lump. Surgical breast biopsy increases the tissue damage, is more costly, and is currently the only available method for women with nonpalpable or small lesions.

An excisional biopsy removes the lump or suspicious tissue mass entirely. The procedure is comparable to a lumpectomy and is performed when the lump is smaller than approximately an inch in diameter. An excisional biopsy is typically performed on an outpatient basis and the woman goes home the same day.

An incisional biopsy removes a portion or cross-section of the lump. This procedure is performed under a local anesthetic as well and is recommended for lumps larger than an inch in diameter. Fully 80 percent of women in the United States who undergo surgical breast biopsies do *not* have cancer.

You should consult with your health-care provider about the procedure being considered and ask whether there will be a change to the breast itself. Obviously, this depends on the type of procedure, the size of the lump, and the location of the lump. You have a right to know what to expect! Remember, most lumps are benign.

Treatment   Research regarding the most effective treatment for breast cancer is ongoing. The treatment prescribed by the **oncologist** should be based on the most current research. Treatment will be based on the stage of cancer and the woman's preference for **lumpectomy** or **mastectomy.** Lumpectomy is the local removal of the lump, some tissue surrounding it, and lymph nodes under the arm. Partial (segmental) mastectomy entails the removal of the cancer and surrounding breast tissue, the lining over the chest muscles below the tumor, and some lymph nodes under the arm. A simple mastectomy (total) is removal of the entire breast and some lymph nodes under the arm. A modified radical mastectomy is removal of the entire breast, some lymph nodes under the arm, the lining over the chest muscles, and occasionally some part of the chest wall muscles. A radical mastectomy is the removal of the entire breast, chest muscles, and all the lymph nodes under the arm.[31] These procedures can be complemented by radiation therapy, chemotherapy, and hormonal therapy in combination or alone. A new treatment protocol under study for special cases of breast cancer is high-dose chemotherapy with bone marrow transplant or stem cell rescue.[32] Now see *Viewpoint:* "Lumpectomy or Mastectomy" and *Her Story:* "Arlette."

Viewpoint

Lumpectomy or Mastectomy?

Regaining control of your own life after the diagnosis of cancer is important. One of the first decisions facing a woman diagnosed with breast cancer is whether to have a lumpectomy or mastectomy. The literature regarding these procedures is mixed and further study is needed. Researchers at the University of Pittsburgh conducted a large study of intraductal breast cancer and concluded that lumpectomy with radiation was an acceptable strategy. They assigned women to one of two treatments, surgery without radiation and surgery with follow-up **radiotherapy.** Women who had surgery alone had a recurrence rate of 16 percent with half being invasive cancers. Women who had surgery with radiotherapy had a recurrence rate of 10 percent with 3 percent being invasive cancers. They concluded that lumpectomy with follow-up radiotherapy is effective.

Other researchers cautioned that further research is needed and if these women had opted for mastectomy, the recurrences probably would not have happened. However, 95 percent of the women did well with the less aggressive lumpectomy, rather than mastectomy. What information would you need to make this decision? What factors are most important to you?

Her Story

Arlette

Arlette is a healthy, active 52-year-old nurse practitioner. She discovered two breast masses on her routine mammogram. Nothing was noticeable on breast self-examination. Further testing including biopsies by her health-care provider determined these to be ductal carcinoma. Arlette interviewed several surgeons, looking for one who would involve her in the decisions regarding treatment. After reviewing all the options, she and her surgeon agreed that bilateral modified radical mastectomies would be the treatment of choice for her. Having used relaxation tapes with several of her clients, Arlette asked a therapist friend to make an audiotape to use during the surgery. The tape was played during the surgery not only for Arlette, but for the entire surgical team. The tape gave suggestions that she would relax and not subconsciously resist the surgery, that all would go smoothly, recovery would be rapid and

without complications. This extensive surgery usually lasts about 5 hours, but Arlette's surgery was completed in 2½ hours with minimal bleeding. She recovered quickly and returned home within a few days after surgery. Her aftercare consisted of mild chemotherapy, physical therapy to assist with recovery of her range of motion, and psychotherapy to facilitate the changes she needed to make in her lifestyle. She was back to work in a few weeks. Three years later she is cancer free. The experience precipitated many changes in her life including a complete job change and leaving an abusive, long-term relationship. Arlette continues to use meditation, massage, acupuncture, and most of all, she has learned to listen to her body. She has been heard to say, "Cancer is one of the best things that ever happened to me."

Breast Reconstruction A woman who has a mastectomy has an additional choice to make. Should she choose breast reconstruction surgery or wear a breast form or prosthesis? New methods and materials have made it possible for women to choose breast reconstruction. However, a number of factors should be considered. Breast reconstruction has some of the same risks and problems as breast implants (discussed in chap. 12 on consumerism). Breast reconstruction provides physical form to the breasts, but sensation is lost. If a woman is interested in breast reconstruction, she should inform her surgeon who consults with a plastic surgeon responsible for the breast reconstruction.

Breast reconstruction can be completed at the time of the mastectomy unless too little skin tissue or blood supply remains in the breast area. In that case, additional reconstruction will occur gradually until the skin is stretched enough to implant a permanent prosthesis. Breast reconstruction consists of inserting a silicone gel or saline-filled implant under the skin to create a breast-shaped mound or using body tissue from another site to rebuild the breast, and possibly the nipple and surrounding areola.[33]

Uterine Cancer

Cervical and endometrial cancer are the two major types of uterine cancer. Cervical cancer is nearly 100

percent curable and endometrial cancer is nearly 94 percent curable when detected early. Ovarian and uterine cancer, even though only 13 percent of the cancers of women, are exceeded only by lung, breast, and colon cancers, as causes of cancer deaths in women. On January 1, 1993, cervical carcinoma was added to the case definition as one of the AIDS-defining illnesses.

---

cyst—a closed sac in or under the skin containing liquid or semisolid material.

oncologist (on **coll** agist)—a physician who specializes in cancer care; can range from a physician who specializes in a particular kind of cancer to a particular cell type of cancer.

lumpectomy—surgical removal of breast tumor with limited removal of surrounding tissue.

mastectomy—surgical removal of one or both breasts; can range from removal of breast tissue to removal of chest muscles and lymph nodes.

radiotherapy—high-energy radiation therapy using X rays or gamma rays to treat cancer; also called radiation therapy.

Risk and Protective Factors Women who are at greatest risk for cervical cancer include those who had histories of early and continued sexual activity (with multiple partners); those with genital herpes; those infected with the human papillomavirus (transmitted from the male during intercourse and causing genital warts); those with frequent cervical infections; cigarette smoking, and low socioeconomic status.

Endometrial cancer is most common in women over the age of 50. The endometrium is the lining of the uterus. Those who are at higher risk for endometrial cancer include those with infertility problems or ovulation failure, family history of endometrial cancer, never having children, estrogen replacement therapy for two years without progesterone, or late menopause (after age 55). Women who have a combination of high blood pressure, diabetes, and obesity are also at higher risk. Tamoxifen-induced endometrial cancer tends to be more invasive and aggressive than other natural-caused endometrial cancer.

Early Detection Early warning signs for cervical cancer include dysplasia (precancerous changes in the cells), detected by regular Pap smears. Specific symptoms of cervical cancer may include: a watery, pink or brown vaginal discharge, spotting after intercourse or douching, or irregular bleeding. The Pap test is rarely effective in detecting endometrial cancer. An annual pelvic exam by a health-care provider is recommended for women aged 40 and over.

Abnormal bleeding for young women is any change in their regular cycle. Abnormal bleeding for women going through menopause might include a heavier than normal flow, a period that lasts longer or comes sooner than expected. Most often, these symptoms do not indicate cancer, but something less serious. Your health-care provider should be contacted to diagnose the problem.

Early detection is essential! The improved survival rates for women with uterine cancers reflect early diagnosis more than improved treatment.

Screening During a pelvic exam, a qualified health-care provider examines the reproductive organs for possible problems. A visual exam explores for signs of infection or injury. A Pap test is performed to extract cells from the cervix in order to detect the presence of abnormalities. A Pap smear will detect abnormal cell changes (dysplasia) several years before cervical cancer occurs. Also, the uterus

and ovaries are palpated to search for growths or tenderness.

The Pap test isn't effective in detecting endometrial cancer, thus, a pelvic exam is essential. If cancer is suspected, endometrial tissue samples can be taken for observation under a microscope. Screening techniques currently being explored include human papillomavirus (HPV) DNA typing, cervicography, loop electrosurgical excision procedure (LEEP), color flow doppler, endometrial sampling, and serum CA-15 measurements.[34]

Treatment Uterine cancer is generally treated by surgery, radiation, hormones, and/or chemotherapy. As yet, the optimal therapy has not been defined. "In precancerous (in situ) stages, changes in the cervix may be treated by cryotherapy (the destruction of cells by extreme cold), by electrocoagulation (the destruction of tissue through intense heat by electric current), or by local surgery."[35]

Ovarian Cancer

A study by the NCI suggests that African American women have a lower risk of ovarian cancer than white women. Nine in 100,000 African American women compared to 14 in 100,000 white women develop ovarian cancer. Ovarian cancer causes more deaths than any other gynecological cancer. It accounts for approximately 18 percent of female reproductive cancers and 4 percent of all cancers in women. Often, the prognosis is poor with a survival rate of less than 40 percent.

Risk and Protective Factors The risk factors for ovarian cancer include being over age 50, a family history of ovarian cancer, a history of irregular menstrual periods, never having children, and previous breast, colon, or endometrial cancer. Current research suggests that women using fertility drugs may increase their risk of ovarian cancer. Pregnancy, breast-feeding, tubal sterilization, and birth control pills appear to reduce the risk of ovarian cancer in women.[36] Although no one is sure why oral contraceptives and tubal sterilization reduce the risk of ovarian cancer, reduction in the number of ovulations a woman has appears to be linked.

Early Detection Hypertension is called the "silent killer." For women, ovarian cancer is also a "silent" killer. By the time the signs and symptoms appear, the ovarian cancer is usually in its later stages. Warning signs include a swollen abdomen (caused by fluid retention), abnormal vaginal bleeding, and persistent digestive disturbances (indigestion or gas).

Screening Ultrasonography, CA-125 radioimmunoassay (CA-125 is a tumor marker in the blood), and physical examinations are used for screening of ovarian cancer. A concern with using these tests for routine screening are the large number of false positives due to insensitivity, thus screening is contraindicated in most women. Only women with hereditary cancer syndrome and a family history of ovarian cancer might benefit from routine screening.[37] Currently, researchers at the University of California, Irvine Clinical Cancer Center are conducting trials on a new blood test that may detect the disease earlier than existing methods.[38]

Treatment Ovarian cancer is the leading cause of death from gynecological malignancy in the United States. Since the death of comedian Gilda Radner, much attention and resources have gone into addressing this disease. Treatment options include surgery, radiation therapy, and drug therapy. Unfortunately, the five-year survival rate remains less than 40 percent despite aggressive cytoreductive surgery and chemotherapy.[39]

Skin Cancer

Skin cancer is the most prevalent and most curable type of cancer found in women. Over 900,000 persons (males and females) are diagnosed with basal and squamous cell skin cancer and 90 percent of these could be prevented by protection from the sun.[40] Basal cell carcinomas are the most common type of malignancy in humans. They are usually raised, hard, reddish lesions with a pearly surface and rarely metastasize. Squamous cell carcinoma is most frequently found on the skin, but is also located in the epithelium of the lungs, anus, cervix, larynx, nose, and bladder. These carcinomas are typically scaly and slightly elevated. They are a relatively, slow-growing malignancy.

Malignant **melanoma** is less common than other types of skin cancer, but more dangerous. Nearly 40,300 people will be diagnosed with melanoma in 1997. Melanoma begins in melanocytes, the cells responsible for producing melanin. Melanin turns darker when exposed to sunlight, thus producing a *suntan* to protect the body from burning. Melanoma

accounts for only 5 percent of all skin cancers, but 75 percent of all skin cancer deaths.[41] In 1994, an estimated 15,000 women were diagnosed with melanoma and 2,600 women died. This skin cancer is twenty times more prevalent in white women than African American women. Melanoma is usually found on the lower legs of white women and on the palms, skin under the nails, and soles of the feet of African American women. Skin cancers are the most frequent secondary lesions in patients with cancers in other sites.

Risk and Protective Factors Severe sunburning during early childhood and excessive exposure to sunlight during adolescence are known risk factors for skin cancer. Other risk factors include fair or lightly pigmented skin, occupational exposure to some products, and family history. The best protective factors to prevent skin cancer are adequate clothing, use of a proper sunscreen with solar protection factor (SPF 15 or higher), and limiting one's exposure to the sun (avoiding midday sun). Sunscreen should be applied at least 15 to 30 minutes before going in the sun, and applied frequently. Ninety percent of skin cancers occur on the parts of the body exposed most to the sun, such as the face, hands, forearms, and ears.

The National Weather Bureau, in cooperation with the Environmental Protection Agency and the Centers for Disease Control, provides sun tanners with an Ultraviolet Index to determine the amount of safe time in the sun. The UV Index is a forecast of the peak amount of UV radiation to reach the earth's surface in a given location when the sun is at its highest peak, during the solar noon hour, from 30 minutes before and after 12 noon. Safeguards under moderate ranges include minimizing exposure during peak times, using sunscreens of SPF 15 or higher, wearing clothing to cover the body, and wearing hats to shade the face and neck. (See *FYI:* "Ultraviolet [UV] Index.")

Early Detection Basal cell cancers first appear as white or gray, small round or oval patches on the skin that are shiny and firm. Squamous cell cancers appear as small, round, and raised areas that are red and

---

melanoma—any of a group of skin cancers made up of melanocytes.

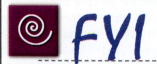

FYI

Ultraviolet (UV) Index

You should know the exposure level for ultraviolet rays and use the appropriate sunscreen. Avoid high and very high levels whenever possible.

Exposure Range	Category
0–2	Minimal
3–4	Low
5–6	Moderate
7–9	High
10–15	Very high

crusty. A sore that won't heal may appear in the middle of a squamous cell cancer. The American Cancer Society[42] recommends the following set of guidelines for detecting melanoma (see Fig. 20.2 and 20.3):

A is for asymmetry

B is for border irregularity

C is for color (change)

D is for a diameter greater than 6 mm ($\frac{1}{4}$ inch)

Screening The best way to become familiar with your skin is to examine it regularly, every six to eight weeks. If a health-care provider thinks you may have skin cancer, a biopsy (a small sample of tissue) will be taken from the area.

Treatment A combination of surgery (90 percent of all cases), radiation therapy, laser therapy, and tissue destruction (either by heat or freezing) are most often used to treat skin cancer. The primary growth and surrounding lymph cells must be removed with malignant melanoma.[43]

Tanning Beds Most modern tanning beds emit predominately UVA radiation, with small amounts of UVB. UVB rays are the harmful rays emitted by the sun, and are particularly important with the reduction in ozone layers. Tanning salon operators point out that UVA rays are not harmful. They suggest that you should only be concerned with UVB rays. They use this difference as a selling point for the safety of tanning beds. They equate a suntan with good health. However, research demonstrates that exposure to UVA leads to increased skin wrinkling, irregu-

FIGURE 20.2 (*A*) Basal cell carcinoma. (*B*) Squamous cell carcinoma.

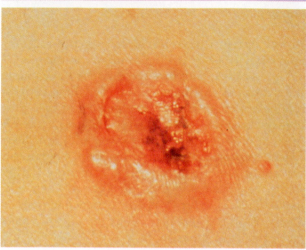

A

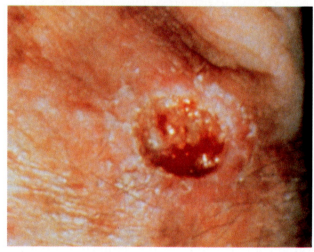

B

lar pigmentation (including deeply pigmented freckles), and systemic immune system suppression. And, tanning in UVA rays does not prepare you for exposure to the UVB rays of the sun. Thus, tanning indoors before spring break does *not* prevent a sunburn. The best way to avoid premature wrinkling and aging of the skin and to prevent skin cancer is to stay away from tanning beds and out of the sun.

Colorectal Cancer

In 1994, an estimated 74,000 new cases of colon and rectal cancer were detected in women and 28,200 women died from the disease. Over 93 percent of

FIGURE 20.3 Guidelines for detecting melanoma.

Asymmetry
One half
unlike the
other half

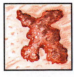

Irregularity
Border
irregular
or poorly
circumscribed

Color
Color varies
from one
area to
another;
shades of tan,
brown, or black

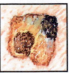

Size
Diameter
larger than
6 mm as a
rule (diameter
of a pencil
eraser)

these cases occurred in individuals over 50 years of age.[44] In 1997, an estimated 64,800 women will get colon and rectal cancer and 27,900 women will die.

Risk and Protective Factors Risk factors include a personal or family history of colorectal cancer, polyps in the colon, or ulcerative colitis. Polyps, masses of tissue that grow inward from the wall of the bowel, are known precursors to colorectal cancer. High-fat and low-fiber diets, physical inactivity, and low intake of fruits and vegetables are possible risk factors.[45]

Early Detection Three simple tests can be used to detect colorectal cancer: (1) stool blood test, (2) digital rectal examination by your health-care provider, and (3) sigmoidoscopy examination. The stool blood test checks the stool for hidden blood, a possible sign of cancer or other internal conditions. A woman prepares a special slide and gives it to her health-care provider. A digital rectal examination is performed to determine the presence of a tumor. If necessary, a fiber-optic sigmoidoscope (a flexible, hollow, lighted tube) is used to examine the rectum and lower colon.

If a woman experiences a persistent change in bowel habits, rectal bleeding, or cramping pain in the abdomen, she should consult her health-care provider immediately. Early detection of cancer in polyps reduces the likelihood of metastasis to other body sites, the need for major surgery, or for a colostomy.

Screening The American Cancer Society has set the following guidelines for colon and rectal cancer detection for any woman without symptoms. A digital rectal examination is recommended for women every year after age 40. A stool blood test should be done yearly and a sigmoidoscopy examination every three to five years after age 50.

Treatment The incidence and mortality rates have declined in recent years as women are being screened earlier and polyps are removed before progression to invasive cancer.[46] If colorectal cancer is found, surgery with a possible follow-up of radiation therapy will occur. Chemotherapy may be effective after surgery in certain colon cancers if the tumor has penetrated the bowel wall.

Many women are afraid that colorectal cancer means living with a colostomy, an insertion in the abdomen for the elimination of body wastes. The American Cancer Society states, "Permanent colostomy (creation of an abdominal opening for elimination of body wastes) is seldom needed for colon cancer and is infrequently required for rectal cancer."[47] Thus, the fear of colostomies should not be a deterrent to early diagnosis.

Health Tips: "Protective Factors to Fight Against Cancer" suggests ways to reduce your risk of cancer.

ACTIONS TO TAKE WHEN CANCER IS DIAGNOSED

When the diagnosis of cancer occurs, a common reaction is to feel like life is out of control. A woman can take a number of steps toward regaining control over her life. First, get more information about the particular cancer. As stated earlier, there are over a hundred different cancers, and each primary site could be one of several different kinds of cancers. Once a woman knows the type of cancer, she can call the National Cancer Institute (1–800–4–CANCER) or the American Cancer Society for more information. NCI provides booklets explaining the cancer, names of oncologists

health tips

Protective Factors to Fight Against Cancer

You can practice these protective factors to reduce your risk of cancer.

- Do not smoke
- Live with a nonsmoker
- Avoid smoke-filled areas
- Maintain your desirable weight
- Eat a wide variety of foods
- Eat in moderation
- Consume fresh fruits and vegetables daily (five servings daily)
- Eat plenty of high-fiber foods
- Limit fat intake (under 20 percent of total calories)
- Limit alcohol consumption

- Consume little or no salt-cured, smoked, or nitrite-cured foods
- Limit exposure to sunlight
- Limit exposure to industrial agents, asbestos, and radon
- Limit exposure to radiation
- If you are 20 to 39 years old, get a cancer-related checkup every three years
- If you are 40 years or older, get a cancer-related checkup annually
- If you are 18 years or older, have an annual Pap test and pelvic exam
- Practice monthly breast self-examination

in the area, sites of clinical trials, and PDQ statements regarding the latest treatments.

Second, get a second opinion before deciding on a particular treatment protocol. Seeking confirmation is reasonable and common. The second oncologist should be informed about the initial diagnosis. She or he will likely be more direct and straightforward with recommendations, particularly because an expert opinion is being solicited, rather than a request for involvement in the patient's progress.

Third, a woman should feel certain about her options. Any questions and responses that are not fully understood should be addressed. If an NCI-designated comprehensive or clinical cancer center is nearby, choose it. The specialists at these centers are most familiar with current treatment protocols and any recent research developments. The primary health-care provider and surgeon should be board certified in cancer care, such as an oncologist or oncology surgeon.

SOCIAL SUPPORT

Social support is a critical factor in recovery from a stressful event such as cancer. Support from family and friends plays a major role in the speed and level of recovery. Unfortunately, women with cancer seem to lose the level of support they enjoyed before the diagnosis of cancer. The fear of cancer causes some people to avoid contact with anyone or anything that reminds them of it. Cancer, compared to other chronic diseases, is a stigmatized condition. In fact, many people still believe that the diagnosis of

cancer is a death sentence. And, a majority also believe that cancer is contagious. Thus, being in the presence of someone with cancer may mean exposing one's self to unnecessary risks.[48]

Women who have undergone a modified radical mastectomy report that their most common concerns are the inability to engage in vigorous physical activity, the fear that the cancer will return, and resentment or worry regarding the quality of care received.[49] Women with chronic diseases such as heart disease feel some control over their destiny, such as when they can modify their diet and increase their physical activity level. This control provides them with a sense of doing something to improve their chance of survival. However, women living with cancer do not have the same opportunity to exhibit control.

The treatment for cancer may preclude women from continuing to engage in social activities. They may not have the same energy level as before and may focus their efforts on necessary tasks such as work and family. Outside activities may need to be curtailed during their period of recovery and social contacts may become lost or less frequent. Cancer survivors who reported energy losses due to treatment also indicated a reduction in discretionary activities and social network size.[50] These reductions may lead to lower levels of emotional and physical support at a time when support is most needed! The American Cancer Society has recognized this need for support and provides several services for women and their families including the following: *Road to*

Recovery, a program that provides transportation to get patients to and from treatment; *Reach to Recovery,* a program of breast cancer survivors who help women and their families deal with breast cancer; *Look Good . . . Feel Good,* a service to help women deal with personal appearance during chemotherapy and radiation treatments, and *I Can Cope,* a cancer education program provided by health-care professionals and community representatives.[51]

COMPLEMENTARY TREATMENT IN CANCER MANAGEMENT

This chapter would not be complete without mention of the complementary therapies used to overcome cancer. When medical therapies do not appear to provide the wanted results (whether by perception or in actuality), women often turn to complementary treatments to supplement the medical therapy. They have read about successes in popular magazines or heard about miracles from friends and family. The American Cancer Society continually reviews current practices, attempting to determine the benefit in the treatment of cancer in human beings. A few of these complementary therapies follow. If you want information regarding the research on these and other therapies, check with the American Cancer Society or the National Institutes of Health for the most current findings.

Magnetic and Electronic Devices

Magnetic and electronic devices use cosmic rays, gamma rays, X rays, light waves, radio waves, and others to cure or slow the progression of cancer. Individuals using electronic devices in complementary therapies appeal to the balancing of life forces, the energy in the body.

Conventional therapies also use a variety of electronic devices, except these procedures have been accepted by the medical community. These devices are used for radiation therapy, magnetic resonance imaging, diagnostic X rays, and others.

Radionic Devices Radionics theorize that radiolike frequencies emitted from pathogens can be used to diagnose and treat diseases. The first radionic device was called the Oscilloclast, which detected diseases by their vibratory rates. Many of the radionic devices used in cancer treatment today are imitations of this model.

Galvanic Devices Galvanic devices are being used by "Energy Medicine," a field using electrodes placed at acupuncture points to measure electrical resistance. Galvanic devices actually measure electrical resistance on the skin and can be influenced by skin moisture and the amount of pressure with which the probe is applied.

Low-Level Output Electrical Devices Low-level output electrical devices are used by some practitioners to treat cancer by passing currents through tumors or to actually diagnose cancer. Scientific experimentation using this procedure with cancer treatment is currently being conducted and these legitimate experimental protocols are registered with the FDA. Fraudulent claims continue to surface with the FDA obtaining injunctions when possible.

Magnetic Devices Many makers of some permanent magnetic devices have been prosecuted by the FDA for false advertising. Electromagnetic devices differ in that they need a power source to activate the magnetism. These devices have not been proven to be effective in cancer treatment.

Color and Light Treatment Devices This therapy theorizes that shining colored light on the body can cure cancer. The FDA secured a permanent injunction against the use of spectrachrome devices but they still find their way into some offices. The use of full-spectrum fluorescent light to prevent cancer has been proposed by some practitioners, however full-spectrum light treatment includes UV light, a known carcinogen for skin cancer.

Food Remedies

Vegetarian Diets A wide array of vegetarian diets have been tried by women with cancer in an effort to slow the progression of the disease. Vegetarians do not eat meat, fish, or poultry, but some will eat products with animal by-products. Vegans consume only foods with plant origin, whereas lacto-vegetarians consume foods with plant origin and dairy products. The Zen macrobiotic diet consists mainly of cereals, such as rice. It is a low-fat, complex carbohydrate diet with no animal products, no refined sugar, and limited fluids. Miso, a soybean product believed to prevent cancer, is a staple of this diet.

Herbal and Vitamin Therapy An array of complementary treatments have been touted, including megavitamin therapy, enzyme therapy, shiitake mushrooms, shark cartilage, Essiac herbs, wheatgrass, coffee enemas, and others.

Hoxsey therapy, a special herbal tonic, evolved when a farmer decided to collect herbs that had healed his cancerous horse. This therapy was banned by the FDA in 1960, but it is still available in Mexico. Shark cartilage therapy evolved because sharks are believed to seldom get cancer. Thus, proponents suggest that shark cartilage should be tested for its cancer inhibiting ability.

Linus Pauling, a Nobel Prize winning chemist, championed the use of vitamin C for a number of ailments. He recommended megadoses of vitamin C and suggested that current RDAs were much too low.

Spiritual and Meditation Practices

Relaxation   A variety of relaxation techniques have been touted as beneficial for women with cancer, not so much as cures but rather as adjuvant therapy. Creative visualization, affirmations, biofeedback, self-hypnosis, humor, art and music therapy, and meditation were discussed in chapter 6.

Acupuncture and Acupressure   Acupuncture is an ancient Chinese form of healing that views that all matter contains Yin/Yang energy. The balancing of life force (qi or "chee") must be maintained for harmony and health, and disease occurs when qi is blocked or flows unevenly. To rebalance qi, fine needles are placed in precisely determined sites to stimulate nerve impulses. These needles are manipulated to increase or decrease the flow of qi. Acupressure treats the whole body by using pressure points to stimulate the harmony of life forces. The points for these techniques are located along twelve meridians, related to the internal organs. Diseases can be diagnosed and cured by addressing the specific points on

JOURNAL ACTIVITY
Complementary Cancer Therapy

Research a complementary treatment approach to cancer. How would you analyze its effectiveness in cancer treatment based on the criteria provided in chapter 12 on consumer health? Would you suggest this complementary treatment to a friend with cancer? Why or why not?

the meridians. Chapter 6 discusses acupressure, a related aspect, and provides further information regarding this technique. Now complete *Journal Activity:* "Complementary Cancer Therapy."

CHOOSING A TREATMENT PLAN

A woman diagnosed with cancer or a recurrence of cancer faces a myriad of decisions, including the choice of medical and complementary treatments. Complementary methods have been touted by too many individuals to be dismissed. Yet, grasping at straws does not provide a sense of control. Knowledge and accurate evaluation of the effectiveness of conventional therapy and alternative treatment protocols is the best method to begin recapturing control. The first step for any woman is to focus on those things most within her control, including becoming more familiar with the treatment options available to her. Deciding whether to follow conventional therapy alone, or a combination of conventional and complementary therapies depends on an accurate diagnosis by an oncologist, and a clear picture of the prognosis for that particular type of cancer. A woman needs to be involved in the process of decision making throughout the treatment and recovery phase. Remember: Early detection is important to your well-being!

Chapter Summary

- Half of all cancers affecting women are cancers of the reproductive system.
- The World Health Organization has identified forty-six body sites and numerous cancers at each site, over a hundred different cancers.
- The warning signs of cancer (CAUTION) are important to know.

- Lifestyle and environmental factors account for most cancer risk.
- The amount of fat a person consumes is a risk factor for some cancers.
- Cigarette smoking accounts for 87 percent of all lung cancer deaths and 30 percent of all cancer deaths.
- Lung cancer is the leading cause of cancer deaths in women.

- Screening mammography complemented by regular breast self-examinations and clinical breast examinations are the best methods for early detection of breast cancer.
- Cervical and endometrial cancer are extremely curable if detected early.
- Skin cancer is the most prevalent and most curable type of cancer found in women.
- Melanoma can be detected by attention to **a**symmetry, **b**order irregularity, **c**olor change, and **d**iameter greater than 6 mm.

- Tanning beds emit UVA rays that contribute to skin wrinkling, irregular pigmentation, and immunosuppression.
- Social support is a critical factor in recovering from cancer.
- Many women explore complementary therapies as an adjunct to conventional health care.
- An important source of information regarding cancer facts, treatment, and physician referrals is 1–800–4–CANCER.

Review Questions

1. What are the seven warning signs of cancer?
2. What are the definitions for the following terms: benign, malignant, metastasis, in situ, and invasive?
3. What are the four most common categories of cancer?
4. What are some of the lifestyle and environmental causes of cancer?
5. What are the leading cancer sites in women based on race and ethnicity?

6. What are the early signs and symptoms for each of the following cancers: lung, breast, uterine, and ovarian?
7. What are the five best preventive measures a woman can practice to reduce the risk of cancer? What criteria did you use to determine these choices?
8. What are some of the complementary therapies a woman might select to supplement conventional therapy?

Resources

Organizations and Hotlines

American Cancer Society
Telephone: (800) ACS–2345.

National Breast Cancer Coalition
P.O. Box 66373
Washington, D.C. 20035
Telephone: (202) 296–7477
Telephone: (202) 265–6854 (fax)
Grassroots advocacy group seeking funds for research and better access to care

American Association of Retired Persons
Lobby for a strong government research program for breast cancer, access to care for all women, and concerns of women with cancer.

The Women's Community Cancer Project
c/o The Women's Center
46 Pleasant Street
Cambridge, MA 02139
Telephone: (617) 354–9888
Established in 1989 to address changes in the social, political, and medical approaches to cancer in women.

National Cancer Institute
Provides up-to-date information about cancer
Telephone: (800) 4–CANCER

Corporate Angel Network, Inc.
Westchester Country Airport, One Loop Road
White Plains, NY 10604
Telephone: (800) 328–4226 (fax)
Telephone: (914) 328–1313
www.corpangelnetwork.org
Attempts to match patients needing to travel by air for cancer treatment with space on corporate airplanes operating on business flights

Gilda Radner Familial Ovarian Cancer Registry
Roswell Park Cancer Institute
New York Department of Health
Elm and Carlton Streets
Buffalo, New York 14263
Telephone: (800) 682–7426

NIH Consensus Program Clearinghouse
P.O. Box 2577
Kensington, MD 20891
Voice Mail: (800) NIH–OMAR
Telephone: (301) 816–2494 (fax)
Telephone: (301) 816–9840 (e-mail)
Up-to-date official consensus statements on a variety of subjects, including cancer

Intercultural Cancer Council
1720 Dryden, Suite C
Houston, TX 77030

Websites

National Cancer Institute
www.nci.nih.gov

American Cancer Society
www.cancer.org

Intercultural Cancer Council
icc.bcm.tmc.edu

Ask NOAH
www.noah.cuny.edu

Memorial Sloan-Kettering Cancer Center
www.mskcc.org

Mayo Clinic
www.mayo.ivi.com

Suggested Readings

Dollinger, M., E. H. Rosenbaum, and G. Cable. 1994. *Everyone's guide to cancer therapy: How cancer is diagnosed, treated, and managed day to day.* Kansas City, MO: Andrews and McMeel, Universal Press Syndicate Company.

Kastner, M., and H. Burroughs. 1993. *Alternative healing: The complete A–Z guide to over 160 different alternative therapies.* LaMesa, CA: Halcyon Publishing.

Lerner, M. 1996. *Choice in healing: Integrating the best of conventional and complementary approaches to cancer.* Cambridge, MA: MIT Press (Trd).

Love, S. 1995. *Dr. Susan Love's breast book.* Reading, MA: Addison-Wesley Longman Publishing Company.

McGinn, K. A., and P. J. Haylock. 1993. *Women's cancers: How to prevent them, how to treat them, how to beat them.* Alameda, CA: Hunter House Inc., Publishers.

Walters, R. 1992. *Options: The alternative cancer therapy book.* Garden City Park, NY: Avery Publishing Group, Inc.

References

1. *Mosby's medical, nursing, and allied health dictionary,* 4th Edition. 1994. St. Louis: Mosby-Year Book, Inc.
2. Dollinger, M., E. H. Rosenbaum, and G. Cable. 1991. *Everyone's guide to cancer therapy: How cancer is diagnosed, treated, and managed day to day.* Kansas City, Mo.: Andrews and McMeel.
3. Ibid.
4. American Cancer Society. 1997. *Cancer facts & figures—1997.* Atlanta, Ga.: American Cancer Society, Inc.
5. Ibid.
6. Ibid.
7. Ibid.
8. Thun, M. J., and others. 1994. Hair dye use and the risk of fatal cancers in U.S. women. *Journal of the National Cancer Institute,* 86: 210.
9. Hair dye study. 1994. *FDA Consumer:* 4.
10. Jackson, J. D. 1992. Are the stray 60-Hz electromagnetic fields associated with the distribution and use of electric power a significant cause of cancer? *Proceedings of the National Academy of Sciences of the United States,* 89: 3508.
11. Hartwell, L. H., and M. B. Kastan. 1994. Cell cycle control and cancer. *Science,* 266: 1821–27.
12. Marx, J. January 21, 1994. How cells cycle toward cancer. *Science,* 263: 319–21.
13. American Cancer Society. Cancer facts & figures—1994.
14. Karp, J. E., and S. Broder. Oncology and hematology. *Journal of the American Medical Association,* 271: 1693.
15. Easton, D. F., T. Bishop, D. Ford, and B. P. Crockford. 1993. Breast cancer linkage consortium. *American Journal of Human Genetics,* 52: 678.
16. Toguchida, J., and others. 1992. Prevalence and spectrum of germlike mutations of the p53 gene among patients with sarcoma. *New England Journal of Medicine,* 326: 1301.
17. Drobnjak, M., and others. 1994. Prognostic implications of p53 nuclear overexpression and high proliferation index of Ki-67 in adult soft-tissue sarcomas. *Journal of the National Cancer Institute,* 86: 549.
18. Cancer facts & figures—1994.
19. Cancer facts & figures—1997.
20. McDougall, J. C. 1994. Lung cancer: To screen or not to screen? *Archives of Internal Medicine,* 154: 945.
21. Flehinger, B. J., M. Kimmell, T. Polyak, and M. R. Melamed. 1993. Screening for lung cancer: The Mayo Lung Project revisited. *Cancer,* 72: 1573.
22. Cancer facts and figures—1997.
23. Cancer facts & figures—1994.
24. Cancer facts & figures—1997.
25. Ibid.
26. Studies spark new tamoxifen controversy. February 26, 1994. *Science News:* 133.
27. Pearson, C. 1994. NCI warns women on tamoxifen of risk of fatal uterine cancer changes in prevention trial consent form too little, too late. *The Network News,* 19: 4.
28. American Cancer Society. 1987. *Facts on breast cancer.* Revised 1991.

29. Segal, M. March, 1994. Mammography facilities must meet quality standards. *FDA Consumer:* 8.

30. GAO Report on Mammography Inspections. January 30, 1997. FDA Talk Papers. Food and Drug Administration, DHHS: Public Health Service.

31. National Cancer Institute's Cancer Information Service. Breast cancer. PDQ capsule summary statement. National Cancer Institute, National Institutes of Health. December, 1996.

32. Cancer facts & figures—1997.

33. American Cancer Society, *Facts on breast cancer.*

34. Averette, H. E., A. Steren, and H. N. Nguyen. 1993. Screening in gynecologic cancers. *Cancer,* 72: 1043.

35. Cancer facts & figures—1994.

36. Whittemore, A. S., R. Harris, J. Itnyre, and the Collaborative Ovarian Cancer Group. 1992. Characteristics relating to ovarian cancer risk: Collaborative analysis of 12 case-control studies, II: Invasive epithelial ovarian cancers in white women. *American Journal of Epidemiology,* 136: 1184–1203.

37. Carlson, K. J., S. J. Skates, and D. E. Singer. 1994. Screening for ovarian cancer. *Annals of Internal Medicine,* 121: 124.

38. Researchers begin trials on new test for cancer. June 13, 1994. *Cancer Researcher Weekly:* 3.

39. Cancer facts & figures—1994.

40. Cancer facts & figures—1997.

41. American Cancer Society. 1988. *Facts on skin cancer.* Revised 1992.

42. Ibid.

43. Cancer facts & figures—1997.

44. Ibid.

45. Ibid.

46. Ibid.

47. Ibid., p.11.

48. Bloom, J. R., K. Grazier, F. Hodge, and W. Hayes. 1991. Factors affecting the use of screening mammography among African American women. *Cancer Epidemiology, Biomarkers, and Prevention,* 1: 75–82.

49. Zemore, R., J. Rinholm, L. Shepel, and M. Richards. 1990. Some social and emotional consequences of breast cancer and mastectomy: A content analysis of 87 interviews. *Journal of Psychosocial Oncology,* 7: 33–45.

50. Bloom, J. R., and L. Kessler. 1994. Emotional support following cancer: A test of the stigma and social activity hypotheses. *Journal of Health and Social Behavior,* 35: 118–33.

51. Cancer facts & figures—1997.

Credits

Chapter 1

p. 3: *But the Difference* in *Listening to Dancing,* Huddersfield, England: Smith/Doorstop Books, 1996, © Janet Fisher; used with permission; **pp. 3, 4, 5:** *photos* by Cynthia K. Chandler.

Chapter 2

p. 17 (Fig. 2.1): Reprinted from *Journal of Counseling and Development,* vol. 71, no. 2, p. 171, 1992 © ACA. Reprinted with permission. No further reproduction authorized without written permission of the American Counseling Association; **p. 23 (Fig. 2.3):** "Maslow's Hierarchy of Needs" from *Motivation and Personality,* 3rd ed. by Abraham H. Maslow. Copyright © 1954, 1987 by Harper & Row, Publishers, Inc. Copyright 1970 by Abraham H. Maslow. Reprinted by permission of Addison Wesley Educational Publishers, Inc; **pp. 18, 20:** *photos* by Cynthia K. Chandler.

Chapter 3

pp. 38, 45, 48, 49, 51: *photos* by Cynthia K. Chandler; **p. 50 (Fig. 3.1):** Source: US Census Bureau; adapted from Postsecondary Education Opportunity, PO Box 127, Iowa City, IA 52244.

Chapter 4

pp. 61–62: From *Educational Gerontology,* vol. 20 (8), pp. 251-254, DK Harris and PS Changas, Taylor & Francis, Inc., Washington, DC. Reproduced with permission. All rights reserved; **pp. 56, 58, 59, 61, 66:** *photos* by Cynthia K. Chandler.

Chapter 5

p. 79 (Assess Yourself): From Cash, T, and Labarge, A: Development of the Appearance Schemas Inventory: A new cognitive body-image assessment. *Cognitive Therapy and Research* 20 (1): 37-50, 1996. Reprinted with permission of Thomas F. Cash, Ph.D., and Plenum Publishing Corporation; **pp. 72, 74, 87:** *photos* by Cynthia K. Chandler.

Chapter 6

p. 92: *Nine to Five* by Dolly Parton (Velvet Apple Music, © 1980). Reproduced with permission; **p. 92 (Fig. 6.2):** From Payne, W, and Hahn, D, *Understanding Your Health,* Dubuque, IA: WCB/McGraw-Hill, 1998;

p. 101 (Assess Yourself): From Chandler, C, and Kolander, C: Quick and effective stress screening. *Human stress: current selected research,* 5, pp. 203-206, 1997. Reproduced with permission; **pp. 92, 94, 109, 113:** *photos* by Cynthia K. Chandler; **p. 111:** *photo* courtesy of The University of North Texas.

Chapter 7

p. 120 (Assess Yourself): Modified from Wardlaw, GM: *Contemporary nutrition: issues and insights,* Dubuque, IA: Brown & Benchmark, 1997; **p. 122:** PhotoDisc; **p. 124 (Fig. 7.1):** US Department of Agriculture/US Department of Health and Human Services, August, 1992; **pp. 129, 130, 131 (Tables 7.1, 7.2, 7.3):** From Wardlaw, GM: *Contemporary nutrition: issues and insights,* Dubuque, IA: Brown & Benchmark, 1997; **p. 135 (Table 7.5):** Modified from Food and Nutrition Board, National Research Council: *Recommended dietary allowances,* ed 10, Washington, DC, 1989, National Academy of Sciences; **p. 139:** PhotoDisc; **p. 143 (Fig. 7.3):** Food and Drug Administration; **p. 144 (Table 7.8):** Reprinted with permission of the Metropolitan Life Insurance Company. Source: Statistical Bulletin.

Chapter 8

pp. 156, 158 (Figs. 8.1, 8.2, 8.3, 8.4): *photos* by James Robinson; **p. 157 (Health Tips):** Modified from Prentice, WE: *Fitness for college and life,* St. Louis: Mosby-Year Book, Inc., 1997 and Fahey, TD, Insel, PM, Roth, WT: *Fit & well: core concepts and labs in physical fitness and wellness,* Mountain View, CA: Mayfield Publishing Co, 1997; **p. 162 (Fig. 8.5) left:** photo by Diana Linsley; **p. 162 (Fig. 8.5) right:** From Payne, WA, and Hahn, DB: *Understanding your health,* Dubuque, IA: WCB/McGraw-Hill Higher Education, 1998, artwork by Jeanne Robertson; **p. 162 (Fig. 8.6):** Adapted from Guthrie, H: *Introductory nutrition,* St. Louis: Mosby-Year Book, Inc., 1989, pp. 205-206, in Payne, WA, and Hahn, DB: *Understanding your health,* Dubuque, IA: WCB/McGraw-Hill Higher Education, 1998; **p. 163 (Table 8.7):** From Payne, WA, and Hahn, DB: *Understanding your health,* Dubuque, IA: WCB/McGraw-Hill Higher Education, 1998; **p. 164 (Journal Activity):** Adapted from Fahey, TD, Insel, PM, Roth,

WT: *Fit & well: core concepts and labs in physical fitness and wellness,* Mountain View, CA: Mayfield Publishing Co, 1997; **p. 167 (FYI):** Adapted from Exercise and women's health, *National women's health report,* 17 (1): 1-3, 7, 1995; **p. 169 (Fig. 8.7):** photo by Kathy Sedovic.

Chapter 9

p. 76 (Fig. 9.1): *photo* by Wolff Communications; **p. 183 (Fig. 9.2):** From Ray, O and Ksir, C: *Drugs, society, and human behavior,* St. Louis: Mosby-Year Book, Inc., 1996, photo by CLG Photographics; **p. 186 (Table 9.2):** Modified from the American Cancer Society for School Health Advocates: *The Advocate* IV (1), 1, 1992. Source: The American Cancer Society and The Centers for Disease Control.

Chapter 10

pp. 198, 202 (Tables 10.2, 10.4): Adapted from Payne, WA, Hahn, DB: *Understanding your health,* Dubuque, IA: WCB/McGraw Hill Higher Education, 1998; **p. 205 (Fig. 10.2),** From Streissguth, A: Teratogenic effects of alcohol in humans and laboratory animals, *Science,* 209:353, July 18, 1980, © 1980 by the AAAS; **pp. 208, 215 (quotes):** Excerpts from *Women Who Run With the Wolves* by Clarissa Pinkola Estés, Ph.D. Copyright © 1992, 1995. All rights including but not limited to performance, derivative, adaptation, musical, audio and recording, illustrative, theatrical, film, pictorial, reprint, and electronic are reserved. Reprinted by kind permission of the author, Dr. Estés, and Ballantine Books, a division of Random House, Inc.

Chapter 12

p. 244 (Fig. 12.2): *photo* by Cynthia K. Chandler; **p. 245 (FYI):** Adapted from What therapists' degrees mean, *Harvard Women's Health Watch,* 111 (10):5, June, 1966; **p. 250 (FYI):** Adapted from Chiropractors, *Consumer Reports,* 59 (6): 383-390, 1994; **p. 257 (FYI):** Adapted from Barrett, S, et al: *Consumer health: a guide to intelligent decisions,* Madison, WI: Brown & Benchmark, 1997; **p. 264 (Fig. 12.3):** Source: US Office of Consumers Affairs: *Consumer Resource Handbook,* Washington, DC, 1997.

Chapter 13

p. 271 (Her Story): Reproduced with permission; **p. 276 (Health Tips):** Reprinted from the brochure "Is Dating Dangerous?" with permission from the American College Health Association, PO Box 28937, Baltimore, MD 21240–8937; **p. 278 (quote):** Excerpted from Wilson, MD, and Daly, M: Who kills whom in spouse killings? On the exceptional sex ratio of spousal homicides in the United States, *Criminology*, 30, November, 1992; **p. 279 (Fig. 13.1):** PhotoDisc; **p. 282 (FYI):** From *Behind closed doors: violence in the American family*, © 1980 by Richard J. Gelles and Murray A. Straus. Reprinted with permission; **p. 290 (poem):** © 1993 Portia Nelson; from *There's a hole in my sidewalk*, Hillsboro, OR: Beyond Words Publishing, Inc. (800) 284-9673.

Chapter 14

p. 298 (Assess Yourself): Modified from Payne, WA and Hahn, DB: Understanding your health, Dubuque, IA: WCB/McGraw-Hill Higher Education, 1998; **p. 303 (FYI):** Adapted from Manning, WD and Landale, NS: Racial and ethnic differences in the role of cohabitation in premarital childbearing, *Journal of Marriage and the Family* 58: 63-77.

Chapter 15

p. 314 (Fig. 15.1): From Payne, WA and Hahn, DB: *Understanding your health*, Dubuque, IA: WCB/McGraw-Hill Higher Education, 1998; **p. 315 (Her Story):** Adapted from Fleeing mutilation, fighting for asylum, *Ms. Magazine*: 12–16, February, 1996; **p. 317 (Fig. 15.2):** From Wardlaw, GM: *Contemporary nutrition: issues and insights*, Dubuque, IA: Brown & Benchmark, 1997; **p. 318 (Fig. 15.3):** Modified from Payne, WA and Hahn, DB: *Understanding your health*, Dubuque, IA: WCB/McGraw-Hill Higher Education, 1998, and the American Cancer Society; **pp. 320, 326 (Figs. 15.4, 15.5):** Modified from Payne, WA and Hahn, DB: *Understanding your health*, Dubuque, IA: WCB/McGraw-Hill Higher Education, 1998, and the American Cancer Society; **p. 324 (Viewpoint),** Adapted from Wartik, N: Is it an illness? *American Health*, April, 1995, p. 67.

Chapter 16

p. 334 (FYI): Reproduced with permission of The Alan Guttmacher Institute from The Alan Guttmacher Institute, *Sex and America's Teenagers*, New York and Washington: AGI, 1994; **pp. 335, 337, 338, 340, 344 (Figs. 16.1, 16.2 bottom, 16.4, 16.7, 16.8 bottom, 16.11):** From Payne, WA and Hahn, DB: *Understanding Your Health*, Dubuque, IA: WCB/McGraw-Hill Higher Education, 1998; **p. 337 (Fig. 16.2 top):** Courtesy, Ortho Pharmaceutical Corp.; **p. 337, 339, 340, 343 (Figs. 16.3, 16.6, 16.8 top, 16.10b):** Laura J. Edwards; **p. 338 (Fig. 16.5):** Courtesy, Wisconsin Pharmacal Company, photo by Diana Linsley; **p. 341 (Health Tips):** Adapted from The American College of Obstetricians and Gynecologists: *Planning for pregnancy, birth and beyond*, Washington, DC, 1995; **p. 341 (Fig. 16.9):** Courtesy, Wyeth-Ayerst Laboratories; **p. 343 (Fig. 16.10a):** Courtesy, Alza Corporation; **p. 347 (FYI):** © May, 1992 Elaine Lissner: Male Contraception Information Project. Statistics in this chart are referenced in *Frontiers in nonhormonal male contraceptive research,* available from MCIP, PO Box 8483, Santa Cruz, CA 95061. Enclose three stamps. This chart may be duplicated and distributed without permission; **p. 348 (FYI):** Reproduced with the permission of The Alan Guttmacher Institute from The Alan Guttmacher Institute, Teen sex and pregnancy, *Facts in Brief*, New York: AGI, 1996; **p. 351 (Assess Yourself):** Sources: Stets, JE and Leik, RK: Attitudes about abortion and varying attitude structures. *Social Science Research* 22: 265–282, 1993, the National Right to Life Committee at www.nrlc.org, and ProChoice at www.choice.org.

Chapter 17

pp. 357, 362, 363 (Figs. 17.1, 17.2, 17.3): From Payne, WA and Hahn, DB: *Understanding your health*, Dubuque, IA: WCB/McGraw-Hill Higher Education, 1998; **pp. 359, 360 (Tables 17.1, 17.2):** American College of Obstetricians and Gynecologists, *You and your baby: prenatal care, labor and delivery, and postpartum care,* (Patient Education Pamphlet No. AB005), Washington, DC © ACOG, April, 1994. Used with permission; **p. 365 (FYI):** WHO. Used with permission; **p. 372 (Assess Yourself):** Adapted from Kazak, A and Linney, JA: Stress, coping, and life change in the single parent family, *American Journal of Community Psychology* 11: 207–220, 1983; **p. 373, 374 (Tables 17.4, 17.5, Journal Activity):** Source: Alvey, KT: *Parent training is prevention*, Department of Health and Human Services: Center for Substance Abuse Prevention.

Chapter 18

p. 380 (Assess Yourself): Reprinted with permission of copyright owner, Ortho Pharmaceutical Corp.; **p. 382 (FYI):** Source: *Sexually transmitted disease surveillance, 1995*, Atlanta: Centers for Disease Control, September, 1996; **pp. 382, 388, 390, 391 (Figs. 18.1, 18.2, 18.3, 18.4, Table 18.1):** Source: Centers for Disease Control and Prevention; **p. 391 (Her Story):** Adapted from Dan Seufert, Associated Press, in *The Courier-Journal*, Louisville, KY, December 1, 1996; **p. 392 (FYI):** Source: *1993 Surveillance Report*, Atlanta: Centers for Disease Control and Prevention; **p. 395 (FYI):** Adapted from American College Health Association; **p. 396 (Health Tips):** Source: Ohio Department of Health: *Women and AIDS,* July, 1991.

Chapter 19

pp. 402, 404, 405, 413 (Figs. 19.1, 19.2, 19.3, 19.4): From Payne, WA and Hahn, DB: *Understanding your health*, Dubuque, IA: WCB/McGraw-Hill Higher Education, 1998; **p. 409 (FYI):** Source: The University of Texas-Houston Health Science Center; **p. 410 (Assess Yourself):** © RISKO, A Heart Health Appraisal, 1994, Copyright American Heart Association, Reproduced with permission; **p. 412 (Health Tips):** © American Heart Association; **p. 414 (Assess Yourself):** Reprinted with permission from the National Osteoporosis Foundation, Washington, DC; **p. 417 (Health Tips):** © American Diabetes Association; **p. 418 (Health Tips):** © Epilepsy Foundation of America. Used with permission. All rights reserved; **p. 418 (Health Tips):** © Arthritis Foundation, Atlanta, Georgia; **p. 420 (FYI):** © *What is lupus?* Lupus Foundation of America, Inc.

Chapter 20

p. 427 (Health Tips): Source: American Cancer Society; **p. 428 (Table 20.1):** American Cancer Society Surveillance Research, 1997, © 1997, American Cancer Society, Inc.; **p. 430 (Table 20.2):** Data source: NCI Surveillance, Epidemiology, and End Results Program, 1996, © 1997, American Cancer Society, Inc.; **p. 435 (FYI):** Source: *New England Journal of Medicine*, December/January, 1996; **pp. 442, 443 (Figs. 20.2, 20.3):** Courtesy, American Academy of Dermatology; artwork by Don O'Connor.

Index

A

Abortion, 346–351
    and adolescents, 347–348
    anti-abortion position, 40–41
    and grief, 349
    lack of access and poor, 346–347
    legal aspects, 346–347, 349–350
    Pro-Choice, 350–351
    Right to Life, 350, 351
    RU-486, 348–349
    vacuum aspiration, 348
Abstinence
    AIDS prevention, 394
    as birth control, 334
Abuse. *See* Violence against women
Accepting parent, 371, 372
Accidents, and alcohol use, 204
Acquaintance rape, 275
    rapist characteristics, 275
Acquaintance violence, 270, 271
Acupressure
    cancer treatment, 446
    stress management, 109
Acupuncture, 248–249
    ailments treated, 248–249
    cancer treatment, 446
    finding acupuncturist, 249
    stress management, 109
Acute stress disorder, 106
Acutrim, 227
Addiction
    to alcohol, 206–207
    cigarette smoking, 181
    cocaine/crack, 232
    and dependency, 207, 220
    detoxification/withdrawal, 207, 220
    to drugs, 220
    heroin, 233
    meaning of, 206
Adjuvant treatment, cancer, 433
Adolescence, 39–46
    abortion in, 346–347
    and autonomy, 44
    birth control, use of, 334
    body image, 41–42
    developmental tasks of, 39
    education, 45–46
    homosexuality, 42–44
    puberty, 39–40
    self-identity, 42
    sexually transmitted diseases (STDs), 380
    social identity, 44–45
    suicide in, 85
    teen pregnancy, 49–50
Adoption, 370
    identity issues, 370
    open and closed, 370

Adrenal glands, 96, 97
Adrenocorticotrophin hormone
    (ACTH), 96, 97
Adult children of alcoholics, 210–211
    negative behaviors of, 211
    roles of children in family, 211
Advertising, 256–259
    analysis of ads, 257
    cigarette ads, 434
    of health-related products, 257
    portrayal of women, 258–259
    techniques of, 257–258
    truth *vs.* hype, 257
Aerobic activities, 154
Affirmative action, 6
African Americans
    and cohabitation, 303
    and heart disease, 407
    and hypertension, 408
    interracial marriage, 303–304
    and ovarian cancer, 440
    and sexually transmitted disease, 382
Agape, 300, 301
Age
    and assisted reproduction, 369
    and breast cancer, 435–436
    and cancer, 430
    and heart disease, 407
    and stress, 102–103
    and stroke, 412
Agoraphobia, 106
Aid for Dependent Children (AFDC), 284
AIDS/HIV, 390–396
    in children, 393–394
    complications of, 392
    definition of, 391
    diagnostic tests, 392–393
    and drug abuse, 234–236
    incidence, by race/ethnicity, 391
    prevention of, 394–396
    risk factors, 390–391
    risky sexual behaviors, 395
    signs of, 392
    specific indications for women, 393
    transmission of, 235, 392
    treatment of, 393
Alcohol
    absorption and women, 197
    absorption of, 196–197
    chemical aspects, 195
    proof, 195
Alcohol dehydrogenase (ADH), 197
Alcoholics Anonymous (AA), 213
    facts about, 214
Alcoholism
    adult children of alcoholics, 210–211
    causation theories, 208–209
    and codependency, 210

    definition of, 208
    disease model, 208–209
    indicators of, 208
    interventions for alcoholic, 209
    prevention, 214–215
Alcoholism treatment, 212–214
    aftercare, 213
    counseling, 213
    drug treatment, 213
    intervention, 212
    lifestyle behavior change, 213
    treatment centers, 213
    twelve-step programs, 213
Alcohol use
    and accidents, 204
    and addiction, 206–207
    behavioral effects, 203
    benefits of moderate use, 202
    blood alcohol concentration (BAC), 196
    and cancer, 431
    classifications by amount, 198
    and college students, 199–200
    detoxification, 207
    and dieting, 202
    diseases related to, 202
    drinking patterns, 198–199
    economic effects, 204
    effects and women, 198
    and ethnic minorities, 203
    gender differences, 198
    and hangover, 196
    heart disease protection, 411
    historical view, 195–196
    hormonal effects, 200–201
    moderation in, 123
    and osteoporosis, 201, 415
    and pregnancy, 205–206
    and rape, 277
    and relationships, 204
    social effects, 203–204
    women's reasons for, 200
Alternative health care, 247–252
    acupuncture, 248–249
    aromatherapy, 252
    for cancer, 445–446
    chiropractic care, 249–250
    growth of, 247–248
    herbalism, 248
    holistic medicine, 251–252
    massage, 250–251, 252
    for menopausal discomforts, 57, 329
    naturopathic medicine, 252
    quackery, 252
    reflexology, 252
Altruistic love, 300
Alveoli, 178, 179
Alzheimer's disease, 421–422
    and caregivers, 422

risk/protective factors, 421
  signs of, 421
  treatment approaches, 421
Amenorrhea, 321
  and overexercise, 167, 415
  stress amenorrhea, 97
Amino acids, essential and nonessential, 126
Amniocentesis, prenatal test, 359
Anatomy of an Illness (Cousins), 248
Androgyny, 38, 296, 297
  and depression, 85
Anger
  fair fights, 310
  inappropriate expression of, 309-310
Angina pectoris, 403-405
  signs of, 404
  treatment of, 404
Angioplasty, 404-405
Anorexia nervosa, 79-80, 147
  diagnostic criteria, 147
  treatment, 147
Anorgasmia, 201
Antabuse, 213
Anterior cruciate ligament, tear and
    exercise, 166
Antidepressants, 223
  types of, 223
Antioxidants, 128
Anxiety disorders, sedative hypnotics for,
    223-224
Aromatherapy, 252
  for stress, 108
Arrhythmia, 406
Arteries, 403
Arthritis, 418-420
  fitness effects, 153
  osteoarthritis, 419
  rheumatoid arthritis, 419
  systemic lupus erythematosus, 419-420
  warning signs, 418
Artificial insemination, 366-367
Aspirin, heart disease protection, 411
Assertiveness
  applications of, 75
  assertive messages, types of, 76
  assertiveness training, 73-75
  elements of, 74
Assisted reproduction. *See* Infertility options
Asymptomatic, meaning of, 380
Atherosclerosis, 403
Athletes (female)
  and amenorrhea, 321, 415
  and osteoporosis, 415
Authoritarian parent, 39
Authoritative parent, 39
Autoinoculation, 384, 385
Autologous bone marrow transplant, 433, 435
Autonomic nervous system, and stress, 96
Autonomy, and adolescent, 44
Avoidance addict, 306

B

Baby-Friendly Hospital Initiative, 364
Bacterial vaginosis, 388-389
  effects of, 388
  signs of, 388
  treatment of, 389

Ballistic stretching, 156
Basal body temperature, fertility awareness,
    336, 337
Basal cell carcinoma, 441
Basal metabolic rate, 146, 147
Battered women, characteristics of,
    280-281
Beauty-related products
  cosmetics, 252-253
  skin care products, 253-254
Behavior
  and needs, 22-23
  and reinforcement/punishment, 22
Behavioral contract, 27-28
Behavior change
  behavioral contract for, 27-28
  field theory, 23-24
  health belief model, 24-25
  planning lifestyle change, 26-28
  self-efficacy, 26
  social cognitive theory, 26
  theory of personal investment, 26
  theory of planned action, 25-26
  theory of reasoned action, 25
  transtheoretical model, 25
Benign tumors, 426, 427
Benzodiazepines, 224
Bioavailability, 221
Biofeedback, stress management, 111
Biophysical profile, prenatal test, 359
Biopsy
  breast cancer, 437-438
  lung cancer, 435
Bipolar disorder, signs of, 83
Birth centers, 363
Birth control, definition of, 333
Birth control methods
  abstinence, 334
  and adolescents, 334
  cervical cap, 339
  condoms, female, 338-339
  condoms, male, 337-338
  DepoProvera, 342
  diaphragm, 339
  emergency contraception, 342
  fertility awareness, 334-335
  intrauterine devices, 342-343
  Norplant, 341
  oral contraceptives, 339-341
  selection of method, 345-346
  spermicides, 336-337
  sterilization, 343-345
  withdrawal, 336
Birth control pills. *See* Oral contraceptives
Birth defects
  and alcohol use in pregnancy, 205-206
  prenatal detection, 358-359
Blaming victim, 280
Blastocyst, 356, 357
Blood pressure, measurement of, 408
Body awareness, of stress/tension, 109-110
Body composition
  and fitness, 158
  measurement of, 158, 161-162
Body dysmorphic disorder (BDD), 77
Body image
  of adolescents, 41-42
  and cosmetic surgery, 46

  and eating disorders, 79-80
  gender differences, 78-79
  and media, 78
  pathology related to, 77
Body mass index (BMI), 162
Bone density, measurement of, 416
Bone marrow transplant research,
    cancer, 433
Brand name, prescription drugs, 221
Braxton Hicks contractions, 360
Breast augmentation, 255-256
  safety measures, 256
  types of procedures, 255-256
Breast augmentation mammoplasty by
    injection (BAMBI), 256
Breast cancer, 435-439
  and alcohol use, 201
  detection of, 436-438
  fitness effects, 153
  and hormone therapy, 224
  post-surgery breast reconstruction, 439
  risk/protective factors, 435-436
  and tamoxifen, 436
  treatment approaches, 438-439
  warning signs, 437
Breastfeeding, 363-364
  benefits of, 36, 37, 364
  and nutrition, 136
  success, steps in, 364
Breast implants, 46, 47
Breasts
  anatomy of, 316, 317
  benign changes, 316-317
  self-examination, 317-318
Breathing, and stress management, 112-113
Bronchiectasis, and cigarette smoking, 178
Bulimia nervosa, 79-80, 147-148
  diagnostic criteria, 147-148
  treatment, 148
Bypass surgery, 404

C

Caffeine
  caffeine-containing products, 188-189
  caffeinism, 190
  chemical aspects, 187-188
  health effects, 189-190
  stimulant effects, 188
Calcium
  and alcohol use, 201
  and caffeine, 189
  and female athletes, 137
  and osteoporosis, 132, 415
  during pregnancy, 135
  sources of, 132
Calendar method, fertility awareness,
    334-335
Calipers, 161, 162
Calories
  and food label, 142
  and physical activity, 136
Cancer
  breast cancer, 435-439
  categories of, 428-429
  colorectal cancer, 442-443
  and ethnic minorities, 428
  in situ vs. invasive, 428

lung cancer, 433–435
  metastasis, 427
  ovarian cancer, 440–441
  positive diagnosis, actions to take,
      443–444
  protective factors, 444
  skin cancer, 441–442
  staging of, 429
  uterine cancer, 439–440
  warning signs, 427
Cancer research
  bone marrow transplant research, 433
  cell cycle research, 432
  gene mutation research, 432
  immunotherapy research, 433
Cancer risk factors
  age, 430
  alcoholism, 431
  cigarette smoking, 179, 430
  diet, 430
  electromagnetic fields, 431
  hair dyes, 431
  passive smoke, 182, 434
  radiation, 431
  substances in cigarettes, 177–178
  sun exposure, 431
  viruses, 431
Cancer treatment
  adjuvant treatment, 433
  alternative treatments, 445–446
  chemotherapy, 433
  choosing treatment plan, 446
  radiotherapy, 438, 439
  social support, value of, 444–445
Candidiasis, 389
  prevention of, 389
  signs of, 389
  treatment of, 389
Capillaries, 403
Carbohydrates, 125–126
  complex, 126
  simple, 125–126
Carcinogens, 430–431
Carcinoma, 428, 429
Cardiovascular disease
  angina pectoris, 403–405
  arrhythmia, 406
  atherosclerosis, 403
  and cigarette smoking, 178–179
  congenital heart disease, 405–406
  congestive heart failure, 406
  endocarditis, 406
  fitness effects, 153
  mitral valve prolapse, 406
  myocardial infarction, 404, 405
  screening for, 412
  silent ischemia, 406
  women excluded from research,
      401, 402
Cardiovascular disease protective factors,
    409–412
  alcohol consumption, 411
  aspirin, 411
  diet, 411
  estrogen, 409, 411
  exercise, 411
Cardiovascular disease risk factors,
    406–409
  cholesterol, high level, 408

cigarette smoking, 407
  diabetes, 408–409
  hypertension, 407–408
  obesity, 409
  physical inactivity, 408
  stress, 409
  unchangeable factors, 407
Cardiovascular endurance, 154–155
  assessment of, 160
  and conditioning, 154–155
  target heart rate, calculation of, 155
Cardiovascular system
  heart, 402
  vascular system, 402–403
Careers
  and educational level, 44–46
  See also Workplace
Caregivers, of Alzheimer's patients, 422
Cataracts, and cigarette smoking, 179–180
Caveat emptor, 257
Cell cycle research, cancer, 432
Cervical cancer
Pap test screening, 323, 440
  warning signs, 440
Cervical cap, 339
Cervicitis, 381
Cervix, 316, 317
  dilation in labor, 360, 362
Cesarean section, 362–363
Chandler, Cleo, 65
Chemotherapy, 433
Child abuse, 38, 271–273
  and adult depression, 83–84
  definition of, 271–272
  emotional abuse, 272
  and later alcoholism, 209
  neglect, 272
  physical abuse, 272
  sexual abuse, 272–273
Childbirth
  birthing options, 360, 362, 363
  cesarean section, 362–363
  hospital deliveries, 362–363
  infant mortality, 364–365
  labor, 360
  maternal mortality, 364–365
  midwives, 360, 362
  positions of woman for, 363
  stages of, 360, 361
Child care, expense of, 48
Childhood, 35–39
  early years and learning, 35
  education, 37
  and family, 39
  gender-role socialization, 37–38
  infancy, 35–36
  mortality in, 36
  nutrition, 36
  physical activity, 36–37
  victimization of children, 38
Children
  and AIDS, 393–394
  having children decisions, 47, 48
  nurturance of, 38
  passive smoke, effects of, 182
  as source of conflict, 309
China
  family planning, 333
  rising cancer rates, 434

Chiropractic care, 249–250
  disorders treated, 250
  finding chiropractor, 250
  training in, 249
Chlamydia, 380–381
  asymptomatic, 380, 381
  and pregnancy, 381
  screening for, 381
  signs of, 381
  treatment, 381
Chocolate, caffeine in, 189
Cholesterol level, and heart disease, 408
Chorionic villus sampling, prenatal test, 359
Cigarette smoking
  addiction of, 181
  cancer risk, 430, 434
  and heart disease, 407
  and osteoporosis, 180, 415
  passive smoking, 181–182, 434
  physical effects of, 178–181
  and pregnancy, 183–184
  prevalence of, 175
  reasons for smoking, 175–176
  smoker's rights, 181
Cilia, 178, 179
Civil Rights Act of 1964, Title VII, 6
Clitoris, 314, 315
Clomid, 366
Cocaine, 231–232
  effects of, 231–232
  pregnancy effects, 230, 232
  withdrawal from, 232
Codependency, characteristics of, 210, 211
Codependency Anonymous (CODA), 213
Coffee
  caffeine in, 187–188
  and calcium loss, 132
Cognitive development, Piaget's theory,
    32–33, 34
Cohabitation, 302–303
  and later marriage, 303
  prevalence of, 302
  racial/ethnic differences, 303
Coitus interruptus, 336, 337
Colas, caffeine in, 188–189
College students
  and alcohol use, 199–200
  and stress, 99–100
Colorectal cancer, 442–443
  early detection, 443
  risk/protective factors, 443
  screening, 443
  signs of, 443
  treatment, 443
Colostrum, 364
Commitment, and dating, 299
Communication, listening in, 75–76
Community, violence prevention
      programs, 289
Companionate love, 300
Complaints about products, 263–264
  information sources, 263
  sample letter, 264
Comprehensive major medical
      insurance, 260
Compulsive exercise, 168–170
Conception, process of, 355–356
Conditioning, principles of, 154–155
Condoms, female, 338–339, 396

Condoms, male, 337-338
 AID prevention, 395
 proper use of, 338
Congenital heart disease, 405-406
Congestive heart failure, 406
Consumer Bill of Rights, 241
 consumer protection laws, 253, 257
 credit reports, 262-263
 FDA assistance, 262
 meaning of, 240
Consumerism
 and advertising, 256-259
 caveat emptor, 256, 257
 complaints about products, 263-264
Consummate love, 300
Contraception. *See* Birth control methods
Contractions in labor, 360
 Braxton Hicks, 360
 true/false labor, 360
Contraction stress test, prenatal test, 359
Contraindications, to drugs, 229
Cool-down, pre-exercise, 159
Corticoids, 96, 97
Cosmetics, 252-253
 categories of, 252
 FDA rules, 253
 safety tips, 253
Cosmetic surgeons, 254
Cosmetic surgery, 46, 254-256
 breast augmentation, 255-256
 cosmetic *vs.* plastic surgeons, 254, 255
 physician for, 254
 types of procedures, 254-255
Counseling, alcoholism treatment, 213
Courage to Heal (Bass and Davis), 286
Crabtree, Melissa, 20
Crack, 231
Credit reports, 262-263
 agencies, list of, 263
 uses of, 263
Crime, and alcohol use, 204
Cross-fiber friction massage, 251
 finding masseur, 251
Cyst, 439

D

Daily hassles, and stress, 100
Date rape, 275-276
 avoidance, guidelines for, 276
Dating, 297-299
 interracial couples, 304
 stages of, 297-299
Death
 end of life arrangements, 66
 grief resolution, 80-82
 infant mortality, 36
 leading causes, 15, 16
 leading causes for children, 36
 leading causes for women, 400
Delirium tremens (DTs), 207
Dependency
 on alcohol, 207
 physical, 207, 220
 psychological, 207, 220
DepoProvera, 339, 342
Depression, 82-86
 antidepressants, 223
 and ethnic minorities, 85

gender differences, 84-85
 and hormones, 84
 meaning of, 82
 positive life changes, effects of, 84
 prevalence of, 82
 and psychosocial stressors, 83-84, 85
 and suicide, 85-86
 types of, 83
Detoxification, from alcohol, 207
Developmental phases
 adolescence, 39-46
 childhood, 35-39
 late adulthood, 59-66
 middle adulthood, 55-58
 young adulthood, 46-49
Developmental theories, exclusion of
  women in, 32-33
Dexatrim, 227
Diabetes
 fitness effects, 153
 gestational diabetes, 417
 and heart disease, 408-409
 insulin-dependent diabetes
  mellitus, 416
 non-insulin-dependent diabetes mellitus,
  416-417
 and stroke, 412
 treatment approaches, 416-417
 warning signs, 417
Diaphragm, 339
Diaphragmatic breathing, 112, 113
Diastolic blood pressure, 408
Diet
 and cancer, 430
 cancer treatment, 445
 heart disease protection, 411
 and osteoporosis, 415
 See also Nutrition
Dietary Reference Intakes (DRIs), 124-125
Dieting
 and alcohol use, 202
 vs. balanced food intake, 145-146
 See also Weight control
Disability, and Social Security payments, 261
Disaccharides, 125
Distress, 95
Diversity, in United States, 5
Divorce, 306
 problems for women, 306
 and remarriage, 306
 statistics on, 47, 306
Domestic violence, 270, 271
 costs related to, 270
 incidence of, 270
Drug abuse
 and HIV infection, 234-236
 and homelessness, 236
 indicators in pregnancy, 231
 and pregnancy, 230-232
 See also Psychoactive drugs
Drugs
 bioavailability of, 221
 contraindications, 229
 legislation related to safety, 220
 over-the-counter (OTC) drugs,
  225-230
 patent medicines, 219-220
 prescription drugs, 220-225
 psychoactive drugs, 230-236

Dysmenorrhea, 166, 320
 and endometriosis, 320
 pain relievers, 320
Dysthymic disorder, signs of, 83

E

Eating disorders, 79-80, 146-148
 anorexia nervosa, 79-80, 147
 bulimia nervosa, 79-80, 147-148
 and osteoporosis, 415
Ectopic pregnancy, 357
Education
 childhood, 37
 as health intervention, 19-21
 and income, 50
 and level of career, 44-46
Egg retrieval, 369
Elder abuse, 63-65
Electromagnetic fields, cancer risk, 431
Electronic therapies, cancer treatment, 445
ELISA test, 392, 393
Embryo, 356, 357
Emotional abuse
 adult women, 273-274
 children, 272
Emotional problems
 of abused children, 272-273
 of abused women, 282
 and counseling/therapy, 86
 depression, 82-86
 eating disorders, 79-80, 146-148
Emotional well-being
 assertiveness training, 73-75
 and communication, 75-76
 and fitness, 153
 and health, 86-87
 image building, 77
 ongoing mindfulness, 72, 73
 and problem solving, 76-77
 resolving grief, 80-82
 self-esteem enhancement, 80
Emphysema, and cigarette smoking, 178
Employment, and stress, 101-102
Empty calorie foods, 126
Empty-nest syndrome, 57
Endarterectomy, 413
Endocarditis, 406
Endocrine system, and stress, 96
Endogenous factors, 16, 17
Endometriosis, 320
Endometrium, 316, 317
Environment
 environmental stress, 105
 protective practices, 20
Epidemiological studies, 121
Epidemiology, 21
Epilepsy, 417-418
 first aid interventions, 418
 and pregnancy, 418
Epinephrine, 96, 97
Episiotomy, 315, 363
Equal Employment Opportunity
  Commission (EEOC), 6
Equal Rights Amendment (ERA), 6
Ergonomics, 106
Erikson's theory
 stages in, 34
 women in, 32

Erotic love, 300, 301
Estraderm, 225
Estrogen
    and alcohol use, 201
    and female athletes, 321
    heart disease protection, 409
    and menstrual cycle, 319
    natural sources of, 329
Estrogen replacement therapy (ERT),
    alternative to, 224–225
Ethnic bias, in health research, 3–4
Ethnic minorities
    and AIDS, 391, 392
    and alcohol use, 203
    and cancer, 428
    cohabitation by, 303
    and depression, 85
    interracial couples, 303–304
    and sexually transmitted diseases, 382
    and stress, 102
    and stroke risk, 412
Ethyl alcohol, 195
Eustress, 95
Exercise
    stress management, 109
    See also Fitness; Fitness activities
Exogenous factors, 16, 17
External affair, effects on relationship, 307

F

Fair Packaging and Labeling Act, 257
Fallopian tubes, 316
Family
    and childhood, 39
    and gender-role socialization, 38
    and middle age, 56–57
    parenting styles, 39
    and young adulthood, 47–48
Family planning, 332–333
    access to methods, 333
    in China and India, 333
Fastin, 223
Fat, dietary, 127
    calculating intake, 122
    and food label, 142
    forms of, 127
    hidden fats, 127
Fatuous love, 300
Federal government, Medicare/Medicaid,
    260, 261
Federal legislation
    on abortion, 346, 350
    for abused women, 289–290
    against sex discrimination, 6
    on birth control, 333
    FDA regulations, cosmetics, 253, 262
    on mammography, 437
Federal Trade Commission (FTC), 257
Fee-for-service insurance plan, 260
Feminine Mystique, The (Friedan), 248
Femininity, 296, 297
Fermentation, alcohol, 195
Fertility awareness, 334–335
    basal body temperature, 336
    calendar method, 334–335
    symptothermal method, 336
Fertility drugs, 366
Fetal alcohol effects (FAE), 205

Fetal alcohol syndrome (FAS), 205
Fiber
    and food label, 142
    vs. laxatives, 228
Fibrocystic breast disease, and caffeine
    intake, 189–190
Field theory, behavior change, 23–24
Fight-or-flight response, stress, 95
Financial problems
    effects on relationships, 307–308
    spending differences in couples, 308
Financial status
    financial goal setting, 50
    financial stress, 103–104
    late adulthood, 64
    middle adulthood, 57
    retirement planning, 64
    young adulthood, 49
Fitness
    assessment of, 160–162
    benefits of, 152–154
    and body composition, 158
    and cardiovascular endurance, 154–155
    diseases prevented by, 153
    and flexibility, 155–157
    heart disease protection, 411
    and muscular strength/endurance,
        157–158
Fitness activities
    adherence to program, 165
    aerobic activities, 154
    beginning program, 163–165
    compulsive exercise, 168–170
    injuries during, 165–166
    martial arts, 154
    and menstrual cycle, 166–167
    pre-exercise evaluation, 163
    in pregnancy, 167–168
    stretching, 155–157
    and warmup/cool-down, 159
    and weight control, 170–171
    weight training, 157–158
Flexibility, 155–157
    assessment of, 161
    and stretching, 155–157
Folacin, during pregnancy, 134–135
Follicle stimulating hormone (FSH), and
    menstrual cycle, 319
Food additives, 138–140
    safety factors, 139
Food and Drug Administration (FDA), 220
    assistance for consumers, 262
    and cosmetics, 253
    over-the-counter drugs, 226
    products regulated by, 262
Food cravings
    and menstruation, 40
    and stress, 108
Food Guide Pyramid, 123–124
Food labeling, 141–143
    example of label, 143
    terms used, 142
Force-field analysis, 24, 25
Foster care, 370
Free radicals, 128
    and cigarette smoke, 182
Freudian theory
    exclusion of women in, 32
    psychosexual stages, 33

G

Gamete intrafallopian transfer (GIFT), 369
Gay men. See Homosexuality
Gender bias
    in developmental theories, 32–33
    earnings, 49, 103–104
    in health research, 3–4
    heart disease diagnosis/treatment, 412
Gender differences
    alcohol use, 198
    body image, 78–79
    depression, 84–85
    views of sex, 308
Gender role
    androgyny, 38, 296
    masculinity/femininity, 295–296
Gender-role socialization
    and depression, 85
    process of, 37–38
Gene mutation research, cancer, 432
General adaptation syndrome (GAS), 96
Generalized anxiety disorder, 106
Generic name, prescription drugs, 220–221
Genetic factors
    alcoholism, 208
    breast cancer, 435
Gestational diabetes, 417
Gilligan's theory, moral development, 33, 35
Global view
    life expectancy for women, 15
    wellness, 19
Goals
    in middle age, 57–58
    in young adulthood, 48–49
Gonorrhea, 382–383
    and pregnancy, 383
    screening for, 382
    signs of, 382
    treatment of, 383
Gray Panthers, 65
Grief
    and abortion, 349
    resolution of, 80–82
    stages of, 81–82

H

Hair dyes, cancer risk, 431
Hangover, 196
Hashish, 232–233
Healing process, abused women, 285–287
Health, and emotions, 86–87
Health assessment quizzes
    Appearance Schemas Inventory (ASI), 79
    cancer risk assessment, 432
    for drinking problem, 210
    facts on aging quiz, 61–62
    folacin containing foods, 136
    food choices, 120
    food quiz, 141
    heart disease risk, 410
    osteoporosis risk assessment, 414
    personal health inventory, 11
    potential for smoking, 177
    stress checklist, 101
    wellness rating, 18
Health belief model, behavior change,
    24–25

Health-care delivery, 245–246
Health care providers
    categories of, 242
    mental health therapists, 244–245
    midwives, 243–244
    nurse practitioner, 243
    physicians, 242–245
    physician's assistant, 243
    selection guidelines, 242
    unprofessionalism, reporting, 245
Health foods, 138, 139
Health insurance, 259–261
    components of good plan, 260–261
    types of plans, 260
    and uninsured, 260
Health interventions
    education, 19–21
    prevention, 21
    treatment, 21–22
Health maintenance organizations (HMOs),
    260, 261
Health practices, health/safety tips, 8
Health promotion, components of, 3
Health research
    absence of women in, 3–4, 7
    cultural issues, 3–4
    female-oriented research, 7
*Healthy People 2000: Midcourse Review
    and 1995 Revisions,* 10
*Healthy People 2000: National Health
    Promotion and Disease Prevention
    Objectives,* 9–10
    objectives, 15, 33, 55, 71, 93, 120, 153,
        175, 195, 220, 241, 269, 315, 333,
        355, 379, 401, 427
Heart, normal functioning of, 402
Heart disease. *See* Cardiovascular disease
Heme iron, 132–133
Hemodialysis, 386, 387
Hepatitis B, 386–387
    and pregnancy, 387
    risk factors, 386
    signs of, 387
    transmission of, 386
    vaccination for, 387
Herbal remedies, 248
    cancer treatment, 445–446
    for stress, 108
Heroin, 233–235
    effects of, 233–234
    pregnancy effects, 234
Herpes simplex virus, 384–385
    control of, 384
    and pregnancy, 385
    prevention of, 384–385
    signs of, 384
Hierarchy of needs, 22–23
Hill, John, 278
Hispanics
    and cohabitation, 303
    and sexually transmitted
        disease, 382
HIV. *See* AIDS/HIV
Holistic medicine, 251–252
    concerns about, 251
    features of, 251
Home health tests, 246
    accuracy of, 246, 247
    categories of, 246

    common tests, 246
    pregnancy tests, 356–357
Homelessness, and drug abuse, 236
Homeostasis, 96, 97, 207, 220
    stress effects, 96
Homophobia, 43, 278, 279
    meaning of, 278, 279
    violence against lesbians, 278
Homosexuality
    and adolescents, 42–44
    and assisted reproduction, 367
    difficulties in relationships, 304
    lesbian couples, 304
    physical intimacy, 308
    raising children, 304
    violence against gays/lesbians, 278
Hormone replacement therapy (HRT),
        224–225, 327–328
    decision making about, 327
    drugs for, 224–225
    indications for, 224
    osteoporosis, 224, 415
    pros/cons of, 224, 327–328
    side effects, 328
    studies on, 328
Hormones
    and alcohol use, 200–201
    and depression, 84
    and menopause, 56
    and menstrual cycle, 319
    and menstruation, 39–40
    and migraine headaches, 99
    and overexercise, 170
    and stress, 96, 99
Hospitals, for childbirth, 362–363
Hot flashes, 327
Household tasks, as source of conflict, 309
Human papilloma virus, 385–386
    and cancer risk, 386
    and pregnancy, 386
    signs of, 386
    treatment of, 386
Humegon, 366
Hydrostatic weighing, 162
Hymen, 315
Hypertension, 407–408
    and African Americans, 408
    and heart disease, 407–408
    measurement of blood pressure, 408
    risk factors, 408
    and stroke, 412
Hypogonadism, and osteoporosis, 415
Hypothalamus, 96, 97

I

Identity
    self-identity in adolescence, 42
    social identity, 44–45
Image building, 77
Immunotherapy research, cancer, 433
Income, and educational level, 50
India, family planning, 333
Infancy, 35–36
    infant mortality, 36
    nutrition, 36
    talking to infant, 35
Infant mortality, and childbirth, 364–365
Infatuation, 299

Infertility, 365–370
    causes of, 367
    primary and secondary, 365, 366
Infertility options
    adoption, 370
    and age, 369
    artificial insemination, 366–367
    donor eggs, 369
    egg retrieval, 369
    fertility drugs, 366
    foster children, 370
    gamete intrafallopian transfer (GIFT), 369
    intracytoplasmic sperm injection
        (ICSI), 369
    and multiple births, 369–370
    surrogacy, 368
    in vitro fertilization (IVF), 368–369
Infidelity, as source of conflict, 307
Information sharing, and dating, 297
Injuries, exercise injuries, 166
Insulin-dependent diabetes mellitus, 416
Interracial couples, 303–304
Intervention, for alcoholic, 212
Intimacy
    and dating, 298–299
    definition of, 298, 299
Intracytoplasmic sperm injection
        (ICSI), 369
Intrauterine devices, 342–343
Intrauterine growth retardation, and
        cocaine use in pregnancy, 232
Iron, 132–133
    deficiency and vegetarians, 137
    and female athletes, 137
    functions of, 132
    heme iron, 132–133
    nonheme iron, 133
    during pregnancy, 134
Ischemia
    and angina, 403–404
    silent, 406
Isokinetic weight training, 157, 158
Isometric weight training, 157, 158
Isotonic weight training, 157, 158

J

Jaundice, 387
Job training, sources for, 285

K

Keach, Aletha, 63
Ketones, 126, 127
Kohlberg's theory, exclusion of women in, 33
Kuhn, Maggie, 65

L

Labels
    food labels, 141–143
    over-the-counter (OTC) drugs, 229
    prescription drugs, 221
Labia majora, 314, 315
Labia minora, 314, 315
Labor, contractions, 360, 361
Late adulthood, 59–66
    depression in, 85
    elder abuse, 63–65

end of life arrangements, 66
family in, 60, 62
financial status, 64
Medicare/Medicaid, 261
physical status, 60
sexuality, 63
sexual response, 325–326
social activities, 65
stressors in, 65–66
wise crone, 60, 63
Laxatives, 227–228
alternatives to, 228
effects of habitual use, 228
Lesbians. *See* Homosexuality
Leukemia, 428, 429
and cigarette smoking, 180
Life expectancy, for women,
global view, 15
Lifestyle, change. *See* Behavior change
Light treatment, cancer treatment, 445
Lincoln, Mary, 6
Lipids, 127
Listening, and communicating, 75–76
Living will, 66
Love, 299–300
styles of, 300
triangular theory, 299–300
Love addiction, dynamics in, 306
Low back pain, and exercise, 166
Ludic love, 300, 301
Lumpectomy, 438, 439
Lung cancer, 433–435
early detection, 434
risk/protective factors, 434
screening for, 435
treatment of, 435
Luteinizing hormone (LH), and menstrual
cycle, 319
Lymphoma, 428, 429

M

MacDonald, Jeffery, 278
Macrominerals, 128
Macrophages, 433
Magnetic devices, cancer treatment, 445
Magnetic resonance imaging (MRI), 435
Main-stream smoke, 182, 183
Major depressive disorder, signs of, 83
Major depressive episode, signs of, 83
Major medical insurance, 260
Male contraception
condom, 337–338
myths/facts about, 347
vasectomy, 344–345
Malignant neoplasm, 427
Mammography
false positives, 437
federal regulation, 437
Mammography Quality Standards Act, 437
Manic love, 300, 301
Marijuana, 232–233
active component in, 232–233
effects of, 233
pregnancy effects, 233
Marital rape, 275, 277
Marriage, 47–48, 301–302
interracial couples, 303–304

marital success, prediction of, 302
peer marriage, 302, 303
typologies of, 301–302
Martial arts, 154
Masculinity, 297, 298
Massage, 250–251, 252
cross-fiber friction massage, 251
stress management, 108, 250–251
trigger-point massage, 251
Mastectomy, 438, 439, 444
Maternal mortality, and childbirth, 364–365
Maternal serum screening, prenatal test, 359
Media
and cigarette ads, 176
and physical image, 78
Medicaid, 261
eligibility for, 261
mandated services, 261
Medical check-ups
information for physician, 243
screening tests, 243
Medicare, 261
Parts A and B, 261
Meditation
cancer treatment, 446
stress management, 112
Melanoma, 441
detection of, 442, 443
Melatonin, 229
Menarche, 318–319
Menopause, 326–329
discomforts of, 56
and hormone replacement therapy
(HRT), 327–328
natural remedies for, 57, 329
perimenopause, 327
Menstrual cycle
affecting factors, 336
and alcohol absorption, 197
and hormones, 319
phases of, 319, 320
Menstruation, 318–322
beginning of, 318–319
onset in puberty, 39–40
and physical activity, 166–167
Menstruation-related problems
and alcohol use, 201
amenorrhea, 167, 321
dysmenorrhea, 166, 320
and overexercise, 167, 170
premenstrual syndrome, 323–324
premenstrual syndrome (PMS), 166
and stress, 97
toxic shock syndrome, 322
Mental health therapists, 244–245
academic degrees/licensures, 245
choosing therapist, 244
Metabolic rate, 96, 97
and stress, 96
Metastasis, 427
Methadone
addiction to, 234
pros/cons of, 234
Methylxanthines, 187
Metrodin, 366
Middle adulthood, 55–58
age of, 56
empty-nest syndrome, 57

family in, 56–57
financial goals, 57
menopause, 56
midlife crisis, 58
physical aspects, 55–56
Midlife crisis, 58, 59
Midwives, 360, 362
effectiveness of, 360, 362
role of, 243–244
Migraine headaches, 99
drugs/foods to avoid, 99
Mind/body/spirit connection, 16–17
Minerals, 128, 131, 132–133
calcium, 132
functions of, 128
iron, 132–133
listing of, 131
during pregnancy, 135–136
Mitral valve prolapse, 406
Moisturizers, types of, 253
Monoamine oxidase inhibitors (MAOIs), 223
Monoclonal antibodies, 435
Monogamy, AIDS prevention, 394
Monosaccharides, 125
Monounsaturated fat, 127
Mons pubis, 313
Moral development
Gilligan's theory, 33, 35
Kohlberg's theory, 33
Mother-daughter relationship
adolescence conflicts, 45
tips for resolving issues, 45
Multiple births, and infertility treatment,
369, 370
Multiple sclerosis, 420–421
diagnosis of, 420
signs of, 420
treatment approaches, 420
Murder of women, 277–278
cases of, 278
Muscular strength/endurance
assessment of, 160
and weight training, 157–158
Myocardial infarction, 404, 405

N

Nalmefene, 213
Naltrexone, 213
Nardil, 223
National Adoption Registry, 370
National Organization for Women (NOW), 6
Natural foods, 140–141
Naturopathic medicine, 252
Needs, hierarchy of needs, 22–23
Negative reinforcer, 22, 23
Neglect, child abuse by, 272
Nicotine, in tobacco, 177
Nicotine gum, 185–186
1997 Consumer's Resource Handbook, 263
Nolvadex, 436
Nonheme iron, 133
Non-insulin-dependent diabetes mellitus,
416–417
Nonstress test, prenatal test, 359
Norepinephrine, 96, 97
Norplant, 339, 341
Nurse practitioner, role of, 243

Nurses Health Study, 7
Nurturance, of children, 38
Nutrient density, 126, 127
Nutrients
  carbohydrates, 125-126
  fats, 127
  minerals, 128, 132-133
  needs for physical activity, 137
  phytochemicals, 133
  protein, 126
  vitamins, 128
  water, 133
Nutrition
  breast-feeding, 136
  childhood, 36
  dietary guidelines for Americans,
    121-123
  Dietary Reference Intakes (DRIs), 124-125
  and food additives, 138-140
  Food Guide Pyramid, 123-124
  food labeling, 141-143
  health foods, 138, 139
  infancy, 36
  late adulthood, 60
  natural foods, 140-141
  organic foods, 140
  during pregnancy, 134-136
  Recommended Dietary Allowance
    (RDA), 124, 125
  and stress, 107-108
  vegetarianism, 137-138
  and weight control, 143-146

O

Obesity
  factors related to, 145
  and heart disease, 409
Obsessive-compulsive disorder, 106
Office of Research on Women's Health
    (ORWH), 7
Omnivorous diet, 137
Oncogenes, 433
Oncologist, 438, 439
Ongoing mindfulness, 72, 73
Oral contraceptives, 339-341
  and alcohol use, 201
  and dangers of smoking, 179
  side effects, 340
  types of, 339-340
Organic foods, 140
Orgasm, 325
  dysfunctions of, 325
  faking, 325
Osteoarthritis, 419
Osteopathic doctors, 242-243
Osteoporosis, 414-416
  and alcohol use, 201, 415
  caffeine effects, 189
  causes of, 132
  and cigarette smoking, 180, 415
  and diet, 415
  and eating disorders, 415
  and female athletes, 415
  fitness effects, 153, 414-415
  and hormone therapy, 224, 415
  protective factors, 414-415
  risk factors, 415-416

Our Bodies, Ourselves, 248
Ovarian cancer, 440-441
  early detection, 440-441
  risk/protective factors, 440
  screening, 441
  treatment options, 441
  warning signs, 440-441
Ovaries, 316, 317
Over-the-counter (OTC) drugs, 225-230
  caffeine in, 189
  FDA categories of, 226
  labeling, 229
  laxatives, 227-228
  legislation related to safety, 226
  and pregnancy, 229-230
  reconstructed from prescription
    drugs, 227
  sleep aids, 229
  for weight control, 227
Ovulation, 334-335
Oxidation, 196, 197

P

Panic attack, 106
Pap test, 322-323, 440
  false results, 323
Parenting, roles/responsibilities for
    caregiving, 373
Parenting styles, 39, 372-373
  accepting parent, 372, 373
  permissive parents, 372, 373
  productive/destructive styles, 372
  rejecting parent, 372, 373
  restrictive parents, 372, 373
Passive smoking, 181-182
  cancer risk, 182, 434
Patella femoral knee pain, and exercise, 166
Patent medicines, 219-220
Peer marriage, 302, 303
Peers, positive peers program, 42
Pelvic examination, 322-323
  components of, 322
  Pap test, 322-323
Pelvic inflammatory disease (PID)
  signs of, 387
  treatment of, 388
Perception, and stress, 93-95
Pergonal, 366
Perimenopause, 56, 327
Perineum, 315
Permissive parents, 39, 372, 373
Phen/Fen, 147
Phenylpropanolime (PPA), 227
Phobia, 106
Physical abuse
  adult women, 273
  children, 272
  forms of, 272, 282
Physical activity
  and caloric intake, 136
  and childhood, 36-37
  and late adulthood, 60
  levels of, 136
  and nutrients, 137
  See also Fitness activities
Physical attraction, and dating, 297
Physical dependency, 207

Physicians, 242-245
  and checkups, 243
  oncologist, 438, 439
  osteopathic doctors, 242-243
  plastic and cosmetic surgeons, 254, 255
  training of, 242
Physician's assistant, role of, 243
Phytochemicals, 133
  food sources of, 134
Piaget's theory
  exclusion of women in, 32-33
  stages in, 34
Pituitary gland, 96, 97
Pneumocystis carinii pneumonia, 392
Polysaccharides, 126, 127
Pondimin, 222-223
Positive reinforcer, 22, 23
Post-traumatic stress disorder (PTSD), 106
  and sexual abuse in childhood, 272-273
Poverty, social programs for poor, 4
Pragmatic love, 300, 301
Preferred provider organizations (PPO),
    260, 261
Pregnancy
  and alcohol use, 205-206
  and antiseizure drugs, 418
  and caffeine intake, 189
  childbirth, 360-363
  and chlamydia, 381
  and cigarette smoking, 183-184
  conception, 355-356
  and drug abuse, 230-234
  drug abuse indicators, 231
  early signs, 356
  ectopic pregnancy, 357
  exercise during, 167-168
  fetal development, 357, 358
  gestational diabetes, 417
  and gonorrhea, 383
  and herpes simplex virus, 385
  home tests for, 356-357
  and human papilloma virus, 386
  nutrition during, 134-136
  and over-the-counter (OTC) drugs,
    229-230
  planning for, 354-355
  prenatal care, 357-360
  and syphilis, 383-384
  teen pregnancy, 49-50
Premarin, 224-225
Premenstrual syndrome (PMS), 166, 323-324
  classification as mental illness, 324
  foods to avoid, 40, 323
  signs of, 39-40, 324
  types of, 40
Prenatal care, 357-360
  first visit, 357-358
  special tests, 359
Prescription drugs, 220-225
  antidepressants, 223
  brand name, 221
  generic name, 220-221
  hormone therapy, 224-225
  labeling of, 221
  patient question related to, 222
  sedative hypnotics, 223-224
  side effects, 225
  for weight control, 222-223

Prevention
    alcoholism, 214–215
    as health intervention, 21
    levels of, 21
Primary infertility, 365
Primary prevention, 21
Problem solving, 76–77
    steps in, 77
Pro-Choice, 350–351
Progesterone, and menstrual cycle, 319
Proof, alcohol, 195
Proprioceptive neuromuscular
        facilitation, 156
Protein, 126
    and amino acids, 126
    complete and incomplete, 126
    during pregnancy, 134
    sources of, 126
Prozac, 223
Psychoactive drugs, 230–236
    cocaine, 231–232
    crack, 231
    heroin, 233–235
    marijuana, 232–233
    methadone, 234
    and pregnancy, 230–234
Psychological dependency, 207
Psychoneuroimmunology (Ader), 248
Psychosexual development, Freudian
        theory, 32, 33
Psychosocial development, Erikson's theory,
        32, 34
Psychosomatic disorders
    and stress, 97
    types of, 97
Puberty, 39–40
    age of, 39
    physical changes in, 39–40
Punishment, 22, 23
    and behavior, 22

Q

Quackery
    alternative health care, 252
    meaning of, 252, 253

R

Radiation
    cancer risk, 431
    cancer treatment, 438, 439
Rape, 274–277
    acquaintance rape, 275
    and alcohol use, 203, 204, 277
    after attack, steps to take, 277
    date rape, 275–276
    marital rape, 275, 277
    prevalence of, 275
    and roofies, 235
Rapists, characteristics of, 276
Rebound deficiencies, 136
Recommended Dietary Allowance (RDA),
        124, 125
Reflexology, 252
    stress management, 108–109
Reinforcement, and behavior, 22
Rejecting parent, 372, 373

Relationship problems
    divorce, 306
    external affair, 307
    financial problems, 307–308
    household task responsibilities, 309
    inattentiveness, 309
    love addiction, 306
    resolution of, 309–310
    sex, 308–309
Relationships
    cohabitation, 302–303
    dating, 297–299
    and gender roles, 295–296
    interracial couples, 303–304
    lesbian couples, 304
    love, 299–300
    marriage, 301–302
    and socialization, 296
    success, components of, 301
    success, tasks in, 300–301
Relaxation exercises
    forms of, 110–111
    stress management, 110–111
Relaxation Response, The, 248
Reproductive anatomy
    breasts, 316–318
    external genitalia, 313–315
    internal genitalia, 316
    menopause, 326–329
    menstruation, 318–322
    pelvic exam, 322–323
    pelvic examination, 322–323
Reproductive tract infections, 387–389
    pelvic inflammatory disease (PID),
        387–388
    vaginitis, 388–389
Resiliency, development of, 287
Retirement
    planning for, 64
    retirement benefits, 261–262
    Social Security payments, 64, 261
Rheumatoid arthritis, 419
    signs of, 420
    treatment of, 420
RICE plan, for exercise injuries, 166
Right to Life, 350, 351
Roe v. Wade, 346
Roles of women, and stress, 100–102
Romantic love, 299–300
Roofies, and rape, 235
RU-486, 348–349

S

Safe shelters, for abused women, 284–285
Saline breast implants, 255, 256
Salt, moderation in use, 123
Sarcoma, 428, 429
Saturated fat, 127
Screening tests, routine, 243
Secondary infertility, 365
Secondary prevention, 21
Secondary reinforcer, 22, 23
Sedative hypnotics, 223–224
    types of, 224
Selective serotonin reuptake inhibitor
        (SSRI), 223
Self-caring, elements of, 287–288

Self-efficacy
    and behavior change, 26
    meaning of, 26, 27
Self-esteem
    of battered women, 280–281
    low, origins of, 80
    meaning of, 80
    self-esteem enhancement, 80
Self-examination, breasts, 317–318
Self-identity
    of adolescents, 42
    image building, 77
Senior citizen, 59
Sex, 308–309
    lesbian couples, 308
    response in. *See* Sexual response
    views by men compared to women, 308
Sex discrimination, legislation against, 6
Sexual abuse of children, 272–273
    forms of, 272
    long-term effects, 272–273
Sexual abuse of women
    of lesbian women, 278
    rape, 274–277
    sexual harassment, 278
Sexual dysfunction, 325
    and alcohol use, 201
Sexual harassment, 278–279
    forms of, 278
    steps to take, 278
Sexuality
    adolescents, 49–50
    late adulthood, 63
Sexually transmitted diseases (STDs)
    AIDS, 390–396
    chlamydia, 380–381
    gonorrhea, 382–383
    hepatitis B, 386–387
    herpes simplex virus, 384–385
    human papilloma virus, 385–386
    long-term risks of, 378
    reproductive tract infections from,
        387–389
    and selection of birth control,
        345–346, 395
    syphilis, 383–384
    and teens, 380
Sexual response, 324–326
    and aging, 325–326
    Masters & Johnson's phases, 325, 326
    orgasm, 325
Shin splints, and exercise, 166
Side effects, drugs, 225
Side-stream smoke, 181–182
Silent ischemia, 406
Silicone-gel filled breast implants, 255, 256
Simpson, O.J., 278
Singlehood, 305
Skin cancer, 441–442
    early detection, 441–442
    prevention of, 431, 441, 442
    risk/protective factors, 441
    screening, 442
    treatment for, 442
    types of, 441
Skin care products, 253–254
    moisturizers, 253
    safety tips, 254

Skin-fold measurement, calipers, 161, 162
Sleep, late adulthood, 60
Sleep aids
    natural aids, 230
    over-the-counter (OTC) drugs, 229
Smoking cessation
    nicotine replacement devices, 184–186
    programs for, 184
    relapse prevention, 187
    short/long-term benefits of, 186
    steps in, 186–187
    tips for, 184
    and weight gain, 179
Social behavior, and alcohol use, 203–204
Social cognitive theory, behavior change, 26
Social identity, of adolescents, 44–45
Socialization
    gender-role, 37–38
    and relationships, 296
Social Security, 261
    future view, 64
    information sources on, 261, 262
Social support, and cancer treatment,
        444–445
Sociocultural influences
    awareness of, 71–72
    impact of, 70–71
    types of, 70
Socioeconomic bias, in health field, 4
Spermicides, 336–337
Spina bifida, and folate deficiency,
        134–135
Spiritual beliefs
    health effects, 102
    and resiliency, 287
Sports, women in, 46
Squamous cell carcinoma, 441
Static stretching, 155–156
Stepfamilies, 306
Stereotypes
    women in media, 78
    in workplace, 104–105
Sterilization, 343–345
    tubal ligation, 343–344
    vasectomy, 344–345
Storgic love, 300, 301
Stress
    and age, 102–103
    and college students, 99–100
    and daily hassles, 100
    and depression, 83–84, 85
    destructive effects of, 102
    environmental stress, 105
    and ethnic minorities, 102
    fight-or-flight response, 95
    financial stress, 103–104
    general adaptation syndrome (GAS), 96
    and heart disease, 409
    meaning of, 93
    and multiple roles of women, 100–102
    and nutrition, 107–108
    and perception, 93–95
    physiological response to, 96, 98
    positive stress, 95
    and trauma, 105, 107
Stress management
    acupressure, 109
    acupuncture, 109

aromatherapy, 108
biofeedback, 111
body awareness, 109–110
and breathing, 112–113
exercise, 109
herbal remedies, 108
massage, 108
meditation, 112
reflexology, 108–109
relaxation exercises, 110–111
time management, 109
yoga, 112
Stressors
    categories of, 93
    meaning of, 93
Stress-related disorders
    migraine headaches, 99
    psychological disorders, types of, 106
    psychosomatic disorders, 97
    stress amenorrhea, 97
Stretching
    ballistic stretching, 156
    proprioceptive neuromuscular
        facilitation, 156
    safety tips, 157
    static stretching, 155–156
Stroke
    cause of, 412, 413
    and cigarette smoking, 178–179
    rehabilitation from, 414
    risk factors, 412–413
    treatment approaches, 413
    types of, 412
    warning signs, 412
Sudden infant death syndrome (SIDS)
    and cocaine use, 232
    and heroin use in pregnancy, 234
    and smoking in pregnancy, 183
Sugars
    and food label, 142
    forms of, 123
    simple sugars, 125–126
Suicide
    predictors of, 86
    statistics on, 85–86
Sun exposure
    cancer risk, 431, 441, 442
    UV index, 441, 442
Surrogacy, 368
Symptothermal method, fertility awareness,
        336, 337
Syphilis, 383–384
    phases of, 383
    and pregnancy, 383–384
    signs of, 383
    treatment of, 383
Systemic lupus erythematosus, 419–420
    diagnosis of, 420
    signs of, 419–420
    treatment of, 420
Systolic blood pressure, 408

T

Tamoxifen, and breast cancer, 436
Tanning beds, cancer risk, 442
Tar, in tobacco, 178, 179
Tea, caffeine in, 188

Technology, stress caused by, 103
Tenuate, 223
Tertiary prevention, 21
Tetrahydrocannabinol (THC), 232–233
Theory of personal investment, behavior
        change, 26
Theory of planned action, behavior change,
        25–26
Theory of reasoned action, behavior
        change, 25
Time management, to reduce stress, 109
TNM cancer staging, 429
Tobacco
    carcinogens in, 177–178
    historical view, 174–175
    See also Cigarette smoking
Toxemia, and heroin use in pregnancy, 234
Toxic shock syndrome, 322, 323
Toys, gender-specific toys, 37, 38
Transdermal nicotine patch, 185–186
Trans fat, 127
Transient ischemic attacks (TIAs), 412–413
Transtheoretical model, behavior change, 25
Trauma, and stress, 105, 107
Treatment, as health intervention, 21–22
Triangular theory, love, 299–300
Trichomoniasis, 389
    signs of, 389
    treatment of, 389
Trigger-point massage, 251
Tubal ligation, 343–344
Twelve-step groups
    for adult children of alcoholics, 211
    alcoholism treatment, 213
Twins, conception of, 355–356
Type A personality, 105
Type E woman, 102

U

Ultrasound, prenatal test, 359
United States Pharmacopeia (USP), 220–221
Urethra, 315
Urethritis, 381
Uterine cancer, 439–440
    early warning signs, 440
    risk/protective factors, 440
    screening for, 440
    treatment options, 440
Uterus, 316, 317

V

Vacuum aspiration, 348
Vagina, 316, 317
Vaginal opening, 315
Vaginitis, 388–389
    bacterial vaginosis, 388–389
    candidiasis, 389
    trichomoniasis, 389
Valium, 224
Vascular disease, stroke, 412–414
Vascular system, 402–403
    composition of, 402–403
Vasectomy, 344–345
Vasoconstrictors
    cocaine, 230
    and stress level, 107–108

Vegetarianism, 137–138
    benefits of, 137
    cancer treatment, 445
    guidelines for, 138
    nutritional concerns of, 137–138
Veins, 403
Violence, and stress, 102
Violence against women
    acquaintance violence, 270
    battered women, characteristics of, 280–281
    child abuse, 271–273
    common elements in, 280
    consequences of, 281–283
    cycle of abuse, 274
    development after abuse, 287–288
    domestic violence, 270
    healing process after abuse, 285–286
    historical view, 268–269
    homophobia, 278
    legislation against, 289–290
    murder, 277–278
    physical abuse, 273
    prevalence of, 269, 270
    prevention of abuse, 288–290
    psychological abuse, 273–274
    rape, 274–277
    safety resources for women, 284–285
    sexual harassment, 278–279
    support of friends/family, 286–287
    women who leave, 283–285
    women who stay, 270–271, 283
Violence Against Women Act, 289–290
Viruses, and cancer, 431
Vitamin deficiencies
    rebound deficiencies, 136
    signs of, 130
    and vegetarians, 137–138
Vitamins, 128, 129–130
    antioxidants, 128
    cancer treatment, 446

    fat-soluble, listing of, 129
    functions of, 128
    during pregnancy, 135–136
    water-soluble, listing of, 130
Vitro fertilization (IVF), 368–369
Von Bulow, Claus, 278
Vulva, 313

W

Wage discrimination, 49, 103–104
Warm-up, pre-exercise, 159
Water
    benefits of consumption, 108
    functions in body, 133
    as nutrient, 133
Weight
    height/weight table, 144
    obesity, 145
Weight control, 143–146
    and balanced food intake, 145–146
    and exercise, 170–171
    over-the-counter (OTC) drugs for, 227
    prescription drugs for, 222–223
    and smoking cessation, 180
    tips for, 146
Weight gain, and smoking cessation, 179, 180
Weight training
    forms of, 157
    time factors, 158
Wellness
    dimensions of, 16, 17
    global view, 19
    holistic model, 16, 17
    personal guide to, 18
Western blot test, 392, 393
Wheeler-Lea Amendment, 257
Whole person concept, of wellness, 16–17

Withdrawal
    from alcohol, 207
    birth control, 336
    from cocaine, 232
    from drugs, 220
Woman, origin of word, 268
Women for Sobriety, 213
Women of the year, 1995, 9
Women's Health Initiative (WHI), 7
Women's movement, 6–7
    progression of, 6–7
Workplace
    ergonomics in, 106
    stereotyping women in, 104–105
    wage discrimination, 49, 103–104
Wrinkles, and cigarette smoking, 180

X

Xanax, 224

Y

Yazzie, Angie, 51
Yoga
    goal of, 252
    stress management, 112
Young adulthood, 46–49
    body image in, 46
    having children decisions, 47, 48
    life goals, 48–49
    marriage, 47–48

Z

Zoloft, 223
Zygote, 355, 356

Be Proactive!! Take Control of Your Health!!

The exciting features in *Contemporary Women's Health: Issues for Today and the Future* will empower you to positively impact your health!

- Attractive full-color design and photos draw you in with every turn of the page.

- Up-to-date coverage of the many dimensions of women's health addresses the needs of women from all cultural backgrounds.

- *Health Tips* help you reduce stress, improve your fitness, become a wise health care consumer, and much more.

- *Journal Activities* give you an opportunity to apply your health knowledge to your own life.

- Web sites included in every chapter are your ticket to health information on the Internet.

Contemporary Women's Health: Issues for Today and the Future will be a valuable resource to you year after year as your health needs change.

So . . . begin reading today and take control of your health!

WCB/McGraw-Hill

A Division of The McGraw·Hill Companies

ISBN 0-8151-0626-2

90000

9 780815 106265

www.mhhe.com